KU-018-354

Contents

Acknowledgements

Reviewers of the UK edition

John Clancy, BSc, PGCEA CERT ECBS,
Lecturer in Physiology Applied to Health, University of East Anglia

Pauline Kingston, RGN, MSc., Spec. Practitioner (DN), NP., RNT, PGCert.Med.Ed.
Senior Lecturer, Adult Nursing. Anglia Ruskin University, Cambridge

Alistair Nicholson RGN, RMN, Dip N, Cert Ed, BSc, MSc
Nursing Lecturer, University of Dundee School of Nursing and Midwifery

Paul Warburton MSc, RN, Cert Ed., V300
Senior Lecturer Non-Medical Prescribing Programme Co-ordinator,
Edge Hill University, Lancashire

Adrian Welyczko BSc, RGN, Cert Ed, MA
Senior Lecturer, Adult Nursing, Coventry University

made INCREDIBLY EASY

Nur Pha

Adapted

William

Lecturer
Nursing a
Medicine
Queen's U

and

Deirdre

Lecturer i
and Midw
Health an
University, Belfast

First UK Edition

Wolters Kluwer | Lippincott Williams & Wilkins
Health
Philadelphia • Baltimore • New York • London
Buenos Aires • Hong Kong • Sydney • Tokyo

Staff

Director, Global Publishing
Cathy Peck

Production Director
Chris Curtis

Senior Production Manager
Richard Owen

Production Editor
Sophie Tatzkow

Copy Editor
Amanda Whelan

Proofreader
Ann Stevens

Academic Marketing Executive
Alison Major

Illustrator
Bot Roda

© 2009 by Lippincott Williams & Wilkins. All rights reserved. This book is protected by copyright. No part of it may be reproduced, stored in a retrieval system, or transmitted, in any form or by any means — electronic, mechanical, photocopy, recording, or otherwise — without prior written permission of the publisher.

Printed in the UK by Stephens & George Ltd, Merthyr Tydfil, Wales. Typeset by Macmillan Publishing Solutions, New Delhi, India.

For information, write to Lippincott Williams & Wilkins, 250 Waterloo Road, London SE1 8RD.

British Library Cataloguing in Publication Data. A catalogue record for this book is available from the British Library.

ISBN13 978-1-901831-04-7
ISBN10 1-901831-04-3

Foreword to the UK edition

Learning pharmacology can be overwhelming to nurses and nursing students in today's complex field of health care. Rapidly emerging technology and a clearer understanding of health and disease have raised the bar for nurses in clinical practice. For example, many nurses are now able to prescribe drugs. In fact, the very aspects that have advanced the practice of nursing have given nurses greater responsibility and elevated the standards for the safe delivery of care.

As each aspect of health care expands, drugs are developed to meet the ever-growing demands of the health field. New drugs are being developed at a rapid pace, and some drugs are approved before clinical trials are even complete. Many of these drugs act by novel, and sometimes quite complex, mechanisms and many new drugs are in classes by themselves. Without a solid foundation of the general principles of pharmacology, understanding the actions of new drugs and drug classes is impossible.

Nursing Pharmacology Made Incredibly Easy!, 1*st* *UK Edition* takes a simplified and lighthearted approach to pharmacology that explains its complex concepts in clear, concise, and interesting language, making the information easy to learn and, most important, to remember. Each aspect of how the body processes a drug and the subsequent actions of that drug on the body are discussed in detail, and many are illustrated for clarification.

This valuable resource has been adapted specifically for the UK healthcare system, incorporating current practice and legistation making it more than a basic pharmacology text. Furthermore, the examples of drugs given throughout the text are generic and relate specifically to those currently in use within the UK.

Because of the rapid development of new drugs, nurses returning to nursing after a break often find that they aren't familiar with a multitude of new drugs and drug classes. This requires not only that these nurses learn the specific characteristics of each new drug and drug class, but also that they learn the likelihood of potentially dangerous drug interactions, current issues related to each drug's risk and benefits, and relevant updates from clinical trials. These nurses must seek out opportunities to learn this information, and *Nursing Pharmacology Made Incredibly Easy!*, 1*st* *UK Edition* is an ideal solution for these experienced nurses returning to practice as well as for new learners. It offers:

Prototype pro—common drug prototypes presented by pharmacologic class for all body systems

Pharm function—clear, illustrated explanations about drugs' actions in the body

Before you give that drug—important drug warnings that should be considered before administration

Education edge—important information that should be shared with patients

Memory joggers—clever mnemonics that help reinforce learning.

In addition to these great features, this incredibly informative book includes nursing process information that helps the nurse integrate the concepts into practice. What's more, at the end of each chapter you'll find a *Quick quiz* that tests your knowledge and provides immediate feedback to help you monitor your progress. The appendices are also packed with helpful information, such as definitions, ophthalmic and dermal drugs, together with a list of useful alternative resources.

Staying informed in the ever-expanding field of pharmacology presents a challenge to even the most seasoned nurse. The spectrum of drugs from which a practitioner can choose seems almost limitless, and the increased responsibility and potential for legal liability that nurses face in health care today drives home the importance of a book such as this. The information contained in *Nursing Pharmacology Made Incredibly Easy!*, *1st UK Edition* is useful for both the specialist and the general nurse, the novice and expert alike. Perhaps its most attractive feature is the brevity and clarity of its content. Like all books in the *Incredibly Easy!* series, this book delivers detailed information while maintaining the interest of the reader and makes learning pharmacology fun!

William N. Scott, BSc, MPhil, PhD
Lecturer in Biomedicine
School of Nursing and Midwifery
Faculty of Medicine, Health and Life Sciences
Queen's University, Belfast

Contributors and consultants to the US edition

Melody C Antoon, RN, MSN
Instructor of Nursing
Lamar State College
Port Arthur, Tex.

Christine Frazer, RN, MSN, CNS
Nursing Instructor
Pennsylvania State University
Hershey

Julia A Greenawalt, RNC, MA, MSN
Adjunct Faculty
University of Pittsburgh
School Nurse
Seneca Valley School District
Harmony, Pa.

Nancy Haynes, RN, MN, CCRN
Assistant Professor of Nursing
Saint Luke's College
Kansas City, Mo.

**Patricia Lange-Otsuka, APRN,BC,
EDD, MSN**
Associate Professor of Nursing
Hawaii Pacific University
Kaneohe

Kathy Latch Johnson, RN, MSN
Assistant Professor of Nursing
Baptist College of Health Sciences
Memphis

Linda May-Ludwig, RN, BS, MEd
Practical Nursing Instructor
Canadian Valley Technology Center
El Reno, Okla.

Catherine Todd Magel, RN, BC, EdD
Assistant Professor
Villanova (Pa.) University College of
    Nursing

Patricia O'Brien, RN, BS, MSN, APRN
Family Nurse Practitioner
Associate Professor, Graduate
    Nursing
Winona State University
Rochester, Minn.

Terri M Perkins, RN, MN
Instructor, Associate Degree Nursing
    Program
Bellevue (Wash.) Community College

Dana Reeves, RN, MSN
Assistant Professor
University of Arkansas
Fort Smith

Allison Jones Terry, RN, MSN
Director of Community Certification
State of Alabama Department
    of Mental Health and Mental
    Retardation
Montgomery

Karen Wilkinson, ARNP, MN
Nurse Practitioner, Pain
Management Program
Children's Hospital and Regional
    Medical Center
Seattle

Sharon Wing, RN, MSN
Assistant Professor
Cleveland State University

① Fundamentals of nursing pharmacology

Just the facts

In this chapter, you'll learn:

♦ pharmacology basics
♦ key concepts of pharmacokinetics, pharmacodynamics, and pharmacotherapeutics
♦ key types of drug interactions and adverse reactions
♦ the nursing process.

Pharmacology basics

Pharmacology is the scientific study of the origin, nature, chemistry, effects, and uses of drugs. This knowledge is essential to providing safe and accurate medication administration to your patients.

Three's company

This chapter reviews the three basic concepts of pharmacology:

 pharmacokinetics—the absorption, distribution, metabolism, and excretion of drugs by the body

pharmacodynamics—the biochemical and physical effects of drugs and the mechanisms of drug actions

pharmacotherapeutics—the use of drugs to prevent and treat diseases.

In addition, it discusses other important aspects of pharmacology, including:
- how drugs are named and classified
- how drugs are derived
- how drugs are administered
- how new drugs are developed.

Naming and classifying drugs

Drugs have a specific kind of nomenclature—that is, a drug can go by three different names:
- The *chemical name* is a scientific name that precisely describes the drug's atomic and molecular structure.
- The *generic*, or *nonproprietary*, *name* is an abbreviation of the chemical name.
- The *trade name* (also known as the *brand name* or *proprietary name*) is selected by the drug company selling the product. Trade names are protected by copyright. The symbol ® after a trade name indicates that the name is registered by, and restricted to, the drug manufacturer.

To avoid confusion, it's best to use a drug's generic name because any one drug can have a number of trade names.

Drugs may have many different trade names. To avoid confusion, refer to a drug by its generic name.

Making it official

European legislation has implemented the use of the Recommended International Non-proprietary Name (rINN) for medical substances so that only one official name represents each drug. The official names are listed in the *European Pharmacopeia* and the *British National Formulary*.

Class act

Drugs that share similar characteristics are grouped together as a *pharmacologic class* (or family). Beta-adrenergic blockers are an example of a pharmacologic class.

A second type of drug grouping is the *therapeutic class*, which categorises drugs by therapeutic use. Antihypertensives are an example of a therapeutic class.

A pharmacologic class groups drugs by their shared characteristics. A therapeutic class groups drugs by their therapeutic use.

Where drugs come from

Traditionally, drugs were derived from *natural* sources, such as:
- plants
- animals
- minerals.

Today, however, laboratory researchers have used traditional knowledge, along with chemical science, to develop *synthetic* drug sources. One advantage of chemically developed drugs is that they're free from the impurities found in natural substances. Also, researchers and drug developers can manipulate the molecular structure of substances such as antibiotics so that a slight change in the chemical structure makes the drug effective against different organisms. The first-, second-, third-, and fourth-generation cephalosporins are an example.

Sowing the seeds of drugs

The earliest drug concoctions from plants used everything: the leaves, roots, bulb, stem, seeds, buds, and blossoms. Subsequently, harmful substances often found their way into the mixture.

Active agents

As the understanding of plants as drug sources became more sophisticated, researchers sought to isolate and intensify *active components* while avoiding harmful ones. The active components of plants vary in character and effect:
• *Alkaloids*, the most active components in plants, react with acids to form a salt that's able to dissolve more readily in body fluids. The names of alkaloids and their salts usually end in "-ine"; examples include atropine, caffeine, and nicotine.
• *Glycosides* are naturally occurring active components that are found in plants, and have both beneficial and toxic effects. They usually have names that end in "-in", such as digoxin.
• *Gums* give products the ability to attract and hold water. Examples include seaweed extractions and seeds with starch.
• *Resins*, of which the chief source is pine tree sap, commonly act as local irritants or as laxatives and caustic agents.
• *Oils*, thick and sometimes greasy liquids, are classified as volatile or fixed. Examples of volatile oils, which readily evaporate, include peppermint, spearmint, and juniper. Fixed oils, which aren't easily evaporated, include castor oil and olive oil.

Active components of plant sources include alkaloids, glycosides, gums, resins, and oils.

Aid from animals

The body fluids or glands of animals are also natural drug sources. The drugs obtained from animal sources include:
• *hormones*, such as insulin
• *oils* and *fats* (usually fixed), such as cod-liver oil
• *enzymes*, which are produced by living cells and act as catalysts, such as pancreatin and pepsin
• *vaccines*, which include suspensions of killed, modified, or attenuated microorganisms, or antigenic materials obtained from these.

Many minerals

Metallic and nonmetallic minerals provide various inorganic materials not available from plants or animals. Mineral sources are used as they occur in nature or can be combined with other ingredients. Examples of drugs that contain minerals are iron, iodine, and magnesium salts.

In the lab

Today, most drugs are produced in laboratories. Examples of such drugs include thyroid hormone (from natural sources) and cimetidine (from synthetic sources).

DNA paving the way

Recombinant deoxyribonucleic acid (DNA) research has led to another chemical source of organic compounds. For example, the manipulation and reordering of genetic information enables scientists to develop bacteria that produce insulin for humans.

How drugs are administered

A drug's administration route influences the quantity given and the rate at which the drug is absorbed and distributed. These variables affect the drug's action and the patient's response.

Buccal, sublingual, and translingual

Certain drugs, such as glyceryl trinitrate, are given buccally (in the pouch between the cheek and teeth), sublingually (under the tongue), or translingually (on the tongue) to prevent their destruction or transformation in the stomach or small intestine.

Gastric

The gastric route allows direct administration of a drug into the GI system. This route is used when patients can't ingest the drug orally.

Intradermal

In intradermal administration, drugs are injected into the skin. A needle is inserted at a 10- to 15-degree angle so that it punctures only the skin's surface. This form of administration is used mainly for diagnostic purposes, such as testing for allergies or tuberculosis.

Intramuscular

The Intramuscular (I.M.) route allows drugs to be injected directly into various muscle groups at varying tissue depths. This

Looks like I need to get involved here. The gastric route is used when a patient can't ingest a drug orally.

form of administration provides rapid systemic action and allows for absorption of relatively large doses (up to 5 ml). Aqueous suspensions and solutions in oil as well as drugs that aren't available in oral forms are given I.M.

Intravenous

The Intravenous (I.V.) route allows injection of drugs and other substances directly into the bloodstream through a vein. Appropriate substances to administer I.V. include drugs, fluids, blood or blood products, and diagnostic contrast agents. Administration can range from a single dose to an ongoing infusion that's delivered with great precision.

Oral

Oral administration is usually the safest, most convenient, and least expensive route. Oral drugs are administered to patients who are conscious and able to swallow.

Rectal and vaginal

Suppositories, ointments, creams, or gels may be instilled into the rectum or vagina to treat local irritation or infection. Some drugs applied to the mucosa of the rectum or vagina can also be absorbed systemically.

Respiratory

Drugs that are available as gases or aerosols can be administered into the respiratory system through inhalation. These drugs are rapidly absorbed. In addition, some of these drugs can be self-administered by devices such as the metered-dose inhaler. The respiratory route is also used in emergencies—for example, to administer some injectable drugs directly into the lungs via an endotracheal tube.

Subcutaneous

In subcutaneous administration, small amounts of a drug are injected beneath the dermis and into the subcutaneous tissue, usually in the patient's upper arm, thigh, or abdomen. This allows the drug to move into the bloodstream more rapidly than if given by mouth. Drugs given subcutaneously include nonirritating aqueous solutions and suspensions contained in 0.5 to 2 ml of fluid, such as heparin and insulin.

Talk about going with the flow! I.V. administration puts substances right into the bloodstream.

Topical

The topical route is used to deliver a drug via the skin or a mucous membrane. This route is used for most dermatologic, ophthalmic, otic, and nasal preparations.

Specialised infusions

Drugs may also be given as specialised infusions. They're given directly to a specific site in the patient's body. Types of infusions include:

- epidural infusion—the drug is injected into the epidural space
- intrapleural infusion—the drug is injected into the pleural cavity
- intraperitoneal infusion—the drug is injected into the peritoneal cavity
- intraosseous infusion—the drug is injected into the rich vascular network of a long bone
- intra-articular infusion—the drug is injected into a joint.

New drug development

In the past drugs were found by trial and error. Now, they're developed primarily by systematic scientific research. The Commission on Human Medicines (CHM) carefully monitors new drug development, which can take many years to complete.

Only after reviewing extensive animal studies and data on the safety and effectiveness of the proposed drug does the CHM approve an application for an Investigational New Drug (IND). Of the thousands of novel compounds screened for therapeutic potential each year, less than 0.01% will be released on the open market. (See *Phases of new drug development*.)

On the fast track

Although most INDs undergo all four phases of clinical evaluation mandated by the CHM, a few can receive expedited approval. For example, because of the public health threat posed by acquired immunodeficiency syndrome (AIDS), the CHM and drug companies have agreed to shorten the IND approval process for drugs to treat the disease. This allows doctors to give qualified AIDS patients "Treatment INDs" which aren't yet approved by the CHM.

Sponsors of drugs that reach phase II or III clinical trials can apply for CHM approval of Treatment IND status. When the IND is approved, the sponsor supplies the drug to doctors whose patients meet appropriate criteria. (See *Cheaper and easier*.)

Government can expedite approval of certain investigational drugs if they show promise in treating a significant public health threat.

Phases of new drug development

When the Commission on Human Medicines (CHM) approves an application for an investigational new drug, the drug must undergo clinical evaluation involving human subjects. This clinical evaluation is divided into four phases. Potential therapeutic agents have been extensively studied with respect to aspects of safety, biological activity and therapeutic index prior to entering phase trials.

Phase I

In phase I, the drug is tested on healthy volunteers. Prior to this the drug has been extensivly tested in model systems, but it is worth bearing in mind that the results of such laboratory studies do not always extrapolate to the clinic. The data that is collected relates to tolerability, pharmacokinetic and pharmacodynamic profiles and adverse event details.

Phase II

Phase II involves trials with human subjects who have the disease for which the drug is thought to be effective. This phase is important for the determination of dosing regimes, dose response relationships and to identify the short-term tolerability profile. The phase enables the pharmacological activity of the drug to be demonstrated. Adverse event details continue to be collected.

Phase III

Large numbers of patients in medical research centres receive the drug in phase III. This larger sampling provides information about infrequent or rare adverse effects. Tolerability and efficacy profiles are established. Appropriate doses are identified and adverse event details collated. The CHM approves a new drug application if phase III studies are satisfactory.

Phase IV

Phase IV is voluntary and involves postmarket surveillance of the drug's therapeutic effects at the completion of phase III. The pharmaceutical company receives reports from doctors and other health care professionals about the therapeutic results and adverse reactions of the drug. Some drugs, for example, have been found to be toxic and have been removed from the market after their initial release. The establishment of a safety database is essential for continued surveillance of the drug, post-marketing.

Cheaper and easier

In the past, only a few drugs for acute conditions (such as headaches and colds) were available without prescription. Now, however, the Commission on Human Medicines approves more drugs for over-the-counter use, making the drugs more easily accessible and much less expensive to consumers. Some examples include GI medications, antihistamines, some corticosteroid creams and antiviral agents.

Caution

Unfortunately, the availability of over-the-counter medications may increase the risk of certain drug interactions and certain herbal preparations are known to interfere with the actions of a number of prescribed drugs.

Pharmacokinetics

The term *kinetics* refers to movement. Pharmacokinetics deals with a drug's actions as it moves through the body. Therefore, pharmacokinetics discusses how a drug is:
- absorbed (taken into the body)
- distributed (moved into various tissues)

- metabolised (changed into a form that can be excreted)
- excreted (removed from the body).

This branch of pharmacology is also concerned with a drug's onset of action, peak concentration level, and duration of action.

Absorption

Drug absorption covers the progress of a drug from the time it's administered, through the time it passes to the tissues, until it becomes available for use by the body.

How drugs are absorbed
On a cellular level, drugs are absorbed by several means—primarily through active or passive transport.

No energy required

Passive transport requires no cellular energy because the drug moves from an area of higher concentration to one of lower concentration. It occurs when small molecules diffuse across membranes. Diffusion (movement from a higher concentration to a lower concentration) stops when the drug concentrations on both sides of the membrane are equal. Oral drugs use passive transport; they move from higher concentrations in the GI tract to lower concentrations in the blood stream.

Get active

Active transport requires cellular energy to move the drug from an area of lower concentration to one of higher concentration. Active transport is used to absorb electrolytes, such as sodium and potassium, as well as some drugs, such as levodopa.

Taking a bite out of particles

Pinocytosis is a unique form of active transport that occurs when a cell engulfs a drug particle. Pinocytosis is commonly employed to transport the fat-soluble vitamins (A, D, E, and K).

We're fat soluble, which means we're absorbed through pinocytosis.

Factors affecting absorption

Various factors—such as the route of administration, the amount of blood flow, and the form of the drug—can affect the rate of a drug's absorption.

Fast acting

If only a few cells separate the active drug from systemic circulation, absorption occurs rapidly and the drug quickly reaches therapeutic levels in the body. Typically, drug absorption occurs within seconds or minutes when administered sublingually, I.V., or by inhalation.

Not so fast

Absorption occurs at slower rates when drugs are administered by the oral, I.M., or subcutaneous routes because the complex membrane systems of GI mucosal layers, muscle, and skin delay drug passage.

At a snail's pace

At the slowest absorption rates, drugs can take several hours or days to reach peak concentration levels. A slow rate usually occurs with rectally administered or sustained-release drugs.

Intestinal interference

Several other factors can affect absorption of a drug. For example, most absorption of oral drugs occurs in the small intestine. If a patient has had large sections of the small intestine surgically removed, drug absorption decreases because of the reduced surface area and the reduced time the drug is in the intestine.

Liver-lowered levels

Drugs absorbed by the small intestine are transported to the liver before being circulated to the rest of the body. The liver may metabolise much of the drug before it enters circulation. This mechanism is referred to as the *first-pass effect*. Liver metabolism may inactivate the drug; if so, the first-pass effect lowers the amount of active drug released into the systemic circulation. Therefore, higher drug dosages must be administered to achieve the desired effect.

The process itself, is carried out by a group of enzymes termed Cytochrome P450. One of the main actions of these enzymes is to conjugate a fat soluble drug by making it water soluble for ease of renal excretion. Some drugs pass through the

Sublingual, I.V., or inhaled drugs are usually absorbed faster than rectally administered or sustained-release drugs.

Watch out for my first-pass effect! It lowers the amount of active drug released into the systemic circulation.

liver unchanged and others, called pro-drugs are activated by the action of these enzymes.

More blood, more absorption

Increased blood flow to an absorption site improves drug absorption, whereas reduced blood flow decreases absorption. More rapid absorption leads to a quicker onset of drug action.

For example, the muscle area selected for I.M. administration can make a difference in the drug absorption rate. Blood flows faster through the deltoid muscle (in the upper arm) than through the gluteal muscle (in the buttocks). The gluteal muscle, however, can accommodate a larger volume of drug than the deltoid muscle.

More pain, more stress, less drug

Pain and stress can also decrease the amount of drug absorbed. This may be due to a change in blood flow, reduced movement through the GI tract, or gastric retention triggered by the autonomic nervous system response to pain.

What's cooking?

High-fat meals and solid foods slow the rate at which contents leave the stomach and enter the intestines, delaying intestinal absorption of a drug. However, the absorption of some fat-soluble drugs is enhanced by the presence of a high fat content meal. An example of a drug that behaves in this manner is griseofulvin.

> Watch what your patient eats. High-fat meals and solid food can delay intestinal absorption of a drug.

Form factors

Drug formulation (such as tablets, capsules, liquids, sustained-release formulas, inactive ingredients, and coatings) affects the drug absorption rate and the time needed to reach peak blood concentration levels. For example, enteric-coated drugs are specifically formulated so that they don't dissolve immediately in the stomach. Rather, they release the active ingredient in the small intestine. Liquid forms, however, are readily absorbed in the stomach and at the beginning of the small intestine.

Combo considerations

Combining one drug with another drug, or with food, can cause interactions that increase or decrease drug absorption, depending on the substances involved.

Distribution

Drug distribution is the process by which the drug is delivered to the tissues and fluids of the body. Distribution of an absorbed drug within the body depends on several factors:
- blood flow
- solubility
- protein binding.

Having a large supply of blood has its perks. Drugs distribute to organs like me faster.

Those served first

After a drug has reached the bloodstream, its distribution in the body depends on blood flow. The drug is distributed quickly to those organs with a large supply of blood, including the heart, liver, and kidneys. Distribution to other internal organs, skin, fat, and muscle is slower.

Membrane crossing

The ability of a drug to cross a cell membrane depends on whether the drug is water- or lipid- (fat-) soluble. Lipid-soluble drugs easily cross through cell membranes, whereas water-soluble drugs can't. Lipid-soluble drugs can also cross the blood-brain barrier and enter the brain.

In a bind

As a drug travels through the body, it comes into contact with proteins, such as the plasma protein albumin. The drug can remain free or bind to the protein. The portion of a drug that's bound to a protein is inactive and can't exert a therapeutic effect. Only the free, or unbound, portion remains active. A drug is said to be *highly protein-bound* if more than 80% of it binds to protein.

Metabolism

Drug metabolism, or *biotransformation*, refers to the body's ability to change a drug from its dosage form to a more water-soluble form that can then be excreted. Drugs can be metabolised in several ways:
- Most commonly, a drug is metabolised into inactive metabolites (products of metabolism), which are then excreted.
- Some drugs can be converted to metabolites that are active, meaning they're capable of exerting their own pharmacologic action. These metabolites may undergo further metabolism or may be excreted from the body unchanged.
- Other drugs can be administered as inactive drugs, called *prodrugs*, and don't become active until they're metabolised.

Where the magic happens

Most drugs are metabolised by enzymes in the liver; however, metabolism can also occur in the plasma, kidneys, and membranes of the intestines. Some drugs inhibit or compete for enzyme metabolism, which can cause the accumulation of drugs when they're given together. This accumulation increases the potential for an adverse reaction or drug toxicity.

Metabolism busters

Certain diseases can reduce metabolism. These include liver disease, such as cirrhosis, and heart failure, which reduces circulation to the liver.

In the genes

Genetics allow some people to be able to metabolise drugs rapidly, while others metabolise them more slowly.

In the environment

Environment, too, can alter drug metabolism. For example, if a person is surrounded by cigarette smoke, the rate of metabolism of some drugs may be affected. A stressful environment, such as one involving prolonged illness or surgery, can also change how a person metabolises drugs.

Age effects

Developmental changes can also affect drug metabolism. For example, infants have immature livers that reduce the rate of metabolism, and elderly patients experience a decline in liver size, blood flow, and enzyme production that also slows metabolism.

Excretion

Drug excretion refers to the elimination of drugs from the body. Most drugs are excreted by the kidneys and leave the body through urine. Drugs can also be excreted through the lungs, exocrine glands (sweat, salivary, or mammary glands), skin, and intestinal tract.

Half-life = half the drug

The half-life of a drug is the time it takes for the plasma concentration of a drug to fall to half its original value. In other words, the time it takes for one-half of the drug to be eliminated by the body. Factors that affect a drug's half-life include its rates of

Although most drugs are metabolised in the liver, metabolism can also occur in the plasma, kidneys, and intestines.

absorption, metabolism, and excretion. Knowing how long a drug remains in the body helps determine how frequently a drug should be taken. Some drugs, for example diazepam, have a very long half-life (20-200 hours); others have a relatively short half-life. Naloxone has a half-life typically of 1-2 hours.

A drug that's given only once is eliminated from the body almost completely after four or five half-lives. A drug that's administered at regular intervals, however, reaches a steady concentration (or *steady state*) after about four or five half-lives. Steady state occurs when the rate of drug administration equals the rate of drug excretion.

A drug's half-life is the time it takes for one-half of the drug to be eliminated by the body.

Onset, peak, and duration

In addition to absorption, distribution, metabolism, and excretion, three other factors play important roles in a drug's pharmacokinetics:
• onset of action
• peak concentration
• duration of action.

How long until we see some action?

Onset of action refers to the time interval that starts when the drug is administered and ends when the therapeutic effect actually begins. Rate of onset varies depending on the route of administration and other pharmacokinetic properties.

When does it peak?

As the body absorbs more drug, blood concentration levels rise. The peak concentration level is reached when the absorption rate equals the elimination rate. However, the time of peak concentration isn't always the time of peak response.

A drug's action refers to the interaction between the drug and the body's cellular components.

How long will it last?

The duration of action is the length of time the drug produces its therapeutic effect.

Pharmacodynamics

Pharmacodynamics is the study of the drug mechanisms that produce biochemical or physiologic changes in the body. The interaction at the cellular level between a drug and cellular components, such as the complex proteins that make up the cell membrane, enzymes, or target receptors, represents drug action. The response resulting from this drug action is called the *drug effect*.

Fooling with function

A drug can modify cell function or the rate of function, but a drug can't impart a new function to a cell or target tissue. Therefore, the drug effect depends on what the cell is capable of accomplishing.

A drug can alter the target cell's function by:
* modifying the cell's physical or chemical environment
* interacting with a receptor (a specialised location on a cell membrane or inside a cell).

Stimulating response

An *agonist* is an example of a drug that interacts with receptors. An agonist drug has an attraction, or affinity, for a receptor, and stimulates it. The drug then binds with the receptor to produce its effect. The drug's ability to initiate a response after binding with the receptor is referred to as *intrinsic activity*.

I find you very attractive. Care to engage in some intrinsic activity?

Preventing response

If a drug has an affinity for a receptor but displays little or no intrinsic activity, it's called an *antagonist*. The antagonist prevents a response from occurring.

Antagonists can be competitive or noncompetitive:
* A *competitive antagonist* competes with the agonist for receptor sites. Because this type of drug binds reversibly to the receptor site, administering large doses of an agonist can overcome the antagonist's effects.
* A *noncompetitive antagonist* binds to receptor sites and blocks the effects of the agonist. Administering large doses of the agonist can't reverse its action.

Not so fussy

If a drug acts on a variety of receptors, it's said to be *nonselective* and can cause multiple and widespread effects.

How much do you need?

Drug potency refers to the relative amount of a drug required to produce a desired response. Drug potency is also used to compare two drugs. If drug X produces the same response as drug Y but at a lower dose, then drug X is more potent than drug Y.

Observe the curve

As its name implies, a dose-response curve is used to graphically represent the relationship between the dose of a drug and the response it produces. (See *Dose-response curve.*)

On the dose-response curve, a low dose usually corresponds with a low response. At a low dose, an increase in dose produces only a slight increase in response. With further increases in dose, there's a marked rise in drug response. After a certain point, an increase in dose yields little or no increase in response. At this point, the drug is said to have reached *maximum effectiveness.*

Good effects vs. bad effects

Most drugs produce multiple effects. The relationship between a drug's desired therapeutic effects and its adverse effects is called the drug's *therapeutic index.* It's also referred to as its *margin of safety.*

The therapeutic index usually measures the difference between:
- an effective dose for 50% of the patients treated
- the minimal dose at which adverse reactions occur.

Dose-response curve

This graph shows the drug-response curve for two different drugs. As you can see, at low doses of each drug, a dosage increase results in only a small increase in drug response (for example, from point A to point B). At higher doses, an increase in dosage produces a much greater response (from point B to point C). As the dosage continues to climb, an increase in dose produces very little increase in response (from point C to point D).

This graph also shows that drug X is more potent than drug Y because it results in the same response, but at a lower dose (compare point A to point E).

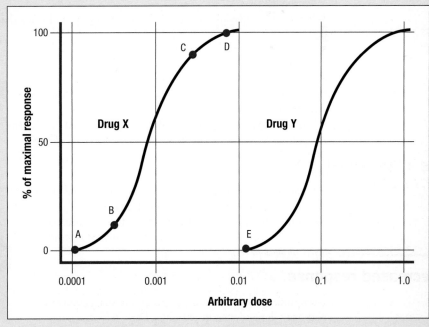

Narrow index = potential danger

A drug with a low or narrow therapeutic index has a narrow range of safety between an effective dose and a lethal one. On the other hand, a drug with a high therapeutic index has a wide range of safety and less risk of toxic effects. It should be emphasised that doubling the dose of a drug does not always double the therapeutic effect but may double the toxic effect. Furthermore, administration above the dose at which the maximum effect is observed will produce no added benefit.

Pharmacotherapeutics

Pharmacotherapeutics is the use of drugs to treat disease. When choosing a drug to treat a particular condition, health care providers consider the drug's effectiveness as well as such factors as the type of therapy the patient will receive.

Pick your therapy

The type of therapy prescribed depends on the severity, urgency, and prognosis of the patient's condition. Therapy types include:
- *acute therapy*, if the patient is critically ill and requires acute intensive therapy
- *empiric therapy*, based on practical experience rather than on pure scientific data
- *maintenance therapy*, for patients with chronic conditions that don't resolve
- *supplemental* or *replacement therapy*, to replenish or substitute for missing substances in the body
- *supportive therapy*, which doesn't treat the cause of the disease but maintains other threatened body systems until the patient's condition resolves
- *palliative therapy*, used for end-stage or terminal diseases to make the patient as comfortable as possible.

It's all personal

A patient's overall health as well as other individual factors can alter their response to a drug. Coinciding medical conditions and personal lifestyle characteristics must also be considered when selecting drug therapy. (See *Factors affecting patient response to a drug*.)

Decreased response...

Certain drugs have a tendency to create drug tolerance and drug dependence in patients. *Drug tolerance* occurs when a patient has a decreased response to a drug over time. The patient then requires larger doses to produce the same response.

> Keep the patient's coinciding medical conditions and lifestyle in mind when selecting drug therapy.

Factors affecting patient response to a drug

Because no two people are alike physiologically or psychologically, patient responses to a drug can vary greatly, depending on such factors as:

- Age: the elderly and very young have less efficient metabolic and removal procesesses and this usually requires a lower than recommended dose.
- Cardiovascular function: the capacity of a drug to reach its target can be reduced by the presence of Peripheral Vascular Disease. An example of this is present in the difficulty in treating infected ulcers in the diabetic patient.
- Diet: some drugs require to be given with or after food and others require to be given on an empty stomach. A drug's absorptive capabilities can be influenced in this way. Furthermore some foods may alter the action of certain drugs. For example, cranberry juice can enhance the effects of coumarin anticoagulants.
- Disease: the presence of disease frequently results in an increased risk of polypharmacy making drug interactions more likely. Some diseases can result in reduced renal function and a reduced capacity for drug elimination.
- Drug interactions: the more drugs prescribed to a patient, the increased risk of drug interaction. A common example of this relates to warfarin, the effects of which can be markedly enhanced by the presence of over-the-counter medicines such as aspirin, or the prolonged use of paracetamol.
- GI function: the absorptive function of the GI tract can be compromised through certain diseases resulting in delayed or reduced uptake of certain drugs.
- Hepatic function: the liver is the main organ of drug metabolism and as such, hepatic disease can seriously inhibit the capacity to detoxify and metabolise drugs.
- Infection: infection raises metabolic rate and hence the speed of drug removal.
- Renal function: the kidneys are the main route of drug excretion and renal disease significantly reduces removal of drugs from the body.
- Gender: there are differences in the way certain drugs affect men and women. Alcohol affects women more strongly than men as gastric alcohol dehydrogenase levels are lower in women resulting in an increased processing time for the drug.
- Body weight: body weight is proportional to the amount of body fat and as many drugs are fat soluble, then there is a greater volume for distribution.
- Genetic differences: as part of our evolutionary processes, our liver has developed the capacity to detoxify many chemicals and the same can be said of drugs. However, we all detoxify drugs at different rates.

...and increased desire

Tolerance differs from *drug dependence*, in which a patient displays a physical or psychological need for the drug. Physical dependence produces withdrawal symptoms when the drug is stopped, whereas psychological dependence is based on a desire to continue taking the drug to relieve tension and avoid discomfort.

Drug interactions

Drug interactions can occur between drugs or between drugs and foods. They can interfere with the results of a laboratory test or produce physical or chemical incompatibilities. The more drugs a patient receives, the greater the chances are that a drug interaction will occur.

Potential drug interactions include:
- additive effects
- potentiation
- antagonistic effects
- decreased or increased absorption
- decreased or increased metabolism and excretion.

Different drugs, similar actions

An *additive* effect can occur when two drugs with similar actions are administered to a patient. The effects are equivalent to the sum of the effects of either drug administered alone in higher doses. Giving two drugs together, such as two analgesics (pain relievers), has these potential advantages:
- Lower doses of each drug can be administered, which can decrease the probability of adverse reactions because higher doses increase the risk of adverse reactions.
- Greater pain control can be achieved than from administration of one drug alone (most likely because of different mechanisms of action).

Empowering effects

A synergistic effect, also called *potentiation*, occurs when two drugs that produce the same effect are given together and one drug potentiates (enhances) the effect of the other drug. This produces greater effects than either drug taken alone.

When two isn't better than one

An *antagonistic* drug interaction occurs when the combined response of two drugs is less than the response produced by either drug alone.

Memory jogger

When a drug is said to be **potentiated** by another drug, the results are more **potent**—the drug goes beyond its original potential.

Altering absorption

Two drugs given together can change the absorption of one or both of the drugs. For example, drugs that change the acidity of the stomach can affect the ability of another drug to dissolve in the stomach. Other drugs can interact and form an insoluble compound that can't be absorbed. Sometimes, an absorption interaction can be avoided by separating the administration of each drug by at least 2 hours.

For some drugs, you can avoid absorption interactions by separating their administration times by at least 2 hours.

Binding battles

After a drug is absorbed, blood distributes it throughout the body as a free drug or one that's bound to plasma protein. When two drugs are given together, they can compete for protein-binding sites, leading to an increase in the effects of one drug as that drug is displaced from the protein and becomes a free, unbound drug.

Turning toxic

Toxic drug levels can occur when a drug's metabolism and excretion are inhibited by another drug, particularly if the drug has a narrow therapeutic index. Some drug interactions affect excretion only.

Tampering with tests

Drug interactions can also alter laboratory tests and can produce changes seen on a patient's electrocardiogram.

Factor in food

Food can alter the therapeutic effects of a drug as well as the rate and amount of drug absorbed from the GI tract, affecting bioavailability (the amount of a drug dose available to the systemic circulation). Dangerous interactions can also occur. For example, when food that contains tyramine (such as aged cheddar cheese) is eaten by a person taking a monoamine oxidase inhibitor (MAOI), hypertensive crisis can occur. Also, grapefruit can inhibit the metabolism of certain drugs and result in toxic blood levels; examples include fexofenadine, albendazole, and ciclosporin.

Patients may need to avoid certain foods when taking drugs. For example, patients taking MAOIs should avoid foods containing tyramine.

Elevating enzymes

Some drugs stimulate enzyme production, increasing metabolic rates and the demand for vitamins that are enzyme cofactors (which must unite with the enzyme in order for the enzyme to function). Drugs can also impair vitamin and mineral absorption.

Adverse drug reactions

A drug's desired effect is called the *expected therapeutic response*. An adverse drug reaction, on the other hand (also called a *side effect* or *adverse effect*), is a harmful, undesirable response. Adverse drug reactions can range from mild reactions that disappear when the drug is stopped to debilitating diseases that become chronic. Adverse reactions can appear shortly after starting a new drug but may become less severe with time.

Due to the dose or the patient?

Adverse drug reactions can be classified as dose-related or patient sensitivity–related. Most adverse drug reactions result from the known pharmacologic effects of a drug and are typically dose-related. These types of reactions can be predicted in most cases.

Dose-related reactions

Dose-related reactions include:
- secondary effects
- hypersusceptibility
- overdose
- iatrogenic effects.

Sedation is an example of a secondary effect.

Secondary effects
A drug typically produces a major therapeutic effect as well as secondary effects that can be beneficial or adverse. For example, morphine used for pain control can lead to two undesirable secondary effects: constipation and respiratory depression. Promethazine used as an antihistamine is accompanied by the adverse reaction of sedation, which is why the drug is also sometimes used as a sleep aid.

Hypersusceptibility
A patient can be hypersusceptible to the pharmacologic actions of a drug. Even when given a usual therapeutic dose, a hypersusceptible patient can experience an excessive therapeutic response.

Hypersusceptibility typically results from altered pharmacokinetics (absorption, metabolism, and excretion), which lead to higher-than-expected blood concentration levels. Increased receptor sensitivity can also increase the patient's response to therapeutic or adverse effects.

Overdose

A toxic drug reaction can occur when an excessive dose is taken, either intentionally or accidentally. The result is an exaggerated response to the drug that can lead to transient changes or more serious reactions, such as respiratory depression, cardiovascular collapse, and even death. To avoid toxic reactions, chronically ill or elderly patients commonly receive lower drug doses.

Iatrogenic effects

Some adverse drug reactions, known as *iatrogenic effects*, can mimic pathologic disorders. For example, such drugs as antineoplastics, aspirin, corticosteroids, and indometacin commonly cause GI irritation and bleeding. Other examples of iatrogenic effects include induced asthma with propranolol and induced deafness with gentamicin.

Patient sensitivity–related adverse reactions

Patient sensitivity–related adverse reactions aren't as common as dose-related reactions. Sensitivity-related reactions result from a patient's unusual and extreme sensitivity to a drug. These adverse reactions arise from a unique tissue response rather than from an exaggerated pharmacologic action. Extreme patient sensitivity can occur as a drug allergy or an idiosyncratic response.

Allergic reaction

A *drug allergy* occurs when a patient's immune system identifies a drug, a drug metabolite, or a drug contaminant as a dangerous foreign substance that must be neutralised or destroyed. Previous exposure to the drug or to one with similar chemical characteristics sensitises the patient's immune system, and subsequent exposure causes an allergic reaction (hypersensitivity).

System-wide damage

An allergic reaction not only directly injures cells and tissues but also produces broader systemic damage by initiating cellular release of vasoactive and inflammatory substances. The allergic reaction can vary in intensity from an immediate, life-threatening anaphylactic reaction with circulatory collapse and swelling of the larynx and bronchioles to a mild reaction with a rash and itching.

Allergic reactions to drugs can range from life-threatening anaphylaxis to a mild rash with itching.

Idiosyncratic response

Some sensitivity-related adverse reactions don't result from the pharmacologic properties of a drug or from an allergy, but are specific to the individual patient. These are called *idiosyncratic responses*. A patient's idiosyncratic response sometimes has a genetic cause.

The nursing process

One of the most significant advances in nursing has been the development of the nursing process. This problem-solving approach to nursing care provides a systematic method of determining the patient's health problems, developing a care plan to address those problems, implementing the plan, and evaluating the plan's effectiveness. The nursing process guides nursing decisions about drug administration to ensure the patient's safety and to meet medical and legal standards.

The five steps of the nursing process are dynamic, flexible, and interrelated. They include:

- assessment
- nursing diagnosis
- planning
- implementation
- evaluation.

> The nursing process guides decisions about drug administration to ensure patient safety and to meet medical and legal standards.

EVALUATION
IMPLEMENTATION
PLANNING
NURSING DIAGNOSIS
ASSESSMENT

Assessment

Assessment involves collecting data that's used to identify the patient's actual and potential health needs, although it may also include the collection of objective data. Often at evaluation, nurses may be required to measure the response to a drug against objective data.

You can obtain data by taking a health history, performing a physical examination, and reviewing pertinent laboratory and diagnostic information. The health history includes documenting drugs and herbal preparations that the patient is taking as well as any allergies.

Nursing diagnosis

Nursing diagnosis can be defined as a "clinical judgment about individual, family, or community responses to actual or potential health problems or life processes."

As such, nursing diagnoses provide the basis for the selection of nursing interventions to achieve outcomes for which the nurse is accountable. Nursing diagnoses need to be individualised for each patient, based on the patient's medical condition and the drugs they are receiving.

Planning

After you establish a nursing diagnosis, you'll develop a written care plan. A written care plan serves as a communication tool among health care team members that helps ensure continuity of care. The plan consists of two parts:

> Your care plan should include expected outcomes and the nursing interventions needed to achieve those outcomes.

📝 patient outcomes, or expected outcomes, which describe behaviour or results to be achieved within a specific time

✌ nursing interventions needed to achieve those outcomes.

These may be based on objective data such as; reduce temperature, increase output, or reduce/increase blood pressure.

Implementation

The implementation phase is when you put your care plan into action. Implementation encompasses all nursing interventions, including drug therapy, that are directed toward meeting the patient's health care needs. While you coordinate implementation, you collaborate with the patient and the patient's family and consult with other caregivers. Implementation can involve a multidisciplinary approach depending on the needs of the patient and family. An important aspect of implementation lies within the realm of good clinical judgement, in tandem with healthcare policies and protocols.

Evaluation

The final step in the nursing process is evaluation. During evaluation, you must determine if the interventions carried out have enabled the patient to achieve the desired outcomes. If you stated the outcome criteria in measurable terms, then you can easily evaluate the extent to which the outcomes were met. This includes evaluating the effectiveness of drug interventions, such as pain relief after the patient received an analgesic. Evaluation is an ongoing process, and reassessment leads to the development of new nursing diagnoses and nursing interventions based on the patient's response to treatment.

Quick quiz

1. How a drug is absorbed or excreted is called:
  A. pharmacodynamics.
  B. pharmacotherapeutics.
  C. pharmacokinetics.
  D. drug interactions.

Answer: C. Pharmacokinetics involves the absorption, distribution, metabolism, and excretion of a drug.

2. What type of drug interaction occurs when two drugs that normally produce the same effect are taken, resulting in an enhanced effect?
  A. Additive effect
  B. Potentiation
  C. Increased absorption
  D. Decreased effect

Answer: B. Potentiation occurs when two drugs that produce the same effect are given together. One drug enhances the effect of the other drug, resulting in greater effects of both drugs.

3. Expected outcomes are defined as:
  A. goals the patient and family ask you to accomplish.
  B. goals that are above the level the patient can realistically reach.
  C. goals that were met by the patient in the past.
  D. goals the patient should reach as a result of planned nursing interventions.

Answer: D. Expected outcomes are realistic, measurable goals for the patient.

Scoring

☆☆☆ If you answered all three questions correctly, fantastic! You obviously know your fundamental pharm facts.

☆☆ If you answered two questions correctly, terrific! You can clearly interact well with this material.

☆ If you answered fewer than two questions correctly, don't have an adverse reaction. You can improve your absorption of this chapter with a quick review.

② Autonomic nervous system drugs

Just the facts

In this chapter, you'll learn:

♦ classes of drugs that affect the autonomic nervous system

♦ uses and actions of these drugs

♦ absorption, distribution, metabolism, and excretion of these drugs

♦ drug interactions and adverse reactions to these drugs.

Cholinergic drugs

Cholinergic drugs promote the action of the neurotransmitter acetylcholine. These drugs are also called *parasympathomimetic drugs* because they produce effects that imitate parasympathetic nerve stimulation.

Mimic or inhibit

There are two major classes of cholinergic drugs:
* *Cholinergic agonists* mimic the action of the neurotransmitter acetylcholine.
* *Anticholinesterase drugs* work by inhibiting the destruction of acetylcholine at cholinergic receptor sites. (See *How cholinergic drugs work.*)

Cholinergic agonists

By directly stimulating cholinergic receptors, cholinergic agonists mimic the action of the neurotransmitter acetylcholine. They include such drugs as:
* acetylcholine (not to be confused with the neurotransmitter)

Simon says, act like an acetylcholine neurotransmitter!

Pharm function

How cholinergic drugs work

Cholinergic drugs fall into one of two major classes: cholinergic agonists and anticholinesterase drugs. Here's how these drugs achieve their effects.

Cholinergic agonists

When a neuron in the parasympathetic nervous system is stimulated, the neurotransmitter acetylcholine is released. Acetylcholine crosses the synapse and interacts with receptors in an adjacent neuron. Cholinergic agonist drugs work by stimulating cholinergic receptors, mimicking the action of acetylcholine.

Anticholinesterase drugs

After acetylcholine stimulates the cholinergic receptor, it's destroyed by the enzyme acetylcholinesterase. Anticholinesterase drugs produce their effects by inhibiting acetylcholinesterase. As a result, acetylcholine isn't broken down and begins to accumulate; therefore, the effects of acetylcholine are prolonged.

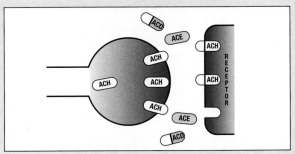

Key:

ACH Acetylcholine   CAD Cholinergic agonist drug   ACE Acetylcholinesterase   ACD Anticholinesterase drug

- bethanechol
- carbachol
- pilocarpine.

Pharmacokinetics

The action and metabolism of cholinergic agonists vary widely and depend on the affinity of the individual drug for muscarinic or nicotinic receptors. For example, the drug acetylcholine poorly penetrates the central nervous system (CNS), and its effects are primarily peripheral, with a widespread parasympathetic action. The drug is rapidly destroyed in the body.

By eyes, mouth, or injection

Cholinergic agonists are usually administered:
- topically, with eye drops
- orally
- by subcutaneous injection.

Subcutaneous injections begin to work more rapidly than oral doses.

N-O to I.M. or I.V.

The cholinergic agonists are rarely administered by I.M. or I.V. injection because they're almost immediately broken down by cholinesterase in the interstitial spaces between tissues and inside the blood vessels. Moreover, they begin to work rapidly and can cause a cholinergic crisis (a drug overdose resulting in extreme muscle weakness and possible paralysis of the muscles used in respiration).

Cholinergic agonists are absorbed rapidly and reach peak levels within 2 hours. Food decreases their absorption. Less than 20% of a cholinergic agonist is protein bound.

Giving cholinergic agonists I.M. or I.V. can cause cholinergic crisis

All summed up

All cholinergic agonists are metabolised by cholinesterase:
- at the muscarinic and nicotinic receptor sites
- in the plasma (the liquid portion of the blood)
- in the liver.

These drugs are excreted by the kidneys.

Pharmacodynamics

Cholinergic agonists work by mimicking the action of acetylcholine on the neurons in certain organs of the body, called *target organs*. When they combine with receptors on the cell membranes of target organs, they stimulate the muscle and produce:
- salivation
- bradycardia (a slow heart rate)
- dilation of blood vessels
- constriction of the pulmonary bronchioles
- increased activity of the GI tract
- increased tone and contraction of the muscles of the bladder
- constriction of the pupils.

Cholinergic agonists stimulate the muscles of target organs.

Pharmacotherapeutics

Cholinergic agonists are used to:
- treat atonic (weak) bladder conditions and postoperative and postpartum urine retention

- treat GI disorders, such as postoperative abdominal distention and GI atony
- reduce eye pressure in patients with glaucoma and during eye surgery
- treat salivary gland hypofunction caused by radiation therapy and Sjögren's syndrome.

Drug interactions

Cholinergic agonists have specific interactions with other drugs. Here are some examples:

- Other cholinergic drugs, particularly anticholinesterase drugs (such as edrophonium, neostigmine, pyridostigmine and rivastigmine) boost the effects of cholinergic agonists and increase the risk of toxicity.
- Anticholinergic drugs (such as atropine, belladonna, homatropine, hyoscine and propantheline) reduce the effects of cholinergic drugs.

Adverse reactions

Because they bind with receptors in the parasympathetic nervous system, cholinergic agonists can produce adverse effects in any organ innervated by the parasympathetic nerves. These adverse effects can include:

- nausea and vomiting
- cramps and diarrhoea
- blurred vision
- decreased heart rate and low blood pressure
- shortness of breath
- urinary frequency
- increased salivation and sweating.

Cholinergic agonists can produce adverse effects in any organ that's supplied with parasympathetic nerves. That includes me!

Nursing process

These nursing process steps are appropriate for patients undergoing treatment with cholinergic agonists.

Assessment

- Assess for disorders in which cholinergic agonists are used, such as myasthenia gravis.
- Assess for urine retention and bladder distention; determine the patient's fluid intake and time and amount of last urination.
- Assess for possible paralytic ileus (paralysis of the small intestine) by checking for bowel sounds and abdominal distention and determining the patient's elimination patterns.

• Assess for disorders that may be aggravated by cholinergic agonists, such as Alzheimer's disease.

Key nursing diagnoses
• Impaired gas exchange related to increased secretions, bronchospasm, or respiratory paralysis.
• Ineffective airway clearance related to increased respiratory secretions.
• Impaired urinary elimination related to cholinergic drug action.

Planning outcome goals
• Effective oxygenation of tissues will be maintained.
• The patient will regain usual patterns of urinary and bowel elimination.
• Therapeutic effects of cholinergic drugs will be observed.
• The patient will demonstrate correct drug administration.

Implementation
• Administer cholinergic drugs as prescribed. Be aware that some drugs, such as bethanechol, should be given before meals.
• Monitor for effects of cholinergic drugs and report adverse reactions.
• Assess for signs of respiratory adequacy, and perform measures to promote adequate gas exchange, such as deep breathing and coughing, suctioning, and proper positioning of the patient.
• Assess for urinary adequacy and signs of urine retention.
• Assist the patient in establishing a drug administration schedule that meets his needs.
• Provide patient teaching. (See *Teaching about cholinergic drugs.*)

Evaluation
• Patient's underlying condition improves.
• Patient maintains a normal respiratory rate.
• Patient maintains a normal voiding pattern.
• Patient regains normal bowel patterns.
• Patient and family demonstrate an understanding of drug therapy.

Anticholinesterase drugs

Anticholinesterase drugs block the action of the enzyme acetylcholinesterase at cholinergic receptor sites, preventing the breakdown of the neurotransmitter acetylcholine. As acetylcholine builds up, it continues to stimulate the cholinergic receptors.

Before giving cholinergic agonists, check for disorders that may be aggravated by these drugs, such as Alzheimer's disease.

Education edge

Teaching about cholinergic drugs

If cholinergic drugs are prescribed, review these points with the patient and caregivers:

- Take the drug as directed on a regular schedule to maintain consistent blood levels of the drug and symptom control.
- Don't chew or crush sustained-release tablets or capsules.
- Take oral cholinergics on an empty stomach to lessen nausea and vomiting and increase the drug's absorption.
- If diarrhoea or vomiting occurs, ensure adequate fluid intake.
- Cholinergic drugs for urine retention act within 60 minutes of taking them. Make sure bathroom facilities are available.
- If taking a cholinergic drug long term, such as for myasthenia gravis, bladder problems, or Alzheimer's disease, wear or carry medical alert identification.
- If indicated, record symptoms of myasthenia gravis and the effects of the drug in a diary, especially if the dosage is adjusted.

- For those with myasthenia gravis, plan rest periods between activities and space activities throughout the day. The goal of therapy is to obtain optimal benefit from the drug using the lowest possible dose with fewest adverse effects. If activity increases, the dosage may need to be increased.
- Report increased muscle weakness, difficulty breathing, recurrence of myasthenia gravis symptoms, and other adverse reactions to the prescriber.
- If dizziness or syncope occurs, lie down and rest, then get up gradually. Ambulation should be supervised.
- Don't take over-the-counter drugs or herbal preparations without first consulting with the prescriber because interactions may occur. For example, remedies such as St. John's wort alter the blood levels of donepezil.

Anticholinesterase drugs are divided into two categories—reversible and irreversible.

Short acting

Reversible anticholinesterase drugs have a short duration of action and include:
- donepezil
- edrophonium
- galantamine
- neostigmine
- pyridostigmine
- rivastigmine

> Anticholinesterase drugs block acetylcholinesterase enzymes from breaking down the neurotransmitter acetylcholine.

Long lasting but limited

Irreversible anticholinesterase drugs have long-lasting effects and are used primarily as toxic insecticides and pesticides or as nerve gas agents in chemical warfare. (Pyridostigmine enhances the effects of antidotes used to counteract nerve agents.)

Pharmacokinetics

Here's a brief rundown of how anticholinesterase drugs move through the body.

Ready to be readily absorbed

Many of the anticholinesterase drugs are readily absorbed from the GI tract, subcutaneous tissue, and mucous membranes.

Poorly absorbed but packs some action

Because neostigmine is poorly absorbed from the GI tract, the patient needs a higher dose when taking this drug orally. The duration of action for an oral dose is longer, however, so the patient doesn't need to take it as frequently.

Need it now?

When a rapid effect is needed, the drug should be given by the I.M. or I.V. route.

Diverse delivery

The distribution of anticholinesterase drugs varies. For example, donepezil is highly bound to plasma proteins, whereas rivastigmine is 40% bound, and galantamine is 18% bound.

Most anticholinesterase drugs are metabolised in the body by enzymes in the plasma and excreted in the urine. Donepezil, galantamine, and rivastigmine, however, are metabolised in the liver but still excreted in urine.

Pharmacodynamics

Anticholinesterase drugs, like cholinergic agonists, promote the action of acetylcholine at receptor sites. Depending on the site and the drug's dose and duration of action, they can produce a stimulant or depressant effect on cholinergic receptors.

How long do the effects go on?

Reversible anticholinesterase drugs block the breakdown of acetylcholine for minutes to hours. The blocking effect of irreversible anticholinesterase drugs can last for days or weeks.

Pharmacotherapeutics

Anticholinesterase drugs have various therapeutic uses. They're used:
* to reduce eye pressure in patients with glaucoma and during eye surgery
* to increase bladder tone
* to improve tone and peristalsis (movement) through the GI tract in patients with reduced motility and paralytic ileus
* to promote muscular contraction in patients with myasthenia gravis
* to diagnose myasthenia gravis (neostigmine and edrophonium are used for this purpose)
* as antidotes to anticholinergic drugs, tricyclic antidepressants, belladonna alkaloids, and opioids
* to treat mild to moderate dementia and enhance cognition in patients with Alzheimer's disease (specifically, donepezil, galantamine, and rivastigmine are used for this purpose).

Anticholinesterase drugs can stimulate or depress cholinergic receptors.

Drug interactions

These interactions can occur with anticholinesterase drugs:
* Other cholinergic drugs, particularly cholinergic agonists (such as bethanechol, carbachol, and pilocarpine), increase the risk of toxic effects when taken with anticholinesterase drugs.
* Carbamazepine, dexamethasone, rifampacin, phenytoin, and phenobarbital may increase elimination rate of donepezil.
* Aminoglycoside antibiotics, anaesthetics, anticholinergic drugs (such as atropine, belladonna, hyoscine and propantheline), magnesium, corticosteroids, and antiarrhythmic drugs (such as procainamide) can reduce the effects of anticholinesterase drugs and can mask early signs of a cholinergic crisis.
* Other drugs with cholinergic-blocking properties, such as tricyclic antidepressants, bladder relaxants, and antipsychotics, can counteract the effects of anticholinesterase drugs.
* The effects of donepezil, and galantamine may be increased when combined with known inhibitors of cytochrome P-450 (CYP450), such as cimetidine and erythromycin.
* Cigarette use increases the clearance (how quickly the drug is excreted from the body) of rivastigmine.

Talk about too much of a good thing! Giving other cholinergics with anticholinesterase drugs increases the risk of toxic effects.

Adverse reactions

Most of the adverse reactions to anticholinesterase drugs result from increased action of acetylcholine at receptor sites. Adverse reactions associated with these drugs include:
* cardiac arrhythmias
* nausea and vomiting
* diarrhoea
* shortness of breath, wheezing, or tightness in the chest

Recognising toxic response

It's difficult to predict adverse reactions to anticholinesterase drugs in a patient with myasthenia gravis because the therapeutic dose varies from day to day. Increased muscle weakness can result from:

- resistance to the drug
- receiving too little anticholinesterase drug
- receiving too much anticholinesterase drug.

Enter edrophonium

Deciding whether a patient is experiencing a toxic drug response (too much drug) or a myasthenic crisis (extreme muscle weakness and severe respiratory difficulties) can be difficult. Edrophonium can be used to distinguish between a toxic drug effect and myasthenic crisis. When edrophonium is used, suction equipment, oxygen, mechanical ventilation, and emergency drugs (such as atropine) must be readily available in case a cholinergic crisis occurs.

- seizures
- headache
- anorexia
- insomnia
- pruritus
- urinary frequency and nocturia.
  (See *Recognising toxic response*.)

Nursing process

These nursing process steps are appropriate for patients undergoing treatment with anticholinesterase drugs.

Assessment

- Assess for disorders in which anticholinesterase drugs are used, such as myasthenia gravis, Alzheimer's disease, glaucoma, and altered bladder function.
- Assess for urine retention and bladder distention, determine the patient's fluid intake, and find out the time and amount of last urination.
- Assess for possible paralytic ileus by checking for bowel sounds and abdominal distention and determining the patient's elimination patterns.

Key nursing diagnoses

- Impaired gas exchange related to bronchospasm or respiratory paralysis.
- Impaired tissue integrity related to effects of anticholinergic drugs.
- Impaired urinary elimination related to anticholinergic drug action.

Planning outcome goals

- Effective oxygenation of tissues will be maintained.

- The patient will regain normal patterns of urinary and bowel elimination.
- Therapeutic effects of anticholinesterase drugs will be observed.
- The patient will demonstrate correct drug administration.

Implementation
- Administer anticholinesterase drugs as prescribed. Give these drugs before meals unless otherwise directed.
- Monitor for effects of anticholinesterase drugs and report adverse reactions.
- Assess for signs of respiratory adequacy and perform measures to promote adequate gas exchange, such as deep breathing and coughing, suctioning, and proper positioning of the patient.
- Assess for urinary adequacy and signs of urine retention.
- Assist the patient in establishing a drug administration schedule that meets their needs.
- Provide patient teaching. (See *Teaching about anticholinesterase drugs.*)

Evaluation
- Patient's underlying condition improves.
- Patient maintains a normal respiratory rate.
- Patient maintains a normal voiding pattern.
- Patient regains normal bowel patterns.
- Patient and family demonstrate an understanding of drug therapy.

When giving anticholinesterase drugs, be sure to promote adequate gas exchange!

Education edge

Teaching about anticholinesterase drugs

If anticholinesterase drugs are prescribed, review these points with the patient and caregivers:

- The drug doesn't alter underlying degenerative disease but can alleviate symptoms.
- Memory improvement may be subtle. A more likely result of therapy is a slower decline in memory loss.
- When used for myasthenia gravis, these drugs relieve ptosis, double vision, difficulty chewing and swallowing, and trunk and limb weakness.
- Take the drug exactly as prescribed. The drug may have to be taken for life.

- Those with myasthenia gravis should wear or carry medical alert identification.
- Immediately report significant adverse effects or changes in overall health status.
- Report the use of anticholinesterase drugs to the health care team before receiving anaesthesia.
- Report episodes of nausea, vomiting, or diarrhoea.
- Consult the prescriber before taking over-the-counter drugs or herbal preparations because these may interact with the anticholinesterase drug.

Anticholinergic drugs

Anticholinergic drugs interrupt parasympathetic nerve impulses in the CNS and autonomic nervous system. They also prevent acetylcholine from stimulating cholinergic receptors.

For muscarinic sites only

Anticholinergic drugs don't block all cholinergic receptors, just the muscarinic receptor sites. Muscarinic receptors are cholinergic receptors that are stimulated by the alkaloid muscarine and blocked by atropine.

Belladonna alkaloids and other derivatives

The major anticholinergic drugs are the belladonna alkaloids:
- atropine (see *Anticholinergic drugs: Atropine.*)
- belladonna
- homatropine
- hyoscine.

> I hate to play favourites, but I prefer muscarinic receptor sites to other receptor sites.

Synthetic string

Synthetic derivatives of belladonna alkaloids (the quaternary ammonium drugs) include:
- glycopyrronium
- propantheline

Third string

The tertiary amines are newer synthetic drugs. They're centrally acting and more selective. They also have fewer adverse effects. Examples of tertiary amines include:
- benzatropine
- dicycloverine
- oxybutynin
- tolterodine
- trihexyphenidyl.

Pharmacokinetics

The belladonna alkaloids are absorbed from the eyes, GI tract, mucous membranes, and skin.

Prototype pro

Anticholinergic drugs: Atropine

Actions

- Competitively antagonises the actions of acetylcholine and other cholinergic agonists at the muscarinic receptors.

Indications

- Symptomatic bradycardia
- Preoperative reduction of secretions and blockage of cardiac vagal reflexes
- Adjunct treatment of peptic ulcer disease
- Functional GI disorders

Nursing considerations

- Monitor for adverse reactions, such as headache, tachycardia, restlessness, dizziness, blurred vision, dry mouth, urinary hesitancy, and constipation.
- Monitor vital signs, cardiac rhythm, urine output, and vision for signs of impending toxicity.
- Constipation may be relieved by stool softeners or bulk laxatives.

GI reliant

The quaternary ammonium drugs and tertiary amines are absorbed primarily through the GI tract, although not as readily as the belladonna alkaloids.

Instant gratification

When administered I.V., anticholinergic drugs such as atropine begin to work immediately. The belladonna alkaloids are distributed more widely throughout the body than the quaternary ammonium derivatives or tertiary amines. The alkaloids readily cross the blood-brain barrier; the other drugs in this class don't.

Ready and able

The belladonna alkaloids have low to moderate binding with serum proteins and are only slightly to moderately protein bound. This means that a moderate to high amount of the drug is active and available to produce a therapeutic response. They're metabolised in the liver and excreted by the kidneys as unchanged drug and metabolites.

Metabolism of the tertiary amines is unknown, but excretion is usually through the kidneys and in faeces.

Each type of drug has its own benefits. For example, the belladonna alkaloids are absorbed more readily through the GI tract and distribute widely, but tertiary amines have fewer adverse effects.

Complicated quaternary kinetics

The quaternary ammonium drugs are a bit more complicated. Hydrolysis occurs in the GI tract and the liver; excretion is in faeces and urine. Dicycloverine metabolism is unknown, but it's excreted equally in faeces and urine.

Pharmacodynamics

Anticholinergic drugs can have paradoxical effects on the body, depending on the dosage, the condition being treated, and the target organ. For example, anticholinergic drugs can produce a stimulating or depressing effect. In the brain, they do both—low drug levels stimulate and high drug levels depress.

Disorder-related dynamics

A patient's disorder can also impact the effects of a drug. Parkinson's disease, for example, is characterised by low dopamine levels that intensify the stimulating effects of acetylcholine. Cholinergic blockers, however, depress this effect. In other disorders, these same drugs stimulate the CNS.

Pharmacotherapeutics

Here's how anticholinergic drugs are used in various GI situations:
• All anticholinergic drugs are used to treat spastic or hyperactive conditions of the GI and urinary tracts because they relax muscles and decrease GI secretions. However, for bladder relaxation and urinary incontinence, the quaternary ammonium compounds, such as propantheline, are the drugs of choice because they cause fewer adverse reactions than the belladonna alkaloids.
• The belladonna alkaloids are used with morphine to treat biliary colic (pain caused by stones in the bile duct).
• Anticholinergic drugs are given by injection before some diagnostic procedures, such as endoscopy or sigmoidoscopy, to relax the GI smooth muscle.

Preop purposes

Anticholinergic drugs such as atropine are given before surgery to:
• reduce oral, gastric, and respiratory secretions
• prevent a drop in heart rate caused by vagal nerve stimulation during anaesthesia.

Brain games

The belladonna alkaloids can affect the brain. For example, when given with the pain medications hyoscine, morphine or pethidine it can cause drowsiness and amnesia. It's also used to treat motion sickness.

Giving anticholinergics by injection before diagnostic procedures relaxes GI smooth muscle.

Heart matters

The belladonna alkaloids also have therapeutic effects on the heart. Atropine is the drug of choice to treat:
• symptomatic sinus bradycardia—when the heart beats too slow, causing low blood pressure or dizziness (See *How atropine speeds heart rate.*)
• arrhythmias resulting from anaesthetics, choline esters, or suxamethonium.

In your eyes

Anticholinergic drugs also are used as cycloplegics, which means they:
• paralyze the ciliary muscles of the eye (used for fine focusing)
• alter the shape of the lens of the eye.
   Furthermore, anticholinergic drugs act as mydriatics to dilate the pupils of the eye, making it easier to measure refractive errors during an eye examination or to perform surgery on the eye.

Antidote-i-ful

The belladonna alkaloids, particularly atropine, are effective antidotes to cholinergic and anticholinesterase drugs. Atropine is the drug of choice to treat poisoning from organophosphate pesticides and can also counteract the effects of the neuromuscular blocking drugs by competing for the same receptor sites.

Belladonna alkaloids can serve as antidotes to certain pesticides and other drugs.

Drug interactions

Because anticholinergic drugs slow the passage of food and drugs through the stomach, drugs remain in prolonged contact with the mucous membranes of the GI tract. This increases the amount of the drug that's absorbed and, therefore, increases the risk of adverse effects.

Effect boosters

Drugs that increase the effects of anticholinergic drugs include:
• disopyramide
• antidyskinetics (such as amantadine)
• antiemetics and antivertigo drugs (such as buclizine and cyclizine)
• antipsychotics (such as haloperidol, phenothiazines, and thioxanthenes)
• orphenadrine
• tricyclic and related antidepressants.

Pharm function

How atropine speeds heart rate

To understand how atropine affects the heart, first consider how the heart's electrical conduction system functions.

Without the drug

When the neurotransmitter acetylcholine is released, the vagus nerve stimulates the sinoatrial (SA) node (the heart's pacemaker) and atrioventricular (AV) node, which controls conduction between the atria and ventricles of the heart. This inhibits electrical conduction and causes the heart rate to slow down.

With the drug

When a patient receives atropine, a cholinergic blocking drug, it competes with acetylcholine for binding with the cholinergic receptors on the SA and AV nodes. By blocking acetylcholine, atropine speeds up the heart rate.

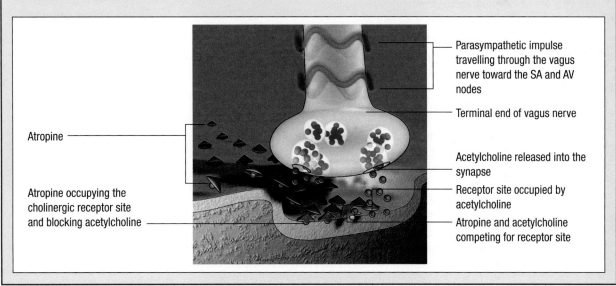

Atropine

Atropine occupying the cholinergic receptor site and blocking acetylcholine

Parasympathetic impulse travelling through the vagus nerve toward the SA and AV nodes

Terminal end of vagus nerve

Acetylcholine released into the synapse

Receptor site occupied by acetylcholine

Atropine and acetylcholine competing for receptor site

Effect busters

Drugs that decrease the effects of anticholinergic drugs include:
- cholinergic agonists (such as bethanechol)
- anticholinesterase drugs (such as neostigmine and pyridostigmine).

And there's more

Here are other drug interactions that can occur:
- The risk of digoxin toxicity increases when digoxin is taken with an anticholinergic drug.

- Opiate-like analgesics further enhance the slow movement of food and drugs through the GI tract when taken with cholinergic blockers.
- The absorption of glyceryl trinitrate tablets placed under the tongue is reduced when taken with a cholinergic blocker.

Adverse reactions

Adverse reactions of anticholinergic drugs are closely related to drug dose. The difference between a therapeutic and a toxic dosage is small with these drugs.

Adverse reactions may include:
- dry mouth
- reduced bronchial secretions
- increased heart rate
- blurred vision
- decreased sweating.

Nursing process

These nursing process steps are appropriate for patients undergoing treatment with anticholinergic drugs.

Assessment
- Assess for conditions in which anticholinergic drugs would be used, such as bradycardia, heart block (a delay or interruption in the conduction of electrical impulses between the atria and ventricles), diarrhoea, and peptic ulcer disease.
- Assess for conditions in which anticholinergic drugs would be contra-indicated, such as glaucoma, myasthenia gravis, prostatic hyperplasia, reflux oesophagitis, or GI obstructive disease.

Key nursing diagnoses
- Urinary retention related to adverse effects on the bladder.
- Constipation related to adverse effects on the GI tract.
- Risk for injury related to adverse drug effects.

Planning outcome goals
- The patient will experience relief of symptoms.
- The patient will remain free from adverse reactions.

Implementation
- Follow dosage recommendations. Some drugs should be given with meals.

Anticholinergics are contraindicated in patients with glaucoma, myasthenia gravis, prostatic hyperplasia, reflux oesophagitis, or GI obstructive disease.

- Monitor vital signs, cardiac rhythm, urine output, and vision for potential drug toxicity.
- Monitor for adverse reactions, such as dry mouth, increased heart rate, and blurred vision.
- Have emergency equipment available to treat new cardiac arrhythmias.
- Help alleviate symptoms if adverse effects occur. For example, provide lozenges and frequent mouth care for patients experiencing dry mouth.
- Provide patient teaching. (See *Teaching about anticholinergic drugs.*)

Evaluation
- Patient's underlying condition improves.
- Patient maintains a normal heart rate.
- Patient maintains a normal voiding pattern.
- Patient regains normal bowel patterns.
- Patient and family demonstrate an understanding of drug therapy.

Education edge

Teaching about anticholinergic drugs

If anticholinergic drugs are prescribed, review these points with the patient and caregivers:

- Take the drug as prescribed; don't take other drugs with the anticholinergic unless prescribed.
- Avoid hazardous tasks if dizziness, drowsiness, or blurred vision occurs.
- The drug may increase sensitivity to high temperatures, resulting in dizziness.
- Avoid alcohol because it may have additive central nervous system effects.
- Drink plenty of fluids and eat a high-fibre diet to prevent constipation.
- Notify the prescriber promptly if confusion, rapid or pounding heartbeat, dry mouth, blurred vision, rash, eye pain, significant change in urine volume, pain on urination, or difficulty urinating occur.
- Women should report planned or known pregnancy.

Adrenergic drugs

Adrenergic drugs are also called *sympathomimetic drugs* because they produce effects similar to those produced by the sympathetic nervous system.

Sort by chemical...

Adrenergic drugs are classified into two groups based on their chemical structure: catecholamines (both naturally occurring as well as synthetic) and noncatecholamines.

...or by action

Adrenergic drugs are also divided by how they act. They can be:
- *direct-acting*, in which the drug acts directly on the organ or tissue innervated (supplied with nerves or nerve impulses) by the sympathetic nervous system
- *indirect-acting*, in which the drug triggers the release of a neurotransmitter, usually noradrenaline (norepinephrine)
- *dual-acting*, in which the drug has direct and indirect actions.
(See *How adrenergics work*.)

Catecholamines

Because of their common basic chemical structure, catecholamines share certain properties—they stimulate the nervous system, constrict peripheral blood vessels, increase heart rate, and dilate the bronchi. They can be manufactured in the body or in a laboratory. Common catecholamines include:
- dobutamine
- dopamine
- adrenaline (epinephrine) and noradrenaline acid tartarate (norepinephrine bitartate)
- noradrenaline (norepinephrine)
- isoprenaline

Pharmacokinetics

Here's an overview of how catecholamines move through the body.

Hard to swallow

Catecholamines can't be taken orally because they're destroyed by digestive enzymes. In contrast, when these drugs are given sublingually (under the tongue), they're rapidly absorbed through the mucous membranes. Any sublingual drug not completely absorbed is rapidly metabolised by swallowed saliva.

Pharm function

How adrenergics work

Adrenergic drugs are distinguished by how they achieve their effect. The illustrations below show the action of direct-, indirect-, and dual-acting adrenergics.

Direct-acting adrenergic action

Direct-acting adrenergic drugs directly stimulate adrenergic receptors.

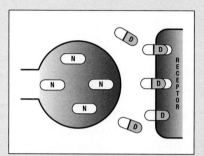

Indirect-acting adrenergic action

Indirect-acting adrenergic drugs stimulate the release of noradrenaline (norepinephrine) from nerve endings into the synapse.

Dual-acting adrenergic action

Dual-acting adrenergic drugs stimulate both adrenergic receptor sites and the release of noradrenaline (norepinephrine) from nerve endings.

Adrenergic drugs can be direct-acting, indirect-acting, or both.

Key:

Noradrenaline (Norepinephrine)   Adrenergic drug

Subcutaneous vs. Intramuscular

Subcutaneous absorption of catecholamines is slowed because these drugs cause the blood vessels around the injection site to constrict. I.M. absorption is more rapid because less constriction of local blood vessels occurs.

Catecholamines are widely distributed in the body. They're metabolised and inactivated predominantly in the liver but can also be metabolised in the GI tract, lungs, kidneys, plasma, and tissues.

Main exit

Catecholamines are excreted primarily in urine; however, a small amount of isoproterenol is excreted in faeces and some adrenaline (epinephrine) is excreted in breast milk.

Pharmacodynamics

Catecholamines are primarily direct-acting. When catecholamines combine with alpha-adrenergic receptors or beta-adrenergic receptors, they cause either an excitatory or inhibitory effect. Typically, activation of alpha-adrenergic receptors generates an excitatory response except for intestinal relaxation. Activation of the beta-adrenergic receptors mostly produces an inhibitory response except in the cells of the heart, where noradrenaline (norepinephrine) produces excitatory effects.

Catecholamines can't be taken orally because they're destroyed by digestive enzymes.

More work for the heart

The clinical effects of catecholamines depend on the dosage and the route of administration. Catecholamines are potent inotropes—they make the heart contract more forcefully. As a result, the ventricles of the heart empty more completely with each heartbeat, increasing the workload of the heart and the amount of oxygen it needs to do this harder work.

Catecholamines make me need more oxygen.

Step up the beat

Catecholamines also produce a positive chronotropic effect, which means they cause the heart to beat faster. That's because pacemaker cells in the sinoatrial (SA) node of the heart depolarise at a faster rate. As catecholamines cause blood vessels to constrict and blood pressure to rise, heart rate can fall as the body tries to compensate and prevent an excessive rise in blood pressure.

All fired up

Catecholamines can cause the Purkinje fibers (an intricate web of fibers that carry electrical impulses into the ventricles of the heart) to fire spontaneously, possibly producing abnormal heart rhythms, such as premature ventricular contractions and fibrillation.

Adrenaline (epinephrine) is more likely than noradrenaline (norepinephrine) to produce this spontaneous firing.

Pharmacotherapeutics

How adrenergic drugs are used depends on which receptors they stimulate and to what degree. Adrenergic drugs can affect:

- alpha-adrenergic receptors
- beta-adrenergic receptors
- dopamine receptors.

Most adrenergics produce their effects by stimulating alpha-adrenergic receptors and beta-adrenergic receptors. These drugs mimic the action of noradrenaline (norepinephrine) and adrenaline (epinephrine).

Of the catecholamines:

- noradrenaline (norepinephrine) has the greatest pure alpha activity
- dobutamine and isoprenaline have only beta-related therapeutic uses
- adrenaline (epinephrine) stimulates alpha-adrenergic receptors and beta-adrenergic receptors
- dopamine primarily exhibits dopaminergic activity (it acts on sympathetic nervous system receptors that are stimulated by dopamine).

Helping hypotension

Catecholamines that stimulate alpha-adrenergic receptors are used to treat low blood pressure (hypotension). As a rule, catecholamines work best when used to treat hypotension caused by:

- relaxation of the blood vessels (also called a *loss of vasomotor tone*)
- blood loss (such as from haemorrhage).

Rhythm makers

Catecholamines that stimulate beta$_1$-adrenergic receptors are used to treat:

- bradycardia
- heart block
- low cardiac output.

Increasing response

Because they're believed to make the heart more responsive to defibrillation (using an electrical current to terminate a deadly arrhythmia), beta$_1$-adrenergic drugs are used to treat:

- ventricular fibrillation (quivering of the ventricles resulting in no pulse)
- asystole (no electrical activity in the heart)
- cardiac arrest.

Catecholamines that stimulate alpha-adrenergic receptors are used to treat hypotension.

Breathing better with beta$_2$ activity

Catecholamines that exert beta$_2$-adrenergic activity are used to treat:
- acute and chronic bronchial asthma
- emphysema
- bronchitis
- acute hypersensitivity (allergic) reactions to drugs.

More blood for the kidneys

Dopamine, which stimulates dopaminergic receptors, is used in low doses to improve blood flow to the kidneys because it dilates the renal blood vessels.

Home grown vs. manufactured

The effects of catecholamines produced by the body differ somewhat from the effects of manufactured catecholamines. Manufactured catecholamines have a short duration of action, which can limit their therapeutic usefulness.

Catecholamines with beta$_2$-adrenergic activity treat respiratory disorders, such as bronchial asthma and bronchitis.

Drug interactions

Drug interactions involving catecholamines can be serious:
- Alpha-adrenergic blockers, such as phentolamine, can produce hypotension.
- Adrenaline (epinephrine) may cause hyperglycaemia. Diabetic patients receiving adrenaline (epinephrine) may require an increased dose of insulin or oral antidiabetics.
- Beta-adrenergic blockers, such as propranolol, can lead to bronchial constriction, especially in patients with asthma.
- Other adrenergic drugs can produce additive effects, such as hypertension (high blood pressure) and arrhythmias, and enhance adverse effects.
- Tricyclic antidepressants can lead to hypertension.

Adverse reactions

Adverse reactions to catecholamines include:
- restlessness
- anxiety
- dizziness
- headache
- palpitations
- cardiac arrhythmias
- hypotension
- hypertension and hypertensive crisis
- stroke
- angina

- increased glucose levels
- tissue necrosis and sloughing (if a catecholamine given I.V. leaks into the surrounding tissue).

Nursing process

These nursing process steps are appropriate for patients undergoing treatment with catecholamines.

Assessment
- Assess the patient's condition before therapy and regularly thereafter.
- Continuously monitor electrocardiogram (ECG), blood pressure, pulmonary artery wedge pressure, cardiac condition, and urine output.
- Monitor electrolyte levels.
- Throughout therapy, assess for adverse reactions, drug interactions, and acidosis, which decreases effectiveness of dopamine.
- After dopamine is stopped, watch closely for a sudden drop in blood pressure.
- Assess the patient's and family's knowledge of drug therapy.

Key nursing diagnoses
- Decreased cardiac output related to underlying condition
- Ineffective tissue perfusion (cerebral, cardiopulmonary, and renal) related to underlying condition.
- Risk for injury related to drug-induced adverse reactions.
- Acute pain related to headache.
- Deficient knowledge related to drug therapy.

Planning outcome goals
- Cardiac output will be maintained.
- Effective tissue perfusion will be maintained.
- The risk for injury will be minimised.
- The patient's pain will decrease.
- The patient will demonstrate an understanding of the purpose and intended effect of therapy.

Implementation
- Before starting catecholamines, correct hypovolaemia with plasma volume expanders.
- Give cardiac glycosides before catecholamines; cardiac glycosides increase atrioventricular (AV) node conduction and patients with atrial fibrillation may develop rapid ventricular rate.
- Administer drug using a central venous catheter or large peripheral vein. Adjust the infusion according to the prescription and the patient's condition. Use an infusion pump.
- Dilute the concentrate for injection before administration, according to pharmacy guidelines.

Sometimes the order of drug administration matters. For example, cardiac glycosides should be given before catecholamines.

- Watch for irritation and infiltration; extravasation can cause an inflammatory response.
- Don't give catecholamines in the same I.V. line as other drugs; be aware of incompatibilities. For example, dobutamine is incompatible with heparin, hydrocortisone, penicillin and entacapone.
- Don't mix dobutamine or dopamine with sodium bicarbonate injection or phenytoin because the drug is incompatible with alkaline solutions.
- Change I.V. sites regularly to avoid phlebitis.
- Provide patient teaching.

Evaluation
- Patient regains adequate cardiac output (evidenced by stable vital signs, normal urine output, and clear mental status).
- Patient regains adequate cerebral, cardiopulmonary, and renal tissue perfusion.
- Patient doesn't experience injury as a result of drug-induced adverse reactions.
- Patient's headache is relieved with analgesic administration.
- Patient and family demonstrate an understanding of drug therapy.

Don't mix me up! Catecholamines shouldn't be administered in the same I.V. line as other drugs.

Noncatecholamines

Noncatecholamine adrenergic drugs have many therapeutic uses because of the various effects these drugs can have on the body, including:
- local or systemic constriction of blood vessels (phenylephrine)
- nasal and eye decongestion and dilation of the bronchioles (ephedrine, formoterol, isoprenaline, salbutamol, salmeterol, and terbutaline)
- smooth-muscle relaxation (terbutaline).

Pharmacokinetics
Absorption of noncatecholamines depends on the route of administration:
- Inhaled drugs, such as salbutamol, are gradually absorbed from the bronchi of the lungs and result in lower drug levels in the body.
- Oral drugs are absorbed well from the GI tract and are distributed widely in the body fluids and tissues.
- Some noncatecholamine drugs (such as ephedrine) cross the blood-brain barrier and can be found in high concentrations in the brain and cerebrospinal fluid (fluid that moves through and protects the brain and spinal canal).

Metabolism and inactivation of noncatecholamines occur primarily in the liver but can also occur in the lungs, GI tract, and other tissues.

Inhaled noncatecholamines are gradually absorbed, providing low drug levels to the body.

Exit time varies

These drugs and their metabolites are excreted primarily in urine. Some, such as inhaled salbutamol, are excreted within 24 hours; others, such as oral salbutamol, within 3 days. Acidic urine increases excretion of many noncatecholamines; alkaline urine slows excretion.

Pharmacodynamics

Noncatecholamines can be direct-acting, indirect-acting, or dual-acting (unlike catecholamines, which are primarily direct-acting).
- Direct-acting noncatecholamines that stimulate alpha activity receptors include phenylephrine. Those that selectively stimulate beta$_2$ activity receptors include salbutamol and terbutaline.
- Indirect-acting noncatecholamines exert their effect by indirect action on adrenergic receptors.
- Dual-acting noncatecholamines include the vasoconstrictor sympathomimetic, ephedrine.

Pharmacotherapeutics

Noncatecholamines stimulate the sympathetic nervous system and produce various effects on the body. Metaraminol for example, causes vasoconstriction and is used to treat hypotension in cases of severe shock. Terbutaline is used to stop preterm labour. It's important to become familiar with each individual drug, including its indication, route, dose, and administration technique. Monitor the patient closely for therapeutic effect and tolerance.

Drug interactions

Here are a few examples of how other drugs may interact with noncatecholamines:
- Anaesthetics (general) and halogenated hydrocarbons can cause arrhythmias. Hypotension can also occur if these drugs are taken with noncatecholamines that have predominantly beta$_2$ activity, such as ritodrine and terbutaline.
- Monoamine oxidase inhibitors can cause severe hypertension and even death.
- Oxytocic drugs that stimulate the uterus to contract can be inhibited when taken with terbutaline. When taken with other noncatecholamines, oxytocic drugs can cause hypertensive crisis or a stroke.
- Tricyclic antidepressants can cause hypertension and arrhythmias.
- Drugs that alkalinise urine such as acetazolamide and sodium bicarbonate, slow excretion of noncatecholamine drugs, prolonging their action.

Adverse reactions

Adverse reactions to noncatecholamines may include:
- headache
- restlessness

- anxiety or euphoria
- irritability
- trembling
- drowsiness or insomnia
- light-headedness
- incoherence
- seizures
- hypertension or hypotension
- palpitations
- bradycardia or tachycardia
- irregular heart rhythm
- cardiac arrest
- cerebral haemorrhage
- tingling or coldness in the arms or legs
- pallor or flushing
- angina
- changes in heart rate and blood pressure in a pregnant woman and her foetus.

Keep in mind that noncatecholamines can change heart rate and blood pressure in a pregnant woman and her foetus.

Nursing process

These nursing process steps are appropriate for patients undergoing treatment with noncatecholamines.

Assessment
- Obtain a baseline assessment of the patient's respiratory status, and assess it frequently throughout therapy.
- Assess for adverse reactions and drug interactions.
- Assess the patient's and family's knowledge of drug therapy.

Key nursing diagnoses
- Impaired gas exchange related to underlying respiratory condition.
- Risk for injury related to drug-induced adverse reactions.
- Deficient knowledge related to drug therapy.

Planning outcome goals
- Adequate gas exchange will be maintained.
- The risk of injury will be minimised.
- The patient will show understanding of the purpose and intended effect of drug therapy.

Implementation
- If using the inhalation route, wait at least 2 minutes between doses if more than one dose is prescribed. If a corticosteroid inhaler also is used, first have the patient use the bronchodilator, wait 5 minutes, and then have the patient use the corticosteroid inhaler. This permits the bronchodilator to open air passages for maximum corticosteroid effectiveness.
- Give the injectable form (terbutaline) in the lateral deltoid area. Protect the injection from light. Don't use the drug if it's discoloured.

Education edge

Teaching about noncatecholamines

If noncatecholamines are prescribed, review these points with the patient and caregivers:

- Stop the drug immediately if paradoxical bronchospasm occurs.
- Follow these instructions for using a metered-dose inhaler:
  - Clear the nasal passages and throat.
  - Breathe out, expelling as much air from the lungs as possible.
  - Place the mouthpiece well into the mouth and inhale deeply as the dose is released.
  - Hold your breath for several seconds, remove the mouthpiece, and exhale slowly.
  - Wait at least 2 minutes before repeating the procedure if more than one inhalation is prescribed.
- Avoid accidentally spraying the inhalant form into the eyes (may temporarily blur vision).
- Reduce intake of foods and herbs containing caffeine, such as coffee, cola, and chocolate, when using a bronchodilator.
- Check pulse rate before and after using the bronchodilator. Call the prescriber if pulse rate increases more than 20 to 30 beats/minute.

- Notify the prescriber immediately if bronchospasms develop during therapy.
- Instruct the patient to use the aerosol form 15 minutes before exercise to prevent exercise-induced bronchospasm as indicated.
- Provide patient teaching. (See *Teaching about noncatecholamines*.)

Evaluation
- Patient's respiratory signs and symptoms improve.
- Patient has no injury from adverse drug reactions.
- Patient and family demonstrate an understanding of drug therapy.

Adrenergic blocking drugs

Adrenergic blocking drugs, also called *sympatholytic drugs*, are used to disrupt sympathetic nervous system function. These drugs work by blocking impulse transmission (and thus sympathetic nervous system stimulation) at adrenergic neurons or adrenergic receptor sites. Their action at these sites can be exerted by:
- interrupting the action of adrenergic drugs
- reducing available noradrenaline (norepinephrine)
- preventing the action of cholinergic drugs.

We're adrenergic blocking drugs. We block impulse transmissions from adrenergic neurons and receptor sites.

Classified information

Adrenergic blocking drugs are classified according to their site of action as:

- alpha-adrenergic blockers (also called *alpha blockers*)
- beta-adrenergic blockers (also called *beta blockers*).

Alpha-adrenergic blockers

Alpha-adrenergic blockers work by interrupting the actions of the catecholamines adrenaline (epinephrine) and noradrenaline (norepinephrine) at alpha receptors. This results in:

- relaxation of the smooth muscle in the blood vessels
- increased dilation of blood vessels
- decreased blood pressure.
  Drugs in this class include:
- ergotamine
- phenoxybenzamine
- phentolamine
- terazosin
- doxazosin
- prazosin (see *Alpha-adrenergic blockers: Prazosin*).

Prototype pro

Alpha-adrenergic blockers: Prazosin

Actions

- Inhibits alpha-adrenergic receptors, causing arterial and venous dilation that reduces peripheral vascular resistance.

Indications

- Mild to moderate hypertension.

Nursing considerations

- Monitor for adverse reactions, such as dizziness, first-dose syncope, palpitations, or nausea.
- Monitor pulse rate and blood pressure frequently.
- Advise the patient to rise slowly and to avoid abrupt position changes.

Two actions in one

Ergotamine is a mixed alpha agonist and antagonist; at high doses, it acts as an alpha-adrenergic blocker.

Pharmacokinetics

The action of alpha-adrenergic blockers in the body isn't well understood. Most of these drugs are absorbed erratically when given orally and more rapidly and completely when given sublingually. Alpha-adrenergic blockers vary considerably in their onset of action, peak concentration levels, and duration of action.

Pharmacodynamics

Alpha-adrenergic blockers work in one of two ways:
• They interfere with or block the synthesis, storage, release, and reuptake of noradrenaline (norepinephrine) by neurons.
• They antagonise adrenaline (epinephrine), noradrenaline (norepinephrine), or adrenergic drugs at alpha-receptor sites.

Alpha-adrenergic blockers include drugs that block stimulation of alpha$_1$ receptors and drugs that may block alpha$_2$ stimulation.

More flow, less pressure

Alpha-adrenergic blockers occupy alpha-receptor sites on the smooth muscle of blood vessels. (See *How alpha-adrenergic blockers affect peripheral blood vessels*.) This prevents catecholamines from occupying and stimulating the receptor sites. As a result, blood vessels dilate, increasing local blood flow to the skin and other organs. The decreased peripheral vascular resistance (resistance to blood flow) helps to decrease blood pressure.

Watch your patient's tone

The therapeutic effect of an alpha-adrenergic blocker depends on the sympathetic tone (the state of partial constriction of blood vessels) in the body before the drug is administered. For instance, when the drug is given with the patient lying down, only a small change in blood pressure occurs. In this position, the sympathetic nerves release very little noradrenaline (norepinephrine).

On the other hand, when a patient stands up, noradrenaline (norepinephrine) is released to constrict the veins and shoot blood back up to the heart. If the patient receives an alpha-adrenergic blocker, however, the veins can't constrict and blood pools in the legs. Because blood return to the heart is reduced, blood pressure drops. This drop in blood pressure that occurs when a person stands up is called *orthostatic hypotension*.

Memory jogger

To help you remember the effects of catecholamines on alpha and beta receptors, remember that **A** stands for **a**lpha (and **a**ctivation, suggesting an excitatory response), and **B** stands for **b**eta (or **b**anished, which suggests an inhibitory effect). However there are some exceptions to this rule.

My job is to block alpha receptor sites so that catecholamines can't occupy them. Sorry, catecholamine. This seat is taken.

Pharm function

How alpha-adrenergic blockers affect peripheral blood vessels

By occupying alpha-receptor sites, alpha-adrenergic blocking drugs cause blood vessel walls to relax. This leads to dilation of blood vessels and reduced peripheral vascular resistance (the pressure that blood must overcome as it flows in a vessel).

One result: Orthostatic hypotension

These effects can cause orthostatic hypotension, a drop in blood pressure that occurs when changing position from lying down to standing. Redistribution of blood to the dilated blood vessels of the legs causes hypotension.

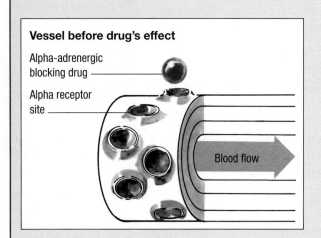

Vessel before drug's effect

Alpha-adrenergic blocking drug

Alpha receptor site

Blood flow

Vessel dilated as a result of drug's effect

Alpha-adrenergic blocking drug

Increased blood flow

Pharmacotherapeutics

Because alpha-adrenergic blockers cause smooth muscles to relax and blood vessels to dilate, they increase local blood flow to the skin and other organs and reduce blood pressure. As a result, they're used to treat:

- hypertension
- peripheral vascular disorders (disease of the blood vessels of the extremities), especially those in which spasm of the blood vessels causes poor local blood flow, such as Raynaud's disease (intermittent pallor, cyanosis, or redness of fingers), acrocyanosis (symmetrical mottled cyanosis [bluish colour] of the hands and feet), and frostbite
- pheochromocytoma (a catecholamine-secreting tumour causing severe hypertension)
- vascular headaches (ergotamine).

Thanks alpha-adrenergic blockers for helping me dilate!

Drug interactions

Many drugs interact with alpha-adrenergic blockers, producing a synergistic or exaggerated effect that may lead to such conditions as severe hypotension or vascular collapse.

Here are some examples of interactions that can occur:
• Prazosin taken with diuretics, propranolol, or other beta-adrenergic blockers results in increased frequency of syncope with loss of consciousness.
• Doxazosin or terazosin taken with clonidine results in decreased clonidine effects.
• Terazosin taken with antihypertensives may cause excessive hypotension.

These effects are specific to ergotamine:
• Caffeine and macrolide antibiotics can increase the effects of ergotamine.
• Dopamine increases the pressor (rise in blood pressure) effect.
• Glyceryl trinitrate can produce hypotension due to excessive dilation of blood vessels.
• Adrenergic drugs, including many over-the-counter drugs, can increase the stimulating effects on the heart. Hypotension with rebound hypertension can occur.

Adverse reactions

Most adverse reactions associated with alpha-adrenergic blockers are caused primarily by dilation of the blood vessels. They include:
• orthostatic hypotension or severe hypertension
• bradycardia or tachycardia
• oedema
• difficulty breathing
• light-headedness
• flushing
• arrhythmias
• angina or heart attack
• spasm of the blood vessels in the brain
• a shocklike state.

Although alpha-adrenergic blockers are commonly used to dilate blood vessels, sometimes this effect can lead to adverse reactions such as orthostatic hypotension.

Nursing process

These nursing process steps are appropriate for patients undergoing treatment with alpha-adrenergic blockers.

Assessment
• Obtain vital signs, especially blood pressure.
• Assess for adverse reactions.
• Assess the patient's and family's knowledge of drug therapy.

Key nursing diagnoses
- Decreased cardiac output related to hypotension.
- Ineffective (peripheral) tissue perfusion related to vasoconstriction.
- Acute pain related to headache.
- Excess fluid volume related to fluid retention.
- Deficient knowledge related to drug therapy.

Planning outcome goals
- Adequate cardiac output will be demonstrated.
- Peripheral tissue perfusion will improve, as evidenced by adequate circulatory checks and pulses.
- The patient will state that pain is decreased.
- Fluid volume status will remain adequate, as demonstrated by adequate blood pressure, urine output, and cardiac parameters.

The patient's blood pressure indicates whether his fluid volume is remaining stable.

Implementation
- Give drugs at bedtime to minimise dizziness or light-headedness.
- Begin therapy with a small dose to avoid syncope with first dose.
- Give ergotamine during the prodromal stage of a headache or as soon as possible after onset.
- Don't give sublingual tablets with food or drink.
- Provide patient teaching.

Evaluation
- Patient maintains adequate cardiac output.
- Patient maintains adequate tissue perfusion to limbs throughout therapy.
- Patient's headache is relieved.
- Patient has no oedema.
- Patient and family demonstrate an understanding of drug therapy. (See *Teaching about alpha-adrenergic blockers.*)

Beta-adrenergic blockers

Beta-adrenergic blockers, the most widely used adrenergic blockers, prevent stimulation of the sympathetic nervous system by inhibiting the action of catecholamines at beta-adrenergic receptors.

Some are picky, others aren't

Beta-adrenergic blockers are selective or nonselective. Nonselective beta-adrenergic blockers affect:
- beta$_1$ receptor sites (located mainly in the heart)
- beta$_2$ receptor sites (located in the bronchi, blood vessels, and uterus).

Education edge

Teaching about alpha-adrenergic blockers

If alpha-adrenergic blockers are prescribed, review these points with the patient and caregivers:

- Don't rise suddenly from a lying or sitting position.
- Avoid hazardous tasks that require mental alertness until the full effects of the drug are known.
- Alcohol, excessive exercise, prolonged standing, and heat exposure intensify adverse effects.
- Report dizziness or irregular heartbeat.
- Don't eat, drink, or smoke while the sublingual tablet is dissolving.

- Don't increase the drug dosage without first consulting the prescriber.
- Avoid prolonged exposure to cold weather whenever possible. Cold may increase adverse reactions to ergotamine.
- If receiving long-term ergotamine therapy, check for and report coldness in the limbs or tingling in the fingers or toes. Severe vasoconstriction may result in tissue damage.

Nonselective beta-adrenergic blocking drugs include carvedilol, labetalol, levobunolol, penbutolol, pindolol, sotalol, nadolol, propranolol, and timolol. (Carvedilol and labetalol also block alpha$_1$ receptors.)

Selective beta-adrenergic blockers primarily affect just the beta$_1$-adrenergic sites. They include acebutolol, atenolol, betaxolol, bisoprolol, esmolol, and metoprolol tartrate.

Part blocker, part stimulator

Some beta-adrenergic blockers, such as pindolol and acebutolol, also have intrinsic sympathetic activity. This means that instead of attaching to beta receptors and blocking them, these beta-adrenergic blockers attach to beta receptors and stimulate them. These drugs are sometimes classified as *partial agonists*.

Pharmacokinetics

Beta-adrenergic blockers are usually absorbed rapidly from the GI tract. They are protein-bound to some extent. Some beta-adrenergic blockers are absorbed more completely than others.

Reach the peak faster: Go I.V.

The onset of action of beta-adrenergic blockers is primarily dose- and drug-dependent. The time it takes to reach peak concentration levels depends on the route

When it comes to beta-adrenergic blockers, you can't beat me to peak levels!

of administration. Beta-adrenergic blockers given I.V. reach peak levels much more rapidly than when given by mouth.

Beta-adrenergic blockers are distributed widely in body tissues, with the highest concentrations found in the heart, liver, lungs, and saliva.

The liver is key

With the exception of nadolol and atenolol, beta-adrenergic blockers are metabolised in the liver. They're excreted primarily in urine, as metabolites or in unchanged form, but can also be excreted in faeces and bile with some secretion in breast milk.

Pharmacodynamics

Beta-adrenergic blockers have widespread effects in the body because they produce their blocking action not only at adrenergic nerve endings but also in the adrenal medulla.

Heart effects

Effects on the heart include increased peripheral vascular resistance, decreased blood pressure, decreased force of heart contractions, decreased oxygen consumption by the heart, slowed conduction of impulses between the atria and ventricles of the heart, and decreased cardiac output (the amount of blood pumped by the heart each minute). (See *How beta-adrenergic blockers work*.)

Blocking beta$_1$

Some of the effects of beta-adrenergic blocking drugs depend on whether the drug is classified as selective or nonselective. Selective beta-adrenergic blockers, which preferentially block beta$_1$ receptor sites, reduce stimulation of the heart. They're commonly referred to as *cardioselective beta-adrenergic blockers*.

Blocking beta$_1$ and beta$_2$

Nonselective beta-adrenergic blockers, which block both beta$_1$ and beta$_2$ receptor sites, not only reduce stimulation of the heart but also cause the bronchioles of the lungs to constrict. Therefore, nonselective beta-adrenergic blockers can cause bronchospasm in patients with chronic obstructive lung disorders. This adverse effect isn't seen when nonselective beta-adrenergic blockers are given at lower doses.

Pharmacotherapeutics

Beta-adrenergic blockers are used to treat many conditions and are under investigation for use in many more. As mentioned earlier,

Pharm function

How beta-adrenergic blockers work

By occupying beta-receptor sites, beta-adrenergic blockers prevent catecholamines such as arenaline (epinephrine) or noradrenaline (norepinephrine) from occupying these sites and exerting their stimulating effects. This illustration shows the effects of beta-adrenergic blockers on the heart, lungs, and blood vessels.

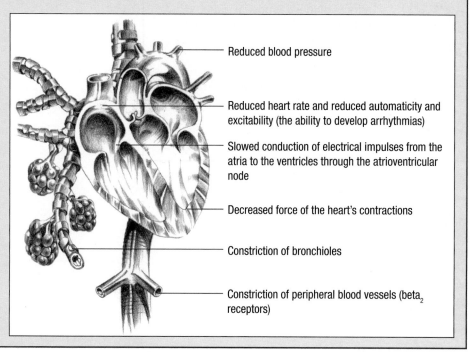

Reduced blood pressure

Reduced heart rate and reduced automaticity and excitability (the ability to develop arrhythmias)

Slowed conduction of electrical impulses from the atria to the ventricles through the atrioventricular node

Decreased force of the heart's contractions

Constriction of bronchioles

Constriction of peripheral blood vessels (beta$_2$ receptors)

their clinical usefulness is based largely (but not exclusively) on how they affect the heart. (See *Are beta-adrenergic blockers underused in elderly patients?*)

Taken to heart

Beta-adrenergic blockers can be prescribed after a heart attack to prevent another heart attack or to treat:
- angina (chest pain)
- hypertension
- hypertrophic cardiomyopathy (a disease of the heart muscle)
- supraventricular arrhythmias (irregular heartbeats that originate in the atria, SA node, or AV node).

Are beta-adrenergic blockers underused in elderly patients?

Research has clearly shown that using a beta-adrenergic blocker after a heart attack reduces the risk of death and another heart attack. Even so, these drugs aren't being prescribed for elderly patients.

What one study found

One study found that only 34% of patients were prescribed a beta-adrenergic blocker after discharge from hospital following a heart attack. The least likely patients to receive beta-adrenergic blockers include the very sick and elderly patients.

Why?

The chief investigator of a study that looked at the use of beta-adrenergic blockers in elderly patients believes that many prescribers fear the adverse effects of these drugs on older patients. The study suggested that a beta-adrenergic blocker can be given safely to an elderly patient after a heart attack if the lowest effective dose of a selective beta-adrenergic blocker is prescribed.

Very versatile

Beta-adrenergic blockers are also used to treat:
- anxiety
- cardiovascular symptoms associated with thyrotoxicosis (overproduction of thyroid hormones)
- essential tremor
- migraine headaches
- open-angle glaucoma
- pheochromocytoma.

Drug interactions

Many drugs can interact with beta-adrenergic blocking drugs to cause potentially dangerous effects. Some of the most serious effects include cardiac depression, arrhythmias, respiratory depression, severe bronchospasm, and severe hypotension that can lead to vascular collapse. Here are some others:
- Increased effects or toxicity can occur when digoxin, calcium channel blockers (primarily verapamil), and cimetidine are taken with beta-adrenergic blockers.
- Decreased effects can occur when antacids, calcium salts, barbiturates, anti-inflammatories (such as indometacin and salicylates), are taken with beta-adrenergic blockers.

Beta-adrenergic blockers may affect how much antidiabetic drug you need.

- The requirements for insulin and oral antidiabetic drugs can be altered when taken with beta-adrenergic blockers.
- Potential lidocaine toxicity can occur when it's taken with beta-adrenergic blockers.
- The ability of theophylline to produce bronchodilation is impaired by nonselective beta-adrenergic blockers.
- Clonidine taken with a nonselective beta-adrenergic blocker can result in life-threatening hypertension during clonidine withdrawal.
- Sympathomimetics and nonselective beta-adrenergic blockers can cause hypertension and reflex bradycardia.

Adverse reactions
Beta-adrenergic blockers generally cause few adverse reactions; the adverse reactions that do occur are drug- or dose-dependent and include:
- hypotension
- bradycardia
- peripheral vascular insufficiency
- AV block
- heart failure
- bronchospasm
- diarrhoea or constipation
- nausea
- vomiting
- abdominal discomfort
- anorexia
- flatulence
- rash
- fever with sore throat
- spasm of the larynx
- respiratory distress (allergic response).

If your patient is undergoing surgery, make sure you tell the anaesthetist that the patient is taking a beta-adrenergic blocker.

Nursing process
These nursing process steps are appropriate for patients undergoing treatment with beta-adrenergic blockers.

Assessment
- Assess the patient's condition before therapy and regularly thereafter.
- Assess respiratory status, especially in a patient with chronic obstructive pulmonary disease or asthma because of the potential risk of bronchospasm.
- Check apical pulse rate daily; alert the prescriber about extremes, such as a pulse rate below 60 beats/minute.
- Monitor blood pressure, ECG, and heart rate and rhythm frequently; be alert for progression of AV block or bradycardia.

- If the patient has heart failure, weigh regularly and watch for weight gain of more than 2.5 kg per week.
- Observe diabetic patients for sweating, fatigue, and hunger. Signs of hypoglycaemic shock are masked.
- Be alert for adverse reactions and drug interactions.
- Assess the patient's and family's knowledge of drug therapy.

Key nursing diagnoses
- Risk for injury related to adverse CNS effects.
- Excess fluid volume related to oedema.
- Decreased cardiac output related to bradycardia or hypotension.
- Deficient knowledge related to drug therapy.

Planning outcome goals
- The patient's chances for injury will be diminished.
- The patient will experience normal fluid volume as shown by adequate urine output and blood pressure.

Implementation
- Before any surgical procedure, notify the anaesthetist that the patient is taking a beta-adrenergic blocker.
- Keep glucagon nearby in case it's prescribed to reverse beta-adrenergic blocker overdose.
- Check the apical pulse before giving drug; if it's slower than 60 beats/minute, withhold the drug and call the prescriber immediately.
- Give the drug with meals because food may increase absorption.
- For I.V. use, give the drug undiluted and by direct injection, unless recommended otherwise by a pharmacy.

Evaluation
- Patient remains free from injury.
- Patient has no signs of oedema.
- Patient maintains normal blood pressure and heart rate.
- Patient and family demonstrate an understanding of drug therapy. (See *Teaching about beta-adrenergic blockers*.)

Education edge

Teaching about beta-adrenergic blockers

If beta-adrenergic blocking drugs are prescribed, review these points with the patient and caregivers:

- Take the drug exactly as prescribed, even if signs or symptoms are relieved.
- Don't stop the drug suddenly. This can worsen angina or precipitate myocardial infarction.
- Take the oral form of the drug with meals to enhance absorption.

- Don't take over-the-counter drugs or herbal remedies without medical consent.
- Be aware of potential adverse reactions and report unusual effects of the drug.
- Avoid performing hazardous activities until central nervous system effects of the drug are known.

Quick quiz

1. Which effect is expected when using cholinergic agonists?
   A. dry mouth
   B. tachycardia
   C. pupil dilation
   D. increased bladder tone

Answer: D. Effects of cholinergic agonists include increased tone and contraction of bladder muscles, salivation, bradycardia, dilated blood vessels, constricted pulmonary bronchioles, increased activity of the GI tract, and constricted pupils.

2. Which drug would the nurse give to a patient experiencing symptomatic sinus bradycardia?
   A. atropine
   B. belladonna
   C. digoxin
   D. propranolol

Answer: A. Atropine is the drug of choice to treat symptomatic sinus bradycardia.

3. Which finding indicates that a patient is having an adverse reaction to catecholamines?
    A. nausea and vomiting
    B. diarrhoea
    C. decreased glucose levels
    D. palpitations

Answer: D. Adverse reactions to catecholamines include palpitations, restlessness, anxiety, dizziness, headache, cardiac arrhythmias, hypotension, hypertension and hypertensive crisis, stroke, angina, and increased glucose levels.

4. Which of the following drugs is a catecholamine?
    A. dopamine
    B. salbutamol
    C. prazosin
    D. labetalol

Answer: A. Dopamine is a catecholamine.

5. Which noncatecholamine is dual-acting?
    A. salbutamol
    B. phenylephrine
    C. ephedrine
    D. terbutaline

Answer: C. Ephedrine is a dual-acting noncatecholamine.

6. Which drug causes toxicity in a patient taking a beta-adrenergic blocker?
    A. an antacid
    B. rifampacin
    C. a nonsteroidal anti-inflammatory drug
    D. digoxin

Answer: D. Increased effects or toxicity can occur when digoxin, calcium channel blockers (primarily verapamil), and cimetidine are taken with beta-adrenergic blockers.

Scoring

★★★ If you answered all six questions correctly, super! Your receptors must really be stimulated by this information.

★★ If you answered four or five questions correctly, good work! You have no reason to be nervous about working with autonomic nervous system drugs.

★ If you answered fewer than four questions correctly, no need to agonise over it. Assess your trouble spots and plan some time for review.

3 Neurologic and neuromuscular drugs

Just the facts

In this chapter, you'll learn:

♦ classes of drugs used to treat neurologic and neuromuscular disorders

♦ uses and actions of these drugs

♦ absorption, distribution, metabolism, and excretion of these drugs

♦ drug interactions and adverse reactions to these drugs.

Skeletal muscle relaxants

There are two main classes of skeletal muscle relaxants: centrally acting and direct acting.

Skeletal muscle relaxants relieve musculoskeletal pain or spasms and severe musculoskeletal spasticity (stiff, awkward movements). They're used to treat acute, painful musculoskeletal conditions and muscle spasticity associated with multiple sclerosis (MS—a progressive demyelination of the white matter of the brain and spinal cord that causes widespread neurologic dysfunction), cerebral palsy (a motor function disorder caused by neurologic damage), stroke (reduced oxygen supply to the brain that results in neurologic deficits), and spinal cord injuries (injuries to the spinal cord that can result in paralysis or death).

This chapter discusses the two main classes of skeletal muscle relaxants: centrally acting and direct acting.

Breaking the cycle

Exposure to severe cold, lack of blood flow to a muscle, or overexertion can send sensory impulses from the posterior sensory nerve fibres to the spinal cord and the higher levels of the central nervous system (CNS). These sensory impulses can cause reflex (involuntary) muscle contractions or spasms from trauma, epilepsy, hypocalcaemia (low calcium levels), or muscular disorders. This muscle contraction further stimulates the sensory receptors to a more intense contraction, establishing a cycle. Centrally acting muscle relaxants are believed to break this cycle by acting as CNS depressants.

> Skeletal muscle relaxants like me can help break your cycle of spasticity.

Centrally acting agents

Centrally acting skeletal muscle relaxants are used to treat acute muscle spasms caused by such conditions as:

- anxiety
- inflammation
- pain
- trauma.
    Examples of these drugs include:
- carisoprodol
- methocarbamol
- orphenadrine
- tizanidine.
    Centrally acting skeletal muscle relaxants, such as baclofen, diazepam, and tizanidine, are commonly used for intermittent and chronic spasticity.

Pharmacokinetics

Much is still unknown about how centrally acting skeletal muscle relaxants circulate within the body. In general, these drugs are absorbed from the GI tract, widely distributed in the body, metabolised in the liver, and excreted by the kidneys.

Time to go!

When administered orally, these drugs can take from 30 minutes to 1 hour to be effective, with a duration of action of 4 to 6 hours.

> I'm an agent of the CAA: Centrally Acting Agency.

Pharmacodynamics

Although their precise mechanism of action is unknown, the centrally acting drugs don't relax skeletal muscles directly or depress neuronal conduction, neuromuscular transmission, or muscle excitability. Rather, centrally acting drugs are known to be CNS depressants. The skeletal muscle relaxant effects that they cause are likely related to their sedative effects.

Pharmacotherapeutics

Patients receive centrally acting skeletal muscle relaxants to treat acute, painful musculoskeletal conditions. They're usually prescribed along with rest and physical therapy.

Drug interactions

Centrally acting skeletal muscle relaxants interact with other CNS depressants (including alcohol, opioids, barbiturates, anticonvulsants, tricyclic antidepressants, and antianxiety drugs), causing increased sedation, impaired motor function, and respiratory depression. In addition, some of these drugs have other interactions, such as those given here:

• Orphenadrine can enhance the effects of cholinergic blocking drugs.
• Methocarbamol can antagonise the cholinergic effects of the anticholinesterase drugs used to treat myasthenia gravis.
• Orphenadrine can reduce the effects of phenothiazines.

Add it up!

• Tizanidine combined with diuretics, central alpha-adrenergic agonists, or antihypertensives may increase hypotensive drug effects.
• Concurrent use of tizanidine with other CNS depressants may cause additive CNS depression.
• Hormonal contraception agents may reduce the clearance of tizanidine, necessitating a dose reduction.

Adverse reactions

Long-term use of centrally acting muscle relaxants can result in physical and psychological dependence. Abrupt cessation of these drugs can cause severe withdrawal symptoms.

Adverse reactions can also occur when a patient is taking these drugs. Common reactions include dizziness and drowsiness. Severe reactions that can occur include allergic reactions, arrhythmias, and bradycardia. Less common reactions include abdominal distress, ataxia, constipation, diarrhoea, heartburn, nausea, and vomiting.

Nursing process

These nursing process steps are appropriate for patients undergoing treatment with centrally acting skeletal muscle relaxants.

Assessment

• Obtain a history of the patient's pain and muscle spasms and reassess regularly thereafter.
• Monitor the patient for hypersensitivity reactions.

Be sure to take the necessary steps to ensure safe administration of these drugs.

- Assess the degree of relief obtained to help the prescriber determine when the dosage can be reduced.
- Closely monitor complete blood count (CBC) results.
- Watch for orthostatic hypotension in a patient receiving methocarbamol.
- Assess compliance of a patient receiving long-term therapy.
- Evaluate the patient's and family's understanding of drug therapy.

Key nursing diagnoses
- Risk for injury related to drug-induced adverse reactions.
- Acute pain related to underlying disorder.
- Deficient knowledge related to drug therapy.

Planning outcome goals
- The patient's risk of injury will be minimised.
- The patient will acknowledge decreased discomfort after administration of medication.
- The patient and family will confirm an understanding of the medication's purpose and intended effect.

Implementation
- After long-term therapy (unless the patient has severe adverse reactions), avoid stopping carisoprodol abruptly to prevent withdrawal symptoms, such as insomnia, headache, nausea, and abdominal pain.
- Institute safety precautions, as needed.
- Give oral forms of these drugs with meals or milk to prevent GI distress.
- Obtain a prescription for mild analgesics to relieve drug-induced headache.
- Avoid abrupt discontinuation to reduce withdrawal symptoms, such as returning spasticity, hypotension, paraesthesia, and muscle rigidity.

Evaluation
- Patient doesn't experience injury as a result of drug-induced drowsiness.
- Patient reports that pain and muscle spasms have ceased with drug therapy.
- Patient complies with therapy, as evidenced by pain relief or improvement of spasticity.
- Patient and family state an understanding of drug therapy. (See *Teaching about skeletal muscle relaxants*.)

Education edge

Teaching about skeletal muscle relaxants

Review this information regarding skeletal muscle relaxants with the patient and their family:

- Take the drug exactly as prescribed. Don't stop baclofen or carisoprodol suddenly after long-term therapy to avoid withdrawal symptoms.
- Avoid hazardous activities that require mental alertness until the central nervous system effects of the drug are known. Drowsiness is usually transient.
- Avoid alcohol or other depressants during therapy.
- Follow the prescriber's advice regarding rest and physical therapy.
- Try to space out activities throughout the day and allow rest periods to avoid fatigue, weakness, and drowsiness. If adverse effects become too severe, consult with a prescriber.
- Change positions slowly to help avoid dizzy spells. If dizziness occurs, avoid driving, operating dangerous machinery, or performing delicate tasks.
- Take the drug with food or milk to prevent GI distress.
- Report urinary hesitancy with baclofen therapy.
- Be aware that urine may be discoloured when taking methocarbamol.
- Regular medical follow-up is necessary to evaluate the effects of this drug

Direct-acting agents

Dantrolene is a direct-acting skeletal muscle relaxant. Although dantrolene has therapeutic effects similar to those of the centrally acting drugs, it works through a different mechanism of action.

In the head

Dantrolene is most effective for spasticity of cerebral origin. Because the drug produces muscle weakness, the benefits of dantrolene administration in a patient with borderline strength are questionable.

Pharmacokinetics
Although the peak drug concentration of dantrolene occurs within about 5 hours after ingestion, the patient may not notice any therapeutic benefit for a week or more. Dantrolene is absorbed

slowly and incompletely (but consistently) from the GI tract and is highly plasma protein–bound. This means that only a small portion of the drug is available to produce a therapeutic effect.

Hepatic interference

Dantrolene is metabolised by the liver and excreted in urine. The elimination half-life in a healthy adult is about 9 hours. Because dantrolene is metabolised in the liver, its half-life can be prolonged in a patient with impaired liver function.

Pharmacodynamics

Dantrolene is chemically and pharmacologically unrelated to other skeletal muscle relaxants. It acts directly on muscle to interfere with calcium ion release from the sarcoplasmic reticulum and weaken the force of contractions. At therapeutic concentrations, dantrolene has little effect on cardiac or intestinal smooth muscle.

Pharmacotherapeutics

Dantrolene can be used to help manage several types of spasticity but is most effective in patients with:
- cerebral palsy
- MS
- spinal cord injury
- stroke.

Anaesthesia antidote

Dantrolene is also used to treat and prevent malignant hyperthermia. This rare but potentially fatal complication of anaesthesia is characterised by skeletal muscle rigidity and high fever. (See *How dantrolene reduces muscle rigidity*.)

Drug interactions

CNS depressants can increase the depressive effects of dantrolene and result in sedation, lack of coordination, and respiratory depression. In addition, dantrolene may have other drug interactions:
- Oestrogens, when given with dantrolene, can increase the risk of liver toxicity.
- I.V. verapamil shouldn't be administered if giving dantrolene as it may result in cardiovascular collapse.
- Alcohol may increase CNS depression when taken with dantrolene.

Pharm function

How dantrolene reduces muscle rigidity

Dantrolene appears to decrease the number of calcium ions released from the sarcoplasmic reticulum (a structure in muscle cells that controls muscle contraction and relaxation by releasing and storing calcium). The lower the calcium level in the muscle plasma or myoplasm, the less energy produced when calcium prompts interaction of the muscle's actin and myosin filaments (responsible for muscle contraction). Less energy means a weaker muscle contraction.

Reducing rigidity, halting hyperthermia

By promoting muscle relaxation, dantrolene prevents or reduces the rigidity that contributes to the life-threatening body temperatures of malignant hyperthermia.

Adverse reactions

Because its major effect is on the muscles, dantrolene has a lower incidence of adverse CNS reactions. However, high therapeutic doses are toxic to the liver. Common adverse effects of dantrolene include drowsiness, dizziness, malaise, and muscle weakness. More serious adverse effects include bleeding, seizures, and hepatitis.

Nursing process

These nursing process steps are appropriate for patients undergoing treatment with direct-acting skeletal muscle relaxants.

Assessment

- Obtain a history of the patient's pain and muscle spasms before therapy and reassess regularly thereafter.
- Monitor the patient for hypersensitivity reactions.
- Assess the degree of relief obtained to help the prescriber determine when the dosage can be reduced.
- Monitor CBC results closely and monitor liver function tests.
- Assess compliance of a patient receiving long-term therapy.
- Evaluate the patient's and family's understanding of drug therapy.

Key nursing diagnoses

- Risk for injury related to drug-induced adverse reactions.
- Acute pain related to underlying disorder.
- Deficient knowledge related to drug therapy.

Planning outcome goals

• The patient's risk of injury will be minimised.
• The patient will acknowledge decreased discomfort after administration of medication.
• The patient and family will confirm an understanding of the medication's purpose and intended effect.

Implementation

• Institute safety precautions as needed.
• If hepatitis, severe diarrhoea, severe weakness, or sensitivity reactions occur, withhold the dose and notify the prescriber.
• Give the oral form of the drug with meals or milk to prevent GI distress.
• Obtain a prescription for a mild analgesic to relieve drug-induced headache.
• Avoid abrupt discontinuation to prevent return of symptoms, such as spasticity, paraesthesia, and muscle rigidity.

Evaluation

• Patient doesn't experience injury as a result of drug-induced drowsiness.
• Patient reports that pain and muscle spasms have ceased with drug therapy.
• Patient complies with therapy, as evidenced by pain relief or improvement of spasticity.
• Patient and family state an understanding of drug therapy. (See *Teaching about skeletal muscle relaxants*.)

Other skeletal muscle relaxants

Two additional drugs used as skeletal muscle relaxants are diazepam and baclofen. Because diazepam is primarily used as an antianxiety drug, this section discusses only baclofen. (See *Diazepam as a skeletal muscle relaxant*.)

Pharmacokinetics

Baclofen is absorbed rapidly from the GI tract. It's distributed widely (with only small amounts crossing the blood-brain barrier), undergoes minimal liver metabolism, and is excreted primarily unchanged in urine.

It can take hours to weeks before the patient notices beneficial effects of baclofen. The elimination half-life of baclofen is 2.5 to 4 hours.

Pharm function

Diazepam as a skeletal muscle relaxant

Diazepam is a benzodiazepine drug that's used to treat acute muscle spasms as well as spasticity caused by chronic disorders. It seems to work by promoting the inhibitory effect of the neurotransmitter gamma-aminobutyric acid on muscle contraction. Other uses of diazepam include treating anxiety, alcohol withdrawal, and seizures.

The negatives: Sedation and tolerance

Diazepam can be used alone or in conjunction with other drugs to treat spasticity, especially in patients with spinal cord lesions and, occasionally, in patients with cerebral palsy. It's also helpful in patients with painful, continuous muscle spasms who aren't too susceptible to the drug's sedative effects. Unfortunately, diazepam's use is limited by its central nervous system effects and the tolerance that develops with prolonged use.

Pharmacodynamics

It isn't known exactly how baclofen works. Chemically similar to the neurotransmitter gamma-aminobutyric acid (GABA), baclofen probably acts in the spinal cord. It reduces nerve impulses from the spinal cord to skeletal muscle, decreasing the number and severity of muscle spasms and the associated pain.

Elasticity vs. spasticity

Because baclofen produces less sedation than diazepam and less peripheral muscle weakness than dantrolene, it's the drug of choice to treat spasticity.

Pharmacotherapeutics

Baclofen's major clinical use is for paraplegic or quadriplegic patients with spinal cord lesions, most commonly caused by MS or trauma. For these patients, baclofen significantly reduces the number and severity of painful flexor spasms. Unfortunately, however, baclofen doesn't improve stiff gait, manual dexterity, or residual muscle function.

Baclofen can be administered intrathecally for patients who are unresponsive to oral baclofen or who experience intolerable adverse effects. After a positive response to a bolus dose, an implantable port for chronic therapy can be placed. Extreme caution should be taken to avoid abrupt discontinuation of intrathecal baclofen.

Avoid abrupt discontinuation of intrathecal baclofen treatment.

CAUTION!

Prototype pro

Skeletal muscle relaxants: Baclofen

Actions

- Unknown
- Appears to reduce the transmission of impulses from the spinal cord to skeletal muscle
- Relieves muscle spasms

Indications

- Spasticity in multiple sclerosis and spinal cord injury
- Can be administered intrathecally for the management of severe spasticity in the patient who doesn't respond to or can't tolerate oral baclofen therapy

Nursing considerations

- Give with meals or milk to prevent GI distress.
- Avoid abrupt discontinuation of intrathecal baclofen as this can result in high fever, altered mental status, exaggerated rebound spasticity, and muscle rigidity that, in rare cases, may progress to rhabdomyolysis, multiple organ system failure, and death.
- If intrathecal baclofen is delayed, treatment with a gamma-aminobutyric acid agonist or I.V. benzodiazepines may prevent potentially fatal sequelae.

No abrupt endings

Abrupt withdrawal of intrathecal baclofen has resulted in high fever, altered mental status, exaggerated rebound spasticity, and muscle rigidity that—in rare cases—has progressed to rhabdomyolysis, multiple organ system failure, and death. (See *Skeletal muscle relaxants: Baclofen*.)

Drug interactions

Baclofen has few drug interactions:
- The most significant drug interaction is an increase in CNS depression when baclofen is administered with other CNS depressants, including alcohol.
- Analgesia can be prolonged when fentanyl and baclofen are administered together.
- Lithium carbonate and baclofen taken together can aggravate hyperkinesia (an abnormal increase in motor function or activity).
- Tricyclic antidepressants and baclofen taken together can increase muscle relaxation.

Adverse reactions

The most common adverse reaction in the patient receiving baclofen is transient drowsiness. Some less common effects include nausea, fatigue, vertigo, hypotonia, muscle weakness, depression, and headache.

Nursing process

These nursing process steps are appropriate for patients undergoing treatment with the skeletal muscle relaxant baclofen.

Assessment
- Obtain a history of the patient's pain and muscle spasms before therapy and reassess regularly thereafter.
- Monitor the patient for hypersensitivity reactions.
- Assess the degree of relief obtained to help the prescriber determine when the dosage can be reduced.
- Monitor CBC results closely.
- Assess compliance of a patient receiving long-term therapy.
- Evaluate the patient's and family's understanding of drug therapy.

Key nursing diagnoses
- Risk for injury related to drug-induced adverse reactions.
- Acute pain related to underlying disorder.
- Deficient knowledge related to drug therapy.

Planning outcome goals
- The patient's risk of injury will be minimised.
- The patient will acknowledge decreased discomfort after administration of the medication.
- The patient and family will confirm an understanding of the medication's purpose and intended effect.

Implementation
- Institute safety precautions as needed. Watch for an increased risk of seizures in the patient with a seizure disorder. Seizures have been reported during overdose and withdrawal of intrathecal baclofen as well as in the patient maintained on therapeutic doses. Monitor the patient carefully and institute seizure precautions.
- Give the oral forms of the drug with meals or milk to prevent GI distress.
- Obtain a prescription for a mild analgesic to relieve drug-induced headache.
- Don't administer an intrathecal injection by the I.V., I.M., subcutaneous, or epidural route.
- Avoid any abrupt discontinuation of intrathecal baclofen. Early symptoms of baclofen withdrawal include return of baseline spasticity, pruritus, hypotension, and paraesthesia. Symptoms that have occurred include high fever, altered mental status, exaggerated rebound

spasticity, and muscle rigidity that—in rare cases—has advanced to rhabdomyolysis, multiple organ system failure, and death.

Evaluation
- Patient doesn't experience injury as a result of drug-induced drowsiness.
- Patient reports that pain and muscle spasms have ceased with drug therapy.
- Patient complies with therapy, as evidenced by pain relief or improvement of spasticity.
- Patient and family state an understanding of drug therapy. (See *Teaching about skeletal muscle relaxants*.)

Neuromuscular blocking drugs

Neuromuscular blocking drugs relax skeletal muscles by disrupting the transmission of nerve impulses at the motor end plate (the branching terminals of a motor nerve axon). (See *How neuromuscular blocking drugs work*.)

Relax, reduce, and manage

Neuromuscular blockers have three major clinical indications:
- to relax skeletal muscles during surgery
- to reduce the intensity of muscle spasms in drug-induced or electrically induced seizures
- to manage patients who are fighting the use of a ventilator to help with breathing.

Polar opposites

There are two main classes of natural and synthetic drugs used as neuromuscular blockers—nondepolarising and depolarising.

Nondepolarising blocking drugs

Nondepolarising blocking drugs, also called *competitive* or *stabilising* drugs, are derived from curare alkaloids and synthetically similar compounds. They include:
- atracurium
- cisatracurium
- mivacurium
- pancuronium
- rocuronium
- vecuronium.

Pharm function

How neuromuscular blocking drugs work

The motor nerve axon divides to form branching terminals called *motor end plates*. These are enfolded in muscle fibres, but separated from the fibres by the synaptic cleft.

Competing with contraction

A stimulus to the nerve causes the release of acetylcholine into the synaptic cleft. There, acetylcholine occupies receptor sites on the muscle cell membrane, depolarising the membrane and causing muscle contraction. Neuromuscular blocking agents act at the motor end plate by competing with acetylcholine for the receptor sites or by blocking depolarisation.

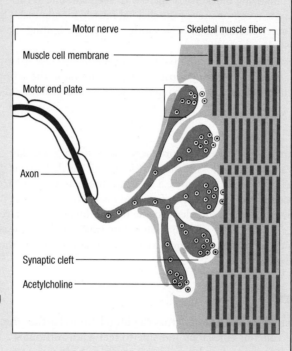

Pharmacokinetics

Because nondepolarising blockers are poorly absorbed from the GI tract, they're administered parenterally. The I.V. route is preferred because the action is more predictable.

Quick distribution

Nondepolarising blockers are distributed rapidly throughout the body. Some drugs, such as pancuronium, rocuronium, and vecuronium, are partially metabolised in the liver. After I.V. administration, atracurium undergoes rapid metabolism by a physiologic process known as *Hofmann elimination* and by enzymatic hydrolysis; it's also partially metabolised in the liver. Mivacurium is hydrolysed by plasma pseudocholinesterase.

These drugs are excreted primarily in urine, and some, such as cisatracurium and vecuronium, are also excreted in faeces.

Pharmacodynamics

Nondepolarising blockers compete with acetylcholine at the cholinergic receptor sites of the skeletal muscle membrane. This blocks acetylcholine's neurotransmitter action, preventing the muscle from contracting.

The effect can be counteracted by anticholinesterase drugs, such as neostigmine or pyridostigmine, which inhibit the action of acetylcholinesterase, the enzyme that destroys acetylcholine.

Paralysis pattern

The initial muscle weakness produced by these drugs quickly changes to a flaccid (loss of muscle tone) paralysis that affects the muscles in a specific sequence. The first muscles to exhibit flaccid paralysis are those of the eyes, face, and neck. Next, the limb, abdomen, and trunk muscles become flaccid. Finally, the intercostal muscles (between the ribs) and diaphragm (the breathing muscle) are paralysed. Recovery from the paralysis usually occurs in the reverse order.

Conscious and aware

Because these drugs don't cross the blood-brain barrier, the patient remains conscious and able to feel pain. Although the patient is paralysed, he's aware of what's happening to him and can experience extreme anxiety. However, they can't communicate their feelings. For this reason, an analgesic or antianxiety drug should be administered along with a neuromuscular blocker.

Pharmacotherapeutics

Nondepolarising blockers are used for intermediate or prolonged muscle relaxation to:
- ease the passage of an endotracheal (ET) tube (a tube placed in the trachea)
- decrease the amount of anaesthetic required during surgery
- facilitate realigning broken bones and dislocated joints
- paralyse the patient who needs ventilatory support, but who fights the ET tube and mechanical ventilation
- prevent muscle injury during electroconvulsive therapy (ECT) (passage of an electric current through the brain to treat depression) by reducing the intensity of muscle spasms.

Remember that the patient can't move but is conscious and can hear conversations and feel pain. As a result, they may become anxious.

Drug interactions

Several drugs alter the effects of nondepolarising neuromuscular blockers:

• Aminoglycoside antibiotics and anaesthetics potentiate or exaggerate the neuromuscular blockade.

• Drugs that alter serum levels of the electrolytes calcium, magnesium, or potassium also alter the effects of nondepolarising blockers.

• Anticholinesterases (neostigmine, pyridostigmine, and edrophonium) antagonise nondepolarising blockers and are used as antidotes.

• Drugs that can increase the intensity and duration of paralysis when taken with a nondepolarising blocking drug include inhalation anaesthetics, aminoglycosides, clindamycin, polymyxin, verapamil, quinine derivatives, ketamine, lithium, nitrates, thiazide diuretics, tetracyclines, and magnesium salts.

• Drugs that can cause decreased neuromuscular blockade when taken with a nondepolarising blocking drug include carbamazepine, hydantoins, ranitidine, and theophylline. Corticosteroids may result in prolonged muscle weakness.

Adverse reactions

A patient taking nondepolarising drugs may experience these adverse reactions:

• apnea
• hypotension
• skin reactions
• bronchospasm
• excessive bronchial and salivary secretions.

A patient taking pancuronium may also experience tachycardia, cardiac arrhythmias, and hypertension.

Nursing process

These nursing process steps are appropriate for patients undergoing treatment with nondepolarising muscle relaxants.

Assessment

• Assess the patient's condition before therapy and regularly thereafter.

• Monitor the patient's baseline electrolyte determinations (electrolyte imbalance can increase neuromuscular effects) and vital signs.

• Measure the patient's fluid intake and output; renal dysfunction may prolong the duration of action because 25% of the drug is unchanged before excretion.

- Nerve stimulator and train-of-four monitoring (a procedure in which electrodes are applied to the skin and electrical stimulation is delivered to measure the degree of neuromuscular blockade) are recommended to confirm the antagonism of neuromuscular blockade and recovery of muscle strength. Before attempting pharmacologic reversal with neostigmine, you should see some evidence of spontaneous recovery.
- Monitor the patient's respirations closely until fully recovered from the neuromuscular blockade, as evidenced by tests of muscle strength (hand grip, head lift, and ability to cough).
- Assess the patient's skin for pressure areas and breakdown.
- Assess for incomplete closure of the eyelids (neuromuscular blockade results in loss of corneal reflex and blocks the action of eye muscles).
- Be alert for adverse reactions and drug interactions.
- Evaluate the patient's and family's knowledge of drug therapy.

The patient's vital signs should remain normal while they are on drug therapy.

Key nursing diagnoses
- Ineffective health maintenance related to condition.
- Ineffective breathing pattern related to the drug's effect on respiratory muscles.
- Deficient knowledge related to drug therapy.

Planning outcome goals
- The patient's vital signs will remain within normal parameters while they are on drug therapy.
- The patient's respiratory function will be maintained as evidenced by adequate arterial blood gas (ABG) values and ventilatory parameters.
- The patient and family will confirm an understanding of the medication's purpose and intended effect.

Implementation
- Administer sedatives or general anaesthetics before neuromuscular blockers. Neuromuscular blockers don't reduce consciousness or alter the pain threshold. Give analgesics for pain. Note that general anaesthetics should only be administered by qualified personnel, such as anaesthetists.
- Neuromuscular blockers should be used only by personnel skilled in airway management.
- Mix the drug only with fresh solutions; precipitates form if alkaline solutions, such as barbiturate solutions, are used. Vecuronium may be given by rapid I.V. injection or diluted to be titrated in a drip form. Reconstituted solutions should be stored at 4°C.
- Allow suxamethonium effects to subside before giving pancuronium.
- Store the drug in a refrigerator. Don't store it in plastic containers or syringes, although plastic syringes may be used for administration.

Education edge

Teaching about neuromuscular blocking drugs

If neuromuscular blocking drugs are prescribed, make sure to tell the patient what you're going to do before administering care. Review these points with the patient and caregivers:

- The drug causes complete paralysis; therefore, expect to be unable to move or speak while receiving the drug. This experience can be very frightening.
- Expect to be unable to breathe (assistance will be provided).
- Expect to be aware of what's going on. The drug doesn't affect level of consciousness.

A reassuring word

The patient will be able to see, hear, and feel, and will be aware of their surroundings. Make sure to explain all events, and reassure the patient and their family.

- Tell the patient that someone will be with them at all times to try to anticipate their needs and explain what's going on.
- Assure the patient that they will be monitored at all times.
- Tell the patient that pain and anti-anxiety medication will be provided, if appropriate.
- Tell the patient that eyedrops will be administered or their eyes may be covered to prevent drying of the corneas.

- Have emergency respiratory support equipment (ET equipment, ventilator, oxygen, atropine, edrophonium, adrenaline (epinephrine), and neostigmine) immediately available.
- Provide skin care and turning to prevent skin breakdown.
- Provide eye care, such as administering lubricating eyedrops and patching and taping eyelids, during neuromuscular blockade.
- When spontaneous recovery starts, drug-induced neuromuscular blockade may be reversed with an anticholinesterase (such as neostigmine or edrophonium), usually given with an anticholinergic such as atropine.

Evaluation
- Patient's condition improves.
- Patient maintains adequate ventilation with mechanical assistance.
- Patient and family state an understanding of drug therapy. (See *Teaching about neuromuscular blocking drugs.*)

Depolarising blocking drugs

Suxamethonium is the only therapeutic depolarising blocking drug. Although it's similar to the nondepolarising blockers in its therapeutic effect, its mechanism of action differs. Suxamethonium acts like acetylcholine, but it isn't immediately inactivated by cholinesterase. It's the drug of choice when short-term muscle relaxation is needed.

Pharmacokinetics

Because suxamethonium is absorbed poorly from the GI tract, the I.V. route is the preferred administration method; the I.M. route can also be used if necessary.

Suxamethonium is hydrolysed in the liver and plasma by the enzyme pseudocholinesterase, producing a metabolite with a nondepolarising blocking action. It's excreted by the kidneys; a small amount is done so unchanged.

Pharmacodynamics

After administration, suxamethonium is rapidly metabolised, although at a slower rate than acetylcholine. As a result, suxamethonium remains attached to receptor sites on the skeletal muscle membrane for a longer period. This prevents repolarisation of the motor end plate and results in muscle paralysis.

Pharmacotherapeutics

Suxamethonium is the drug of choice for short-term muscle relaxation such as that needed during intubation and ECT.

Drug interactions

The action of suxamethonium is potentiated by a number of anaesthetics and antibiotics. In contrast to their interaction with nondepolarising blockers, anticholinesterases increase suxamethonium blockade.

Adverse reactions

The primary adverse reactions to suxamethonium include:
- prolonged apnea
- hypotension.

Genetics increases the risk

The risk associated with suxamethonium is increased with certain genetic predispositions, such as a low pseudocholinesterase level and the tendency to develop malignant hyperthermia.

Because suxamethonium is absorbed poorly from the GI tract, the I.V. route is used most often.

Nursing process

These nursing process steps are appropriate for patients receiving treatment with depolarising muscle relaxants.

Assessment
* Assess the patient's condition before therapy and regularly thereafter.
* Monitor the patient's baseline electrolyte determinations (electrolyte imbalance can increase neuromuscular effects) and vital signs.
* Measure the patient's fluid intake and output; renal dysfunction may prolong the duration of action because 25% of the drug is unchanged before excretion.
* Nerve stimulator and train-of-four monitoring are recommended to confirm the antagonism of the neuromuscular blockade and recovery of muscle strength.
* Monitor the patient's respirations closely until fully recovered from neuromuscular blockade, as evidenced by tests of muscle strength (handgrip, head lift, and ability to cough).
* Be alert for adverse reactions and drug interactions.
* Evaluate the patient's and family's knowledge of drug therapy.

Key nursing diagnoses
* Ineffective health maintenance related to the condition.
* Ineffective breathing pattern related to the drug's effect on respiratory muscles.
* Deficient knowledge related to drug therapy.

Planning outcome goals
* The patient's vital signs will remain within normal parameters while receiving drug therapy.
* The patient's respiratory function will be maintained as evidenced by adequate arterial blood gas (ABG) values and ventilatory parameters.
* The patient's family will confirm an understanding of the medication's purpose and intended effect.

Implementation
* Suxamethonium is the drug of choice for short procedures (less than 3 minutes) and for orthopaedic manipulations; use caution in the treatment of fractures or dislocations.
* Administer sedatives or general anaesthetics before neuromuscular blockers. Neuromuscular blockers don't reduce consciousness or alter pain threshold. Give analgesics for pain. Note that general anaesthesia and suxamethonium should only be

administered by personnel skilled in airway management, such as anaesthetists.
• Allow suxamethonium effects to subside before giving pancuronium.
• Have emergency respiratory support equipment (ET equipment, ventilator, oxygen, atropine, edrophonium, (adrenaline) epinephrine, and neostigmine) available for immediate use.
• For I.V. use, to evaluate the patient's ability to metabolise suxamethonium, give a test dose after they have been anaesthetised. A normal response (no respiratory depression or transient depression for up to 5 minutes) indicates that the drug may be given. Don't give subsequent doses if the patient develops respiratory paralysis sufficient to permit ET intubation.
• For I.M. use, give deep I.M., preferably high into the deltoid.
• Store the injectable form at 4°C. Store the powder form at room temperature in a tightly closed container and use it immediately after reconstitution. Don't mix with alkaline solutions (thiopental sodium, sodium bicarbonate, or barbiturates).
• Reversing drugs shouldn't be used. Unlike what happens with nondepolarising drugs, giving neostigmine or edrophonium with suxamethonium may worsen neuromuscular blockade.
• Continuous infusions of suxamethonium are not advised; this may reduce response or prolong muscle relaxation and apnea.

Evaluation
• Patient's condition improves.
• Patient maintains adequate ventilation with mechanical assistance.
• Patient and family state an understanding of drug therapy. (See *Teaching about neuromuscular blocking drugs*.)

Antiparkinsonian drugs

Drug therapy is an important part of the treatment of Parkinson's disease, a progressive neurologic disorder characterised by four cardinal features:
• muscle rigidity (inflexibility)
• akinesia (loss of voluntary muscle movement)
• tremors at rest
• disturbances of posture and balance.

Upsetting the balance

Reduction of dopamine in the corpus striatum disturbs the normal balance between two neurotransmitters, acetylcholine and dopamine. This results in a relative excess of acetylcholine. The excessive excitation caused by cholinergic activity creates the movement disorders of Parkinson's disease.

Defect in the dopamine pathway...

Parkinson's disease affects the extrapyramidal system, which influences movement. The extrapyramidal system includes the corpus striatum, globus pallidus, and substantia nigra of the brain. In Parkinson's disease, dopamine deficiency occurs in the basal ganglia, the dopamine-releasing pathway that connects the substantia nigra to the corpus striatum.

Other culprits

Parkinsonism can also result from drugs, encephalitis, neurotoxins, trauma, arteriosclerosis, or other neurologic disorders and environmental factors.

Bringing back balance

The goal of drug therapy is to provide symptom relief and maintain the patient's independence and mobility. This can be achieved by correcting the imbalance of neurotransmitters in one of several ways, including:
- inhibiting cholinergic effects (with anticholinergic drugs)
- enhancing the effects of dopamine (with dopaminergic drugs)
- inhibiting catechol *O*-methyltransferase (COMT) with COMT-inhibiting drugs.

> Drug therapy to correct the imbalance of neurotransmitters in patients with Parkinson's disease can help maintain mobility.

Anticholinergic drugs

Anticholinergic drugs are sometimes called *parasympatholytic drugs* because they inhibit the action of acetylcholine at special receptors in the parasympathetic nervous system. Anticholinergics used to treat Parkinson's disease include synthetic tertiary amines, such as benzatropine, procyclidine, and trihexyphenidyl.

Pharmacokinetics

Typically, anticholinergic drugs are well absorbed from the GI tract and cross the blood-brain barrier to their action site in the brain. Most are metabolised in the liver, at least partially, and are excreted by the kidneys as metabolites or unchanged drug. The exact distribution of these drugs is unknown.

Benzatropine is a long-acting drug with a duration of action of up to 24 hours in some patients. For most anticholinergics, half-life is undetermined.

Pharmacodynamics

High acetylcholine levels produce an excitatory effect on the CNS, which can cause parkinsonian tremors. Patients with Parkinson's disease take anticholinergic drugs to inhibit the action of acetylcholine at receptor sites in the central and autonomic nervous systems, thus reducing tremors.

Pharmacotherapeutics

Anticholinergics are used to treat all forms of parkinsonism. They're most commonly used in the early stages of Parkinson's disease, when symptoms are mild and don't have a major impact on the patient's lifestyle. These drugs effectively control sialorrhoea (excessive flow of saliva) and are about 20% effective in reducing the incidence and severity of akinesia and rigidity.

Early on

Anticholinergics can be used alone or with amantadine in the early stages of Parkinson's disease.

Later on

Anticholinergics can be given with levodopa during the later stages of Parkinson's disease to further relieve symptoms.

Drug interactions

Interactions can occur when certain medications are taken with anticholinergics:
• Amantadine can cause increased anticholinergic adverse effects.
• The absorption of levodopa can be decreased, which can lead to worsening of parkinsonian signs and symptoms.
• Antipsychotics (such as the phenothiazines and haloperidol) decrease the effectiveness of anticholinergics and antipsychotics. The incidence of anticholinergic adverse effects can also be increased.
• Over-the-counter cough and cold preparations, diet aids, and analeptics (drugs used to stay awake) increase anticholinergic effects.
• Alcohol increases CNS depression.

Be aware that OTC cough and cold preparations, diet aids, and analeptics increase anticholinergic effects.

Adverse reactions

Mild, dose-related adverse reactions to anticholinergics are seen in 30% to 50% of patients. Dry mouth may be a dose-related reaction to trihexyphenidyl.

Common complaints

Some common adverse reactions to anticholinergic drugs include:
- confusion
- restlessness
- agitation and excitement
- drowsiness or insomnia
- tachycardia
- palpitations
- constipation
- nausea and vomiting
- urine retention
- increased intraocular pressure (IOP), blurred vision, pupil dilation, and photophobia.

Can't help it if you're sensitive

Sensitivity-related reactions to anticholinergics can include hives and allergic rashes.

Senior sensitivity

Among elderly patients, increased sensitivity to anticholinergic drugs may occur. Signs and symptoms include mental confusion, agitation and, possibly, psychotic symptoms such as hallucinations.

Nursing process

These nursing process steps are appropriate for patients undergoing treatment with anticholinergic drugs.

Assessment
- Obtain a baseline assessment of the patient's impairment.
- Monitor drug effectiveness by regularly checking body movements for signs of improvement; keep in mind that the full effect of the drug may take 2 to 3 days.
- Monitor the patient for adverse reactions and be alert for drug interactions. Some adverse reactions may result from atropine-like toxicity and are dose related.
- Monitor the patient's vital signs, especially during dosage adjustments.
- Evaluate the patient's and family's understanding of drug therapy.

Key nursing diagnoses
• Impaired physical mobility related to dyskinetic movements.
• Risk for injury related to adverse CNS effects.
• Urinary retention related to anticholinergic effects on the bladder.
• Deficient knowledge related to drug therapy.

Planning outcome goals
• The patient will exhibit improved mobility with a reduction in muscle rigidity, akinesia, and tremors.
• The patient's risk of injury will be reduced.
• The patient's voiding pattern won't change.
• The patient and family will confirm an understanding of drug therapy.

Implementation
• Administer the drug with food to prevent GI irritation.
• Adjust the dosage according to the patient's response and tolerance.
• Never withdraw the drug abruptly; reduce the dose gradually.
• Institute safety precautions.
• Provide ice cubes, drinks, or sugarless hard sweets to relieve dry mouth. Increase fluid and fibre intake to prevent constipation, as appropriate.
• Notify the prescriber about urine retention and be prepared to catheterise the patient, if necessary.
• Give the drug at bedtime if the patient receives a single daily dose.

Evaluation
• Patient remains free from injury.
• Patient has no change in voiding pattern.
• Patient's sleep pattern isn't altered during amantadine therapy.
• Patient and family state an understanding of drug therapy. (See *Teaching about antiparkinsonian drugs*.)

Dopaminergic drugs

Dopaminergics include drugs that are chemically unrelated. Dopaminergic drugs increase the effects of dopamine at receptor sites and are useful in treating symptoms of Parkinson's disease. Examples include:
• levodopa, the metabolic precursor to dopamine
• co-careldopa, a combination drug composed of carbidopa and levodopa
• amantadine, an antiviral drug with dopamine activity
• bromocriptine and pergolide, ergot-type dopamine agonists

Education edge

Teaching about anti-parkinsonian drugs

If anti-parkinsonian drugs are prescribed, review these points with the patient and caregivers:

- Take the drug exactly as prescribed and don't stop the drug suddenly.
- Take the drug with food to prevent GI upset. Don't crush or break tablets, especially catechol *O*-methyltransferase (COMT) inhibitors, and take them at the same time as co-carledopa.
- To relieve dry mouth, take sips of water, suck on sugarless sweets.
- Avoid hazardous tasks if adverse central nervous system effects occur. Also avoid alcohol use during therapy.
- Use caution when standing after a prolonged period of sitting or lying down because dizziness may occur, especially early in therapy.
- Report severe or persistent adverse reactions. Also report

any uncontrolled movements of the body, chest pain, palpitations, depression or mood changes, difficulty voiding, or severe or persistent nausea or vomiting. With COMT inhibitors, hallucinations, increased dyskinesia, nausea, and diarrhoea may occur.

- Don't take vitamins, herbal products, or over-the-counter preparations without consulting a health care provider.
- Be aware that COMT inhibitors may cause urine to turn brownish-orange.
- Tell all health care providers about the drug therapy.
- Avoid overexertion even when beginning to feel better.
- Obtain regular medical follow-up, which is necessary to evaluate the effects of this drug.

- ropinirole and pramipexole, two non-ergot-type dopamine agonists
- selegiline, a type B MAO inhibitor.

Pharmacokinetics

Like anticholinergic drugs, dopaminergic drugs are absorbed from the GI tract into the bloodstream and delivered to their action site in the brain. The body absorbs most levodopa, co-careldopa, pramipexole, or amantadine from the GI tract after oral administration, but only about 28% of bromocriptine is absorbed. Absorption of levodopa is slowed and reduced when it's ingested with food. In some patients, levodopa can significantly interact with foods. Dietary amino acids can decrease levodopa's effectiveness by competing with it for absorption from the intestine and slowing its transport to the brain. The body can absorb a significant amount of pergolide, although how much is absorbed isn't fully known. About 73% of an oral dose of selegiline is absorbed.

Levodopa is widely distributed in body tissues, including those in the GI tract, liver, pancreas, kidneys, salivary glands, and skin. Co-careldopa and pramipexole are also widely distributed. Amantadine is distributed in saliva, nasal secretions, and breast milk. Bromocriptine and pergolide are highly protein bound. The distribution of selegiline is unknown.

Each drug is different

Dopaminergic drugs are metabolised extensively in various areas of the body and are eliminated by the liver, the kidneys, or both. Here are more specifics about the metabolism and excretion of dopaminergic drugs:

• Large amounts of levodopa are metabolised in the stomach and during the first pass through the liver. It's metabolised extensively and excreted by the kidneys.

• Carbidopa isn't metabolised extensively. The kidneys excrete approximately one-third of it unchanged within 24 hours. (See *Antiparkinsonian drugs: Carbidopa and levodopa.*)

• Amantadine, ropinirole, and pramipexole are excreted by the kidneys largely unchanged.

• Almost all of a bromocriptine dose is metabolised by the liver to pharmacologically inactive compounds and primarily eliminated in faeces; only a small amount is excreted in urine.

• After pergolide is metabolised, it's excreted by the kidneys.

• Selegiline is metabolised to amphetamine, methamphetamine, and N-desmethylselegiline (the major metabolite), which are eliminated in urine.

Pharmacodynamics

Dopaminergic drugs act in the brain to improve motor function in one of two ways: by increasing the dopamine concentration or by enhancing the neurotransmission of dopamine.

Getting the job done

Levodopa is inactive until it crosses the blood-brain barrier and is converted to dopamine by enzymes in the brain, increasing dopamine concentrations in the basal ganglia. Carbidopa enhances levodopa's effectiveness by blocking the peripheral conversion of L-dopa, thus permitting more levodopa to be transported to the brain.

The other dopaminergic drugs have various mechanisms of action:

• Amantadine's mechanism of action isn't clear. It's thought to release dopamine from intact neurons, but it may also have nondopaminergic mechanisms.

• Bromocriptine, ropinirole, and pramipexole stimulate dopamine receptors in the brain, producing effects similar to those of dopamine.

Prototype pro

Antiparkinsonian drugs: co-careldopa

Actions

- Improves voluntary movement

Levodopa

- Chemical effect of levodopa unknown; thought to be carboxylated (addition of a carboxyl group) to dopamine, countering depletion of striatal dopamine in extrapyramidal centres

Carbidopa

- Inhibits peripheral decarboxylation (removal of a carboxyl group) of levodopa without affecting levodopa's metabolism within the central nervous system, making more levodopa available to be decarboxylated to dopamine in the brain

Indications

- Idiopathic Parkinson's disease
- Postencephalitic parkinsonism
- Symptomatic parkinsonism resulting from carbon monoxide or manganese intoxication

Nursing considerations

- If the patient is being treated with levodopa, discontinue the drug at least 8 hours before starting co-careldopa.
- The dosage should be adjusted according to the patient's response and tolerance.
- Withhold the dose and notify the prescriber if the patient's vital signs or mental status change significantly. A reduced dosage or discontinuation may be necessary.
- Monitor the patient for adverse effects, such as choreiform, dystonic, dyskinetic movements; involuntary grimacing; head movements; myoclonic jerks; ataxia; suicidal tendencies; hypotension; dry mouth; nausea and vomiting; signs and symptoms of haematologic disorders; and hepatoxicity.
- A patient on long-term therapy should be tested for acromegaly and diabetes.

- Pergolide directly stimulates postsynaptic dopamine receptors in the CNS.
- Selegiline can increase dopaminergic activity by inhibiting MAO activity (type B) or by other mechanisms.

Pharmacotherapeutics

The choice of therapy is highly individualised and is determined by the patient's symptoms and level of disability. A patient with mild Parkinson's disease with predominantly symptoms of tremor is commonly given anticholinergics or amantadine. Selegiline is indicated for extending the duration of levodopa by blocking its breakdown; it has also been used in early Parkinson's disorder because of its

> # Levodopa toxicity? Or worsening of Parkinson's disease?
>
> Levodopa is commonly used to treat Parkinson's disease; however, this use isn't without controversy. Initially, levodopa is very effective in controlling symptoms. But after several years, the effects of the drug sometimes don't last as long (the *wearing-off effect*) or lead to sharp fluctuations in symptoms (the *on-off phenomenon*).
>
> ## Low doses? Or later?
>
> Some prescribers feel that levodopa should be used early (when diagnosis is made) in low doses. Others believe in starting later in the course of the disease (when symptoms compromise function). Those who advocate starting early feel that fluctuations in response to levodopa are from the progression of Parkinson's disease and not from the effects of levodopa. Some prescribers are even concerned that levodopa accelerates the progression of Parkinson's disease by providing a source of free radicals that contribute to the degeneration of dopaminergic neurons.

neuroprotective properties and potential to slow the progression of Parkinsonism. Usually, dopaminergic drugs are used to treat the patient with severe Parkinson's disease or the patient who doesn't respond to anticholinergics alone. Levodopa is the most effective drug used to treat Parkinson's disease; however, it loses its effectiveness after 3 to 5 years. (See *Levodopa toxicity? Or worsening of Parkinson's disease?*)

When fluctuations in response to levodopa occur, dosage adjustments and increased frequency of administration may be tried. Alternatively, adjunctive therapy, such as dopamine agonists, selegiline, amantadine, or a COMT inhibitor may be added. Controlled-release formulations of co-careldopa may be helpful in managing the wearing-off effect or delayed-onset motor fluctuations.

Add carbidopa, reduce levodopa

When carbidopa is given with levodopa, the dosage of levodopa can be reduced, decreasing the risk of GI and cardiovascular adverse effects. Levodopa is almost exclusively combined with carbidopa as the standard therapy for Parkinson's disease.

Tapered treatment

Some dopaminergic drugs, such as amantadine, levodopa, pramipexole, and bromocriptine, must be gradually tapered to avoid precipitating parkinsonian crisis (sudden marked clinical deterioration) and possible life-threatening complications (including a syndrome with muscle rigidity, elevated body temperature, tachycardia, mental changes, and increased serum creatine kinase [CK] resembling neuroleptic malignant syndrome).

Drug interactions

Dopaminergic drugs can interfere with many other drugs, causing potentially fatal reactions. Here are some examples:
*   The effectiveness of levodopa can be reduced when taking pyridoxine (vitamin B$_6$), phenytoin, benzodiazepines, and papaverine.
*   Concomitant use with a type A MAO inhibitor, such as tranylcypromine, increases the risk of hypertensive crisis.
*   Antipsychotics, such as phenothiazines, and haloperidol, can reduce the effectiveness of levodopa and pergolide.
*   Amantadine may potentiate anticholinergic adverse effects of anticholinergic drugs, such as confusion and hallucinations, and can reduce the absorption of levodopa.
*   Pethidine taken with selegiline at higher than recommended doses can cause a fatal reaction.

Adverse reactions

Adverse reactions to dopaminergic drugs vary with the drug prescribed.

Levodopa

Adverse effects of levodopa include:
*   nausea and vomiting
*   orthostatic hypotension
*   anorexia
*   neuroleptic malignant syndrome
*   arrhythmias
*   irritability
*   confusion.

Levodopa can cause arrhythmias. Why me?

Amantadine

Adverse effects of amantadine include orthostatic hypotension and constipation.

Bromocriptine

Adverse effects of bromocriptine include:
*   persistent orthostatic hypotension
*   ventricular tachycardia
*   bradycardia
*   worsening angina.

Pergolide

Adverse effects of pergolide include:

- confusion
- dyskinesia
- hallucinations
- nausea.

Pramipexole/ropinirole

Adverse effects of pramipexole/ropinirole include:

- orthostatic hypotension
- dizziness
- confusion
- insomnia.

Nursing process

These nursing process steps are appropriate for patients undergoing treatment with dopaminergic drugs.

Assessment

- Assess the patient's underlying condition before therapy and regularly thereafter; therapeutic response usually follows each dose and disappears within 5 hours, but may vary considerably.
- Monitor drug effectiveness by regularly checking body movements for signs of improvement; the full effect of the drug may take 2 to 3 days.
- Monitor the patient for adverse reactions and be alert for drug interactions. Some adverse reactions may result from atropine-like toxicity and are dose-related. Immediately report muscle twitching and blepharospasm (twitching of the eyelids), which may be early signs of drug overdose.
- Monitor the patient's vital signs, especially during dosage adjustments.
- Evaluate the patient's and family's understanding of drug therapy.

Key nursing diagnoses

- Impaired physical mobility related to dyskinetic movements.
- Risk for injury related to adverse CNS effects.
- Disturbed thought processes related to drug-induced CNS adverse reactions.
- Deficient knowledge related to drug therapy.

Planning outcome goals

- The patient will exhibit improved mobility with reduction in muscle rigidity, akinesia, and tremors.
- The patient's risk of injury will be reduced.

- The patient's voiding pattern won't change.
- The patient and family will confirm an understanding of drug therapy.

Implementation
- Administer the drug with food to prevent GI irritation.
- The dosage should be adjusted by the prescriber according to the patient's response and tolerance.
- Never withdraw the drug abruptly; reduce the dose gradually.
- Withhold the dose and notify the prescriber if the patient's vital signs or mental status change significantly. A reduced dosage or discontinuation may be necessary.
- Institute safety precautions.
- Provide ice cubes, drinks, or sugarless sweets to relieve dry mouth. Increase fluid and fibre intake to prevent constipation, as appropriate.
- Give the drug at bedtime if the patient receives a single daily dose.
- If the patient is being treated with levodopa, discontinue the drug at least 8 hours before starting co-careldopa.
- Treat a patient with open-angle glaucoma with caution. Monitor them closely, watch for a change in intra-occular pressure (IOP), and arrange for periodic eye exams.
- A patient receiving long-term therapy should be tested regularly for diabetes and acromegaly and should have periodic tests of liver, renal, and haematopoietic function.

> Patient and family understanding is important with any type of drug therapy.

Evaluation
- Patient remains free from injury.
- Patient remains mentally alert.
- Patient exhibits improved mobility with a reduction of muscular rigidity and tremor.
- Patient and family state an understanding of drug therapy.

(See *Teaching about antiparkinsonian drugs*.)

COMT inhibitors

COMT inhibitors are used as adjunctive treatments to co-careldopa in the management of a patient with Parkinson's disease who experiences "wearing off" at the end of the dosing interval.

Choice of two

Two COMT inhibitors are currently available:
- tolcapone
- entacapone.

Pharmacokinetics

Tolcapone and entacapone are rapidly absorbed by the GI tract, and absolute bioavailability of each agent is 65% and 35%, respectively. Both drugs are highly bound to albumin and, therefore, have limited distribution to the tissues. They're almost completely metabolised in the liver to inactive metabolites and are excreted in urine.

Pharmacodynamics

Tolcapone and entacapone are selective and reversible inhibitors of COMT, the major metabolising enzyme for levodopa in the presence of a decarboxylase inhibitor such as carbidopa. Inhibition of COMT alters the pharmacokinetics for levodopa, leading to sustained plasma levels of levodopa. This results in more sustained dopaminergic stimulation in the brain and improvement in the signs and symptoms of Parkinson's disease.

Pharmacotherapeutics

Tolcapone or entacapone may be added to co-careldopa in a patient who experiences wearing-off symptoms at the end of a dosing interval or random on-off fluctuations in response to co-careldopa. COMT inhibitors have no antiparkinsonian effect when used alone and should always be combined with co-careldopa. Addition of a COMT inhibitor commonly necessitates a decrease in the dose of co-careldopa, particularly in the patient receiving extreme doses of levodopa.

Not too fast

Rapid withdrawal of COMT inhibitors may lead to parkinsonian crisis and may cause a syndrome of muscle rigidity, high fever, tachycardia, confusion, and elevated serum CK similar to neuroleptic malignant syndrome. A slow tapering of the dosage is suggested to avoid rapid withdrawal.

> Combining COMT inhibitors with co-carledopa may reduce wearing-off symptoms at the end of a dosing interval.

Drug interactions

COMT inhibitors can interfere with many drugs. Here are some examples:
• COMT inhibitors shouldn't be used concurrently with type A MAO inhibitors, but may be used with selegiline.
• Significant arrhythmias may result when COMT inhibitors are combined with catecholamine drugs (dopamine, dobutamine, adrenaline (epinephrine), methyldopa, noradrenaline (norepinephrine)).
• The use of COMT inhibitors with CNS depressants (benzodiazepines, tricyclic antidepressants, antipsychotics, ethanol,

opioid analgesics, and other sedative hypnotics) may cause additive CNS effects.
• Entacapone chelates iron and, therefore, iron absorption may be decreased.
• Due to MAO inhibition, COMT inhibitors shouldn't be taken concomitantly with linezolid.
• Fibrotic complications have been associated with the use of entacapone and bromocriptine or pergolide.
• Drugs that interfere with glucuronidation (erythromycin, colestyramine, rifampacin and probenecid) may decrease entacapone elimination.
• When using COMT inhibitors for a patient on dopaminergic therapy, the potential for orthostatic hypotension may be increased.

Adverse reactions
Common adverse reactions to COMT inhibitors include:
• nausea
• dyskinesia
• diarrhoea
• brown-orange urine discolouration (entacapone)
• hyperkinesia or hypokinesia.
  Less common adverse reactions include:
• orthostatic hypotension
• syncope
• dizziness
• fatigue
• abdominal pain
• constipation
• vomiting
• dry mouth
• back pain
• diaphoresis.

You bet your life!

Life-threatening reactions to COMT inhibitors include acute liver failure. Due to this risk, tolcapone should be used only in a patient with Parkinson's disease who experiences fluctuations in levodopa response and doesn't respond to or isn't an appropriate candidate for other adjunctive therapies. The patient should be advised of the risks of liver injury, and written informed consent should be obtained before drug administration. Liver function tests should be obtained at baseline and every 2 weeks for the first year, every 4 weeks for the next 3 months, and every 8 weeks thereafter.

Nursing process

These nursing process steps are appropriate for patients undergoing treatment with COMT inhibitors.

Assessment

- Assess the patient's hepatic and biliary function before starting therapy.
- Monitor the patient's blood pressure closely. Watch for orthostatic hypotension.
- Monitor the patient for hallucinations.
- Evaluate the patient's and family's knowledge of drug therapy.

Key nursing diagnoses

- Impaired physical mobility related to presence of parkinsonism.
- Disturbed thought processes related to drug-induced adverse reactions.
- Deficient knowledge related to drug therapy.

Planning outcome goals

- The patient's physical mobility will improve.
- The patient will be alert and able to confirm orientation adequately.
- The patient and family will confirm an understanding of drug therapy.

Implementation

- The drug can be given with immediate or sustained-release co-careldopa and can be taken with or without food.
- The drug should be used only with co-careldopa; no anti-parkinsonian effects will occur when the drug is given as monotherapy.
- Co-careldopa dosage requirements are usually lower when given with entacapone; the co-careldopa dose should be lowered or the dosing interval should be increased to avoid adverse effects.
- Keep in mind that the drug may cause or worsen dyskinesia despite a reduced levodopa dosage.
- Watch the patient for onset of diarrhoea, which usually begins 4 to 12 weeks after therapy starts, but may begin as early as the first week or as late as many months.
- Rapid withdrawal or abrupt reduction in the dosage could lead to signs and symptoms of Parkinson's disease; it may also lead to hyperpyrexia and confusion, a symptom complex resembling neuroleptic malignant syndrome. Discontinue the drug slowly and monitor the patient closely. Adjust other dopaminergic treatments.

- Observe for urine discolouration.
- Rarely, rhabdomyolysis has occurred with drug use.

Evaluation
- Patient exhibits improved physical mobility.
- Patient maintains normal thought processes.
- Patient and family state an understanding of drug therapy. (See *Teaching about antiparkinsonian drugs.*)

Anticonvulsant drugs

Anticonvulsant drugs inhibit neuromuscular transmission. They can be prescribed for:
- long-term management of chronic epilepsy (recurrent seizures)
- short-term management of acute isolated seizures not caused by epilepsy such as seizures after trauma or brain surgery.

In addition, some anticonvulsants are used in the emergency treatment of status epilepticus (a continuous seizure state).

Try one, then another, before together

Treatment of epilepsy should begin with a single drug, increasing the dosage until seizures are controlled or adverse effects become problematic. Generally, a second alternative should be tried as monotherapy before considering combination therapy. Choice of drug treatment depends on the seizure type, the drug's characteristics, and the patient's preferences.

Class discussion

Anticonvulsants can be categorised into several major classes:
- hydantoins
- barbiturates
- iminostilbenes
- benzodiazepines
- carboxylic acid derivatives
- 1 (amino-methyl) cyclohexane acetic acid
- phenyltriazine
- carboxamide
- sulphamate substitute derivatives of monosaccharides
- succinimides
- sulphonamides.

Anticonvulsants can be categorised into several major classes.

Hydantoins

The two most commonly prescribed anticonvulsant drugs—phenytoin and fosphenytoin—belong to the hydantoin class.

Pharmacokinetics
The pharmacokinetics of these two hydantoins is different for each.

Phenytoin fits in slowly

Phenytoin is absorbed slowly after oral and I.M. administration. It's distributed rapidly to all tissues and is highly (90%) protein bound. Phenytoin is metabolised in the liver. Inactive metabolites are excreted in bile and then reabsorbed from the GI tract. Eventually, however, they're excreted in urine.

Fosphenytoin for the short-term

Fosphenytoin is indicated for short-term I.M. or I.V. administration. It's widely distributed throughout the body, is highly (90%) protein bound, and is metabolised by the liver and excreted in urine.

Pharmacodynamics
In most cases, the hydantoin anticonvulsants stabilise nerve cells to keep them from getting overexcited. Phenytoin appears to work in the motor cortex of the brain, where it stops the spread of seizure activity. The pharmacodynamics of fosphenytoin are thought to mimic those of phenytoin.

Also got heart

Phenytoin is also used as an antiarrhythmic drug to control irregular heart rhythms, with properties similar to those of procainamide.

Pharmacotherapeutics
Because of its effectiveness and relatively low toxicity, phenytoin is the most commonly prescribed anticonvulsant and one of the drugs of choice to treat:
*   complex partial seizures (also called *psychomotor* or *temporal lobe seizures*)
*   tonic-clonic seizures.
    The enzyme system responsible for the metabolism of phenytoin is saturable. A change in dose can result in disproportional changes in serum concentration. (See *Anticonvulsants: Phenytoin.*)

The most commonly prescribed anticonvulsants are phenytoin and fosphenytoin.

Prototype pro

Anticonvulsants: Phenytoin

Actions

- Stabilises neuronal membranes and limits seizure activity by either increasing efflux or decreasing influx of sodium ions across cell membranes in the motor cortex during generation of nerve impulses.

Indications

- Control of tonic-clonic and complex partial seizures.
- Status epilepticus.
- Prevention of and treatment for seizures during neurosurgery.

Nursing considerations

- Monitor the patient for adverse effects, such as ataxia, slurred speech, mental confusion, nystagmus, blurred vision, gingival hyperplasia, nausea, vomiting, haematologic disorders, hepatitis, Stevens-Johnson syndrome, and hirsutism.
- Don't withdraw the drug suddenly; seizures may occur.
- Monitor drug levels, following prescribed dosage changes: therapeutic levels range from 10 to 20 mcg/ml.

Resistance is futile

Phenytoin and fosphenytoin are the long-acting anticonvulsants of choice to treat status epilepticus after initial I.V. benzodiazepines.

Drug interactions

Hydantoins interact with several drugs. Here are some drug interactions of major to moderate clinical significance:
- The effect of phenytoin is reduced when taken with phenobarbital, diazoxide, theophylline, carbamazepine, rifampicin, antacids, and sucralfate.

Oral interference

- Enteral tube feedings may interfere with the absorption of oral phenytoin. Stop feedings for 2 hours before and after phenytoin administration.
- The effect of phenytoin is increased and the risk of toxicity increases when phenytoin is taken with allopurinol, cimetidine, disulfiram, fluconazole, isoniazid, omeprazole, sulphonamides, oral anticoagulants, chloramphenicol, valproic acid, and amiodarone.

• The effect of the following drugs is reduced when taken with an hydantoin anticonvulsant: oral anticoagulants, levodopa, amiodarone, corticosteroids, doxycycline, methadone, metyrapone, theophylline, thyroid hormone, hormonal contraceptives, valproic acid, ciclosporine, and carbamazepine.

Adverse reactions

Adverse reactions to hydantoins include:
• drowsiness
• ataxia
• irritability and restlessness
• headache
• nystagmus
• dizziness and vertigo
• dysarthria
• nausea and vomiting
• abdominal pain
• anorexia
• depressed atrial and ventricular conduction
• ventricular fibrillation (in toxic states)
• bradycardia, hypotension, and cardiac arrest (with I.V. administration)
• hypersensitivity reactions.

Nursing process

These nursing process steps are appropriate for patients undergoing treatment with hydantoin anticonvulsant drugs.

Assessment

• Monitor the patient's response to the prescribed drug and serum levels, as indicated.
• Assess the patient's condition before therapy and regularly thereafter.
• Monitor the patient's blood levels; the therapeutic level is 10 to 20 mcg/ml.
• Monitor CBC and calcium level every 6 months.
• Periodically monitor hepatic function.
• Check the patient's vital signs, blood pressure, and electrocardiography (ECG) during I.V. administration.
• Monitor the patient for adverse reactions.
• Assess the patient's compliance with therapy at each follow-up visit.
• Monitor the patient for increased seizure activity; mononucleosis may decrease the phenytoin level.
• Evaluate the patient's and family's knowledge of drug therapy.

Bradycardia, hypotension, and cardiac arrest can occur with I.V. administration of hydantoins.

Key nursing diagnoses
- Risk for injury related to adverse reactions.
- Impaired physical mobility related to sedation.
- Deficient knowledge related to drug therapy.
- Noncompliance related to long-term therapy.

Planning outcome goals
- Risk to the patient will be minimised.
- The patient will be able to perform activities of daily living (ADLs).
- The patient and family will confirm an understanding of drug therapy.

Implementation
- Administer oral forms with food to reduce GI irritation.
- Phenytoin binds with tube feedings, thus decreasing the absorption of the drug. Turn off tube feedings for 2 hours before and after giving phenytoin, according to your facility's policy.
- If using as an infusion, don't mix the drug with glucose 5% in water because phenytoin will precipitate. Clear I.V. tubing first with normal saline solution. Mix with normal saline solution if necessary and infuse over 30 to 60 minutes with an in-line filter.
- Avoid giving phenytoin by I.V. push into veins on the back of the hand to avoid discolouration known as *purple glove syndrome*. Inject into larger veins or a central venous catheter, if available.
- Discard 4 hours after preparation for I.V. administration.
- Don't give phenytoin I.M. unless dosage adjustments are made. The drug may precipitate at the site, cause pain, and be erratically absorbed.
- Expect to adjust the dosage according to the patient's response.
- Administer safety precautions if the patient has an adverse CNS reaction.

Evaluation
- Patient sustains no injury from adverse reactions.
- Patient is free from seizure activity.
- Patient maintains physical mobility.
- Patient complies with therapy and has no seizures.
- Patient and family state an understanding of drug therapy. (See *Teaching about anticonvulsants*.)

Barbiturates

Formerly one of the most widely used anticonvulsants, the long-acting barbiturate phenobarbital is now used less frequently because

Education edge

Teaching about anticonvulsants

If anticonvulsants are prescribed, review these points with the patient and caregivers:

- Take the drug exactly as prescribed and don't stop the drug without medical supervision. The drug must be taken regularly to be effective.
- Take the drug with food to reduce GI upset and loss of appetite. Eating small, frequent meals can help.
- Don't change brands or dosage forms.
- Avoid hazardous activities that require mental alertness if adverse central nervous system reactions occur.
- Wear or carry medical identification at all times.
- Record and report any seizure activity while taking the drug.
- Don't stop the drug abruptly. If for some reason the patient is unable to continue taking the drug, notify the health care provider at once; the drug must be slowly withdrawn when it's discontinued.

- Try to space activities throughout the day and allow rest periods to avoid fatigue, weakness, and drowsiness. Take safety precautions and avoid driving or operating dangerous machinery if these conditions occur.
- Report persistent or bothersome adverse effects to the prescriber.
- Perform oral hygiene and see a dentist for regular examinations, especially if taking phenytoin or its derivatives.
- Be aware that phenytoin may discolour urine pink, red, or red-brown.
- Don't take over-the-counter medications or herbal preparations without first consulting with a health care provider.
- Be aware that heavy alcohol use may diminish the drug's benefit.
- Regular medical follow-up, possibly including blood tests, is necessary to help evaluate the effects of the drug.

of its sedative effects. Phenobarbital is sometimes used for long-term treatment of epilepsy and is prescribed selectively for treatment of status epilepticus if hydantoins aren't effective.

Other choices

Primidone, a structural analog of phenobarbital that's closely related chemically to the barbiturate-derivative anticonvulsants, is also used in the chronic treatment of epilepsy.

Pharmacokinetics

Each barbiturate has a slightly different set of pharmacokinetic properties.

Phenobarbital for the long haul

Although absorbed slowly, phenobarbital is well absorbed from the GI tract. Peak plasma concentration levels occur 8 to 12 hours after a single dose. The drug is 20% to 45% bound to serum proteins and to a similar extent to other tissues, including the brain. The liver metabolises about 75% of a phenobarbital dose, and 25% is excreted unchanged in urine.

Primidone evens out

Approximately 60% to 80% of a primidone dose is absorbed from the GI tract, and it's distributed evenly among body tissues. The drug is protein bound to a small extent in the plasma. Primidone is metabolised by the liver to two active metabolites, phenobarbital and phenylethylmalonamide (PEMA). Approximately 15% to 25% of primidone is excreted unchanged in urine, 15% to 25% is metabolised to phenobarbital, and 50% to 70% is excreted in urine as PEMA.

Pharmacodynamics

Barbiturates exhibit anticonvulsant action at doses below those that produce hypnotic effects. For this reason, the barbiturates usually don't produce addiction when used to treat epilepsy. Barbiturates elevate the seizure threshold by decreasing postsynaptic excitation.

Pharmacotherapeutics

The barbiturate anticonvulsants are effective alternative therapy for:
- partial seizures
- tonic-clonic seizures
- febrile seizures.

Barbiturates can be used alone or with other anticonvulsants. I.V. phenobarbital is also used to treat status epilepticus. The major disadvantage of using phenobarbital for status epilepticus is a delayed onset of action when an immediate response is needed. Barbiturate anticonvulsants are ineffective in treating absence seizures.

"Ph" before "pr"

In general, because of monitoring, costs, and dosing frequency, phenobarbital is tried before primidone. Primidone may be effective in a patient who doesn't respond to phenobarbital.

Drug interactions

Here are some drug interactions of barbiturates:
• The effects of barbiturates can be reduced when taken with rifampicin.
• The risk of toxicity increases when phenobarbital is taken with CNS depressants, valproic acid, chloramphenicol, cimetidine, or phenytoin.
• The metabolism of corticosteroids, cimetidine, or phenytoin can be enhanced with phenobarbital therapy, leading to decreased effects. Evening primrose oil may increase anticonvulsant dosage requirements.

Reduced rates

In addition, the effects of many drugs can be reduced when taken with a barbiturate, including such drugs as beta-adrenergic blockers, corticosteroids, digoxin, oestrogens, doxycycline, oral anticoagulants, hormonal contraceptives, phenothiazine, metronidazole, tricyclic antidepressants, theophylline, ciclosporine, carbamazepine, felodipine, and verapamil.

Adverse reactions

Adverse reactions to phenobarbital include:
• drowsiness
• lethargy
• dizziness
• nystagmus, confusion, and ataxia (with large doses)
• laryngospasm, respiratory depression, and hypotension (when administered I.V.).

And then some

Primidone can cause the same CNS and GI adverse reactions as phenobarbital. It can also cause acute psychoses, hair loss, impotence, and osteomalacia.

As a group

Both barbiturate anticonvulsants can produce hypersensitivity rashes and other rashes, lupuslike syndrome (an inflammatory disorder), and enlarged lymph nodes.

Nursing process

These nursing process steps are appropriate for patients undergoing treatment with barbiturate anticonvulsant drugs.

Assessment
• Monitor the patient's response to the prescribed drug and serum levels, as indicated.
• Assess the patient's condition before therapy and regularly thereafter.
• Monitor the patient's blood level closely, as indicated.
• Monitor the patient for adverse reactions.
• Assess the patient's compliance with therapy at each follow-up visit.

Key nursing diagnoses
• Risk for injury related to adverse reactions.
• Impaired physical mobility related to sedation.
• Noncompliance related to long-term therapy.

Planning outcome goals
• Risk of injury to the patient will be minimised.
• The patient will be able to perform ADLs.
• The patient and family will confirm an understanding of drug therapy.

Implementation
• Administer oral forms of the drug with food to reduce GI irritation.
• I.V. phenobarbital is reserved for emergency treatment; monitor the patient's respirations closely and don't give more than 60 mg/minute. Have resuscitation equipment available.
• Don't stop the drug abruptly because seizures may worsen. Call the prescriber immediately if adverse reactions occur.
• Give the I.M. injection deeply. Superficial injection may cause pain, sterile abscess, and tissue sloughing.
• Expect to adjust the dosage according to the patient's response.
• Administer safety precautions if the patient has adverse CNS reactions.

Evaluation
• Patient sustains no trauma from adverse reactions.
• Patient maintains physical mobility.
• Patient complies with therapy and has no seizures.

Iminostilbenes

Carbamazepine is the most commonly used iminostilbene anticonvulsant. It effectively treats:

- partial and generalised tonic-clonic seizures
- mixed seizure types
- complex partial seizures (first choice of treatment).

Pharmacokinetics

Carbamazepine is absorbed slowly from the GI tract, is metabolised in the liver by the cytochrome P-450 isoform 3A4 (CYP3A4), and is excreted in urine. Carbamazepine is distributed rapidly to all tissues; 75% to 90% is bound to plasma proteins. The half-life varies greatly.

Pharmacodynamics

Carbamazepine's anticonvulsant effect is similar to that of phenytoin. The anticonvulsant action of the drug can occur because of its ability to inhibit the spread of seizure activity or neuromuscular transmission in general.

Pharmacotherapeutics

Carbamazepine is the drug of choice, in adults and children, for treating:

- generalised tonic-clonic seizures
- simple and complex partial seizures.

More than a seizure server

Carbamazepine also relieves pain when used to treat trigeminal neuralgia (tic douloureux, characterised by excruciating facial pain along the trigeminal nerve) and may be useful in some psychiatric disorders, such as bipolar affective disorder and intermittent explosive disorder. Carbamazepine may increase absence or myoclonic seizures and isn't recommended for treatment for these types of seizures.

Drug interactions

Carbamazepine can reduce the effects of several drugs, including oral anticoagulants, haloperidol, bupropion, lamotrigine, tricyclic antidepressants, hormonal contraceptives, doxycycline, theophylline, and valproic acid.

Other drug interactions can also occur:

- Increased carbamazepine levels and toxicity can occur with cimetidine, danazol, diltiazem, erythromycin, isoniazid, selective

serotonin reuptake inhibitors (SSRIs), ketoconazole, valproic acid, and verapamil.
• Lithium and carbamazepine taken together increase the risk of toxic neurologic effects.
• Carbamazepine levels can decrease when taken with barbiturates, or phenytoin.
• Plantain may inhibit GI absorption.

Adverse reactions
Occasionally, serious haematologic toxicity occurs. Because carbamazepine is related structurally to the tricyclic antidepressants, it can cause similar toxicities and affect behaviours and emotions. Hives and Stevens-Johnson syndrome (a potentially fatal inflammatory disease) can occur. Rashes are the most frequent hypersensitivity response.

Nursing process
These nursing process steps are appropriate for patients undergoing treatment with iminostilbene anticonvulsant drugs.

Assessment
• Assess the patient's seizure disorder or trigeminal neuralgia before therapy and regularly thereafter.
• Obtain baseline determinations of urinalysis, blood urea nitrogen level, liver function, CBC, platelet and reticulocyte counts, and iron level. Reassess regularly.
• Monitor drug level and drug effects closely; therapeutic level is 4 to 12 mcg/ml.
• Monitor the patient's response to the prescribed drug and serum levels, as indicated.
• Monitor the patient for adverse reactions.
• Assess the patient's compliance with therapy at each follow-up visit.

Key nursing diagnoses
• Risk for injury related to adverse reactions.
• Impaired physical mobility related to sedation.
• Noncompliance related to long-term therapy.

Planning outcome goals
• Risk of injury to the patient will be minimised.
• The patient will be able to perform ADLs.

- The patient and family will confirm an understanding of drug therapy.

Implementation
- Administer oral forms with food to reduce GI irritation. Give the drug in divided doses, when possible, to maintain a consistent blood level.
- Shake an oral suspension well before measuring the dose.
- When giving the drug by nasogastric tube, mix the dose with an equal volume of water, normal saline solution, or 5% glucose in water. Flush the tube with 100 ml of diluent after administering the dose.
- Expect to adjust the dosage according to the patient's response.
- Administer safety precautions if the patient has adverse CNS reactions.
- Never suddenly discontinue the drug when treating seizures or status epilepticus.
- Notify the prescriber immediately if adverse reactions occur.

Evaluation
- Patient sustains no injury from adverse reactions.
- Patient maintains physical mobility.
- Patient complies with therapy and has no seizures.

Benzodiazepines

The four benzodiazepine drugs that provide anticonvulsant effects are:
- diazepam (in the parenteral form)
- clonazepam
- lorazepam.

Only one for ongoing treatment

Only clonazepam is recommended for long-term treatment of epilepsy. Diazepam is restricted to acute treatment of status epilepticus and rectally for repetitive seizures. I.V. lorazepam is considered the drug of choice for acute management of status epilepticus.

Pharmacokinetics
The patient can receive benzodiazepines orally, parenterally or, in special situations, rectally. These drugs are absorbed rapidly and almost completely from the GI tract, but are distributed at

Clonazepam is the only benzodiazepine drug recommended for the long-term treatment of epilepsy.

different rates. Protein binding of benzodiazepines ranges from 85% to 90%.

Benzodiazepines are metabolised in the liver to multiple metabolites and are then excreted in urine. The benzodiazepines readily cross the placenta and are excreted in breast milk.

Pharmacodynamics

Benzodiazepines act as:
- anticonvulsants
- antianxiety agents
- sedative-hypnotics
- muscle relaxants.

Their mechanism of action is poorly understood.

Pharmacotherapeutics

Each of the benzodiazepines can be used in slightly different ways:
- Clonazepam is used to treat absence (petit mal), atypical absence (Lennox-Gastaut syndrome), atonic, and myoclonic seizures.
- Diazepam isn't recommended for long-term treatment because of its potential for addiction and the high serum concentrations required to control seizures.
- I.V. lorazepam is currently considered the benzodiazepine of choice for status epilepticus.
- I.V. diazepam is used to control status epilepticus. Because diazepam provides only short-term effects of less than 1 hour, the patient must also be given a long-acting anticonvulsant, such as phenytoin or phenobarbital, during diazepam therapy.
- Diazepam rectal gel is approved for the treatment of repetitive seizures and has reduced the incidence of recurrent seizures in children.

Drug interactions

When benzodiazepines are taken with CNS depressants, sedative and other depressant effects become enhanced. This can cause motor skill impairment, respiratory depression, and even death at high doses.

Cimetidine and hormonal contraceptives, taken with a benzodiazepine drug, can also cause excessive sedation and CNS depression.

Adverse reactions

The most common adverse reactions to benzodiazepines include:

- drowsiness
- confusion
- ataxia
- weakness
- dizziness
- nystagmus
- vertigo
- fainting
- dysarthria
- headache
- tremor
- glassy-eyed appearance.

These are the most common adverse reactions to benzodiazepines.

Around the less common bend

Less common adverse reactions include respiratory depression and decreased heart rate (with high doses and with I.V. diazepam) as well as rash and acute hypersensitivity reactions.

Nursing process

These nursing process steps are appropriate for patients undergoing treatment with benzodiazepine anticonvulsant drugs.

Assessment

- Obtain a history of the patient's underlying condition before therapy and reassess regularly thereafter.
- Monitor the patient's respiratory rate every 5 to 15 minutes and before each repeated I.V. dose.
- Periodically monitor liver, kidney, and haematopoietic function studies in a patient receiving repeated or prolonged therapy.
- Monitor the patient's response to prescribed drug and serum levels, as indicated.
- Monitor the patient for adverse reactions.
- Assess the patient's compliance with therapy at each follow-up visit.

Key nursing diagnoses

- Risk for injury related to adverse reactions.
- Impaired physical mobility related to sedation.
- Noncompliance related to long-term therapy.

Planning outcome goals
- Risk of injury to the patient will be minimised.
- The patient will be able to perform ADLs.
- The patient and family will confirm an understanding of drug therapy.

Implementation
- Administer oral forms of the drug with food to reduce GI irritation. If an oral concentrate solution is used, dilute the dose immediately before administering. Use water, juice, carbonated drinks, or mix with semisolid foods.
- Avoid use of diazepam rectal gel for more than five episodes per month or one episode every 5 days.
- If giving the I.V. form of diazepam, administer no more than 5 mg/minute and inject directly into a vein or watch the insertion site closely.
- Have emergency resuscitation equipment and oxygen at the bedside when giving these drugs I.V.
- Use I.M. forms only when the I.V. and oral routes aren't applicable; I.M. forms aren't recommended because absorption is variable and injection is painful.
- Don't store parenteral diazepam solutions in plastic syringes.
- Expect to adjust the dosage according to the patient's response.
- Administer safety precautions if the patient has adverse CNS reactions.

Evaluation
- Patient sustains no trauma from adverse reactions.
- Patient maintains physical mobility.
- Patient complies with therapy and has no seizures.

Carboxylic acid derivatives

The drugs in this class are:
- valproate
- valproic acid.

Pharmacokinetics
Valproic acid is converted rapidly to valproic acid in the stomach. Valproic acid is a hepatic enzyme inhibitor. It's absorbed well, strongly protein bound, and metabolised in the liver. Metabolites and unchanged drug are excreted in urine.

Valproic acid readily crosses the placental barrier and also appears in breast milk.

Keep in mind that valproic acid crosses the placental barrier and appears in breast milk.

Pharmacodynamics

The mechanism of action for valproic acid remains unknown. It's thought to increase levels of GABA, an inhibitory neurotransmitter, as well as having a direct-membrane stabilising effect. (See *Happy accident*.)

Pharmacotherapeutics

Valproic acid is prescribed for long-term treatment of:
- absence seizures
- myoclonic seizures
- tonic-clonic seizures
- partial seizures.

Baby blues

Valproic acid may also be useful for neonatal seizures. However, it must be used cautiously in children younger than 2 years old, particularly those receiving multiple anticonvulsants, those with congenital metabolic disorders or hepatic disease, those with severe seizures and mental retardation, and those with organic brain disease. For these patients, the drug carries a risk of potentially fatal liver toxicity (usually within the first 6 months of treatment). This risk limits the use of valproic acid as a drug of choice for seizure disorders.

Drug interactions

Here are the most significant drug interactions associated with valproic acid:
- Cimetidine, aspirin, and erythromycin may increase levels of valproic acid.
- Carbamazepine, lamotrigine, phenobarbital, primidone, and phenytoin, may decrease levels of valproic acid.
- Valproic acid may decrease the effects of lamotrigine, phenobarbital, primidone, benzodiazepines, CNS depressants, warfarin, and zidovudine.

Adverse reactions

Rare, but deadly, liver toxicity has occurred with valproic acid use. The drug should be used with caution in the patient who has a history of liver disease. Paediatric patients younger than 2 years old are at considerable risk for developing hepatotoxicity. Most other

Pharm function

Happy accident

The anticonvulsant properties of valproic acid were actually discovered when it was being used as a vehicle for other compounds being tested for anticonvulsant properties. Structurally, valproic acid is unlike other anticonvulsants. Its mechanism of action isn't completely understood.

The use of valproic acid for seizures in children aged 2 and younger should be limited due to the risk of potentially fatal liver toxicity.

adverse reactions to valproic acid are tolerable and dose-related. These include:

* nausea and vomiting
* diarrhoea or constipation
* sedation
* dizziness
* ataxia
* headache
* muscle weakness
* increased blood ammonia.

Nursing process

These nursing process steps are appropriate for patients undergoing treatment with carboxylic acid derivative anticonvulsant drugs.

Assessment
* Assess the patient's condition before therapy and regularly thereafter.
* Monitor the level of the drug in the blood (therapeutic level is 50 to 100 mcg/ml).
* Monitor liver function studies, platelet counts, and prothrombin time before starting the drug and periodically thereafter.
* Monitor the patient's response to the drug, especially for adverse reactions.
* Be aware that the drug may produce false-positive test results for ketones in urine.
* Assess the patient's compliance with therapy at each follow-up visit.

Key nursing diagnoses
* Risk for injury related to adverse reactions.
* Impaired physical mobility related to sedation.
* Noncompliance related to long-term therapy.

Planning outcome goals
* The risk of injury to the patient will be minimised.
* The patient will be able to perform ADLs.
* The patient and family will confirm an understanding of drug therapy.

Implementation
* Administer oral forms of the drug with food to reduce GI irritation. Don't give the syrup form to a patient who needs sodium restriction. Check with the prescriber.

Reducing the patient's risk of injury is an important planning goal.

- Dilute the drug with at least 50 ml of a compatible diluent (glucose 5% in water, saline solution, Ringer-Lactate solution) if injecting I.V. and give over 1 hour. Don't exceed 20 mg/minute.
- Avoid sudden withdrawal, which may worsen seizures.
- Expect to adjust the dosage according to the patient's response. In elderly patients, a reduced starting dose is suggested, with slower dosage increases.
- Administer safety precautions if the patient has adverse CNS reactions to the drug.
- Monitor closely for hepatotoxicity because it may follow nonspecific symptoms, such as malaise, fever, and lethargy.

Evaluation
- Patient sustains no injury from adverse reactions.
- Patient maintains physical mobility.
- Patient complies with therapy and has no seizures.

1 (aminomethyl) cyclohexane acetic acid

The 1 (aminomethyl) cyclohexane acetic acid drug class includes the drug gabapentin. This drug was designed to be a GABA agonist, but its exact mechanism of action is unknown. It's approved as adjunctive therapy for partial seizures in adults with epilepsy and in children aged 3 and older. Gabapentin has also been used for the treatment of pain, tremors associated with MS, bipolar disorder, migraine prophylaxis, and Parkinson's disease.

Pharmacokinetics
Gabapentin is readily absorbed in the GI tract. Bioavailability isn't dose-proportional; as the dose increases, the bioavailability decreases. Gabapentin isn't metabolised and is excreted exclusively by the kidneys. The patient with renal impairment requires dosage reduction.

Pharmacodynamics
The exact mechanism of action of gabapentin isn't known. Originally designed as a GABA agonist, it doesn't appear to act at the GABA receptor, affect GABA uptake, or interfere with GABA transaminase. Rather, gabapentin appears to bind to a carrier protein and act as a unique receptor, resulting in elevated GABA in the brain.

Pharmacotherapeutics

Gabapentin is used as adjunctive therapy in adults and children aged 3 and older with partial and secondarily generalised seizures. Like carbamazepine, gabapentin may worsen myoclonic seizures.

Drug interactions

Antacids and cimetidine may affect gabapentin concentration.

Adverse reactions

Adverse reactions to gabapentin commonly include:

- fatigue
- somnolence
- dizziness
- ataxia
- leucopenia.

Not so common

Some less common reactions include:

- oedema
- weight gain
- hostility
- emotional lability
- nausea and vomiting
- bronchitis
- viral infection
- fever
- nystagmus
- rhinitis
- diplopia
- tremor.

Nursing process

These nursing process steps are appropriate for patients undergoing treatment with 1 (aminomethyl) cyclohexane acetic acid anticonvulsant drugs.

Assessment

- Assess the patient's disorder before therapy and regularly thereafter.
- Monitor the patient's serum levels and response to the prescribed drug, as indicated.
- Monitor the patient for adverse reactions.
- Assess the patient's compliance with therapy at each follow-up visit.

If your patient is seeing two of you, they may be experiencing diplopia as an adverse reaction to gabapentin.

Key nursing diagnoses
- Risk for injury related to adverse reactions.
- Impaired physical mobility related to sedation.
- Noncompliance related to long-term therapy.

Planning outcome goals
- The risk to the patient will be minimised.
- The patient will be able to perform ADLs.
- The patient and family will confirm an understanding of drug therapy.

Implementation
- Administer oral forms of the drug with food to reduce GI irritation.
- Expect to adjust the drug dosage according to the patient's response.
- Administer safety precautions if the patient has adverse CNS reactions to the drug. Administer the first dose at bedtime to minimise drowsiness, dizziness, fatigue, and ataxia.
- Withdraw the drug gradually over 1 week to minimise seizure risk. Don't suddenly withdraw other anticonvulsants in the patient starting gabapentin therapy.

Evaluation
- Patient sustains no injury from adverse reactions.
- Patient maintains physical mobility.
- Patient complies with therapy and has no seizures.

Phenyltriazine

Lamotrigine belongs to the phenyltriazine drug class and is chemically unrelated to other anticonvulsants. It is approved for adjunctive therapy in adults with partial seizures and in children older than aged 2 with generalised seizures or Lennox-Gastaut syndrome.

Pharmacokinetics

Lamotrigine is well absorbed by the body at a rapid rate. It's metabolised by the liver and excreted by the kidneys. Clearance increases in the presence of other enzyme-inducing anticonvulsant drugs. The drug isn't significantly bound to plasma proteins.

Pharmacodynamics

The precise mechanism of action of lamotrigine is unknown, but is thought to involve a use-dependent blocking effect on sodium channels, resulting in inhibition of the release of excitatory neurotransmitters, glutamate, and aspartate.

Pharmacotherapeutics

Lamotrigine is approved for adjunctive therapy in adults and children older than aged 2 with generalised seizures or Lennox-Gastaut syndrome. It may also be used for conversion to monotherapy in adults. Lamotrigine appears effective for many types of generalised seizures, but can worsen myoclonic seizures. Lamotrigine may also lead to improvement in the patient's mood.

Drug interactions

- Carbamazepine, phenytoin, phenobarbital, primidone, and paracetamol may result in decreased lamotrigine effects.
- Valproic acid may decrease the clearance of lamotrigine and the steady-state level of lamotrigine.
- Lamotrigine may produce additive effects when combined with folate inhibitors.

Adverse reactions

Adverse reactions to lamotrigine commonly include:
- dizziness
- ataxia
- somnolence
- headache
- diplopia
- nausea
- vomiting
- rash.

Don't be rash

Several types of rash may occur with lamotrigine use, including Stevens-Johnson syndrome. This generalised, erythematous, morbilliform rash usually appears in the first 3 to 4 weeks of therapy and is usually mild to moderate, but may be severe. Patients should be warned to contact their prescriber immediately if rash or signs or symptoms of hypersensitivity syndrome develop. The risk of rash may be increased by starting at high doses, by rapidly increasing doses, or using with valproic acid.

Discontinue lamotrigine at the first sight of a rash.

Nursing process

These nursing process steps are appropriate for patients undergoing treatment with phenyltriazine anticonvulsant drugs.

Assessment
- Obtain a history of the patient's seizure disorder before therapy.
- Evaluate the patient for reduction in seizure frequency and duration after therapy begins. Check the adjunct anticonvulsant's level periodically.
- Monitor the patient's serum levels and response to the prescribed drug, as indicated.
- Monitor the patient for adverse reactions.
- Assess the patient's compliance with therapy at each follow-up visit.

Key nursing diagnoses
- Risk for injury related to adverse reactions.
- Impaired physical mobility related to sedation.
- Noncompliance related to long-term therapy.

Planning outcome goals
- Risk to the patient will be minimised.
- The patient will be able to perform ADLs.
- The patient and family will confirm an understanding of therapy.

Implementation
- Administer oral forms of the drug with food to reduce GI irritation.
- The dosage should be lowered if the drug is added to a multidrug regimen that includes valproic acid.
- A lowered maintenance dosage should be used in a patient with severe renal impairment.
- Don't stop the drug abruptly. Abrupt withdrawal increases the risk of seizures. Instead, drug withdrawal should be tapered over at least 2 weeks.
- A rash may be life threatening. Stop the drug and notify the prescriber at the first sign of a rash.
- Administer safety precautions if the patient has adverse CNS reactions.

Evaluation
- Patient sustains no injury from adverse reactions.
- Patient maintains physical mobility.
- Patient complies with therapy and has no seizures.

Carboxamide

Oxcarbazepine, a carboxamide, is chemically similar to carbamazepine, but causes less induction of liver enzymes. Oxcarbazepine is useful as adjunctive therapy or monotherapy in adults for partial seizures and in children as adjunctive therapy for partial seizures.

Pharmacokinetics

Oxcarbazepine is completely absorbed and extensively metabolised via liver enzymes to the 10-monohydroxy metabolite (MHD) that's responsible for its pharmacologic activity. It's excreted primarily by the kidneys. The half-life of MHD is about 9 hours. Unlike carbamazepine, oxcarbazepine doesn't induce its own metabolism.

Pharmacodynamics

The precise mechanism of oxcarbazepine and MHD is unknown, but antiseizure activity is thought to occur through blockade of sodium-sensitive channels, which prevents seizure spread in the brain.

Pharmacotherapeutics

Oxcarbazepine is approved for adjunctive therapy of partial seizures in adults and children older than aged 6, and as monotherapy in adults. As with carbamazepine, it's also effective for generalised seizures, but may worsen myoclonic and absence seizures.

Drug interactions

Carbamazepine, phenytoin, phenobarbital, valproic acid, and verapamil may decrease the levels of active MHD. Oxcarbazepine may decrease the effectiveness of hormonal contraceptives and felodipine. Reduced dosages are necessary in the patient with renal impairment (clearance less than 30 ml/minute) and in the patient at risk for renal impairment (such as an elderly patient).

Adverse reactions

Adverse reactions to oxcarbazepine commonly include:
- somnolence
- dizziness
- diplopia
- ataxia

Quiz the patient about a history of hypersensitivity to carbamazepine.

- nausea
- vomiting
- abnormal gait
- tremor
- aggravated seizures
- abdominal pain.
  Some less common reactions include:
- agitation
- confusion
- hypotension
- hyponatraemia
- rhinitis
- speech disorder
- back pain
- upper respiratory tract infection.
  About 20% to 30% of patients who have had an allergic reaction to carbamazepine will experience a hypersensitivity reaction to oxcarbazepine.

Nursing process

These nursing process steps are appropriate for patients undergoing treatment with carboxamide anticonvulsant drugs.

Assessment

- Question the patient about a history of hypersensitivity reactions to carbamazepine (25% to 30% of affected patients may develop hypersensitivity to oxcarbazepine).
- Obtain a history of the patient's underlying condition before therapy, and reassess it regularly thereafter.
- Monitor the patient's serum levels and response to the prescribed drug, as indicated.
- Monitor the patient for adverse reactions.
- Assess the patient's compliance with therapy at each follow-up visit.

Key nursing diagnoses

- Risk for injury related to adverse reactions.
- Impaired physical mobility related to sedation.
- Noncompliance related to long-term therapy.

Planning outcome goals

- Risk to the patient will be minimised.
- The patient will be able to perform ADLs.
- The patient and family will confirm an understanding of drug therapy.

Implementation
- Withdraw the drug gradually to minimise the risk of increased seizure frequency.
- Correct hyponatraemia, as needed.
- For an oral suspension, shake well before administration. It can be mixed with water or may be swallowed directly from the syringe. It can be taken without regard to food. Oral suspensions and tablets may be interchanged at equal doses.
- Expect to adjust the dosage according to the patient's response.
- Administer safety precautions if the patient has adverse CNS reactions.

Evaluation
- Patient sustains no injury from adverse reactions.
- Patient maintains physical mobility.
- Patient complies with therapy and has no seizures.

Sulfamate-substituted monosaccharides

Sulfamate-substituted monosaccharide is structurally distinct from other anticonvulsant drug classes. The effect is to block the spread of seizures rather than to raise the threshold (like other anticonvulsant drugs). This class of drugs is derived from the natural monosaccharide D-fructose. Topiramate is a newer anticonvulsant drug in this class.

Pharmacokinetics
Topiramate is rapidly absorbed by the body. It's partially metabolised in the liver and excreted mostly unchanged in urine. For the patient with renal impairment (creatinine clearance less than 70 ml/minute), the dosage of topiramate is reduced.

Pharmacodynamics
Topiramate is believed to act by blocking voltage-dependent sodium channels, enhancing the activity of GABA receptors and antagonising glutamate receptors.

Pharmacotherapeutics
Topiramate is approved as adjunctive therapy for partial and primary generalised tonic-clonic seizures in adults and children older than aged 2 and for children with Lennox-Gastaut syndrome. It may also prove beneficial for other types of seizures and as monotherapy.

Drug interactions

Carbamazepine, phenytoin, and valproic acid may cause decreased topiramate levels. Topiramate may decrease the efficacy of hormonal contraceptives and may decrease valproic acid levels. CNS depressants may be potentiated when combined with topiramate.

Adverse reactions

Psychomotor slowing, difficulty finding words, impaired concentration, and memory impairment are common and may require stopping the drug. Low starting doses and slow titration may minimise these effects.

Other common adverse reactions to topiramate include:

- drowsiness
- dizziness
- headache
- ataxia
- nervousness
- confusion
- paraesthesia
- weight gain
- diplopia.

Serious but uncommon adverse reactions include:

- secondary angle-closure glaucoma
- liver failure
- hypohidrosis
- hyperthermia
- heat stroke
- renal calculi.

Nursing process

These nursing process steps are appropriate for patients undergoing treatment with sulfamate-substituted monosaccharide anticonvulsant drugs.

Assessment

- Assess the patient's seizure disorder before therapy and regularly thereafter.
- Carefully monitor the patient taking topiramate in conjunction with other antiepileptic drugs; dosage adjustments may be needed to achieve an optimal response.
- Monitor the patient's serum levels and response to the prescribed drug, as indicated.
- Monitor the patient for adverse reactions.
- Assess the patient's compliance with therapy at each follow-up visit.

Key nursing diagnoses
- Risk for injury related to adverse reactions.
- Impaired physical mobility related to sedation.
- Noncompliance related to long-term therapy.

Planning outcome goals
- Risk to the patient will be minimised.
- The patient will be able to perform ADLs.
- The patient and family will confirm an understanding of drug therapy.

Implementation
- Administer oral forms of the drug with food to reduce GI irritation.
- Expect to adjust the dosage according to the patient's response.
- Administer safety precautions if the patient has adverse CNS reactions.
- The patient with renal insufficiency requires reduced doses. For the patient on haemodialysis, supplemental doses may be needed to avoid rapid drops in drug levels during prolonged treatment.
- Discontinue the drug if an ocular adverse event occurs, characterised by acute myopia and secondary angle-closure glaucoma.

Evaluation
- Patient sustains no injury from adverse reactions.
- Patient maintains physical mobility.
- Patient complies with therapy and has no seizures.

Succinimides

The succinimide, ethosuximide, is used for the management of absence seizures and is considered the drug of choice for this indication.

Pharmacokinetics
The succinimides are readily absorbed from the GI tract, metabolised in the liver, and excreted in urine. Metabolites are believed to be inactive. The elimination half-life of ethosuximide is about 60 hours in adults and 30 hours in children.

Ethosuximide is considered the drug of choice for absence seizures.

Pharmacodynamics

Ethosuximide raises the seizure threshold; it suppresses the characteristic spike-and-wave pattern by depressing neuronal transmission in the motor cortex and basal ganglia. It's indicated for absence seizures.

Pharmacotherapeutics

The only indication for ethosuximide is the treatment of absence seizures. It's the treatment of choice for this type of seizure disorder, but may be used in combination with valproic acid for difficult-to-control absence seizures.

Drug interactions

Ethosuximide may interact with concurrently administered anticonvulsant drugs. Carbamazepine may induce the metabolism of ethosuximide. Valproic acid may increase or decrease levels of ethosuximide. It can elevate serum phenytoin levels.

Adverse reactions

Ethosuximide is generally well tolerated and causes few adverse reactions. The most common effects include anorexia, nausea, and vomiting (in up to 40% of cases). Other common adverse effects include:
- drowsiness and fatigue
- lethargy
- dizziness
- hiccups
- headaches
- mood changes.

Rarely, blood dyscrasias, rashes (including Stevens-Johnson syndrome and erythema multiforme, lupuslike syndrome), and psychotic behavior can occur.

Nursing process

These nursing process steps are appropriate for patients undergoing treatment with succinimide anticonvulsant drugs.

Assessment

- Monitor the patient's serum levels and response to the prescribed drug, as indicated.
- Monitor the patient for adverse reactions.
- Assess the patient's compliance with therapy at each follow-up visit.

Key nursing diagnoses
- Risk for injury related to adverse reactions.
- Impaired physical mobility related to sedation.
- Noncompliance related to long-term therapy.

Planning outcome goals
- The risk to the patient will be minimised.
- The patient will be able to perform ADLs.
- The patient and family will confirm an understanding of drug therapy.

Implementation
- Administer oral drug forms with food to reduce GI irritation.
- Expect to adjust the dosage according to the patient's response.
- Administer safety precautions if the patient has adverse CNS reactions.

Evaluation
- Patient sustains no injury from adverse reactions.
- Patient maintains physical mobility.
- Patient complies with therapy and has no seizures.

Sulphonamides

Sulphonamides are a group of compounds consisting of amides of sulphanilic acid. They're known for their bacteriostatic effects; they interfere with the functioning of the enzyme necessary for bacteria metabolism, growth, and multiplication. Zonisamide, a sulphonamide, is approved for the adjunctive treatment of partial seizure in adults.

Pharmacokinetics
Peak concentrations of zonisamide occur within 2 to 6 hours of administration. The drug is widely distributed and is extensively bound to erythrocytes. Zonisamide is metabolised by the CYP3A4 enzyme in the liver and is excreted in urine, primarily as the parent drug and the glucuronide metabolite. Low doses should be initiated in elderly patients due to the possibility of renal impairment.

Pharmacodynamics
The precise mechanism of zonisamide is unknown, but it's believed to involve stabilisation of neuronal membranes and suppression of neuronal hypersensitivity.

Pharmacotherapeutics

Zonisamide is approved only as adjunctive therapy for partial seizures in adults. Despite its limited indication, it has demonstrated usefulness in other types of seizure activity (infantile spasms and myoclonic, generalised, and atypical absence seizures).

Drug interactions

Drugs that induce liver enzymes (such as phenytoin, carbamazepine, or phenobarbital) increase the metabolism and decrease the half-life of zonisamide. Concurrent use of zonisamide with drugs that inhibit or induce CYP3A4 can be expected to increase or decrease the serum concentration of zonisamide. Zonisamide isn't an inducer of CYP3A4, so it's unlikely to affect other drugs metabolised by the CYP3A4 system.

Adverse reactions

Common adverse reactions to zonisamide include:
- somnolence
- dizziness
- confusion
- anorexia
- nausea
- diarrhoea
- weight loss
- rash.

Slow she goes

Slow titration of the dosage and administration with meals may decrease the incidence of adverse reactions.

Serious sides

More serious adverse reactions that have been associated with zonisamide include:
- Stevens-Johnson syndrome
- toxic epidermal necrolysis
- psychosis
- aplastic anaemia
- agranulocytosis
- oligohidrosis, hyperthermia, and heatstroke (in children).
  Zonisamide is contraindicated in patients with allergies to sulphonamides. Zonisamide requires effective contraception during and for 4 weeks after treatment, if there is a risk of pregnancy occurring; its disposition in breast milk is unknown. The safety and

effectiveness of the drug in children younger than aged 16 hasn't been established. The use of zonisamide in patients with renal clearances of less than 50 ml/minute isn't recommended.

Nursing process

These nursing process steps are appropriate for patients undergoing treatment with sulphonamide anticonvulsant drugs.

Assessment
- Obtain a history of the patient's underlying condition before therapy and reassess it regularly thereafter.
- Monitor the patient's body temperature, especially during the summer, because decreased sweating may occur (especially in children aged 17 and younger), resulting in heat stroke and dehydration.
- Monitor the patient's renal function periodically.
- Monitor the patient's serum levels and response to the prescribed drug, as indicated.
- Monitor the patient for hypersensitivity or adverse reactions.
- Assess the patient's compliance with therapy at each follow-up visit.

Key nursing diagnoses
- Risk for injury related to adverse reactions.
- Impaired physical mobility related to sedation.
- Noncompliance related to long-term therapy.

Planning outcome goals
- Risk to the patient will be minimised.
- The patient will be able to perform ADLs.
- The patient and family will confirm an understanding of drug therapy.

Implementation
- The drug may be taken with or without food. Don't bite or break the capsule.
- Use cautiously in the patient with hepatic or renal disease; slower adjustments and more frequent monitoring may be required. If the glomerular filtration rate is less than 50 ml/minute, don't use the drug.

The safety and effectiveness of zonisamide in children younger than aged 16 hasn't been established.

• Reduce doses or discontinue the drug gradually; abrupt withdrawal of the drug may cause increased frequency of seizures or status epilepticus.
• Increase the patient's fluid intake and urine output to help prevent renal calculi, especially if predisposing factors are present.
• Expect to adjust the drug dosage according to the patient's response.
• Administer safety precautions if the patient has adverse CNS reactions.

Evaluation
• Patient sustains no injury from adverse reactions.
• Patient maintains physical mobility.
• Patient complies with therapy and has no seizures.

Antimigraine drugs

A migraine, an episodic headache disorder, is one of the most common primary headache disorders, affecting an estimated 15 percent of the UK adult population. A migraine is usually described as a unilateral headache pain that's pounding, pulsating, or throbbing. It may be preceded by an aura. Other symptoms typically associated with a migraine are sensitivity to light or sound, nausea, vomiting, and constipation or diarrhoea.

Current theories suggest that the symptoms of migraines are due to vasodilation or to the release of vasoactive and proinflammatory substances from nerves in an activated trigeminal system.

So many choices

Treatment for migraines is targeted at altering an attack after it's under way (abortive and symptomatic treatment) or preventing the attack before it begins. The choice of therapy depends upon the severity, duration, frequency, and degree of disability the headache creates, as well as the patient's characteristics. Abortive treatments may include analgesics (aspirin and paracetamol), nonsteroidal anti-inflammatory drugs (NSAIDs), ergotamine, 5-HT agonists, and other miscellaneous agents (such as isometheptene combinations, metoclopramide, and corticosteroids). Prophylactic therapy includes beta-adrenergic blockers, tricyclic antidepressants, valproic acid, and NSAIDs, amongst others.

Memory jogger

How can you tell if it's a migraine or a headache? Look at the **PAIN** to see if the patient has these key symptoms:

Pain

Aura

Irritated by light

Nausea.

5-HT agonists

The 5-HT agonists, commonly known as the *triptans*, are the treatment of choice for moderate to severe migraine. Drugs in this class include:

- almotriptan
- eletriptan
- frovatriptan
- naratriptan
- rizatriptan
- sumatriptan
- zolmitriptan.

This chapter is giving me a migraine!

Pharmacokinetics

When comparing the triptans, key pharmacokinetic features are onset of effect and duration of action. Most triptans have a half-life of approximately 2 hours; almotriptan and eletriptan have half-lives of 3 to 4 hours, naratriptan has a half-life of about 6 hours, and frovatriptan has the longest half-life (25 hours) and the most delayed onset of action.

Freedom of choice

All of the triptans are available in an oral formulation. Rizatriptan is available in a rapid-dissolve tablet, and sumatriptan is also available in an injectable and intranasal formulation. The injectable form of sumatriptan has the most rapid onset of action.

Pharmacodynamics

Triptans are specific serotonin 5-HT$_1$ receptor agonists that result in cranial vessel constriction, and inhibition and reduction of the inflammatory process along the trigeminal nerve pathway. These actions may abort or provide symptomatic relief for a migraine. Triptans are effective in controlling the pain, nausea, and vomiting associated with migraines.

Pharmacotherapeutics

The choice of a triptan depends on patient preferences for dosage form (if nausea and vomiting are present), presence of recurrent migraine, and formulary restrictions. A patient experiencing nausea and vomiting may prefer injectable or intranasal sumatriptan. Recurrent migraines may respond better to triptans with longer half-lives, such as frovatriptan and naratriptan; however, these drugs have delayed onset of effects. Two newer triptans, almotriptan and eletriptan, have rapid onset and an intermediate half-life.

Pharm function

Contra-triptans

Triptans are contraindicated in patients with ischaemic heart disease (such as angina pectoris, history of myocardial infarction, or documented silent ischaemia) and in patients who have symptoms or findings consistent with ischaemic heart disease, coronary artery vaso-spasm (including Prinzmetal's variant angina), or other significant underlying cardiovascular conditions.

No strokes allowed

Triptans shouldn't be prescribed for patients with cerebrovascular syndromes (such as strokes of any type or transient ischaemic attacks) or for patients with peripheral vascular disease, including, but not limited to, ischaemic bowel disease. Triptans also shouldn't be given to patients with uncontrolled hypertension or to patients with hemiplegic or basilar migraines.

Not for the faint of heart

Triptans aren't recommended for use in the patient who has coronary artery disease (CAD) or risk factors for CAD (such as hypertension, hypercholesterolaemia, smoking, obesity, diabetes, a strong family history of CAD, or a surgically or physiologically menopausal woman, or a male over aged 40) unless a cardiovascular evaluation provides satisfactory evidence that the patient is reasonably free from underlying cardiovascular disease. If a triptan is used for a patient who has any of these risk factors, it's strongly recommended that the first dose be administered in a physician's office or other medically staffed and equipped facility.

It's further suggested that intermittent, long-term users of 5-HT agonists or those who have or acquire risk factors undergo periodic cardiac evaluation.

Triptans have many contraindications and should not be used in patients with certain conditions. (See *Contra-triptans*.)

More than 3 in 30

The safety of treating an average of more than three migraine attacks in a 30-day period hasn't been established.

Drug interactions

These drug interactions are possible when taking triptans:
• The administration of a triptan within 24 hours of treatment with another 5-HT$_1$ agonist, ergotamine-containing or ergot-type

medication, may cause prolonged vasospastic reactions. The use of ergot-containing medications and 5-HT agonists within 24 hours of each other should be avoided.

• Eletriptan shouldn't be used within at least 72 hours of treatment with the following potent CYP3A4 inhibitors: ketoconazole, itraconazole, clarithromycin, ritonavir, and nelfinavir or other drugs that have demonstrated potent CYP3A4 inhibition.

• Almotriptan, rizatriptan, sumatriptan, and zolmitriptan shouldn't be used with or within 2 weeks of discontinuing an MAO inhibitor.

• Although rare, SSRIs, such as citalopram, fluoxetine, fluvoxamine, paroxetine, and sertraline, have been reported to cause weakness, hyperreflexia, and incoordination when co-administered with 5-HT$_1$ agonists. Monitor the patient closely if concomitant treatment with a triptan and an SSRI is clinically warranted. This reaction has also been reported with co-administration of a triptan and sibutramine.

• The bioavailability of frovatriptan is 30% higher in a patient taking oral forms of hormonal contraceptives.

• Propranolol increases the bioavailability of zolmitriptan, rizatriptan, frovatriptan, and eletriptan.

Adverse reactions

Adverse reactions to triptans include:
• tingling
• warm or hot sensations or flushing
• nasal and throat discomfort
• visual disturbances
• paraesthesia
• dizziness
• weakness and fatigue
• somnolence
• chest pain or pressure
• neck or throat pain
• jaw pain or pressure
• dry mouth
• dyspepsia
• nausea
• sweating
• injection site reaction (subcutaneous sumatriptan)
• taste disturbances (intranasal sumatriptan).

The heart takes part

Serious cardiac events, including acute myocardial infarction, arrhythmias, and death, have been reported within a few hours after taking triptans. However, the incidence of these events is considered extremely low.

Nursing process

These nursing process steps are appropriate for patients undergoing treatment with triptans.

Assessment

• Assess the patient's condition before and during drug therapy. These drugs aren't intended for the patient with ischaemic heart disease or hemiplegic or basilar migraines.
• Obtain a list of the patient's medication intake within 24 hours to prevent drug interactions. Use caution when giving the drug to a patient who's taking an MAO inhibitor or a CYP-450 3A4 or 2D6 inhibitor. Don't give the drug with other serotonin agonist or ergotamine derivatives.
• Be alert for adverse reactions.
• Monitor the ECG in a patient with risk factors for coronary artery disease (CAD) or with symptoms similar to those of CAD, such as chest or throat tightness, pain, and heaviness.
• Evaluate the patient's and family's knowledge of drug therapy.

Key nursing diagnoses

• Acute pain related to the presence of an acute migraine attack.
• Risk for injury related to drug-induced interactions.
• Deficient knowledge related to drug therapy.

Planning outcome goals

• The patient will state that pain is decreased.
• Risk of injury to the patient will be reduced.
• The patient and family will confirm an understanding of drug therapy.

Implementation

• Give the dose as soon as the patient complains of migraine symptoms.
• Reduce the dosage in a patient with poor renal or hepatic function.
• Repeat the dose as prescribed and as needed, and monitor the patient for effect.
• Don't give more than two doses within 24 hours.

Education edge

Teaching about migraine drugs

If migraine drugs are prescribed, review these points with the patient and caregivers:

- Take the drug exactly as prescribed, such as only when having a migraine, and to repeat the dosage as per the prescriber's instructions. Tell the patient not to exceed the prescribed dosage.
- Avoid possible migraine triggers, such as cheese, chocolate, citrus fruits, caffeine, and alcohol.
- Don't take other medicines, over-the-counter preparations, or herbal preparations without first consulting with the prescriber. Drug interactions can occur.
- Immediately report adverse reactions (chest, throat, jaw, or neck tightness, pain, or heaviness) to the prescriber and discontinue use of the drug until further notice.
- Use caution when driving or operating machinery while taking migraine drugs.

Evaluation
- Patient's symptoms are alleviated and the patient is free from pain.
- Patient won't develop serious complications from drug interactions.
- Patient and family state an understanding of drug therapy. (See *Teaching about migraine drugs*.)

Ergotamine preparations

Ergotamine and its derivatives may be used as abortive or symptomatic therapy for migraines.

The most common preparations used for migraines include:
- ergotamine— sublingual (SL) or oral tablet or suppository (combined with caffeine)

Pharmacokinetics

Ergotamine is incompletely absorbed from the GI tract. Peak plasma concentrations, following subcutaneous injection, occur within 45 minutes, and 90% of the dose is plasma protein bound.

Ergotamine is metabolised in the liver, and 90% of the metabolites are excreted in bile; traces of unchanged drug are excreted in urine.

Pharmacodynamics

Ergotamine derivative antimigraine effects are believed to be due to a blockade of neurogenic inflammation. They also act as partial agonists or antagonists at serotonin, dopaminergic, and alpha-adrenergic receptors, depending on their site. Ergotamine preparations commonly need to be prescribed with antiemetic preparations when used for migraines.

Pharmacotherapeutics

Ergotamine preparations are used to prevent or treat vascular headaches, such as migraines, migraine variants, and cluster headaches.

Drug interactions

These drug interactions can occur in a patient taking ergotamine preparations:

• Propranolol and other beta-adrenergic blockers close the natural pathway for vasodilation in the patient receiving ergotamine preparations, resulting in excessive vasoconstriction and cold extremities.

• The patient may be at increased risk for weakness, hyperflexion, and incoordination when ergotamine preparations are used with SSRIs.

• Sumatriptan may cause an additive effect when taken with ergotamine derivatives, increasing the risk of coronary vasospasm. Don't give an ergotamine preparation within 24 hours of administering a triptan.

• Drugs inhibiting CYP3A4 enzymes (such as erythromycin, clarithromycin, ritonavir, nelfinavir, indinavir, and azole-derivative antifungal agents) may alter the metabolism of ergotamine, resulting in increased serum concentrations of ergotamine. This increases the risk of vasospasm and cerebral or peripheral ischaemia. These drugs shouldn't be used together.

• Vasoconstrictors may cause an additive effect when given with ergotamine preparations, increasing the risk of high blood pressure.

When prescribed for migraines, an ergotamine preparation is commonly accompanied by an antiemetic.

Adverse reactions

Adverse reactions to ergotamine derivatives include:

- nausea
- vomiting
- numbness
- tingling
- muscle pain
- leg weakness
- itching.

Prolonged administration of ergotamine derivatives may result in ergotism, gangrene, and rebound headaches.

Nursing process

These nursing process steps are appropriate for patients undergoing treatment with ergotamine preparations.

Assessment

- Assess the patient for coronary, cerebral, or peripheral vascular disease, hypertension, and liver or kidney disease. These are contraindications to the use of ergotamine preparations.
- Assess the patient's condition before and during drug therapy.
- Be alert for adverse reactions and drug interactions.
- Be alert for ergotamine rebound or an increase in the frequency and duration of headaches, which may occur if the drug is discontinued suddenly.
- Monitor the ECG in a patient with risk factors for CAD or with symptoms similar to those of CAD, such as chest or throat tightness, pain, and heaviness.
- Evaluate the patient's and family's knowledge of drug therapy.

Key nursing diagnoses

- Acute pain related to the presence of an acute migraine attack.
- Risk for injury related to drug-induced interactions.
- Deficient knowledge related to drug therapy.

Planning outcome goals

- The patient will acknowledge a decrease in pain.
- Risk of injury to the patient will be reduced.
- The patient and family will confirm an understanding of drug therapy.

Implementation

- Give the dose as soon as the patient complains of migraine symptoms.
- Avoid prolonged administration and don't exceed the recommended dosage.

• Don't give sublingual tablets with food or drink while tablets are dissolving. Sublingual tablets are preferred during the early stage of an attack because of their rapid absorption.
• Monitor the patient for signs of vasoconstriction and report them to the prescriber.

Evaluation

• Patient's symptoms are alleviated and they are free from pain.
• Patient won't develop serious complications from drug interactions.
• Patient and family state an understanding of drug therapy.

Quick quiz

1. A 15-year-old patient has a tonic-clonic seizure disorder and is prescribed phenytoin. Which term best describes the absorption rate of oral phenytoin?
  A. Rapid
  B. Slow
  C. Erratic
  D. Moderate

Answer: B. Phenytoin is absorbed slowly through the GI tract. It's absorbed much more rapidly when administered I.V.

2. An 11-year-old patient develops myoclonic seizures. Which potential adverse reaction makes it unlikely that valproic acid will be prescribed for this patient?
  A. Liver toxicity
  B. CNS sedation
  C. Respiratory depression
  D. Hyperthermia

Answer: A. When administered to children and patients taking other anticonvulsants, valproic acid carries a risk of potentially fatal liver toxicity.

3. Anticonvulsants fall into several major classes, including:
  A. anticholinergics.
  B. quinolones.
  C. succinimides.
  D. dopaminergics.

Answer: C. The major classes of anticonvulsants are succinimides, hydantoins, barbiturates, benzodiazepines, and sulphonamides.

4. A 48-year-old patient has been prescribed trihexyphenidyl for her Parkinson's disease. Which adverse reaction to this drug can be dose-related?

    A. Excessive salivation
    B. Dryness of mouth
    C. Bradycardia
    D. Constipation

Answer: B. Dry mouth may be a dose-related adverse effect of trihexyphenidyl therapy.

5. Which antiparkinsonian drug is associated with the on-off phenomenon and the wearing-off effect?

    A. Amantadine
    B. Benzatropine
    C. Levodopa
    D. Pramipexole

Answer: C. Levodopa is associated with the on-off phenomenon (sharp fluctuations in symptoms) and wearing-off effect (shorter duration of the drug's effect) in patients taking the drug for many years. For this reason, some prescribers believe the drug should be given in lower doses or started later in the course of the disorder.

6. The effectiveness of levodopa can be reduced when taking:

    A. pyridoxine.
    B. amantadine.
    C. bromocriptine.
    D. pramipexole.

Answer: A. Levodopa's effectiveness can be reduced when taking pyridoxine (vitamin B_{12}), phenytoin, benzodiazepines, and papaverine.

7. Barbiturate anticonvulsants are effective in treating all of these seizure types, except:

    A. partial seizures.
    B. tonic-clonic seizures.
    C. febrile seizures.
    D. absence seizures.

Answer: D. Barbiturate anticonvulsants are effective in treating partial, tonic-clonic, and febrile seizures. They're an ineffective treatment for absence seizures.

Scoring

☆☆☆ If you answered all seven questions correctly, marvellous! Your knowledge has a rapid onset and long duration.

☆☆ If you answered five or six questions correctly, congratulations! You obviously answered these questions about neurologic drugs logically.

☆ If you answered fewer than five questions correctly, don't worry. Just give yourself another dose of this chapter and recheck the results.

4 Pain medications

Just the facts

In this chapter, you'll learn:

♦ classes of drugs used to control pain

♦ uses and actions of these drugs

♦ absorption, distribution, metabolism, and excretion of these drugs

♦ drug interactions and adverse reactions to these drugs.

Drugs and pain control

Drugs used to control pain range from mild, over-the-counter (OTC) preparations, such as paracetamol, to potent general anaesthetics. Drug classes in this category include:
- nonopioid analgesics, antipyretics, and nonsteroidal anti-inflammatory drugs (NSAIDs)
- opioid agonist and antagonist drugs
- anaesthetic drugs.

Nonopioid analgesics, antipyretics, and NSAIDs

Nonopioid analgesics, antipyretics, and NSAIDs are a broad group of pain medications. In addition to pain control, they also produce antipyretic (fever control) and anti-inflammatory effects. They can be used alone or as adjuvant medications. These drugs have a ceiling effect (where an increasing dose has a progressively smaller incremental response) and no physical dependence is associated with them.

The drug classes included in this group are:
• salicylates (especially aspirin), which are widely used
• the para-aminophenol derivative paracetamol
• NSAIDs.

Salicylates

Salicylates are among the most commonly used pain medications. They're used to control pain and reduce fever and inflammation.

Cheap, easy, and reliable

Salicylates usually cost less than other analgesics and are readily available without a prescription. Aspirin is the most commonly used salicylate for anti-inflammatory drug therapy.

Other salicylates include:
• choline salicylate
• diflunisal

We're the number one salicylate for reducing inflammation in adults.

Pharmacokinetics

Taken orally, salicylates are partially absorbed in the stomach, but are primarily absorbed in the upper part of the small intestine. The pure and buffered forms of aspirin reabsorb readily, but for sustained-release and enteric-coated salicylate preparations, food or antacids in the stomach delay absorption. Salicylates given rectally have a slower, more erratic absorption. Enteric-coated products are slowly absorbed and not suitable for acute effects. They cause less GI bleeding and may be better suited for long-term therapy such as for arthritis. Absorption after rectal administration is slow and variable, depending on how long the suppository is retained.

Excellent distribution

Salicylates are distributed widely throughout body tissues and fluids, including breast milk. In addition, they easily cross the placenta. The liver metabolises salicylates extensively into several metabolites. The kidneys excrete the metabolites and some unchanged drug.

I'm great at metabolising salicylates into metabolites!

Pharmacodynamics

The different effects of salicylates stem from their separate mechanisms of action. They relieve pain primarily by inhibiting the synthesis of prostaglandin. (Recall that prostaglandin is a chemical mediator that sensitises nerve cells to pain.) In addition, they may reduce inflammation by inhibiting prostaglandin synthesis and release that occurs during inflammation.

Increase sweating, reduce temperature

Salicylates reduce fever by stimulating the hypothalamus, and producing peripheral blood vessel dilation and increased sweating. This promotes heat loss through the skin and cooling by evaporation. Also, because prostaglandin E increases body temperature, inhibiting its production lowers a fever.

Bonus effect

One salicylate, aspirin, inhibits platelet aggregation (the clumping of platelets to form a clot) permanently by interfering with the production of thromboxane A_2, a substance necessary for platelet aggregation. Unlike aspirin, NSAIDs' effects on platelet aggregation are temporary. As a result, aspirin can be used to enhance blood flow during myocardial infarction (MI) and to prevent an event such as recurrent MI.

Pharmacotherapeutics

Salicylates are primarily used to relieve pain and reduce fever. However, they don't effectively relieve visceral pain (pain from the organs and smooth muscle) or severe pain from trauma. They can also be used to reduce an elevated body temperature in conjunction with relieving headache and muscle ache. When used to reduce inflammation in rheumatic fever, rheumatoid arthritis, and osteoarthritis, salicylates can provide considerable relief within 24 hours.

How low can you go?

No matter what the clinical indication, the main guideline of salicylate therapy is to use the lowest dose that provides relief. This reduces the likelihood of adverse reactions. (See *Salicylate warning*.)

Drug interactions

Because salicylates are highly protein bound, they can interact with many other protein-bound drugs by displacing those drugs from sites to which they normally bind. This increases the serum concentration of the unbound active drug, causing increased pharmacologic effects (the unbound drug is said to be *potentiated*). For example, these drug interactions may occur:
• Oral anticoagulants, heparin, methotrexate, oral antidiabetic agents, and insulin are among the drugs that have increased effects or risk of toxicity when taken with salicylates.

Before you give that drug!

Salicylate warning

Before administering salicylates to a patient, be aware of its risks to special populations:

• *Children and teenagers:* Avoid the use of aspirin and salicylates to treat flulike symptoms or chickenpox because Reye's syndrome may develop.
• *Surgical patients:* If possible, discontinue aspirin 1 week before surgery because of the risk of postoperative bleeding.
• *Asthmatics:* Be aware that these patients are more likely to develop bronchospasm, urticaria, angioedema, or shock when salicylates are administered.

- Probenecid, sulfinpyrazone, and spironolactone may have decreased effects when taken with salicylates.
- Corticosteroids may decrease plasma salicylate levels and increase the risk of ulcers.
- Alkalinising drugs and antacids may reduce salicylate levels.
- The antihypertensive effects of angiotensin-converting enzyme (ACE) inhibitors and beta-adrenergic blockers (commonly called *beta blockers*) may be reduced when these drugs are taken concomitantly with salicylates.
- NSAIDs may have reduced therapeutic effects and an increased risk of GI effects when taken with salicylates.

Adverse reactions

The most common adverse reactions to salicylates include gastric distress, nausea, vomiting, and bleeding tendencies. (Choline magnesium is a salicylate that doesn't increase bleeding time.) Other adverse reactions include:
- hearing loss (when taken for prolonged periods)
- diarrhoea
- thirst
- sweating
- tinnitus
- confusion
- dizziness
- impaired vision
- hyperventilation (rapid breathing)
- Reye's syndrome (when given to children with chickenpox or flulike symptoms).

Nursing process

These nursing process steps are appropriate for patients undergoing treatment with salicylates.

Assessment

- Assess the patient's level of pain and inflammation before therapy begins and evaluate drug effectiveness after administration.
- Monitor the patient for signs and symptoms of bleeding. Assess bleeding time if scheduled to undergo surgery.
- Monitor the patient's ophthalmic and auditory function before drug therapy and periodically thereafter to detect toxicity.
- Periodically monitor CBC, platelet count, prothrombin time (PT), and hepatic and renal function to detect abnormalities.

- Be alert for adverse reactions and drug interactions. Watch for bronchospasm in the patient with aspirin hypersensitivity, rhinitis or nasal polyps, or asthma.
- During long-term therapy, monitor serum salicylate levels. A therapeutic level in a patient with arthritis is 10 to 30 mg/dl.
- Evaluate the patient's and family's knowledge of drug therapy.

Key nursing diagnoses
- Acute pain related to the underlying process.
- Risk for injury related to adverse reactions.
- Deficient knowledge related to drug therapy.

Planning outcome goals
- The patient will acknowledge a reduction in pain.
- No serious complications will occur while the patient is on drug therapy.
- The patient and family will demonstrate an understanding of the purpose and intended effect of drug therapy.

Implementation
- Give aspirin with food, milk, antacids, or a large glass of water to reduce GI reactions.
- If the patient has trouble swallowing the drug, crush tablets or mix them with food or fluid. Don't crush enteric-coated aspirin.
- Hold the dose and notify the prescriber if bleeding, salicylism (salicylate poisoning, characterised by tinnitus or hearing loss), or adverse GI reactions occur.
- Stop aspirin 5 to 7 days before elective surgery, as prescribed.

Evaluation
- Patient states that pain is relieved.
- Patient remains free from adverse GI effects throughout drug therapy.
- Patient and family state an understanding of drug therapy.
(See *Teaching about salicylates*.)

Paracetamol

Paracetamol is an OTC drug that produces analgesic and antipyretic effects. It appears in many products designed to relieve pain and symptoms associated with colds and influenza.

Pharmacokinetics
Paracetamol is absorbed rapidly and completely from the GI tract. It's also absorbed well from the mucous membranes of the rectum.

Be sure not to crush enteric-coated aspirin because these drugs are made to protect the lining of the stomach.

Education edge

Teaching about salicylates

If salicylates are prescribed, review these points with the patient and caregivers:

- For the patient receiving high-dose prolonged treatment, maintain adequate fluid intake and watch for petechiae (dicoloured spots on the surface of the skin caused by ruptured blood vessels), bleeding gums, and signs of GI bleeding. Use a soft toothbrush.
- Be aware that various over-the-counter (OTC) preparations contain aspirin. Because numerous drug interactions are possible when taking aspirin, check with a prescriber or pharmacist before taking herbal preparations or OTC medications containing aspirin.
- Avoid alcohol consumption during drug therapy.
- Restrict caffeine intake during drug therapy.

- Take the drug as directed to achieve the desired effect. Know that the benefits of drug therapy may not be noticeable for 2 to 4 weeks.
- Take the drug with food or milk to prevent GI upset.
- Don't chew enteric-coated products.
- Notify the prescriber about severe or persistent adverse reactions.
- Be sure to safely store medications in the home. Aspirin is a leading cause of poisoning in children. Keep aspirin and other drugs out of children's reach. Use child-resistant containers in households with children.
- If salicylate therapy will be long-term, be sure to follow the prescriber's instructions for monitoring laboratory values, especially blood urea nitrogen and creatinine levels, liver function, and complete blood count.

It's widely distributed in body fluids and readily crosses the placenta. After the liver metabolises paracetamol, it's excreted by the kidneys and, in small amounts, in breast milk. However, it is considered safe for use in pregnancy.

Pharmacodynamics

Paracetamol reduces pain and fever but, unlike salicylates, it does not significantly affect inflammation or platelet function. It may potentiate the effects of warfarin and increase international normalised ratio values with long term use.

Mystery theatre

The pain-control effects of paracetamol aren't well understood. It may work in the central nervous system (CNS) by inhibiting prostaglandin synthesis and in the peripheral nervous system in some unknown way. It reduces fever by acting directly on the heat-regulating centre in the hypothalamus.

Pharmacotherapeutics

Paracetamol is used to reduce fever and relieve headache, muscle ache, and general pain. In addition, the Arthritis Research Campaign has indicated that paracetamol is an effective pain reliever for some types of arthritis.

Child's play

Paracetamol is the drug of choice to treat fever and flu-like symptoms in children.

Paracetamol is commonly used to treat fever and flu-like symptoms in children.

Drug interactions

Paracetamol can produce these drug interactions:
- It may slightly increase the effects of oral anticoagulants, such as warfarin, and thrombolytic drugs.
- The risk of liver toxicity is increased when phenytoin, barbiturates, carbamazepine, and isoniazid are combined with paracetamol. This risk is also increased with chronic alcohol use.
- The effects of lamotrigine, loop diuretics, and zidovudine may be reduced when taken with paracetamol.

Adverse reactions

Most patients tolerate paracetamol well. Unlike the salicylates, paracetamol rarely causes gastric irritation or bleeding tendencies. However, it may cause liver toxicity, and the total daily dose should be monitored.

Other adverse reactions include:
- skin rash
- hypoglycaemia
- neutropenia.

Nursing process

These nursing process steps are appropriate for patients undergoing treatment with paracetamol.

Assessment

- Assess the patient's level of pain and inflammation before therapy begins and evaluate drug effectiveness after administration.
- Assess the patient's medication history. Many OTC products and combination prescription pain products contain paracetamol and must be considered when calculating the total daily dosage.
- Be alert for adverse reactions and drug interactions.
- Evaluate the patient's and family's knowledge of drug therapy.

Key nursing diagnoses
- Acute pain related to underlying process.
- Risk for injury related to adverse reactions.
- Deficient knowledge related to drug therapy.

Planning outcome goals
- The patient will acknowledge a reduction in pain.
- No serious complications will occur while the patient is on drug therapy.
- The patient and family will demonstrate an understanding of the purpose and intended effect of drug therapy.

Implementation
- Administer the liquid form of the drug to children and other patients who have difficulty swallowing.
- Use the rectal route in small children and other patients for whom oral administration isn't feasible.

Evaluation
- Patient states that pain is relieved.
- Patient remains free from adverse effects throughout drug therapy.
- Patient and family state an understanding of drug therapy.
(See *Teaching about paracetamol.*)

Nonselective NSAIDs

As their name suggests, nonsteroidal anti-inflammatory drugs, or NSAIDs, are typically used to combat inflammation. Their anti-inflammatory action equals that of aspirin. They also have analgesic and antipyretic effects.

Nonselective NSAIDs inhibit prostaglandin synthesis by blocking two enzymes know as cyclooxygenase-1 (COX-1) and cyclooxygenase-2 (COX-2). These drugs (called *COX-1* and *COX-2 inhibitors*) include indometacin, ibuprofen, diclofenac, etodolac, fenoprofen, flurbiprofen, ketoprofen, ketorolac, mefenamic acid, meloxicam, nabumetone, naproxen, piroxicam, and sulindac.

Selective NSAIDs selectively block COX-2 enzymes, thereby inhibiting prostaglandin synthesis. This selective inhibition of COX-2 produces the analgesic and anti-inflammatory effects without causing the adverse GI effects associated with COX-1 inhibition by nonselective NSAIDS. (See *NSAIDs: Ibuprofen.*)

Pharmacokinetics
All NSAIDs (nonselective and selective) are absorbed in the GI tract. They're mostly metabolised in the liver and excreted primarily by the kidneys.

Education edge

Teaching about paracetamol

If paracetamol is prescribed, review these points with the patient and caregivers:

- Consult a prescriber before giving the drug to children younger than aged 2.
- Be aware that the drug is for short-term use only. A prescriber should be consulted if that drug is to be administered to children for more than 5 days or to adults for more than 10 days.
- Don't use the drug for marked fever (over 39.5° C), fever persisting longer than 3 days, or recurrent fever, unless directed by a prescriber.

- Be aware that high doses or unsupervised long-term use can cause liver damage. Excessive ingestion of alcoholic beverages may increase the risk of hepatotoxicity.
- Keep track of daily paracetamol intake, including over-the-counter and prescription medications. Don't exceed the total recommended dose of paracetamol per day because of the risk of hepatotoxicity.
- Be aware that the drug is found in breast milk in low levels (less than 1% of the dose). The drug is safe for short-term therapy as long as the recommended dose isn't exceeded.

Pharmacodynamics

Inflammatory disorders produce and release prostaglandins from cell membranes, resulting in pain. Nonselective NSAIDs produce their effects by inhibiting prostaglandin synthesis and cyclooxygenase activity. NSAIDs inhibit both isoenzymes of cyclooxygenase, COX-1 and COX-2, which convert arachidonic acid into prostaglandins. COX-1 produces prostaglandins that maintain the stomach lining, whereas COX-2 produces prostaglandins that mediate an inflammatory response. Therefore, COX-1 inhibition is associated with NSAID-induced GI toxicity, whereas COX-2 inhibition alleviates pain and inflammation.

Pharmacotherapeutics

NSAIDs are primarily used to decrease inflammation. They're also used to relieve pain, but are seldom prescribed to reduce fever. (See *Nonselective NSAIDs warning*.)

Prototype pro

NSAIDs: Ibuprofen

Actions

- Interferes with the prostaglandins involved in pain; appears to sensitise pain receptors to mechanical stimulation or to other chemical mediators (such as bradykinin and histamine)
- Inhibits synthesis of prostaglandins peripherally and possibly centrally
- Inhibits prostaglandin synthesis and release during inflammation
- Suppresses prostaglandin synthesis in the central nervous system, causing an antipyretic effect

Indications

- Rheumatoid arthritis
- Osteoarthritis
- Juvenile arthritis
- Mild to moderate pain
- Fever

Nursing considerations

- Monitor the patient for adverse effects, such as bronchospasm, Stevens-Johnson syndrome, haematologic disorders, and aseptic meningitis.
- Keep in mind that it may take 1 to 2 weeks to achieve full anti-inflammatory effects.
- Be aware that the drug may mask the signs and symptoms of infection.

All in favour?

The following conditions respond favorably to treatment with NSAIDs:
- ankylosing spondylitis (an inflammatory joint disease that first affects the spine)
- moderate to severe rheumatoid arthritis (an inflammatory disease of peripheral joints)
- osteoarthritis (a degenerative joint disease) in the hip, shoulder, or other large joints
- osteoarthritis accompanied by inflammation
- acute gouty arthritis (urate deposits in the joints)
- dysmenorrhoea (painful menstruation)
- migraines
- bursitis
- tendonitis
- mild to moderate pain.

Before you give that drug!

Nonselective NSAIDs warning

Before administering a nonsteroidal anti-inflammatory drug (NSAID) to a patient, be aware of its risks to special populations:

- *Children:* Some NSAIDs aren't recommended for use in children.
- *Elderly people:* The risk of ulcers increases with age.
- *Pregnant women:* Ketoprofen, naproxen, flurbiprofen, and diclofenac have not shown adverse effects in animal studies. There are adequate well controlled studies in pregnant women which suggest the drugs present no risk to the foetus in any trimester. Etodolac, ketorolac, meloxicam, nabumetone, oxaprozin, and piroxicam have shown adverse effects in animals. Although there are no adequate and controlled studies in humans, the potential benefits may warrant the use of these drugs in pregnant women, despite potential risks. Most NSAIDs are excreted in breast milk. In general, nonselective NSAIDs shouldn't be administered to nursing mothers.

Drug interactions

Many drugs can interact with NSAIDs, especially with indometacin, piroxicam, and sulindac. Because they're highly protein bound, NSAIDs are likely to interact with other protein-bound drugs. Drugs such as fluconazole, phenobarbital, rifampicin, ritonavir, and salicylates affect NSAIDs; whereas NSAIDs affect oral anticoagulants, aminoglycosides, ACE inhibitors, beta-adrenergic blockers, digoxin, and others.

Adverse reactions

All NSAIDs produce similar adverse reactions, which can include:
- abdominal pain and bleeding
- anorexia
- diarrhoea
- nausea
- ulcers
- liver toxicity
- drowsiness
- headache
- dizziness
- confusion
- tinnitus
- vertigo
- depression
- bladder infection
- blood in urine

- hypertension
- heart failure
- pedal oedema.

Nursing process

These nursing process steps are appropriate for patients undergoing treatment with nonselective NSAIDs.

Assessment

- Obtain an assessment of the patient's underlying condition before starting drug therapy.
- Assess the patient's level of pain and inflammation before therapy begins and evaluate drug effectiveness after administration.
- Monitor the patient for signs and symptoms of bleeding. Assess bleeding time if they are expected to undergo surgery.
- Monitor the patient's ophthalmic and auditory function before and periodically during therapy to detect toxicity.
- Monitor CBC, platelet count, PT, and hepatic and renal function periodically to detect abnormalities.
- Be alert for adverse reactions and drug interactions. Watch for bronchospasm in the patient with aspirin hypersensitivity, rhinitis or nasal polyps, or asthma.
- Evaluate the patient's and family's knowledge of drug therapy.

Key nursing diagnoses

- Risk for injury related to adverse reactions.
- Acute pain related to the underlying condition.
- Deficient knowledge related to drug therapy.

Planning outcome goals

- The patient will acknowledge a reduction in pain.
- No serious complications will occur while the patient is on drug therapy.
- The patient and family will demonstrate an understanding of the purpose and intended effect of drug therapy.

Implementation

- Administer oral NSAIDs with 240 ml of water to ensure adequate passage into the stomach. Have the patient sit up for 15 to 30 minutes after taking the drug to prevent it from lodging in the oesophagus.
- As needed, crush tablets or mix with food or fluid to aid swallowing.
- Give the drug with meals or milk or administer it with antacids to reduce adverse GI reactions.

Education edge

Teaching about NSAIDs

If nonsteroidal anti-inflammatory drugs (NSAIDs) are prescribed, review these points with the patient and caregivers:

- Take the drug as directed to achieve the desired effect. Be aware that the benefits of some types of therapy may not be achieved for 2 to 4 weeks.
- Take the drug with meals or milk to reduce adverse GI reactions.
- Don't exceed the recommended daily dose, don't give the drug to children younger than aged 12, and don't take the drug for extended periods without consulting a prescriber.
- Be aware that using the drug with aspirin, alcohol, or corticosteroids may increase the risk of adverse GI effects.
- Recognise and report signs and symptoms of GI bleeding, such as

dark-coloured stools, blood in urine, and unusual bleeding (for example, in the gums).
- Avoid alcohol during drug therapy.
- Use sunblock, wear protective clothing, and avoid prolonged exposure to sunlight during therapy.
- If taking the medication as long-term therapy, check with the prescriber about the need for monitoring of laboratory values, especially blood urea nitrogen and creatinine levels, liver function, and complete blood count.
- Notify the prescriber about severe or persistent adverse reactions.
- Don't take other medications, over-the-counter products, or herbal products without first consulting with a prescriber.

- Notify the prescriber if the drug is ineffective.
- If renal or hepatic abnormalities occur, stop the drug and notify the prescriber.

Evaluation
- Patient states that pain is relieved
- Patient remains free from adverse effects throughout drug therapy.
- Patient and family state an understanding of drug therapy. (See *Teaching about NSAIDs*.)

Selective NSAIDs

Prostaglandins produced by COX-2 are associated with pain and inflammation. The selective NSAIDs (also called COX-2 inhibitor drugs) are NSAIDs that selectively block COX-2, relieving pain and inflammation. They have fewer adverse effects, such as stomach damage, than nonselective NSAIDs. Celecoxib is one of the more common selective NSAIDs.

Pharmacokinetics

The selective NSAIDs are highly protein bound, primarily to albumin, and are extensively distributed into the tissues. Peak levels occur within 3 hours, and steady plasma states can be expected in 5 days, if given in multiple doses. These drugs are metabolised in the liver, with less than 3% unchanged and excreted in urine and faeces.

Pharmacodynamics

Selective NSAIDs produce their effects by selectively blocking the COX-2 enzyme, thereby inhibiting prostaglandin synthesis.

Less than the rest

This selective inhibition of COX-2 produces analgesic and anti-inflammatory effects without the adverse GI effects associated with COX-1 inhibition by nonselective NSAIDs. However, some degree of COX-1 inhibition still occurs.

Pharmacotherapeutics

Selective NSAIDs are primarily used to provide analgesia and to decrease inflammation. They're particularly useful in the treatment of osteoarthritis, rheumatoid arthritis, acute pain, primary dysmenorrhea, and familial adenomatous polyposis.

Drug interactions

Because selective NSAIDs are metabolised by the liver, drug interactions have been identified for all agents. For example:
*   Selective NSAIDs decrease the clearance of lithium, which can result in lithium toxicity.
*   They reduce the antihypertensive effects of ACE inhibitors and diuretics.
*   When taken with warfarin, increased PT levels and bleeding complications can occur.
*   They interact with herbal preparations that increase the risk of bleeding, such as dong quai, feverfew, garlic, ginger, ginkgo, horse chestnut, and red clover.

Adverse reactions

These adverse reactions may occur with selective NSAIDs:
*   dyspepsia
*   nausea and vomiting
*   GI ulcers (to a lesser degree than with nonselective NSAIDs)

- hypertension
- fluid retention
- peripheral oedema
- dizziness
- headache.

Nursing process

These nursing process steps are appropriate for patients undergoing treatment with selective NSAIDs (COX-2 inhibitors).

Assessment

- Obtain an assessment of the patient's underlying condition before starting drug therapy.
- Obtain an accurate list of the patient's allergies. If they are allergic to or has anaphylactic reactions to sulphonamides, aspirin, or other NSAIDs, they may also be allergic to selective NSAIDs.
- Assess the patient's level of pain and inflammation before therapy begins and evaluate drug effectiveness after administration.
- Monitor the patient for signs and symptoms of bleeding. Assess bleeding time if he requires surgery.
- Monitor the patient's ophthalmic and auditory function before therapy and periodically thereafter to detect toxicity.
- Periodically monitor CBC, platelet count, PT, and hepatic and renal function to detect abnormalities.
- Closely monitor the patient on celecoxib for signs or symptoms of MI. This drug has been linked to a relatively high risk of heart attacks.
- Evaluate the patient's and family's knowledge of drug therapy.

Woe is me! Celecoxib has been linked to a relatively high risk of heart disease.

Key nursing diagnoses

- Risk for injury related to adverse reactions.
- Acute pain related to the underlying condition.
- Deficient knowledge related to drug therapy.

Planning outcome goals

- The patient will acknowledge a reduction in pain.
- No serious complications will occur while the patient is on drug therapy.
- The patient and family will demonstrate an understanding of the purpose and intended effect of drug therapy.

Implementation

- Although the drug can be given without regard to meals, food may decrease GI upset.

Education edge

Teaching about selective NSAIDs

If selective nonsteroidal anti-inflammatory drugs (NSAIDs), or cyclooxygenase-2 (COX-2) drugs, are prescribed, review these points with the patient and caregivers:

- Report a history of allergic reactions to sulphonamides, aspirin, or other NSAIDs before starting therapy.
- Immediately report to the prescriber signs of GI bleeding (such as bloody vomitus, blood in urine or stool, and black, tarry stools), rash, and unexplained weight gain or oedema.
- Notify the prescriber if you become pregnant or are planning to become pregnant while taking this drug.
- Take the drug with food if stomach upset occurs.
- Be aware that all NSAIDs, including COX-2 inhibitors, may adversely affect the liver. Signs and symptoms of liver toxicity include nausea, fatigue, lethargy, itching, jaundice, right upper quadrant tenderness, and flu-like symptoms. Stop therapy and seek immediate medical advice if any of these signs and symptoms develops.
- Be aware that it may take several days to feel consistent pain relief.
- Don't take other medications, over-the-counter products, or herbal remedies unless first approved by the prescriber.
- Inform all health care providers that you're taking this medication.
- Avoid or minimise alcoholic beverages because alcohol increases gastric irritation and the risk of bleeding.

- Before starting treatment, be sure to rehydrate the patient.
- Although the drug may be used with low aspirin dosages, the combination may increase the risk of GI bleeding.
- NSAIDs such as celecoxib can cause fluid retention; closely monitor the patient who has hypertension, oedema, or heart failure.
- Notify the prescriber if the drug is ineffective.

Evaluation
- Patient states that pain is relieved.
- Patient remains free from adverse effects throughout drug therapy.
- Patient and family state an understanding of drug therapy.
(See *Teaching about selective NSAIDs*.)

Opioid agonists and antagonists

The word *opioid* refers to any derivative of the opium plant or any synthetic drug that imitates natural narcotics. Opioid agonists (also called *narcotic agonists*) include opium derivatives and synthetic drugs with similar properties. They're used to relieve or decrease pain without causing the person to lose consciousness. Some opioid agonists also have antitussive and antidiarrhoeal effects.

Anta-dote

Opioid antagonists aren't pain medications. They block the effects of opioid agonists and are used to reverse adverse drug reactions, such as respiratory and CNS depression produced by those drugs. Unfortunately, by reversing the analgesic effect, they also cause the patient's pain to recur.

Having it both ways

Some opioid analgesics, called *mixed opioid agonist-antagonists*, have agonist and antagonist properties. The agonist component relieves pain, and the antagonist component decreases the risk of toxicity and drug dependence. These mixed opioid agonist-antagonists reduce the risk of respiratory depression and drug abuse.

Opioid agonists

Opioid agonists include:
- codeine
- fentanyl
- hydromorphone hydrochloride
- pethidine hydrochloride
- methadone hydrochloride
- morphine sulphate (including morphine sulphate sustained-release tablets and intensified oral solution)
- oxycodone
- remifentanil.

Gold standard

Morphine sulphate is the standard against which the effectiveness and adverse reactions of other pain medications are measured. (See *Opioid agonists: Morphine.*)

Pharmacokinetics

Opioid agonists can be administered by any route, although inhalation administration is uncommon. Oral doses are absorbed

Prototype pro

Opioid agonists: Morphine

Actions

- Acts on opiate receptors in the central nervous system

Indications

- Pain

Nursing considerations

- Monitor the patient for adverse effects, such as sedation, euphoria, seizures, dizziness, nightmares, bradycardia, shock, cardiac arrest, nausea, constipation, vomiting, thrombocytopenia, and respiratory depression.
- Keep an opioid antagonist (naloxone) and resuscitation equipment available.

readily from the GI tract. Transmucosal and intrathecal opiates are fast acting. Opioid agonists administered I.V. provide the most rapid (almost immediate) and reliable pain relief. The subcutaneous and I.M. routes may result in delayed absorption, especially in patients with poor circulation.

Opioid agonists are distributed widely throughout body tissues. They have a relatively low plasma protein-binding capacity (30% to 35%).

Liver lovers

These drugs are metabolised extensively in the liver. For example, pethidine is metabolised to norpethidine, a toxic metabolite with a longer half-life than pethidine. This metabolite accumulates in renal failure and may lead to CNS excitation. Administration of pethidine for more than 48 hours increases the risk of neurotoxicity and seizures from a buildup of norpethidine.

Metabolites are excreted by the kidneys. A small amount is excreted in faeces through the biliary tract.

Pharmacodynamics

Opioid agonists reduce pain by binding to opiate receptor sites in the peripheral nervous system and the CNS. When these drugs stimulate the opiate receptors, they mimic the effects of endorphins (naturally occurring opiates that are part of the body's own pain relief system). This receptor-site binding produces the therapeutic effects of analgesia and cough suppression as well as adverse reactions, such as respiratory depression and constipation. (See *How opioid agonists control pain*.)

Smooth operator

Opioid agonists, especially morphine, affect the smooth muscle of the GI and genitourinary tracts (the organs of the reproductive and urinary systems). This causes contraction of the bladder and ureters and slows intestinal peristalsis (rhythmic contractions that move food along the digestive tract), resulting in constipation, a common adverse reaction to opiates.

A fine line

These drugs also cause blood vessels to dilate, especially in the face, head, and neck. In addition, they suppress the cough centre in the brain, producing antitussive effects and causing constriction of the bronchial muscles. Any of these effects can become adverse reactions

Pharm function

How opioid agonists control pain

Opioid agonists, such as pethidine, inhibit pain transmission by mimicking the body's natural pain control mechanisms.

Where neurons meet

In the dorsal horn of the spinal cord, peripheral pain neurons meet central nervous system (CNS) neurons. At the synapse, the pain neuron releases substance P (a pain neurotransmitter). This agent helps transfer pain impulses to the CNS neurons that carry the impulses to the brain.

Taking up Space

In theory, the spinal interneurons respond to stimulation from the descending neurons of the CNS by releasing endogenous opiates. These opiates bind to the peripheral pain neuron to inhibit release of substance P and to retard the transmission of pain impulses.

Stopping substance P

Synthetic opiates supplement this pain-blocking effect by binding with free opiate receptors to inhibit the release of substance P. Opiates also alter consciousness of pain, but how this mechanism works remains unknown.

if produced in excess. For example, if the blood vessels dilate too much, hypotension can occur.

Pharmacotherapeutics

Opioid agonists are prescribed to relieve severe pain in acute, chronic, and terminal illnesses. They're sometimes prescribed to control diarrhoea and suppress coughing. Methadone is used for temporary maintenance of opioid addiction. Opioids such as fentanyl and remifentanil are used for the induction and maintenance of general anaesthesia.

Cardio-assistance

Morphine relieves shortness of breath in the patient with pulmonary oedema (fluid in the lungs) or left-sided heart failure (inability of the heart to pump enough blood to meet the body's needs). It does this by dilating peripheral blood vessels, keeping more blood in the periphery, and decreasing cardiac preload, thus reducing myocardial workload overall.

Drug interactions

Drugs that can affect opioid analgesic activity include amitriptyline, protease inhibitors, diazepam and rifampicin. Taking tricyclic antidepressants, phenothiazines, or anticholinergics with opioid agonists may cause severe constipation and urine retention. Drugs that may be affected by opioid analgesics include carbamazepine, warfarin, beta-adrenergic blockers and calcium channel blockers. The use of opioid agonists with other substances that decrease respiration, such as alcohol, sedatives, hypnotics, and anaesthetics, increases the patient's risk of severe respiratory depression. (See *Opioid agonists warning*.)

Adverse reactions

One of the most common adverse reactions to opioid agonists is decreased rate and depth of breathing that worsens as the dose of narcotic is increased. This may cause periodic, irregular breathing or trigger asthmatic attacks in a susceptible patient.

Other adverse reactions include:
- flushing
- orthostatic hypotension
- pupil constriction.

Before you give that drug!

Opioid agonists warning

Before administering medications, be aware that morphine sulphate (MSO_4) can be confused with magnesium sulphate ($MgSO_4$). Write out the medication in full to avoid confusion.

Opioid agonists have been reported to have adverse effects in animals. However, there are no adequate controlled studies in pregnant women which detail adverse effects. Most opiod agonists appear in breast milk; most prescribers recommend waiting 4 to 6 hours after ingestion to breast-feed.

Pethidine's list

With pethidine administration, these adverse reactions can occur:
- tremors
- palpitations
- tachycardia
- delirium
- neurotoxicity and seizures (if administered for more than 48 hours).

Watch out! pethidine can cause tremors, palpitations, tachycardia, and delirium.

Nursing process

These nursing process steps are appropriate for patients undergoing treatment with opioid agonists.

Assessment
- Obtain a baseline assessment of the patient's pain and reassess frequently to determine drug effectiveness.
- Evaluate the patient's respiratory status before each dose; watch for a respiratory rate below the patient's baseline level and for restlessness, which may be compensatory signs of hypoxia. Respiratory depression may last longer than the analgesic effect.
- Monitor the patient for other adverse reactions.
- Monitor the patient for tolerance and dependence. The first sign of tolerance to opioids is usually a shortened duration of effect.

Key nursing diagnoses
- Acute pain related to the underlying condition.
- Ineffective breathing pattern related to depressive effect on respiratory system.
- Deficient knowledge related to drug therapy.

Planning outcome goals
- The patient will acknowledge a reduction in pain.
- Throughout therapy, the patient will maintain adequate breathing function.
- The patient and family will demonstrate an understanding of the purpose and intended effect of drug therapy.

Implementation
- Keep resuscitative equipment and a narcotic antagonist (naloxone) available.
- Give the I.V. drug by slow injection, preferably in diluted solution. Rapid I.V. injection increases the risk of adverse effects.

Education edge

Teaching about opioid agonists

If opioid agonists are prescribed, review these points with the patient and caregivers:

- Take the drug exactly as prescribed. Call the prescriber if you don't experience the desired effect or if you experience significant adverse reactions.
- Be careful when getting out of bed and walking. Avoid hazardous activities until the drug's effects are known.
- Avoid alcohol while taking opioid agonists because it causes additive central nervous system depression.
- To prevent constipation, increase fibre in the diet and use a stool softener.
- Breathe deeply, cough, and change position every 2 hours to avoid respiratory complications.
- Report continued pain.

- Give I.M. or subcutaneous (S.C.) injections cautiously to a patient with a decreased platelet count and to a patient who's chilled, hypovolaemic, or in shock; decreased perfusion may lead to drug accumulation and toxicity. Rotate injection sites to avoid induration.
- Carefully note the strength of the solution when measuring a dose. Oral solutions of varying concentrations are available.
- For maximum effectiveness, give the drug on a regular dosage schedule rather than as needed.
- Institute safety precautions.
- Encourage a postoperative patient to turn, cough, and breathe deeply every 2 hours to avoid atelectasis.
- If GI irritation occurs, give oral forms of the drug with food.
- Be aware that withdrawal symptoms, including tremors, agitation, nausea, and vomiting, may occur if the drug is stopped abruptly. Monitor the patient with these symptoms carefully and provide supportive therapy.

Evaluation

- Patient states that pain is relieved.
- Patient maintains adequate ventilation, as evidenced by normal respiratory rate and rhythm and pink skin colour.
- Patient and family state an understanding of drug therapy.
(See *Teaching about opioid agonists*.)

Mixed opioid agonist-antagonists

Mixed opioid agonist-antagonists are given to relieve pain while reducing toxic effects and dependency. Examples include:

- buprenorphine hydrochloride
- pentazocine hydrochloride (combined with pentazocine lactate, naloxone hydrochloride, aspirin, or paracetamol).

Originally, mixed opioid agonist-antagonists appeared to have less abuse potential than the pure opioid agonists. However, pentazocine has reportedly caused dependence. This class of drugs isn't recommended for use in patients with chronic pain who are taking other opioid agonists.

Pharmacokinetics

Absorption of mixed opioid agonist-antagonists occurs rapidly from parenteral sites. These drugs are distributed to most body tissues and cross the placenta. They're metabolised in the liver and excreted primarily by the kidneys.

Pharmacodynamics

The exact mechanism of action of mixed opioid agonist-antagonists isn't known. However, researchers believe that these drugs weakly antagonise the effects of morphine, pethidine, and other opiates at one of the opioid receptors. They also exert agonistic effects at other opioid receptors.

In no rush

Buprenorphine binds with receptors in the CNS, altering the perception of and the emotional response to pain through an unknown mechanism. It seems to release slowly from binding sites, producing a longer duration of action than the other drugs in this class.

Putting up resistance

Pentazocine, acts on the pulmonary circulation, increasing pulmonary vascular resistance (resistance in the blood vessels of the lungs that the right ventricle must pump against). As a result it increases blood pressure and the workload of the heart.

Pharmacotherapeutics

Mixed opioid agonist-antagonists are used as analgesia during childbirth as well as postoperatively.

Argh! Pentazocine increases my workload!

Independence day

Mixed opioid agonist-antagonists are sometimes prescribed in place of opioid agonists because they have a lower risk of drug dependence. Mixed opioid agonist-antagonists also are less likely to cause respiratory depression and constipation, although they can produce some adverse reactions.

Drug interactions

Increased CNS depression and an additive decrease in respiratory rate and depth may result if mixed opioid agonist-antagonists are administered to a patient taking other CNS depressants, such as barbiturates and alcohol.

Clean and sober?

The patient with a history of opioid abuse shouldn't receive any mixed opioid agonist-antagonists because they can cause withdrawal symptoms.

Adverse reactions

The most common adverse reactions to opioid agonist-antagonists include nausea, vomiting, light-headedness, sedation, and euphoria.

Nursing process

These nursing process steps are appropriate for patients undergoing treatment with an opioid agonist-antagonist.

Assessment
• Obtain a baseline assessment of the patient's pain and reassess frequently to determine drug effectiveness.
• Evaluate the patient's respiratory status before each dose; watch for a respiratory rate below the baseline level and watch for restlessness, which may be a compensatory sign of hypoxaemia. Respiratory depression may last longer than the analgesic effect.
• Monitor the patient for other adverse reactions.
• Monitor the patient for tolerance and dependence. The first sign of tolerance to opioids is usually a shortened duration of effect.

Key nursing diagnoses
• Acute pain related to the underlying condition.
• Ineffective breathing pattern related to depressive effect on respiratory system.
• Deficient knowledge related to drug therapy.

A patient with a history of opioid abuse shouldn't receive opioid agonist-antagonists. Withdrawal symptoms may result.

CAUTION!

Planning outcome goals
- The patient will acknowledge a reduction in pain.
- Throughout therapy, the patient will maintain an adequate breathing pattern.
- The patient and family will demonstrate an understanding of the purpose and intended effect of drug therapy.

Implementation
- Keep resuscitative equipment and an opioid antagonist (naloxone) available. Naloxone won't completely reverse respiratory depression caused by buprenorphine overdose; mechanical ventilation may be necessary. Doxapram and larger-than-usual doses of naloxone may also be prescribed.
- Give the I.V. form of the drug by slow injection, preferably in diluted solution. Rapid I.V. injection increases the risk of adverse effects.
- Institute safety precautions.
- Encourage a postoperative patient to turn, cough, and breathe deeply every 2 hours to avoid atelectasis.
- Be aware that the drug may precipitate withdrawal syndrome in a opioid-dependent patient. Withdrawal symptoms—including tremors, agitation, nausea, and vomiting—may occur if the drug is stopped abruptly. If dependence occurs, withdrawal symptoms may appear up to 14 days after the drug is stopped. Monitor a patient with these symptoms carefully and provide supportive therapy.

Evaluation
- Patient states that pain is relieved.
- Patient maintains adequate ventilation, as evidenced by normal respiratory rate and rhythm and pink skin colour.
- Patient and family state an understanding of drug therapy.

Opioid antagonists

Opioid antagonists attach to opiate receptors, but don't stimulate them, and have a greater attraction for opiate receptors than opioids do. As a result, they prevent opioid drugs, encephalins, and endorphins from producing their effects.

Opioid antagonists include:
- naloxone hydrochloride
- naltrexone hydrochloride.

Pharmacokinetics
Naloxone is administered subcutaneously, I.M., or I.V. Naltrexone is administered orally in tablet form. Both drugs are metabolised by the liver and excreted by the kidneys.

Pharmacodynamics

In a process known as *competitive inhibition*, opioid antagonists block the effects of opioids by occupying the opiate receptor sites, displacing opioids attached to opiate receptors and blocking further opioid binding at these sites.

Pharmacotherapeutics

Naloxone is the drug of choice for managing an opioid overdose. It reverses respiratory depression and sedation and helps stabilise the patient's vital signs within seconds after administration.

Because naloxone also reverses the analgesic effects of opioid drugs, a patient who was given an opioid drug for pain relief may complain of pain or even experience withdrawal symptoms.

Kicking the habit

Naltrexone is used along with psychotherapy or counselling to treat drug abuse. It's only given, however, to a patient who has gone through a detoxification program to remove all opioids from the body. A patient who still has opioids in the body may experience acute withdrawal symptoms if given naltrexone.

Drug interactions

Naloxone produces no significant drug interactions. Naltrexone will cause withdrawal symptoms if given to a patient who's receiving an opioid agonist or who's an opioid addict.

Adverse reactions

Naltrexone can cause several adverse reactions, including:
- oedema
- hypertension
- palpitations
- phlebitis
- shortness of breath
- anxiety
- depression
- disorientation
- dizziness
- headache
- nervousness
- anorexia
- diarrhoea or constipation
- nausea and vomiting
- thirst
- urinary frequency
- liver toxicity.

It's tough out there for us opioids. The competitive inhibition of opioid antagonists can keep me from doing my job.

Naltrexone can cause nausea and vomiting.

Watch the wake-up

Naloxone may cause nausea, vomiting and, occasionally, hypertension and tachycardia. An unconscious patient returned to consciousness abruptly after naloxone administration may hyperventilate and experience tremors.

Nursing process

These nursing process steps are appropriate for patients undergoing treatment with an opioid antagonist.

Assessment
- Assess the patient's opioid use before therapy.
- Assess the drug's effectiveness regularly throughout therapy.
- Monitor the patient's respiratory depth and rate. The duration of the opioid may exceed that of naloxone, causing relapse into respiratory depression.
- Monitor the patient's hydration status if adverse GI reactions occur.
- Evaluate the patient's and family's knowledge of drug therapy.

Key nursing diagnoses
- Ineffective health maintenance related to opioid use.
- Risk for deficient fluid volume related to drug-induced adverse GI reactions.
- Deficient knowledge related to drug therapy.

Planning outcome goals
- The patient will demonstrate improved health as evidenced by maintenance of vital signs within normal parameters.
- The patient will maintain adequate hydration as evidenced by adequate urine output.
- The patient and family will demonstrate an understanding of the purpose and intended effect of drug therapy.

Implementation
- Provide oxygen, ventilation, and other resuscitation measures when the drug is used in the management of acute opiate overdose, and when the patient has severe respiratory depression.
- Keep in mind that these drugs are effective in reversing respiratory depression only when caused by opioids. When they're used for this purpose, monitor the patient for tachypnea.
- Be prepared to give continuous I.V. naloxone infusion to control adverse effects of epidural morphine.

Evaluation
* Patient responds well to drug therapy.
* Patient maintains adequate hydration.
* Patient and family state an understanding of drug therapy.

Anaesthetic drugs

Anaesthetic drugs can be divided into three groups—general anaesthetics, local anaesthetics, and topical anaesthetics.

Inhale or inject?

General anaesthetic drugs are further subdivided into two main types, those given by inhalation and those given I.V.

Inhalation anaesthetics

Commonly used general anaesthetics given by inhalation include:
* desflurane
* sevoflurane
* isoflurane
* nitrous oxide.

Pharmacokinetics

The absorption and elimination rates of anaesthetics are governed by their solubility in blood. Inhalation anaesthetics enter the blood from the lungs and are distributed to other tissues. Distribution is most rapid to organs with high blood flow, such as the brain, liver, kidneys, and heart. Inhalation anaesthetics are eliminated primarily by the lungs; sevoflurane is also eliminated by the liver. Metabolites are excreted in urine.

Pharmacodynamics

Inhalation anaesthetics work primarily by depressing the CNS, producing loss of consciousness, loss of responsiveness to sensory stimulation (including pain), and muscle relaxation. They also affect other organ systems.

Pharmacotherapeutics

Inhalation anaesthetics are used for surgery because they offer more precise and rapid control of depth of anaesthesia than injection anaesthetics. These anaesthetics, which are liquids at room temperature, require a vaporiser and special delivery system for safe use.

My high blood flow means that anaesthetics can make their way to me more quickly.

Of the inhalation anaesthetics available, desflurane, isoflurane, and nitrous oxide are the most commonly used.

Stop signs

Inhalation anaesthetics are contraindicated in a patient with known hypersensitivity to the drug, a liver disorder, or malignant hyperthermia (a potentially fatal complication of anaesthesia characterised by skeletal muscle rigidity and high fever). They require cautious use in a pregnant or breast-feeding patient.

Drug interactions

The most important drug interactions involving inhalation anaesthetics are with other CNS, cardiac, or respiratory-depressant drugs. These drug combinations can cause CNS depression, cardiac arrhythmias, or respiratory depression, resulting in compromised patient status.

Adverse reactions

The most common adverse reaction to inhalation anaesthetics is an exaggerated patient response to a normal dose. Malignant hyperthermia, characterised by a sudden and usually lethal increase in body temperature, is a serious and unexpected reaction to inhalation anaesthetics. It occurs in the genetically susceptible patient only, and may result from a failure in calcium uptake by muscle cells. The skeletal muscle relaxant dantrolene is used to treat this condition.

Waking up

After surgery, a patient may experience reactions similar to those seen with other CNS depressants, including depression of breathing and circulation, confusion, sedation, nausea, vomiting, ataxia, and hypothermia.

Nursing process

These nursing process steps are appropriate for patients undergoing treatment with anaesthetic drugs.

Assessment
• Assess the patient's use of prescription, nonprescription, and herbal remedies, especially within the past 3 days.
• Assess drug allergies and risk factors for complications of anaesthesia and surgery (cigarette smoking, obesity, limited exercise or activity, and chronic cardiovascular, respiratory, renal, or other disease processes)

• Assess the patient's vital signs, laboratory data, and their physical condition to establish baseline measurements for monitoring changes.

Key nursing diagnoses
• Risk for injury related to impaired sensory perception from anaesthetic or sedative drugs.
• Risk for ineffective breathing pattern related to respiratory depression.
• Deficient knowledge related to drug therapy.

Planning outcome goals
• The risk of injury to the patient will be minimised.
• While taking medication, the patient will maintain adequate ventilation and breathing pattern.
• The patient and family will demonstrate an understanding of the purpose and intended effect of drug therapy.

Interventions
• Explain the preoperative and expected postoperative phases of the recovery period.
• Review postoperative recovery requirements, such as deep breathing exercises, coughing, leg exercises, early ambulation, maintaining fluid balance, and urine output.
• Monitor the patient's vital signs, level of consciousness (LOC), respiratory and cardiovascular status, and laboratory results, as indicated.
• Monitor the patient's response to pain medication.

Evaluation
• Patient remains free from major complications.
• Patient maintains adequate ventilation.
• Patient and family understand the use of anaesthetic drugs.

I.V. anaesthetics

I.V. anaesthetics are usually used as general anaesthesia when anaesthesia is needed for only a short period, such as with outpatient surgery. They're also used to promote rapid induction of anaesthesia or to supplement inhalation anaesthetics.

Main options

The drugs used as I.V. anaesthetics are:
• barbiturates (thiopental)
• benzodiazepines (midazolam)

I.V. administration promotes rapid induction of anaesthetics.

- dissociatives (ketamine)
- hypnotics (etomidate, propofol)
- opiates (fentanyl).

Pharmacokinetics

I.V. anaesthetic agents are lipid soluble and are well distributed throughout the body, crossing the placenta and entering breast milk. These drugs are metabolised in the liver and excreted in urine.

Pharmacodynamics

Opiates work by occupying sites on specialised receptors scattered throughout the CNS and modifying the release of neurotransmitters from sensory nerves entering the CNS. Ketamine appears to induce a profound sense of dissociation from the environment by acting directly on the cortex and limbic system of the brain.

Getting sleepy

Barbiturates, benzodiazepines, and etomidate seem to enhance responses to the CNS neurotransmitter gamma-aminobutyric acid. This inhibits the brain's response to stimulation of the reticular activating system, the area of the brain stem that controls alertness. Barbiturates also depress the excitability of CNS neurons.

Pharmacotherapeutics

Because of the short duration of action of I.V. anaesthetics, they're used in shorter surgical procedures, including outpatient surgery.

Loner or helper

Barbiturates are used alone in surgery that isn't expected to be painful and as adjuncts to other drugs in more extensive procedures.

Benzodiazepines produce sedation and amnesia, but not pain relief. Etomidate is used to induce anaesthesia and to supplement low-potency inhalation anaesthetics such as nitrous oxide. The opiates provide pain relief and supplement other anaesthetic drugs.

Drug interactions

I.V. anaesthetics, particularly ketamine, can produce many drug interactions:

- Verapamil enhances the anaesthetic effects of etomidate, producing respiratory depression and apnea.
- Giving ketamine and nondepolarising drugs together increases neuromuscular effects, resulting in prolonged respiratory depression.
- Using barbiturates or opioids with ketamine may prolong recovery time after anaesthesia.

- Ketamine plus theophylline may promote seizures.
- Ketamine and thyroid hormones may cause hypertension and tachycardia (rapid heart rate).

Adverse reactions

Adverse reactions to injection anaesthetics vary by drug.

Ketamine

Ketamine can produce these adverse effects:
- prolonged recovery
- irrational behaviour
- excitement
- disorientation
- delirium or hallucinations
- increased heart rate
- hypertension
- excess salivation
- tearing
- shivering
- increased cerebrospinal fluid and eye pressure
- seizures.

How sad. Ketamine can cause irrational behavior, excessive salivation, and tearing.

Propofol

Propofol can cause:
- respiratory depression
- hiccups
- coughing
- muscle twitching.

Thiopental

Thiopental can cause:
- respiratory depression
- hiccups
- coughing
- muscle twitching
- depressed cardiac function and peripheral dilation.

Etomidate

Etomidate can cause:
- hiccups
- coughing
- muscle twitching.

Fentanyl

Fentanyl can cause:
- CNS and respiratory depression
- hypoventilation
- arrhythmias.

Midazolam

Midazolam can cause:
- CNS and respiratory depression
- hypotension
- dizziness.

Nursing process

These nursing process steps are appropriate for patients undergoing treatment with I.V. anaesthetics.

Assessment
- Assess the use of prescription, nonprescription, and herbal remedies, especially within the past 3 days.
- Assess the patient's drug allergies and risk factors for complications of anaesthesia and surgery (cigarette smoking, obesity, limited exercise or activity, and chronic cardiovascular, respiratory, renal, or other disease processes).
- Assess the patient's vital signs, laboratory data, and their physical condition to establish baseline measurements for monitoring changes.

Key nursing diagnoses
- Risk for injury related to impaired sensory perception from anaesthetic or sedative drugs.
- Risk for ineffective breathing pattern related to respiratory depression.
- Deficient knowledge related to drug therapy.

Planning outcome goals
- The risk of injury to the patient will be minimised.
- While taking the medication, the patient will maintain adequate ventilation and breathing pattern.
- The patient and family will demonstrate an understanding of the purpose and intended effect of drug therapy.

Interventions
- Explain expectations for the preoperative and postoperative phases of the recovery period.

- Review postoperative recovery requirements, such as deep-breathing exercises, coughing, leg exercises, early ambulation, maintaining fluid balance, and urine output.
- Monitor the patient's vital signs, LOC, respiratory and cardiovascular status, and laboratory results, as indicated.
- Monitor the patient's response to pain medication.

Evaluation
- Patient remains free from major complications.
- Patient maintains adequate ventilation.
- Patient and family state an understanding of drug therapy.

Local anaesthetics

Local anaesthetics are administered to prevent or relieve pain in a specific area of the body. In addition, these drugs are commonly used as an alternative to general anaesthesia for elderly or debilitated patients.

Chain gang

Local anaesthetics may be classified as:
- amide drugs (with nitrogen in the molecular chain, such as bupivacaine, ropivacaine, lidocaine, levobupivicaine, mepivacaine, prilocaine)
- ester drugs (with oxygen in the molecular chain, such as procaine, chloroprocaine, tetracaine). (See *Amide and ester examples*.)

Pharmacokinetics
Absorption of local anaesthetics varies widely, but distribution occurs throughout the body. Esters and amides undergo different types of metabolism, but both yield metabolites that are excreted in urine.

Pharmacodynamics
Local anaesthetics block nerve impulses at the point of contact in all kinds of nerves. For example, they can accumulate and cause the nerve cell membrane to expand. As the membrane expands, the cell loses its ability to depolarise, which is necessary for impulse transmission.

Pharmacotherapeutics
Local anaesthetics are used to prevent and relieve pain caused by medical procedures, diseases, or injuries. They're used for severe pain that topical anaesthetics or analgesics can't relieve.

Local anaesthetics are typically a safer choice than general anaesthesia for elderly patients.

When a general won't do

Local anaesthetics are usually preferred to general anaesthetics for surgery in elderly or debilitated patients or in patients with disorders that affect respiratory function, such as chronic obstructive pulmonary disease and myasthenia gravis.

Combining and coordinating

For some procedures, a local anaesthetic is combined with a drug, such as adrenaline (epinephrine), that constricts blood vessels. Vasoconstriction helps control local bleeding and reduces absorption of the anaesthetic. Reduced absorption prolongs the anaesthetic's action at the site and limits its distribution and CNS effects.

Drug interactions

Local anaesthetics produce few significant interactions with other drugs, but can produce adverse reactions.

Adverse reactions

Dose-related CNS reactions include anxiety, apprehension, restlessness, nervousness, disorientation, confusion, dizziness, blurred vision, tremors, twitching, shivering, and seizures. Dose-related cardiovascular reactions may include myocardial depression, bradycardia (slow heart rate), arrhythmias, hypotension, cardiovascular collapse, and cardiac arrest.

All the rest

Local anaesthetic solutions that contain vasoconstrictors, such as adrenaline (epinephrine), can also produce CNS and cardiovascular reactions, including anxiety, dizziness, headache, restlessness, tremors, palpitations, tachycardia, angina, and hypertension.

Nursing process

These nursing process steps are appropriate for patients undergoing treatment with local anaesthetics.

Assessment
• Assess the patient's drug allergies and risk factors for complications of anaesthesia and surgery (cigarette smoking, obesity, limited exercise or activity, and chronic cardiovascular, respiratory, renal, or other disease processes).
• Assess the patient's vital signs, laboratory data, and their physical condition to establish baseline measurements for monitoring changes.

Amide and ester examples

Amide anaesthetics are local anaesthetics that have nitrogen as part of their molecular makeup. They include:

• bupivacaine hydrochloride
• levobupivacaine
• lidocaine hydrochloride
• mepivacaine hydrochloride
• prilocaine hydrochloride
• ropivacaine hydrochloride.

Give them oxygen

Ester anaesthetics have oxygen, not nitrogen, as part of their molecular makeup. They include:

• procaine hydrochloride
• tetracaine hydrochloride.

Key nursing diagnoses
* Risk for injury related to impaired sensory perception from the drug.
* Acute pain related to the underlying disorder.
* Deficient knowledge related to drug therapy.

Planning outcome goals
* Risk for injury to the patient will be minimised.
* The patient will acknowledge a reduction in pain.
* The patient and family will demonstrate an understanding of the purpose and intended effect of drug therapy.

Interventions
* Explain the purpose of therapy and its intended effect.
* Monitor the patient's vital signs, level of pain, respiratory and cardiovascular status, and laboratory results, as indicated.
* Monitor the patient's response to medication.

Evaluation
* Patient remains free from major complications.
* Patient has reduced pain.
* Patient and family state an understanding of drug therapy.

Topical anaesthetics

Topical anaesthetics are applied directly to intact skin or mucous membranes. All topical anaesthetics are used to prevent or relieve minor pain.

All together now

Some injectable local anaesthetics, such as lidocaine and tetracaine, also are effective topically. In addition, some topical anaesthetics, such as lidocaine, are combined in products.

Pharmacokinetics

Topical anaesthetics produce little systemic absorption, except for the application of procaine to mucous membranes. However, systemic absorption may occur if the patient receives frequent or high-dose applications to the eye or large areas of burned or injured skin.

Tetracaine and other esters are metabolised extensively in the blood and to a lesser extent in the liver. Cinchocaine, lidocaine, and other amides are metabolised primarily in the liver. Both types of topical anaesthetics are excreted in urine.

Pharmacodynamics

Benzocaine, procaine, and pramocaine produce topical anaesthesia by blocking nerve impulse transmission. They accumulate in the nerve cell membrane, causing it to expand and lose its ability to depolarise, thus blocking impulse transmission. Cinchocaine, lidocaine, and tetracaine may block impulse transmission across nerve cell membranes.

Drowning out input

The aromatic compounds, such as benzyl alcohol and oil of cloves, appear to stimulate nerve endings. This stimulation causes counterirritation that interferes with pain perception.

Putting on the deep freeze

Ethyl chloride spray superficially freezes the tissue, stimulating the cold sensation receptors and blocking the nerve endings in the frozen area. Menthol selectively stimulates the sensory nerve endings for cold, causing a cool sensation and some local pain relief.

Pharmacotherapeutics

Topical anaesthetics are used to:
- relieve or prevent pain, especially minor burn pain
- relieve itching and irritation
- anaesthetise an area before an injection is given
- numb mucosal surfaces before a tube, such as a urinary catheter, is inserted
- alleviate sore throat or mouth pain when used in a spray or solution. Tetracaine also is used as a topical anaesthetic for the eye.

Benzocaine is used with other drugs in several ear preparations.

Drug interactions

Few interactions with other drugs occur with topical anaesthetics because they aren't absorbed well into the systemic circulation.

Adverse reactions

Topical anaesthetics can cause several adverse reactions, depending on the specific drug:
- Any topical anaesthetic can cause a hypersensitivity reaction, including a rash, itching, hives, swelling of the mouth and throat, and breathing difficulty.
- Benzyl alcohol can cause topical reactions such as skin irritation.
- Freezing agents, such as ethyl chloride, may produce frostbite at the application site.

Some topical anaesthetics stimulate a cooling sensation to initiate local pain relief.

Nursing process

These nursing process steps are appropriate for patients undergoing treatment with topical anaesthetics.

Assessment

- Assess the patient's underlying condition and need for drug therapy.
- Assess the patient's vital signs, laboratory data, level of pain, and their physical condition to establish baseline measurements for monitoring changes.

Key nursing diagnoses

- Risk for injury related to impaired sensory perception from drug therapy.
- Acute pain related to the underlying process.
- Deficient knowledge related to drug therapy.

Planning outcome goals

- The risk of injury will be minimised.
- The patient will acknowledge a reduction in pain.
- The patient and family will demonstrate an understanding of the purpose and intended effect of drug therapy.

Interventions

- Explain the purpose of therapy and its intended effect.
- Monitor the patient's vital signs, level of pain, respiratory and cardiovascular status, and laboratory results, as indicated.
- Monitor the patient's response to pain medication.

Evaluation

- Patient remains free from major complications.
- Patient states pain is lessened with drug therapy.
- Patient and family state an understanding of drug therapy.

(See *Teaching about topical anaesthetics*.)

Quick quiz

1. How does the topical anaesthetic benzocaine relieve sunburn pain?
   A. It numbs the skin surface, decreasing the perception of pain.
   B. It freezes the skin, which prevents nerve impulse transmission.
   C. It blocks nerve impulse transmission by preventing nerve cell depolarisation.
   D. It occupies sites on specialised receptors, modifying the release of neurotransmitters.

Answer: C. Benzocaine prevents nerve cell depolarisation, thus blocking nerve impulse transmission and relieving pain.

2. Which adverse reaction is a patient most likely to experience after receiving general anaesthesia for surgery?
   A. Nausea and vomiting
   B. Seizures
   C. Cyanosis
   D. Increased heart rate

Answer: A. After surgery involving general anaesthesia, a patient is most likely to experience adverse reactions similar to those produced by other CNS depressant drugs, including nausea and vomiting.

3. Before administering buprenorphine hydrochloride, the nurse asks a patient if he has used opioids. Administering a mixed opioid agonist-antagonist to a patient dependent on opioid agonists may cause which reaction?
   A. Hypersensitivity reaction
   B. Constipation
   C. Urinary incontinence
   D. Withdrawal symptoms

Answer: D. Because they can counteract the effects of opioid agonists, mixed opioid agonist-antagonists can cause withdrawal symptoms in the patient who's dependent on opioid agonists.

4. The drug commonly prescribed to treat an opioid overdose is:
   A. pethidine.
   B. naloxone.
   C. pentazocine.
   D. naltrexone.

Answer: B. Naloxone is the drug of choice for managing an opioid overdose.

5. What are the most common adverse reactions to aspirin?
   A. Increased rate and depth of respirations
   B. Nausea, vomiting, and GI distress
   C. Dizziness and vision changes
   D. Bladder infection

Answer: B. Aspirin most commonly produces adverse GI reactions, such as nausea, vomiting, and GI distress.

6. Desflurane is which type of anaesthetic?
   A. General
   B. Local
   C. Topical
   D. I.V.

Answer: A. Desflurane is a commonly used general anaesthetic that's administered by inhalation.

7. A topical anaesthetic can be used:
    A. as an alternative to general anaesthesia for an elderly or debilitated patient.
    B. to numb a mucosal surface before tube insertion.
    C. when anaesthesia is needed for only a short period.
    D. to prevent or relieve pain in a specific area.

Answer: B. Topical anaesthetics are used to numb mucosal surfaces as well as relieve or prevent pain, relieve itching and irritation, anaesthetise an area for an injection, and alleviate sore throat or mouth pain.

Scoring

☆☆☆ If you answered all seven questions correctly, bravo! You're a pain medication powerhouse.

☆☆ If you answered five or six questions correctly, fabulous! For you, this chapter was painless.

☆ If you answered fewer than five questions correctly, hey, don't give up! Remember: No pain, no gain.

5 Cardiovascular drugs

Just the facts

In this chapter, you'll learn:

♦ classes of drugs used to treat cardiovascular disorders

♦ uses and varying actions of these drugs

♦ absorption, distribution, metabolism, and excretion of these drugs

♦ drug interactions and adverse reactions to these drugs.

Drugs and the cardiovascular system

Components of the cardiovascular system include the heart, arteries, veins, and lymphatics. These structures transport life-supporting oxygen and nutrients to cells, remove metabolic waste products, and carry hormones from one part of the body to another. Because this system performs such vital functions, any problem with the heart or blood vessels can seriously affect a person's health.

Types of drugs used to improve cardiovascular function include:
- inotropic drugs
- antiarrhythmic drugs
- anti-anginal drugs
- antihypertensive drugs
- diuretics
- antilipemic drugs.

Inotropic drugs

Inotropic drugs influence the contractility of muscular tissue. As a result, they increase the force of the heart's contractions (this is known as a *positive inotropic effect*). Cardiac glycosides and phosphodiesterase (PDE) inhibitors are two types of inotropic drugs.

In slow motion

Cardiac glycosides also slow the heart rate (a negative chronotropic effect) and slow electrical impulse conduction through the atrioventricular (AV) node (a negative dromotropic effect).

Cardiac glycosides

Cardiac glycosides are a group of drugs derived from digitalis, a substance that occurs naturally in foxglove plants. The most commonly used cardiac glycoside is digoxin. (See *Cardiac glycosides: Digoxin.*)

Pharmacokinetics

The intestinal absorption of digoxin varies greatly. Capsules are absorbed most efficiently, followed by the elixir form, and then tablets. Digoxin is distributed widely throughout the body with

Prototype pro

Cardiac glycosides: Digoxin

Actions

- Inhibits sodium-potassium-activated adenosine triphosphate, which regulates the amount of sodium and potassium inside the cell
- Promotes movement of calcium from extracellular to intracellular cytoplasm and strengthens myocardial contraction
- Acts on the central nervous system to enhance vagal tone, slowing contractions through the sinoatrial and atrioventricular nodes and providing an antiarrhythmic effect

Indications

- Heart failure
- Atrial fibrillation and flutter
- Supraventricular tachycardia

Nursing considerations

- Monitor the patient for adverse effects, such as fatigue, agitation, hallucinations, arrhythmias, anorexia, and nausea.
- Withhold the drug if the apical pulse is less than 60 beats/minute, and notify the prescriber.
- Periodically monitor serum potassium and digoxin levels.

highest concentrations in the heart muscle, liver, and kidneys. Digoxin is poorly bound to plasma proteins.

Going out the way it came in

In most patients, a small amount of digoxin is metabolised in the liver and gut by bacteria. This effect varies and may be substantial in some people. Most of the drug is excreted by the kidneys unchanged.

Pharmacodynamics

Digoxin is used to treat heart failure because it boosts intracellular calcium at the cell membrane, enabling stronger heart contractions. Digoxin may also enhance the movement of calcium into the myocardial cells and stimulate the release, or block the reuptake, of noradrenaline (norepinephrine) at the adrenergic nerve terminal.

What nerve!

Digoxin acts on the central nervous system (CNS) to slow the heart rate, thus making it useful for treating supraventricular arrhythmias (an abnormal heart rhythm that originates above the bundle branches of the heart's conduction system), such as atrial fibrillation and atrial flutter. It also increases the refractory period (the period when the cells of the conduction system can't conduct an impulse).

Pharmacotherapeutics

In addition to treating heart failure and supraventricular arrhythmias, digoxin is used to treat paroxysmal atrial tachycardia (an arrhythmia marked by brief periods of tachycardia that alternate with brief periods of sinus rhythm). (See *Load that dose*.)

Drug interactions

Many drugs can interact with digoxin:
• Rifampicin, barbituates, colestyramine, antacids, kaolin, sulfasalazine, neomycin, and metoclopramide reduce the therapeutic effects of digoxin.
• Calcium preparations, verapamil, ciclosporine, tetracycline, clarithromycin, propafenone, amiodarone, spironolactone, hydroxychloroquine, erythromycin, itraconazole, and omeprazole increase the risk of digoxin toxicity.
• Amphotericin B, potassium-wasting diuretics, and steroids taken with digoxin may cause hypokalaemia (low potassium levels) and increase the risk of digoxin toxicity.
• Beta-adrenergic blockers and calcium channel blockers taken with digoxin may cause an excessively slow heart rate and arrhythmias.

Digoxin gives me a real boost.

Load that dose

Because digoxin has a long half-life, a loading dose must be given to a patient who requires immediate drug effects, as in supraventricular arrhythmia. By giving a larger initial dose, a minimum effective concentration of the drug in the blood may be reached faster. *Note:* Loading doses should be avoided in patients with heart failure to avoid toxicity.

• Neuromuscular-blocking drugs, such as suxamethonium, and thyroid preparations, such as levothyroxine, increase the risk of arrhythmias when taken with digoxin.
• St. John's wort, a herbal preparation, can increase levels of digoxin and increase the risk of toxicity.

Adverse reactions

Because cardiac glycosides have a narrow therapeutic index (margin of safety), they may produce digoxin toxicity. To prevent digoxin toxicity, the dosage should be individualised based on the patient's serum digoxin concentration.

Signs and symptoms of digoxin toxicity include:
• nausea and vomiting
• abdominal pain
• diarrhoea
• headache
• irritability
• depression
• insomnia
• confusion
• vision changes
• arrhythmias
• complete heart block.

Nursing process

These nursing process steps are appropriate for patients undergoing treatment with cardiac glycosides.

Assessment
• Obtain a history of the underlying condition before therapy.
• Monitor drug effectiveness by taking the patient's apical pulse for 1 minute before each dose. Evaluate the electrocardiogram (ECG), when requested, and regularly assess the patient's cardiopulmonary status for signs of improvement.
• Monitor digoxin levels (therapeutic blood levels range from 0.5 to 2 ng/ml). Obtain blood for digoxin levels 8 hours after the last oral dose.
• Closely monitor potassium levels.
• Be alert for adverse reactions and drug interactions.

Key nursing diagnoses
• Decreased cardiac output related to underlying condition.
• Risk for injury related to adverse reactions.
• Risk for injury related to digoxin toxicity caused by the drug.
• Deficient knowledge related to drug therapy.

Planning outcome goals
- Cardiac output will improve as evidenced by vital signs, urine output, and level of consciousness.
- Risk for digoxin toxicity will be minimised.
- The patient will demonstrate correct drug administration.

Implementation
- Keep in mind that patients with hypothyroidism are extremely sensitive to glycosides and may need lower doses. Reduce the dosage in patients with impaired renal function.
- Before giving a loading dose, obtain baseline data (heart rate and rhythm, blood pressure, and electrolyte levels) and question the patient about recent use of cardiac glycosides (within the previous 3 weeks). The loading dose is always divided over the first 24 hours unless the clinical situation indicates otherwise.
- Before giving the drug, take the apical pulse for 1 full minute. Record and report to the prescriber significant changes (sudden increase or decrease in pulse rate, pulse deficit, irregular beats, and regularisation of previously irregular rhythm). If these changes occur, check blood pressure and obtain a 12-lead ECG.
- Withhold the drug and notify the prescriber if the pulse rate slows to 60 beats/minute or less.
- Infuse the I.V. form of the drug slowly over at least 5 minutes.
- Withhold the drug for 1 to 2 days before elective cardioversion. Adjust the dose after cardioversion.
- Remember that colestipol and colestyramine bind with the drug in the intestine. Treat arrhythmias with phenytoin I.V. or lidocaine I.V., and treat potentially life-threatening toxicity with specific antigen-binding fragments (such as Digoxin Immune Fab).

Evaluation
- Patient has adequate cardiac output.
- Patient has no digoxin toxicity.
- Patient and family understand drug therapy. (See *Teaching about digoxin*.)

Phosphodiesterase (PDE) inhibitors

PDE inhibitors are typically used for short-term management of heart failure or long-term management in patients awaiting heart transplant surgery. In the UK, two PDE inhibitors (enoximone and milrinone) have been approved for use.

Education edge

Teaching about digoxin

If digoxin is prescribed, review these points with the patient and caregivers:

- Digoxin helps strengthen the heartbeat and relieve ankle swelling, shortness of breath, and fatigue, which can accompany a heart problem.
- Take digoxin and other heart medications as prescribed, usually once daily, at the same time each day.
- Don't miss any doses of the medication.
- Don't take a double dose of the medication if a dose is missed.
- Don't take any over-the-counter medications or herbal remedies without first consulting with your prescriber.
- You will need to have periodic physical examinations, electrocardiograms, and blood tests (for digoxin as well as electrolytes) to see whether changes in dosages are needed.

- Report adverse effects, such as changes in heart rate or rhythm, nausea, vomiting, or vision problems, to your prescriber. These symptoms may mean that your dosage needs to be changed.
- Limit salt intake and be sure to get enough potassium. Follow the diet set by your prescriber, and don't take salt substitutes, such as potassium chloride, without first consulting with your prescriber.
- Use the same brand and type of digoxin all the time because forms and concentrations are different and aren't interchangeable.
- Take your pulse as instructed by your prescriber; count your pulse before each dose. If it's less than 60 beats/minute, call your prescriber.
- Don't crush digoxin capsules. Tablets may be crushed and can be taken with or after meals.
- If taking the liquid form of digoxin, measure accurately to prevent overdosage.

Pharmacokinetics

Enoximone is administered I.V., distributed rapidly, metabolised by the liver, and excreted by the kidneys.

Quick and short

Milrinone is also administered I.V. and is distributed rapidly and excreted by the kidneys, primarily as unchanged drug.

Pharmacodynamics

PDE inhibitors improve cardiac output by strengthening contractions. These drugs are thought to help move calcium into the cardiac cells or to increase calcium storage in the sarcoplasmic reticulum. By directly relaxing vascular smooth muscle, they also decrease peripheral vascular resistance (afterload) and the amount of blood returning to the heart (preload).

By decreasing my afterload and preload, PDE inhibitors certainly lighten my load.

Pharmacotherapeutics

Enoximone and milrinone are used for the management of heart failure in patients who haven't responded adequately to treatment with cardiac glycosides, diuretics, or vasodilators. Prolonged use of these drugs may increase the patient's risk of complications and death. (See *PDE inhibitors warning*.)

Drug interactions

PDE inhibitors may interact with disopyramide, causing hypotension. Because PDE inhibitors reduce serum potassium levels, taking them with a potassium-wasting diuretic may lead to hypokalaemia.

Adverse reactions

Adverse reactions to PDE inhibitors are uncommon, but the likelihood increases significantly with prolonged therapy. Adverse reactions may include:
- arrhythmias
- nausea and vomiting
- headache and fever
- chest pain
- hypokalaemia
- thrombocytopenia
- mild increase in heart rate.

Nursing process

These nursing process steps are appropriate for patients undergoing treatment with PDE inhibitors.

Assessment
- Assess the patient's heart failure before therapy and regularly thereafter.
- Monitor fluid and electrolyte status, blood pressure, heart rate, and kidney function during therapy.
- Monitor the patient's ECG continuously during therapy.
- Be alert for adverse reactions.
- Evaluate the patient's and family's knowledge of drug therapy.

Key nursing diagnoses
- Impaired gas exchange related to presence of heart failure.
- Decreased cardiac output related to drug-induced cardiac arrhythmias.
- Deficient knowledge related to drug therapy.

Before you give that drug!

Phosphodiesterase inhibitors warning

When giving PDE inhibitors, such as milrinone, remember that improvement of cardiac output may result in enhanced urine output. Expect a dosage reduction in diuretic therapy as heart failure improves. Potassium loss may predispose the patient to digoxin toxicity.

Planning outcome goals
- Adequate gas exchange will be achieved as evidenced by arterial blood gas values.
- Cardiac output will improve as evidenced by blood pressure, vital signs, and cardiac monitoring.
- The patient will demonstrate correct drug administration.

Implementation
- Know that milrinone typically is given with digoxin and diuretics.
- Keep in mind that inotropics may aggravate outflow tract obstruction in hypertrophic cardiomyopathy (also known as *idiopathic hypertrophic subaortic stenosis*).
- Prepare I.V. solutions in glucose 5% in water, normal saline solution, or half-normal saline solution.
- If an excessive decrease in blood pressure occurs, discontinue the drug or infuse it more slowly.
- Provide patient teaching.

Evaluation
- Patient exhibits adequate gas exchange as heart failure resolves.
- Drug-induced arrhythmias don't develop during therapy.
- Patient and family understand drug therapy.

Antiarrhythmic drugs

Antiarrhythmic drugs are used to treat arrhythmias (disturbances in the normal heart rhythm).

For better or worse?

Unfortunately, many antiarrhythmic drugs can also worsen or cause the very arrhythmias they're supposed to treat. Therefore, the benefits of this therapy must always be weighed against its risks.
Antiarrhythmics are categorised into four classes:
- I (which includes classes IA, IB, and IC)
- II
- III
- IV.

Class I antiarrhythmics, the largest group of antiarrhythmic drugs, consist of sodium channel blockers. Class I agents are usually subdivided into classes IA, IB, and IC. One drug, adenosine (an AV nodal-blocking agent used to treat paroxysmal supraventricular tachycardia [PSVT]), doesn't fall into any of these classes.

Be aware! Antiarrhythmics can actually worsen the arrhythmias they're prescribed to treat.

The mechanisms of action of antiarrhythmic drugs vary widely, and a few drugs exhibit properties common to more than one class.

Class IA antiarrhythmics

Class IA antiarrhythmics are used to treat a wide variety of atrial and ventricular arrhythmias. Class IA antiarrhythmics include:
- disopyramide phosphate
- procainamide hydrochloride

Pharmacokinetics

When administered orally, class IA drugs are rapidly absorbed and metabolised. Because they work so quickly, sustained-release forms of these drugs are available to help maintain therapeutic levels.

Not so brainy!

These drugs are distributed through all body tissues but do not cross the blood-brain barrier.

All class IA antiarrhythmics are metabolised in the liver and are excreted unchanged by the kidneys.

Pharmacodynamics

Class IA antiarrhythmics control arrhythmias by altering the myocardial cell membrane and interfering with autonomic nervous system control of pacemaker cells. (See *How class I antiarrhythmics work*.)

No (para)sympathy

Class IA antiarrhythmics also block parasympathetic stimulation of the sinoatrial (SA) and AV nodes. Because stimulation of the parasympathetic nervous system causes the heart rate to slow down, drugs that block the parasympathetic nervous system increase the conduction rate of the AV node.

A chain reaction

This increase in conduction rate can produce dangerous increases in ventricular heart rate if rapid atrial activity is present, as in a patient with atrial fibrillation. In turn, the increased ventricular heart rate can offset the ability of the antiarrhythmics to convert atrial arrhythmias to a regular rhythm.

Pharm function

How class I antiarrhythmics work

Class I antiarrhythmics block the sodium channels in the cell membrane during an action potential, which occurs among cardiac cells. This interferes with the conduction of impulses along the cells, producing a more membrane-stabilising effect. The antiarrhythmic agents bind more quickly to the sodium channels that are open or inactive before repolarisation has occurred in the cell. The drugs are most effective on tachycardia-type rhythms.

At phase 0, sodium enters the cell and class IA and IB antiarrhythmics slow the phase of the action potential.

Class 1C antiarrhythmics markedly slow phase 0 as well.

In phase 1 and phase 2, sodium levels equalise.

In phase 3, potassium leaves the cell; class IA antiarrhythmics work on this phase to block sodium channels. The sodium-potassium pump activates, restoring potassium to the inside of the cell and sodium to the outside of the cell.

In phase 4, potassium has left the cell, the cell membrane is impermeable to sodium, and the resting membrane potential is reached. Then the cell cycle begins again.

Action potential curve: Pacemaker cell

Pharmacotherapeutics

Class IA antiarrhythmics are used to treat certain arrhythmias, such as premature ventricular contractions, ventricular tachycardia, atrial fibrillation, atrial flutter, and paroxysmal atrial tachycardia. (See *Class IA antiarrhythmics: Disopyramide phosphate.*)

Prototype pro

Class IA antiarrhythmics: Disopyramide phosphate

Actions

- Causes direct and indirect effects on cardiac tissue
- Decreases automaticity, conduction velocity, and membrane responsiveness
- Prolongs effective refractory period

Indications

- Atrial fibrillation, flutter, and tachycardia
- Premature atrial and ventricular contractions
- Paroxysmal supraventricular tachycardia

Nursing considerations

- Monitor for adverse effects, such as vertigo, headache, arrhythmias, electrocradiogram changes (specifically, a widening QRS complex and prolonged QT interval), hypotension, heart failure, tinnitus, diarrhoea, nausea, vomiting, haematologic disorders, hepatotoxicity, respiratory arrest, angioedema, fever, and cinchonism.
- Frequently monitor pulse and blood pressure.
- Keep in mind that anticoagulation may be performed prior to treatment.

Drug interactions

Class IA antiarrhythmics can interact with other drugs in various ways:

- Disopyramide taken with macrolide antibiotics, such as clarithromycin and erythromycin, increases the risk of QT-interval prolongation, which may lead to an increased risk of arrhythmias, especially polymorphic ventricular tachycardia.
- Disopyramide plus verapamil may produce added myocardial depression and should be avoided in patients with heart failure.
- Other antiarrhythmics, such as beta-adrenergic blockers, increase the risk of arrhythmias.

Adverse reactions

Class IA antiarrhythmics, commonly produce GI symptoms, such as diarrhoea, cramping, nausea, vomiting, anorexia, and bitter taste.

Good news, bad news

Ironically, not only do class IA antiarrhythmics treat arrhythmias, but they can also induce arrhythmias, especially conduction delays that may worsen existing heart blocks.

Nursing process

These nursing process steps are appropriate for patients undergoing treatment with class IA antiarrhythmics.

Assessment
- Assess the patient's arrhythmia before therapy and regularly thereafter.
- Monitor the ECG continuously when therapy starts and when the dosage is adjusted. Specifically, monitor for ventricular arrhythmias and ECG changes (widening QRS complexes and a prolonged QT interval).
- Monitor the patient's vital signs frequently, and assess for signs of toxicity and adverse reactions.
- Measure apical pulse rate and blood pressure before giving the drug.
- Monitor serum drug levels as indicated.
- Monitor blood studies, such as liver function tests, as indicated.
- Be alert for adverse reactions and drug interactions.
- Evaluate the patient's and family's knowledge of drug therapy.

Key nursing diagnoses
- Decreased cardiac output related to arrhythmias or myocardial depression.
- Ineffective cardiopulmonary tissue perfusion related to adverse drug effects.
- Deficient knowledge related to drug therapy.

Planning outcome goals
- Cardiac output will improve as evidenced by stable blood pressure, cardiac monitoring, and adequate urine output.
- Complications from adverse reactions will be diminished.
- The patient will demonstrate correct drug administration.

Implementation
- Don't crush sustained-release tablets.
- Notify the prescriber about adverse reactions.
- Use I.V. forms of these drugs to treat acute arrhythmias.

Have you heard the news? Class IA antiarrhythmics can induce arrhythmias as well as treat them.

Education edge

Teaching about antiarrhythmics

If antiarrhythmics are prescribed, review these points with the patient and caregivers:

- Antiarrhythmic drug therapy helps stop irregular beats in the heart and helps it to beat more effectively.
- It's important to take the drug exactly as prescribed. You may need to use an alarm clock or other reminders if the medication needs to be taken at odd hours around the clock.
- Take your pulse before each dose. Notify your prescriber if your pulse is irregular or less than 60 beats/minute.
- Avoid hazardous activities that require mental alertness if adverse central nervous system reactions occur.
- Limit fluid and salt intake if the prescribed drug causes fluid retention.
- Disopyramide should be taken with food if GI upset occurs.
- Verapamil should be taken on an empty stomach or 1 to 2 hours after a meal.
- Some medications, may require you to limit intake of such foods as citrus juices, milk, and vegetables as well as avoid over-the counter

drugs (such as antacids) that make urine alkaline.
- Report adverse effects, such as constipation or diarrhoea, chest pain, difficulty breathing, ringing in the ears, swelling, unusually slow or fast pulse, sudden irregular pulse, or rash, to your prescriber.
- If tiredness occurs, space activities throughout the day and take periodic rest periods to help conserve energy.
- If nausea, vomiting, or loss of appetite occurs, eat small, frequent meals or take the drug with meals, if appropriate.
- Some medications, such as disopyramide, may make you more sensitive to light, so avoid prolonged exposure to sunlight.
- Avoid over-the-counter medications as well as herbal products unless approved by your prescriber. Many of these drugs and preparations can interfere with the action of antiarrhythmics.
- It's important to follow up with the prescriber to help evaluate heart rhythm and response to the drug.
- Don't stop taking the medication on your own; talk to your prescriber regarding any concerns.

Evaluation
- Patient maintains adequate cardiac output, as evidenced by normal vital signs and adequate tissue perfusion.
- Patient has no serious adverse reactions.
- Patient and family understand drug therapy. (See *Teaching about antiarrhythmics*.)

Class IB antiarrhythmics

Lidocaine and mexiletine are class IB antiarrhythmics, used for treating acute ventricular arrhythmias.

Pharmacokinetics

Lidocaine, is typically administered I.V., while other class IB antiarrhythmics are absorbed well from the GI tract after oral administration.

It's (un)bound to happen

Lidocaine is distributed widely throughout the body, including the brain. Both lidocaine and mexiletine are moderately bound to plasma proteins. (Remember, only the portion of a drug that's unbound can produce a response.)

Class IB antiarrhythmics are metabolised in the liver and excreted in the urine. Mexiletine also is excreted in breast milk.

Pharmacodynamics

Class IB drugs work by blocking the rapid influx of sodium ions during the depolarisation phase of the heart's depolarisation-repolarisation cycle. This results in a decreased refractory period, which reduces the risk of arrhythmias.

Don't worry! Plasma proteins like him can keep some antiarrhythmics occupied but my "unbound" portion will still get the job done.

Make an IB-line for the ventricle

Because class IB antiarrhythmics affect the Purkinje fibers (fibers in the conduction system of the heart) and myocardial cells in the ventricles, they're only used to treat ventricular arrhythmias. (See *Class IB antiarrhythmics: Lidocaine.*)

Prototype pro

Class IB antiarrhythmics: Lidocaine

Actions

- Decreases depolarisation, automaticity, and excitability in the ventricles during diastole by direct action on the tissues, especially the Purkinje network

Indications

- Ventricular arrhythmias

Nursing considerations

- Monitor for adverse effects, such as confusion, tremor, restlessness, seizures, hypotension, new arrhythmias, cardiac arrest, tinnitus, blurred vision, respiratory depression, and anaphylaxis.
- Monitor serum lidocaine levels for toxicity.
- Monitor electrolytes, blood urea nitrogen, and creatinine levels.

Pharmacotherapeutics

Class IB antiarrhythmics are used to treat ventricular ectopic beats, ventricular tachycardia, and ventricular fibrillation.

Drug interactions

Class IB antiarrhythmics may exhibit additive or antagonistic effects when administered with other antiarrhythmics, such as phenytoin, propranolol, and procainamide.

In addition:
- Theophylline plasma levels are increased when theophylline is given with mexiletine.
- Use of a beta-adrenergic blocker or disopyramide with mexiletine may reduce the contractility of the heart.

Adverse reactions

Adverse reactions to class IB antiarrhythmics include:
- drowsiness
- light-headedness
- paraesthesia
- sensory disturbances
- hypotension
- bradycardia.

Adverse reactions to mexiletine also include hypotension, atrioventricular block, bradycardia, confusion, ataxia, and double vision. Mexiletine may produce nausea and vomiting.

In addition, lidocaine toxicity can cause seizures and respiratory and cardiac arrest.

All four classes of antiarrhythmics treat disturbances of heart rhythm. However, combining these drugs can result in adverse drug interactions.

Nursing process

These nursing process steps are appropriate for patients undergoing treatment with class IB antiarrhythmics.

Assessment
- Assess the patient's arrhythmia before therapy and regularly thereafter.
- Monitor the ECG continuously when therapy starts and when the dosage is adjusted. A patient receiving the drug via infusion must be on the cardiac monitor and be attended at all times.
- Monitor the patient's vital signs frequently, especially ECG and blood pressure.
- Assess for adverse reactions and signs of toxicity. As blood levels of lidocaine increase, nervousness, confusion, dizziness, tinnitus, somnolence, paraesthesia, and circumoral numbness may occur. Acute toxicity may result in seizures, cardiovascular collapse, and respiratory arrest.
- Measure apical pulse rate and blood pressure before giving the drug.

- Monitor serum drug levels as indicated. Therapeutic levels for lidocaine are 2 to 5 mcg/ml.
- Monitor blood studies as indicated, such as liver function tests, blood urea nitrogen (BUN), and creatinine levels.
- Evaluate the patient's and family's knowledge of drug therapy.

Key nursing diagnoses
- Decreased cardiac output related to arrhythmias or myocardial depression.
- Risk for injury related to adverse reactions.
- Deficient knowledge related to drug therapy.

Planning outcome goals
- Cardiac output will improve as evidenced by stable blood pressure, cardiac monitoring, and adequate urine output.
- Complications from adverse reactions will be diminished.
- The patient will demonstrate correct drug administration.

Implementation
- Use an infusion-control device to administer the infusion. If giving lidocaine, don't exceed 4 mg/minute; a faster rate greatly increases the risk of toxicity.
- Dilute concentrated forms for I.V. infusion.
- If administering the drug via the I.M. route (alternative route for lidocaine), give in the deltoid area.
- Remember that I. M. injections increase creatine kinase (CK) levels. The CK-MM isoenzyme (which originates in skeletal muscle, not cardiac muscle) level increases significantly in patients who receive an I.M. injection.
- Don't crush sustained-release tablets.
- Be aware that sustained-release and extended-release medications aren't interchangeable.
- Take safety precautions if adverse CNS reactions occur.
- Notify the prescriber about adverse reactions. If signs of lidocaine toxicity occur, stop the drug at once and notify the prescriber. Continued infusion could lead to seizures, cardiovascular collapse, coma, and respiratory arrest.
- Use I.V. forms of these drugs to treat acute arrhythmias. Discontinue the drug and notify the prescriber if arrhythmias worsen or if ECG changes, such as widening QRS complex or substantially prolonged PR interval, are evident.
- Provide patient teaching.

Evaluation
- Patient maintains adequate cardiac output, as evidenced by normal vital signs and adequate tissue perfusion.

- Patient has no serious adverse reactions.
- Patient and family understand drug therapy.

Class IC antiarrhythmics

Class IC antiarrhythmics are used to treat certain severe, refractory (resistant) ventricular arrhythmias. Class IC antiarrhythmics include:
- flecainide acetate
- propafenone hydrochloride
- moracizine (a class I antiarrhythmic drug that shares class IA, IB, and IC properties and is available on a named patient basis).

Pharmacokinetics

After oral administration, class IC antiarrhythmics are absorbed well, distributed in varying degrees, and probably metabolised by the liver. They're excreted primarily by the kidneys, except for propafenone, which is excreted primarily in faeces. (See *Class IC antiarrhythmics: Propafenone.*) After oral administration, about 38% of moracizine is absorbed. It undergoes extensive metabolism, with less than 1% of a dose excreted unchanged in the urine. Moracizine is highly protein bound, leaving only a small portion of the drug free to produce its antiarrhythmic effect.

Pharmacodynamics

Class IC antiarrhythmics primarily slow conduction along the heart's conduction system. Moracizine decreases the fast inward current of sodium ions of the action potential, depressing the depolarisation rate and effective refractory period.

Pharmacotherapeutics

Like class IB antiarrhythmics, class IC antiarrhythmic drugs are used to treat life-threatening ventricular arrhythmias. They're also used to treat supraventricular arrhythmias (abnormal heart rhythms that originate above the bundle branches of the heart's conduction system).

Flecainide and propafenone may also be used to prevent PSVT in patients without structural heart disease. Moracizine is used to manage life-threatening ventricular arrhythmias such as sustained ventricular tachycardia.

Prototype pro

Class IC antiarrhythmics: Propafenone

Actions

- Reduces inward sodium current in Purkinje and myocardial cells
- Decreases excitability, conduction velocity, and automaticity in atrioventricular (AV) nodal, His-Purkinje, and intraventricular tissue
- Prolongs refractory period in AV nodal tissue

Indications

- Ventricular arrhythmias

Nursing considerations

- Administer with food to minimise adverse GI reactions.
- Notify the prescriber if QRS complex increases by more than 25%.
- During use with digoxin, monitor electrocardiogram and digoxin levels frequently.

Drug interactions

Class IC antiarrhythmics may exhibit additive effects when administered with other antiarrhythmics. Here are some other interactions:

- When used with digoxin, flecainide and propafenone increase the risk of digoxin toxicity.
- Cimetidine may increase the plasma level and the risk of toxicity of moracizine.
- Propranolol or digoxin given with moricizine may increase the PR interval.
- Theophylline levels may be reduced in the patient receiving moracizine.
- Propafenone increases the serum concentration and effects of metoprolol and propranolol.

Adverse reactions

Class IC antiarrhythmics can produce serious adverse reactions, including the development of new arrhythmias and aggravation of existing arrhythmias (especially with moracizine). These drugs aren't given to patients with structural heart defects because of a high incidence of resulting mortality. Other cardiovascular adverse reactions include palpitations, shortness of breath, chest pain, heart failure, and cardiac arrest.

Because propafenone has beta-adrenergic blocking properties, it may also cause bronchospasm.

Can't stomach it

GI adverse reactions include abdominal pain, heartburn, nausea, and vomiting.

Nursing process

These nursing process steps are appropriate for patients undergoing treatment with class IC antiarrhythmics.

Assessment

- Assess the patient's arrhythmia before therapy and regularly thereafter.
- Monitor the ECG continuously when therapy starts and when the dosage is adjusted.
- Monitor the patient's vital signs frequently and assess for signs of toxicity and adverse reactions.
- Measure the apical pulse rate and blood pressure before giving the drug.

- Monitor serum drug levels as indicated.
- Monitor blood studies, such as liver function tests, as indicated.
- Be alert for adverse reactions and drug interactions.
- Evaluate the patient's and family's knowledge of drug therapy.

Key nursing diagnoses
- Decreased cardiac output related to arrhythmias or myocardial depression.
- Risk for injury related to adverse reactions.
- Deficient knowledge related to drug therapy.

Planning outcome goals
- Cardiac output will improve as evidenced by stable blood pressure, cardiac monitoring, and adequate urine output.
- Complications from adverse reactions will be diminished.
- The patient will demonstrate correct drug administration.

Implementation
- Don't crush sustained-release tablets.
- Take safety precautions if adverse CNS reactions occur.
- Notify the prescriber about adverse reactions.
- Use I.V. forms of these drugs to treat acute arrhythmias.
- Administer the drug with food to minimise adverse reactions as indicated.
- Notify the prescriber if the PR interval or QRS complex increases by more than 25%. Reduction in dosage may be necessary.
- Monitor the ECG and digoxin levels frequently if used with digoxin.
- Provide patient teaching.

Evaluation
- Patient maintains adequate cardiac output, as evidenced by normal vital signs and adequate tissue perfusion.
- Patient has no serious adverse reactions.
- Patient and family understand drug therapy.

Class II antiarrhythmics

Class II antiarrhythmics are composed of beta-adrenergic antagonists, which are also known as *beta-adrenergic blockers* or *beta blockers*. Beta-adrenergic blockers used as antiarrhythmics include:
- acebutolol
- esmolol
- propranolol.

Pharmacokinetics

Acebutolol and propranolol are absorbed almost entirely from the GI tract after an oral dose. Esmolol, which can only be given I.V., is immediately available throughout the body.

No breaking and entering

Acebutolol and esmolol have low lipid solubility. That means that they can't penetrate the blood-brain barrier (highly fatty cells that act as barriers between the blood and brain). Propranolol has high lipid solubility and readily crosses the blood-brain barrier.

Just a little gets the job done

Propranolol undergoes significant first-pass effect, leaving only a small portion of this drug available to be distributed to the body.

Esmolol is metabolised exclusively by red blood cells (RBCs), with only 1% excreted in the urine. Approximately 50% of acebutolol is excreted in faeces. Propranolol's metabolites are excreted in urine as well.

Pharmacodynamics

Class II antiarrhythmics block beta-adrenergic receptor sites in the conduction system of the heart. As a result, the ability of the SA node to fire spontaneously (automaticity) is slowed. The ability of the AV node and other cells to receive and conduct an electrical impulse to nearby cells (conductivity) is also reduced.

Class II antiarrhythmics also reduce the strength of the heart's contractions. When the heart beats less forcefully, it doesn't require as much oxygen to do its work.

Pharmacotherapeutics

Class II antiarrhythmics slow ventricular rates in patients with atrial flutter, atrial fibrillation, and paroxysmal atrial tachycardia.

Drug interactions

Class II antiarrhythmics can cause a variety of drug interactions:
• Administering class II antiarrhythmics with phenothiazines and other antihypertensive drugs increases the antihypertensive effect.
• Administration with nonsteroidal anti-inflammatory drugs (NSAIDs) can cause fluid and water retention, decreasing the antihypertensive effects of the drug.
• The effects of sympathomimetics may be reduced when taken with class II antiarrhythmics.

Hmph! I know when I'm not needed.

• Beta-adrenergic blockers given with verapamil can depress the heart, causing hypotension, bradycardia, AV block, and asystole.
• Beta-adrenergic blockers reduce the effects of sulphonylureas.
• The risk of digoxin toxicity increases when digoxin is taken with esmolol.

Adverse reactions

Common adverse reactions to class II antiarrhythmics include:
• arrhythmias
• bradycardia
• heart failure
• hypotension
• GI reactions, such as nausea, vomiting, and diarrhoea
• bronchoconstriction.

Nursing process

These nursing process steps are appropriate for patients undergoing treatment with class II antiarrhythmics.

Assessment

• Assess the patient's arrhythmia before therapy and regularly thereafter.
• Monitor the ECG continuously when therapy starts, when dosage is adjusted, and especially during I.V. therapy.
• Monitor the patient's vital signs frequently, and assess for signs of toxicity and adverse reactions.
• Measure the apical pulse rate and blood pressure before giving the drug.
• Monitor serum drug levels as indicated.
• Monitor blood studies, such as liver function tests, as indicated.
• Be alert for adverse reactions and drug interactions.
• Evaluate the patient's and family's knowledge of drug therapy.

Key nursing diagnoses

• Decreased cardiac output related to arrhythmias or myocardial depression.
• Risk for injury related to adverse reactions.
• Deficient knowledge related to drug therapy.

Planning outcome goals

• Cardiac output will improve as evidenced by stable blood pressure, cardiac monitoring, and adequate urine output.
• Complications from adverse reactions will be diminished.
• The patient will demonstrate correct drug administration.

Implementation
- Don't crush sustained-release tablets.
- Take safety precautions if adverse CNS reactions occur.
- Notify the prescriber about adverse reactions.
- Use I.V. forms of these drugs for treating acute arrhythmias; they may be given as loading dose I.V. or diluted with normal saline solution and given by intermittent infusion.
- Check the apical pulse before giving the drug. If extremes in pulse rate are detected, withhold the drug and call the prescriber immediately.
- Administer the drug with meals as indicated.
- Before any surgical procedure, notify the anaesthetist that the patient is receiving this drug.
- Don't discontinue the I.V. abruptly.
- Provide patient teaching.

Evaluation
- Patient maintains adequate cardiac output, as evidenced by normal vital signs and adequate tissue perfusion.
- Patient has no serious adverse reactions.
- Patient and family understand drug therapy.

Class III antiarrhythmics

Class III antiarrhythmics are used to treat ventricular arrhythmias. Drugs in this class include amiodarone and sotalol.

Sotalol is a nonselective (not having a specific affinity for a receptor) beta-adrenergic blocker (class II) that also has class III properties. The class III antiarrhythmic effects are more predominant, especially at higher doses, so sotalol is usually listed as a class III antiarrhythmic.

Pharmacokinetics
The absorption of class III antiarrhythmics varies widely.

Slow but sure

After oral administration, amiodarone is absorbed slowly at widely varying rates. This drug is distributed extensively and accumulates in many sites, especially in organs with a rich blood supply and fatty tissue. It's highly protein bound in plasma, mainly to albumin.

Sotalol is also slowly absorbed, with the amount varying between 60% and 100% with minimal protein binding.

Pharmacodynamics

Although the exact mechanism of action isn't known, class III antiarrhythmics are thought to suppress arrhythmias by converting a unidirectional block to a bidirectional block. They have little or no effect on depolarisation. These drugs slow repolarisation and prolong the refractory period and duration of the action potential.

Pharmacotherapeutics

Class III antiarrhythmics are used for life-threatening arrhythmias. Amiodarone is the first-line drug of choice for ventricular tachycardia and ventricular fibrillation. (See *Class III antiarrhythmics: Amiodarone.*)

Prototype pro

Class III antiarrhythmics: Amiodarone

Actions

- Thought to prolong refractory period and duration of action potential and to decrease repolarisation

Indications

- Life-threatening ventricular arrhythmias
- Suppression of supraventricular tachycardias

Nursing considerations

- Be aware that the drug poses major and potentially life-threatening management problems in patients at risk for sudden death and should be used only in patients with documented, life-threatening, recurrent ventricular arrhythmias who are nonresponsive to adequate doses of other antiarrhythmics, or when alternative drugs can't be tolerated.
- Know that amiodarone can cause fatal toxicities, including hepatic and pulmonary toxicity.
- Be aware that the drug causes vision impairment; most adults taking amiodarone develop corneal microdeposits, and cases of optic neuritis have been reported.
- Administer an oral loading dose in three equal doses; give with meals to decrease GI intolerance.
- Only give the drug I.V. if the patient is closely monitored for cardiac function and resuscitation equipment is available.
- Oral forms of the drug shouldn't be taken with grapefruit juice because it interferes with drug metabolism.

Drug interactions

These drug interactions can occur with class III antiarrhythmics:
- Amiodarone increases procainamide, and phenytoin levels.
- Amiodarone increases the risk of digoxin toxicity.
- Sotalol shouldn't be administered with dolasetron because of an increased risk of life-threatening arrhythmias.
- Severe hypotension may develop when I.V. amiodarone is administered too rapidly.

Adverse reactions

Adverse reactions to class III antiarrhythmics, especially amiodarone, vary widely and commonly lead to drug discontinuation. A common adverse effect is aggravation of arrhythmias.

Other adverse reactions vary by drug:
- Amiodarone may also produce hypotension, nausea, and anorexia. Severe pulmonary toxicity occurs in 15% of patients and can be fatal. Vision disturbances and corneal microdeposits may also occur.
- Sotalol may cause AV block, bradycardia, ventricular arrhythmias, bronchospasm, and hypotension.

Nursing process

These nursing process steps are appropriate for patients undergoing treatment with class III antiarrhythmics.

Assessment
- Assess the patient's arrhythmia before therapy and regularly thereafter.
- Monitor the ECG continuously when therapy starts and when the dosage is adjusted.
- Monitor the patient's vital signs frequently, and assess for signs of toxicity and adverse reactions.
- Measure the apical pulse rate and blood pressure before giving the drug.
- Monitor serum drug levels as indicated.
- Monitor blood studies, such as liver function tests, as indicated.
- Be alert for adverse reactions and drug interactions.
- Evaluate the patient's and family's knowledge of drug therapy.

Key nursing diagnoses
- Decreased cardiac output related to arrhythmias or myocardial depression.
- Risk for injury related to adverse reactions.
- Deficient knowledge related to drug therapy.

Planning outcome goals
- Cardiac output will improve as evidenced by stable blood pressure, cardiac monitoring, and adequate urine output.
- Complications from adverse reactions will be diminished.
- The patient will demonstrate correct drug administration.

Implementation
- During and after administration, proper equipment and facilities, such as cardiac monitoring, intracardiac pacing, a cardioverter-defibrillator, and medication for treatment of sustained ventricular tachycardia, should be available.
- Correct hypokalaemia and hypomagnesaemia before therapy to reduce the risk of arrhythmias.
- Remember that admixtures and approved diluents are chemically and physically stable for 24 hours at room temperature, or 48 hours if refrigerated.
- Don't crush sustained-release tablets.
- Be aware that sustained-release and extended-release medications aren't interchangeable.
- Take safety precautions if adverse CNS reactions occur.
- Notify the prescriber about adverse reactions.
- Use I.V. forms of the drug to treat acute arrhythmias.
- Provide patient teaching.

Evaluation
- Patient maintains adequate cardiac output, as evidenced by normal vital signs and adequate tissue perfusion.
- Patient has no serious adverse reactions.
- Patient states the importance of compliance with therapy.

Class IV antiarrhythmics

Class IV antiarrhythmics are composed of calcium channel blockers. Calcium channel blockers used to treat arrhythmias include verapamil and diltiazem.

One mission

Verapamil and diltiazem are used to treat supraventricular arrhythmias with rapid ventricular response rates (rapid heart rate in which the rhythm originates above the ventricles).

Pharmacokinetics

Class IV antiarrhythmics are rapidly and completely absorbed from the GI tract after oral administration; only about 20% to 35% reaches systemic circulation. About 90% of the circulating drug is bound to plasma proteins. Class IV antiarrhythmics are metabolised in the liver and excreted in the urine as unchanged drug and active metabolites.

Pharmacodynamics

Class IV antiarrhythmics inhibit calcium ion influx across cardiac and smooth muscle cells, thus decreasing myocardial contractility and oxygen demand. They also dilate coronary arteries and arterioles.

Pharmacotherapeutics

This class of drugs is used to relieve angina, lower blood pressure, and restore normal sinus rhythm.

Drug interactions

These drug interactions may occur with class IV antiarrhythmics:
- Furosemide forms a precipitate when mixed with diltiazem injection. Give through separate I.V. lines.
- Anaesthetics may potentiate the effects of medication.
- Ciclosporine levels may be increased by diltiazem, resulting in toxicity; avoid using these drugs together.
- Diltiazem may increase levels of digoxin. Monitor the patient and drug levels.
- Propranolol and other beta-adrenergic blockers may precipitate heart failure or prolong cardiac conduction time with diltiazem and, therefore, should be used together cautiously.
- Antihypertensives may cause hypotension when used with verapamil; monitor blood pressure.
- Disopyramide, propranolol, and other beta-adrenergic blockers may cause heart failure when used with verapamil.
- Verapamil may decrease lithium levels.
- Rifampicin may decrease the effects of verapamil.
- Black catechu may cause additive effects when used with verapamil.

Class IV antiarrhythmics are used to relieve angina, lower blood pressure, and restore normal sinus rhythm.

Don't drink and...

- Verapamil enhances the effect of alcohol; discourage concurrent use.

Adverse reactions

The following adverse effects can occur when taking class IV antiarrhythmics.

Mild effects
- Dizziness
- Headache
- Hypotension
- Constipation
- Nausea
- Rash

Serious effects
- Heart failure
- Bradycardia
- AV block
- Ventricular asystole
- Ventricular fibrillation
- Pulmonary oedema

Nursing process

These nursing process steps are appropriate for patients undergoing treatment with class IV antiarrhythmics.

Assessment
- Obtain a history of the patient's underlying condition before therapy, and reassess regularly thereafter.
- Assess the patient's arrhythmia before therapy and regularly thereafter.
- Monitor the ECG continuously when therapy starts and when the dosage is adjusted.
- Monitor the patient's vital signs frequently, and assess for signs of toxicity and adverse reactions.
- Measure the apical pulse rate and blood pressure before giving the drug.
- Monitor serum drug levels as indicated.
- Monitor blood studies, such as liver function tests, as indicated.
- Be alert for adverse reactions and drug interactions.
- Evaluate the patient's and family's knowledge of drug therapy.

Key nursing diagnoses
- Decreased cardiac output related to arrhythmias or myocardial depression.
- Risk for injury related to adverse reactions.
- Deficient knowledge related to drug therapy.

Planning outcome goals
- Cardiac output will improve as evidenced by stable blood pressure, cardiac monitoring, and adequate urine output.
- Complications from adverse reactions will be diminished.
- The patient will demonstrate correct drug administration.

Implementation
- Don't crush sustained-release tablets.
- Know that sustained-release and extended-release drug forms aren't interchangeable.
- Fluid and sodium intake may need to be restricted to minimise oedema.
- Take safety precautions if adverse CNS reactions occur.
- Notify the prescriber about adverse reactions.
- Use I.V. forms of the drug for treating acute arrhythmias; cardiac monitoring is required during administrations.
- Withhold the dose and notify the prescriber if systolic pressure is below 90 mm Hg or heart rate is less than 60 beats/minute, or follow the prescriber's parameters for withholding the medication.
- Assist the patient with walking because dizziness can occur.
- If the drugs are being used to terminate supraventricular tachycardia, the prescriber may have the patient perform vagal manoeuvers after receiving the drug.
- Provide patient teaching.

Evaluation
- Patient maintains adequate cardiac output, as evidenced by normal vital signs and adequate tissue perfusion.
- Patient has no serious adverse reactions.
- Patient states the importance of compliance with therapy.

Adenosine

Adenosine is an injectable antiarrhythmic drug indicated for acute treatment of PSVT.

Pharmacokinetics

After I.V. administration, adenosine probably is distributed rapidly throughout the body and metabolised inside RBCs as well as in vascular endothelial cells.

Pharmacodynamics

Adenosine depresses the pacemaker activity of the SA node, reducing heart rate and the ability of the AV node to conduct impulses from the atria to the ventricles.

Pharmacotherapeutics

Adenosine is especially effective against reentry tachycardias (when an impulse depolarises an area of heart muscle and returns and repolarises it) that involve the AV node.

Gets the job done

Adenosine is also effective in more than 90% of PSVT cases. It's predominantly used to treat arrhythmias associated with accessory bypass tracts (brief periods of rapid heart rate in which the rhythm's origin is above the ventricle), as in Wolff-Parkinson-White syndrome, a condition in which strands of heart tissue formed during foetal development abnormally connect structures, such as the atria and ventricles, bypassing normal conduction. This condition is also known as a *preexcitation syndrome*.

Drug interactions

Adenosine has various drug interactions:
- Methylxanthines antagonise the effects of adenosine so that larger doses of adenosine may be necessary.
- Dipyridamole and carbamazepine potentiate the effects of adenosine; therefore, smaller doses of adenosine may be necessary.
- When adenosine is administered with carbamazepine, the risk of heart block increases.

Adverse reactions

Adenosine many cause facial flushing, shortness of breath, dyspnea, and chest discomfort.

Nursing process

These nursing process steps are appropriate for patients undergoing treatment with adenosine.

Assessment
• Assess the patient's arrhythmia before therapy and regularly thereafter.
• Monitor the ECG continuously when therapy starts and when the dosage is adjusted.
• Monitor the patient's vital signs frequently, and assess for signs of toxicity and adverse reactions.
• Measure the apical pulse rate and blood pressure before giving the drug.
• Be alert for adverse reactions and drug interactions.
• Evaluate the patient's and family's knowledge of drug therapy.

Key nursing diagnoses
• Decreased cardiac output related to arrhythmias or myocardial depression.
• Risk for injury related to adverse reactions.
• Deficient knowledge related to drug therapy.

Planning outcome goals
• Cardiac output will improve as evidenced by stable blood pressure, cardiac monitoring, and adequate urine output.
• Complications from adverse reactions will be diminished.
• The patient will demonstrate correct drug administration.

Implementation
• If the solution is cold, check for crystals that may form. If crystals are visible, gently warm the solution to room temperature. Don't use unclear solutions.
• Give rapidly for effective drug action. Give directly into the vein, if possible. If an I.V. line is used, inject the drug into the most proximal port and follow with a rapid saline flush to ensure that the drug reaches systemic circulation quickly.
• If ECG disturbances occur, withhold the drug, obtain a rhythm strip, and notify the prescriber immediately.
• Take safety precautions if adverse CNS reactions occur.
• Notify the prescriber about adverse reactions.

Evaluation
• Patient maintains adequate cardiac output, as evidenced by normal vital signs and adequate tissue perfusion.
• Patient has no serious adverse reactions.
• Patient states the importance of compliance with therapy.

Antianginal drugs

Although angina's cardinal symptom is chest pain, the drugs used to treat angina aren't typically analgesics. Rather, antianginal drugs treat angina by reducing myocardial oxygen demand (reducing the amount of oxygen the heart needs to do its work), by increasing the supply of oxygen to the heart, or both. (See *How antianginal drugs work*.)

Pharm function

How antianginal drugs work

Angina occurs when the coronary arteries, the heart's primary source of oxygen, supply insufficient oxygen to the myocardium. This increases the heart's workload, increasing heart rate, preload (blood volume in ventricle at end of diastole), afterload (pressure in arteries leading from ventricle), and force of myocardial contractility. The antianginal drugs relieve angina by decreasing one or more of these four factors. This diagram summarises how antianginal drugs affect the cardiovascular system.

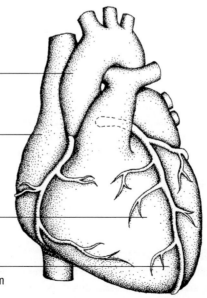

Afterload
Decreased by calcium channel blockers and nitrates

Heart rate
Decreased by beta-adrenergic blockers and some calcium channel blockers

Preload
Decreased by nitrates

Contractility
Decreased by beta-adrenergic blockers and calcium channel blockers

The three classes of antianginal drugs discussed in this section include:
- nitrates (for treating acute angina)
- beta-adrenergic blockers (for long-term prevention of angina)
- calcium channel blockers (used when other drugs fail to prevent angina).

Nitrates

Nitrates are the drugs of choice for relieving acute angina. Nitrates commonly prescribed to treat angina include:
- isosorbide dinitrate
- isosorbide mononitrate
- glyceryl trinitrate.

Pharmacokinetics
Nitrates can be administered in a variety of ways.

All absorbed...

Nitrates given sublingually (under the tongue), buccally (in the pocket of the cheek), as chewable tablets, as lingual aerosols (sprayed onto or under the tongue), are absorbed almost completely because of the rich blood supply of the mucous membranes of the mouth.

...half-absorbed...

Swallowed nitrate capsules are absorbed through the mucous membranes of the GI tract, and only about half the dose enters circulation.

Transdermal nitrates (a patch or ointment placed on the skin) are absorbed slowly and in varying amounts, depending on the quantity of drug applied, the location where the patch is applied, the surface area of skin used, and the circulation to the skin.

...or not absorbed at all

I.V. glyceryl trinitrate, which doesn't need to be absorbed, goes directly into circulation. (See *Nitrates: Glyceryl trinitrate.*)

Pharmacodynamics
Nitrates cause the smooth muscle of the veins and, to a lesser extent, the arteries to relax and dilate. Nitrates work in the following way:
- When the veins dilate, less blood returns to the heart.

Prototype pro

Nitrates: Glyceryl trinitrate

Actions
- Relaxes vascular smooth muscle
- Causes general vasodilation

Indications
- Acute or chronic anginal attacks

Nursing considerations
- Monitor for adverse effects, such as headache, dizziness, orthostatic hypotension, tachycardia, flushing, palpitations, and hypersensitivity reactions.
- Monitor vital signs closely.
- Treat headaches with paracetamol or aspirin.

- This, in turn, reduces the amount of blood in the ventricles at the end of diastole, when the ventricles are full. (This blood volume in the ventricles just before contraction is called *preload*.)
- By reducing preload, nitrates reduce ventricular size and ventricular wall tension (the left ventricle doesn't have to stretch as much to pump blood). This, in turn, reduces the oxygen requirements of the heart.

Lighten the load

The arterioles provide the most resistance to the blood pumped by the left ventricle (called *peripheral vascular resistance*). Nitrates decrease afterload by dilating the arterioles, reducing resistance, easing the heart's workload, and easing the demand for oxygen.

Pharmacotherapeutics

Nitrates are used to relieve and prevent angina.

The short story...

Rapidly absorbed nitrates, such as glyceryl trinitrate, are the drugs of choice for relief of acute angina because they have a rapid onset of action, are easy to take, and are inexpensive.

...or the long one

Longer-acting nitrates, such as the daily glyceryl trinitrate transdermal patch, are convenient and can be used to prevent chronic angina. Oral nitrates are also used because they seldom produce serious adverse reactions.

Drug interactions

These drug interactions may occur with nitrates:
- Severe hypotension can result when nitrates interact with alcohol.
- Sildenafil shouldn't be taken within 24 hours of nitrates because of possible enhanced hypotensive effects.
- Absorption of sublingual nitrates may be delayed when taken with an anticholinergic drug.
- Marked orthostatic hypotension (a drop in blood pressure when a person stands up) with light-headedness, fainting, or blurred vision may occur when calcium channel blockers and nitrates are used together.

Nitrates are used to treat acute angina because of their rapid onset of action.

Adverse reactions

Most adverse reactions to nitrates are caused by changes in the cardiovascular system. The reactions usually disappear when the dosage is reduced.

Headache is the most common adverse reaction. Hypotension may occur, accompanied by dizziness and increased heart rate.

Nursing process

These nursing process steps are appropriate for patients undergoing treatment with nitrates.

Assessment

• Monitor vital signs. With I.V. glyceryl trinitrate, monitor blood pressure and pulse rate every 5 to 15 minutes while adjusting dosage and every hour thereafter.
• Monitor the effectiveness of the prescribed drug.
• Observe for adverse reactions.

Key nursing diagnoses

• Risk for injury related to adverse reactions.
• Excess fluid volume related to adverse cardiovascular effects.
• Deficient knowledge related to drug therapy.

Planning outcome goals

• Risk of injury to the patient will be minimised.
• Fluid volume will remain within normal limits as evidenced by vital signs, cardiac monitoring, and urine output.
• The patient will demonstrate correct drug administration.

Implementation

• Tablets may be given on an empty stomach, either 30 minutes before or 1 to 2 hours after meals. Tell the patient to swallow tablets whole (not chew them).
• Have the patient sit or lie down when receiving the first nitrate dose. Take the patients pulse and blood pressure before giving the dose and when the drug action starts.
• Don't give a beta-adrenergic blocker or calcium channel blocker to relieve acute angina.
• Withhold the dose and notify the prescriber if the patient's heart rate is less than 60 beats/minute or systolic blood pressure is below 90 mm Hg, or follow the prescriber's parameters for withholding the medication.
• Dilute I.V. glyceryl trinitrate with glucose 5% in water, or normal saline solution for injection, using a glass bottle. Avoid the use of I.V. filters because the drug binds to plastic. Special

Education edge

Teaching about anti-anginals

If antianginals are prescribed, review these points with the patient and caregivers:

- It's essential to understand how to use the prescribed form of the drug.
- It's important to take the drug regularly, as prescribed, and to have it accessible at all times.
- Don't discontinue the drug abruptly without your prescriber's approval. Coronary vasospasm can occur.
- If taking nitrates, an additional dose may be required before anticipated stress or at bedtime if angina is nocturnal. Check with your prescriber.
- Use caution when wearing a transdermal patch near a microwave oven. Leaking radiation may heat the metallic backing of the patch and cause burns.
- Avoid alcohol during drug therapy.
- Change to an upright position slowly. Go up and down stairs carefully, and lie down at the first sign of dizziness.

- Store nitrates in a cool, dark place in a tightly closed container. To ensure freshness, replace sublingual tablets every 3 months and remove the cotton wool because it absorbs the drug.
- Store sublingual tablets in their original container or another container specifically approved for this use, and carry the container in a jacket pocket or purse, not in a pocket close to the body.
- As indicated, take your pulse before taking the medication, such as with beta-adrenergic blockers and calcium channel blockers. Withhold the dose and alert your prescriber if your pulse rate is below 60 beats/minute.
- If taking glyceryl trinitrate sublingually, go to the emergency department if three tablets taken 5 minutes apart don't relieve anginal pain.
- Report serious or persistent adverse reactions to your prescriber.

nonabsorbent polyvinyl chloride tubing is available from the manufacturer. Administer the drug with an infusion control device. Concentration shouldn't exceed 400 mcg/ml.

• Administer sublingual glyceryl trinitrate tablets at the first sign of an attack, placing the medication under the tongue until it's completely absorbed. The dose can be repeated every 10 to 15 minutes, up to three doses.

• Place topical ointments on paper as prescribed; then place the paper on a nonhairy area and cover it with plastic. Remove excess ointment from the previous site when applying the next dose.

• Remove a transdermal patch before defibrillation. Aluminium backing on the patch may explode with electric current.

• Be aware that the drug may initially cause headache until tolerance develops or the dosage is minimised.

Evaluation
• Patient sustains no injury from adverse reactions.
• Patient maintains normal fluid balance.
• Patient and family understand drug therapy. (See *Teaching about anti-anginals*.)

Beta-adrenergic antagonists

Beta-adrenergic antagonists (also called *beta-adrenergic blockers*) are used for long-term prevention of angina and are one of the main types of drugs used to treat hypertension. Beta-adrenergic blockers include:

- atenolol
- carvedilol
- metoprolol tartrate
- nadolol
- propranolol hydrochloride.

Prototype pro

Beta$_1$- and beta$_2$-adrenergic blockers: Propranolol

Actions

- Reduces cardiac oxygen demand by blocking catecholamine-induced increases in heart rate, blood pressure, and force of myocardial contraction
- Depresses renin secretion and prevents vasodilation of cerebral arteries
- Relieves anginal and migraine pain, lowers blood pressure, restores normal sinus rhythm, and helps limit myocardial infarction (MI) damage

Indications

- Angina pectoris
- Mortality reduction after MI
- Supraventricular, ventricular, and atrial arrhythmias
- Tachyarrhythmias caused by excessive catecholamine action during anaesthesia, hyperthyroidism, or pheochromocytoma
- Hypertension
- Prevention of frequent, severe, uncontrollable, or disabling migraine or vascular headache
- Essential tremor
- Hypertrophic cardiomyopathy

Nursing considerations

- Check the patient's apical pulse before giving the drug. If you detect extremes in pulse rate, withhold the drug and call the prescriber immediately.
- Give the drug with meals. Food may increase the drug's absorption.
- Before any surgical procedure, notify the anaesthetist that the patient is receiving propranolol. The drug shouldn't be stopped before surgery, especially for patients with cardiovascular disorders or pheochromocytoma.
- Notify the prescriber if the patient develops severe hypotension; a vasopressor may be prescribed.
- Be aware that elderly patients may have increased adverse reactions and may need dosage adjustment.
- Don't stop the drug abruptly.
- For overdose, give I.V. atropine, I.V. isoprenaline or glucagon; refractory cases may require a pacemaker.

Pharmacokinetics

Metoprolol and propranolol are absorbed almost entirely from the GI tract, whereas less than half the dose of atenolol or nadolol is absorbed. These beta-adrenergic blockers are distributed widely. Propranolol is highly protein bound; the other beta-adrenergic blockers are poorly protein bound. (See *Beta$_1$- and beta$_2$-adrenergic blockers: Propranolol* and *Beta$_1$-adrenergic blockers: Metoprolol*.)

Propranolol and metoprolol are metabolised in the liver, and their metabolites are excreted in urine. Atenolol and nadolol aren't metabolised and are excreted unchanged in urine and faeces.

Pharmacodynamics

Beta-adrenergic blockers decrease blood pressure and block beta-adrenergic receptor sites in the heart muscle and conduction system. This decreases heart rate and reduces the force of the heart's contractions, resulting in a lower demand for oxygen.

Pharmacotherapeutics

Beta-adrenergic blockers are indicated for the long-term prevention of angina. Metoprolol may be given I.V. in acute coronary syndrome, followed by an oral dose. Carvedilol and metoprolol are indicated for heart failure. Beta-adrenergic blockers are also first-line therapy for treating hypertension.

Drug interactions

Several drugs interact with beta-adrenergic blockers:
- Antacids delay absorption of beta-adrenergic blockers.
- NSAIDs can decrease the hypotensive effects of beta-adrenergic blockers.
- Lidocaine toxicity may occur when the drug is taken with beta-adrenergic blockers.
- The requirements for insulin and oral antidiabetic drugs can be altered by beta-adrenergic blockers.
- The ability of theophylline to produce bronchodilation is impaired by nonselective beta-adrenergic blockers.

Adverse reactions

Adverse reactions to beta-adrenergic blockers include:
- bradycardia, angina, heart failure, and arrhythmias, especially AV block
- fainting
- fluid retention
- peripheral oedema

Prototype pro

Beta$_1$-adrenergic blockers: Metoprolol

Actions

- Competes with beta-adrenergic agonists for available beta-adrenergic receptor sites

Indications

- Hypertension
- Angina pectoris

Nursing considerations

- Monitor for adverse reactions, such as fatigue, dizziness, bradycardia, hypotension, heart failure, and atrioventricular block.
- Withhold the drug, as prescribed, if the apical pulse is less than 60 beats/minute.
- Monitor blood pressure frequently.

- shock
- nausea and vomiting
- diarrhoea
- significant constriction of the bronchioles.

Not so quick

Suddenly stopping a beta-adrenergic blocker may trigger angina, hypertension, arrhythmias, and acute myocardial infarction (MI).

Nursing process

These nursing process steps are appropriate for patients undergoing treatment with beta-adrenergic blockers.

Assessment

- Assess the patient's arrhythmia before therapy and regularly thereafter.
- Monitor the ECG continuously when therapy starts, when dosage is adjusted, and particularly during I.V. therapy.
- Monitor the patient's vital signs frequently; assess for signs of toxicity and adverse reactions.
- Measure the apical pulse rate and blood pressure before giving the drug.
- Monitor serum drug levels as indicated.
- Monitor blood studies, such as liver function tests, as indicated.
- Be alert for adverse reactions and drug interactions.
- Evaluate the patient's and family's knowledge of drug therapy.

Key nursing diagnoses

- Decreased cardiac output related to arrhythmias or myocardial depression
- Risk for injury related to adverse reactions
- Deficient knowledge related to drug therapy

Planning outcome goals

- Cardiac output will improve as evidenced by stable blood pressure, cardiac monitoring, and adequate urine output.
- Complications from adverse reactions will be diminished.
- The patient will demonstrate correct drug administration.

Implementation

- Don't crush sustained-release tablets.
- Be aware that sustained-released and extended-release medications aren't interchangeable.
- Take safety precautions if adverse CNS reactions occur.
- Notify the prescriber about adverse reactions.

- Use I.V. forms of the drug for treating acute arrhythmias. I.V. forms may be given as a loading dose I.V. or may be diluted with normal saline solution and given by intermittent infusion.
- Check the apical pulse before giving the drug. If extreme pulse rate is detected, withhold the drug and call the prescriber immediately.
- Know that the drug may be given with meals as indicated.
- Before any surgical procedure, notify the anaesthetist that the patient is receiving this drug.
- Don't discontinue I.V. administration abruptly.
- Provide patient teaching.

Evaluation
- Patient maintains adequate cardiac output, as evidenced by normal vital signs and adequate tissue perfusion.
- Patient has no serious adverse reactions.
- Patient states the importance of compliance with therapy.

Calcium channel blockers

Calcium channel blockers are commonly used to prevent angina that doesn't respond to drugs in either of the other anti-anginal classes. Several of the calcium channel blockers are also used as antiarrhythmics and in the treatment of hypertension.

Calcium channel blockers used to treat angina include:
- amlodipine besylate (or alternatively mesylate or maleate; these salts are considered interchangable)
- diltiazem
- nicardipine
- nifedipine
- verapamil.

Pharmacokinetics
When administered orally, calcium channel blockers are absorbed quickly and almost completely. Because of the first-pass effect, however, the bioavailability of these drugs is much lower. Calcium channel blockers are highly bound to plasma proteins.

All calcium channel blockers are metabolised rapidly and almost completely in the liver.

Pharmacodynamics
Calcium channel blockers prevent the passage of calcium ions across the myocardial cell membrane and vascular smooth muscle cells. This causes dilation of the coronary and peripheral arteries, which decreases the force of the heart's contractions and reduces the workload of the heart. (See *How calcium channel blockers work*.)

Pharm function

How calcium channel blockers work

Calcium channel blockers increase myocardial oxygen supply and slow cardiac impulse formation. Apparently, the drugs produce these effects by blocking the slow calcium channel. This action inhibits the influx of extracellular calcium ions across both myocardial and vascular smooth-muscle cell membranes. Calcium channel blockers achieve this blockade without changing serum calcium concentrations.

No calcium = dilation

This calcium blockade causes the coronary arteries (and, to a lesser extent, the peripheral arteries and arterioles) to dilate, decreasing afterload and increasing myocardial oxygen supply.

Putting on the brakes

By preventing arterioles from constricting, calcium channel blockers also reduce afterload, resulting in a decreased oxygen demand of the heart.

Some calcium channel blockers (diltiazem and verapamil) also reduce the heart rate by slowing conduction through the SA and AV nodes. A slower heart rate reduces the heart's need for additional oxygen.

Prototype pro

Calcium channel blockers: Verapamil

Actions

- Inhibits calcium ion influx across the cardiac and smooth-muscle cells
- Reduces myocardial contractility and oxygen demand
- Dilates coronary arteries and arterioles

Indications

- Angina relief
- Decreased blood pressure
- Restoration of normal sinus rhythm

Nursing considerations

- A patient with severely compromised cardiac function or one taking beta-adrenergic blockers should receive lower doses of verapamil.
- Monitor cardiac rhythm and blood pressure during the start of therapy and with dose adjustments.
- Notify the prescriber if signs and symptoms of heart failure occur, such as swelling of the hands and feet and shortness of breath.

Pharmacotherapeutics

Calcium channel blockers are used only for long-term prevention of angina, not for short-term relief of chest pain. Calcium channel blockers are particularly effective for preventing Prinzmetal's angina. (See *Calcium channel blockers: Verapamil.*)

Drug interactions

These drug interactions can occur with calcium channel blockers:
- Calcium salts and vitamin D reduce the effectiveness of calcium channel blockers.
- Nondepolarising blocking drugs may enhance the muscle-relaxant effect when taken with calcium channel blockers.
- Verapamil and diltiazem increase the risk of digoxin toxicity, enhance the action of carbamazepine, and can produce myocardial depression.

Adverse reactions

As with other anti-anginal drugs, cardiovascular reactions are the most common and serious adverse reactions to calcium channel blockers. Possible adverse reactions include orthostatic hypotension, heart failure, hypotension, and arrhythmias, such as bradycardia and AV block. Other possible adverse reactions include dizziness, headache, flushing, weakness, and persistent peripheral oedema.

Nursing process

These nursing process steps are appropriate for patients undergoing treatment with calcium channel blockers.

Assessment
• Obtain a history of the patient's underlying condition before therapy, and reassess regularly thereafter.
• Assess the patient's arrhythmia before therapy and regularly thereafter.
• Monitor the ECG continuously when therapy starts and when the dosage is adjusted.
• Monitor the patient's vital signs frequently, and assess for signs of toxicity and adverse reactions.
• Measure the apical pulse rate and blood pressure before giving the drug.
• Assist the patient with ambulation during the start of therapy because dizziness may occur.
• Advise the patient that fluid and sodium intake may need to be restricted to minimise oedema.
• Monitor serum drug levels as indicated.
• Monitor blood studies, such as liver function tests, as indicated.
• Be alert for adverse reactions and drug interactions.
• Evaluate the patient's and family's knowledge of drug therapy.

Key nursing diagnoses
• Decreased cardiac output related to arrhythmias or myocardial depression.
• Risk for injury related to adverse reactions.
• Deficient knowledge related to drug therapy.

Planning outcome goals
• Cardiac output will improve as evidenced by stable blood pressure, cardiac monitoring, and adequate urine output.
• Complications from adverse reactions will be diminished.
• The patient will demonstrate correct drug administration.

Implementation
• Don't crush sustained-release tablets.
• Be aware that sustained-released and extended-release medications aren't interchangeable.
• Take safety precautions if adverse CNS reactions occur.
• Notify the prescriber about adverse reactions.
• Know that I.V. forms are used for treating acute arrhythmias; cardiac monitoring is required during administration.
• If systolic pressure is below 90 mm Hg or heart rate is below 60 beats/minute, withhold the dose and notify the prescriber or follow the prescriber's parameters for withholding the medication.

- Assist the patient with walking because dizziness can occur.
- If the drug is being used to terminate supraventricular tachycardia, the prescriber may have the patient perform vagal manoeuvres after receiving the drug.
- Provide patient teaching.

Evaluation
- Patient maintains adequate cardiac output, as evidenced by normal vital signs and adequate tissue perfusion.
- Patient has no serious adverse reactions.
- Patient states the importance of compliance with therapy.

Antihypertensive drugs

Antihypertensive drugs are used to treat hypertension, a disorder characterised by elevation in systolic blood pressure, diastolic blood pressure, or both.

Antihypertensive drugs are used to treat hypertension. That makes sense!

A word to the wise

Several classes of drugs have been shown in clinical trials to be effective in treating hypertension. Diuretics, primarily thiazide diuretics, are used as initial therapy in treating most patients with hypertension. (These drugs will be discussed later in the chapter). Other classes of drugs used to treat hypertension include:
- angiotensin-converting enzyme (ACE) inhibitors
- angiotensin-receptor blockers (ARBs)
- beta-adrenergic antagonists
- calcium channel blockers.

If these drugs are ineffective, treatment continues with sympatholytic drugs (other than beta-adrenergic blockers), direct vasodilators, selective aldosterone-receptor antagonists, or a combination of drugs.

Angiotensin-converting enzyme inhibitors

ACE inhibitors reduce blood pressure by interrupting the renin-angiotensin activating system (RAAS). Commonly prescribed ACE inhibitors include:
- captopril
- enalapril

Prototype pro

ACE inhibitors: Captopril

Actions

- Thought to inhibit angiotensin-converting enzyme (ACE), preventing conversion of angiotensin I to angiotensin II (reduced formation of angiotensin II decreases peripheral arterial resistance, thus decreasing aldosterone secretion)

Indications

- Reduction of sodium and water retention
- Blood pressure reduction
- Improved renal function in patients with diabetes

Nursing considerations

- Monitor white blood cell and differential counts before therapy, every 2 weeks for the first 3 months of therapy, and periodically thereafter.
- Give the drug 1 hour before meals because food may reduce drug absorption.
- Withhold the dose and notify the prescriber if the patient develops fever, sore throat, leucopenia, hypotension, or tachycardia.
- Light-headedness and syncope can develop in hot weather, with inadequate fluid intake, vomiting, diarrhoea, and excessive perspiration.

- fosinopril sodium
- lisinopril
- moexipril
- quinapril hydrochloride
- ramipril
- trandolapril.
  (See *ACE inhibitors: Captopril.*)

Pharmacokinetics

ACE inhibitors are absorbed from the GI tract, distributed to most body tissues, metabolised somewhat in the liver, and excreted by the kidneys. Ramipril also is excreted in faeces.

Pharmacodynamics

ACE inhibitors work by preventing the conversion of angiotensin I to angiotensin II. Angiotensin I is a potent vasoconstrictor that increases peripheral resistance and promotes the excretion of aldosterone (which promotes sodium and water retention). As angiotensin II is reduced, arterioles dilate, reducing peripheral vascular resistance.

By reducing aldosterone secretion, ACE inhibitors promote the excretion of sodium and water, reducing the amount of blood the heart needs to pump and reducing blood pressure.

Pharmacotherapeutics

ACE inhibitors may be used alone or in combination with other agents, such as a thiazide diuretic, to treat hypertension. They're commonly used when beta-adrenergic blockers or diuretics are ineffective.

Captopril, enalapril, fosinopril, lisinopril, quinapril, ramipril, and trandolapril are also indicated for use in heart failure for the following situations:
• left ventricular systolic failure (unless contraindicated or intolerant)
• left ventricular systolic dysfunction without symptoms of heart failure
• after acute MI (especially in patients with prior myocardial injury) to reduce mortality
• left ventricular dysfunction (recent or remote) to prevent or delay the development of left ventricular dilation and overt heart failure
• combined use with beta-adrenergic blockers may produce complementary effects
• combined use with diuretics if fluid retention persists.

Multiple MI uses

Lisinopril, ramipril, and trandolapril are also indicated for use in patients who have had an MI to improve survival and to reduce morbidity and mortality in patients with left ventricular dysfunction.

Historically speaking…

Ramipril is also indicated to prevent major cardiovascular events in patients with a history of vascular disease or diabetes. It's also used to reduce overall cardiovascular risk, including death, nonfatal MI, nonfatal stroke, and complications of diabetes.

Drug interactions

ACE inhibitors can cause several different types of interactions with other cardiovascular drugs:
• All ACE inhibitors enhance the hypotensive effects of diuretics and other antihypertensives such as beta-adrenergic blockers. They can also increase serum lithium levels, possibly resulting in lithium toxicity.

• When ACE inhibitors are used with potassium-sparing diuretics, potassium supplements, or potassium-containing salt substitutes, hyperkalaemia may occur.
• ACE inhibitors may interact with other medications, both prescribed and over the counter. For example, patients taking ACE inhibitors should avoid taking NSAIDs. In addition to decreasing the antihypertensive effects of ACE inhibitors, NSAIDs may also alter renal function.

On their own

Captopril, enalapril, and lisinopril may become less effective when administered with NSAIDs. Antacids may impair the absorption of fosinopril, and quinapril may reduce the absorption of tetracycline.

Adverse reactions
ACE inhibitors can cause these adverse reactions:
• headache
• fatigue
• dry, nonproductive, persistent cough
• angioedema
• GI reactions
• increased serum potassium concentrations
• tickling in the throat
• transient elevations of BUN and serum creatinine levels (indicators of kidney function).
They can cause problems with foetal circulation and shouldn't be administered during pregnancy.

Be cautious with captopril

Captopril may cause protein in the urine, reduced neutrophils and granulocytes (types of white blood cells), rash, loss of taste, hypotension, or a severe allergic reaction.

Nursing process
These nursing process steps are appropriate for patients undergoing treatment with ACE inhibitors.

Assessment
• Obtain a baseline blood pressure and pulse rate and rhythm, and recheck regularly.
• Monitor the patient for adverse reactions and drug interactions.
• Monitor the patient's weight and fluid and electrolyte status.
• Assess the patient's underlying condition before therapy and regularly thereafter.

Be sure to monitor the weight of a patient taking ACE inhibitors.

- Monitor laboratory results, including white cell count and differential, potassium level, and renal function (BUN and creatinine clearance levels, urinalysis).
- Monitor the patient's compliance with treatment.
- Observe the patient's tolerance of the drug's therapeutic effects. The dosage may need to be increased.
- Monitor a transdermal patch for dermatitis, and ask the patient about pruritus. Keep in mind that the patch can require several days to take effect and that interim oral therapy may be needed.

Key nursing diagnoses
- Risk for injury related to orthostatic hypotension.
- Risk for injury related to presence of hypertension.
- Deficient knowledge related to drug therapy.

Planning outcome goals
- Blood pressure will be maintained within acceptable limits.
- Risk for injury will be minimised.
- The patient will demonstrate correct drug administration.

Implementation
- If giving orally, administer the drug before meals as indicated.
- Follow the manufacturer's guidelines when mixing and administering parenteral drugs.
- Prevent or minimise orthostatic hypotension by assisting the patient to get up slowly, and by telling the patient not to make sudden movements.
- Maintain the patient's nonpharmacologic therapies, such as sodium restriction, calorie reduction, stress management, and exercise program.
- Keep in mind that drug therapy may be given to lower blood pressure rapidly in some hypertensive emergency situations.
- Know that the dosage is usually adjusted to the patient's blood pressure and tolerance.
- To improve adherence of a transdermal patch, apply an adhesive overlay. Place the patch at a different site each week.
- Remove a transdermal patch before defibrillation to prevent arcing.
- Periodic eye examinations are recommended.

Evaluation
- Patient sustains no trauma from orthostatic hypotension.
- Patient sustains no injury.
- Patient and family understand drug therapy.

Angiotensin II receptor blocking agents

Angiotensin II receptor blocking agents (ARBs) lower blood pressure by inhibiting the vasoconstrictive effects of angiotensin II. Available ARBs include:

- losartan
- valsartan
- irbesartan
- telmisartan
- eprosartan
- olmesartan.

Pharmacokinetics

ARBs have varying pharmacokinetic properties, and all are highly bound to plasma proteins.

Pharmacodynamics

ARBs act by interfering with the RAAS. They selectively block the binding of angiotensin II to the angiotensin II receptors. This prevents the vasoconstricting and aldosterone-secreting effects of angiotensin II (a potent vasoconstrictor), resulting in a blood pressure decrease.

ARBs don't inhibit the production of ACE that's responsible for the conversion of angiotensin I to angiotensin II, nor do they cause a breakdown in bradykinin (a vasodilator). (See *Angiotensin II receptor blockers: Losartan.*)

Pharmacotherapeutics

ARBs may be used alone or in combination with other agents, such as a diuretic, for the treatment of hypertension. Valsartan may also be used as an alternative to ACE inhibitors or for the management of heart failure. Irbesartan and losartan are indicated for patients with type 2 diabetes because of their inherent renal protective effect.

Drug interactions

These drug interactions may occur with ARBs:
- Losartan taken with fluconazole may increase levels of losartan, leading to increased hypotensive effects.
- NSAIDs reduce the antihypertensive effects of ARBs.
- Rifampicin may increase metabolism of losartan, leading to decreased antihypertensive effect.
- Potassium supplements can increase the risk of hyperkalaemia when used with ARBs.

 Prototype pro

Angiotensin II receptor blockers: Losartan

Actions

- Inhibits vasoconstricting and aldosterone-secreting effects of angiotensin II by selectively blocking binding of angiotensin II to receptor sites in many tissues, including vascular smooth muscle and adrenal glands

Indications

- Blood pressure reduction

Nursing considerations

- Monitor blood pressure before therapy and regularly thereafter.
- Regularly assess patient's kidney function (creatinine and blood urea nitrogen levels).

Adverse reactions

Adverse effects of angiotensin II receptor antagonists include:

- headache
- fatigue
- cough and tickling in the throat
- angioedema
- GI reactions
- increased serum potassium
- transient elevations of BUN and serum creatinine levels.

  ARBs shouldn't be used during the second and third trimester of pregnancy; this can result in injury to and death of the foetus.

Nursing process

These nursing process steps are appropriate for patients undergoing treatment with ARBs.

Assessment

- Obtain a baseline blood pressure and pulse rate and rhythm; recheck regularly.
- Monitor the patient for adverse reactions.
- Monitor the patient's weight and fluid and electrolyte status.
- Observe the patient's compliance with treatment.
- Observe the patient's tolerance of the drug, and monitor the drug's therapeutic effects. The dosage may need to be adjusted.
- Monitor a transdermal patch for dermatitis; ask the patient about pruritus. Keep in mind that the patch can require several days to take effect and that interim oral therapy may be needed.

Key nursing diagnoses

- Risk for injury related to orthostatic hypotension.
- Risk for injury related to the presence of hypertension.
- Deficient knowledge related to drug therapy.

Planning outcome goals

- Blood pressure will be maintained within acceptable limits.
- Risk for injury will be minimised.
- The patient will demonstrate correct drug administration.

Implementation

- If giving orally, administer the drug with food or at bedtime, as indicated.
- Follow the manufacturer's guidelines when mixing and administering parenteral drugs.

- Prevent or minimise orthostatic hypotension by assisting the patient to get up slowly, and by telling the patient not to make sudden movements.
- Maintain the patient's nonpharmacologic therapies, such as sodium restriction, calorie reduction, stress management, and exercise program.
- Keep in mind that drug therapy may be given to lower blood pressure rapidly in some hypertensive emergency situations.
- Know that the dosage is usually adjusted to the patient's blood pressure and tolerance.
- To improve adherence of a transdermal patch, apply an adhesive overlay. Place the patch at a different site each week.
- Remove a transdermal patch before defibrillation to prevent arcing.
- If giving once daily, administer in the morning to prevent insomnia.
- Periodic eye examinations are recommended.

Evaluation
- Patient sustains no trauma from orthostatic hypotension.
- Patient sustains no injury.
- Patient and family understand drug therapy.

Beta-adrenergic antagonists

Beta-adrenergic antagonists, or beta-adrenergic blockers, are one of the main types of drugs used to treat hypertension. They're also used for long-term prevention of angina. Beta-adrenergic blockers used for hypertension include:
- acebutolol
- atenolol
- betaxolol
- bisoprolol
- carvedilol
- labetalol
- metoprolol tartrate
- nadolol
- nevbivol
- pindolol
- propranolol hydrochloride
- timolol.

Pharmacokinetics
The pharmacokinetics of beta-adrenergic blockers varies by drug. Acebutolol, betaxolol, labetalol, metoprolol, pindolol, propranolol, and timolol are absorbed almost entirely from the GI tract, whereas

less than half of atenolol or nadolol is absorbed. GI tract absorption of bisoprolol is approximately 80%.

Acebutolol, propranolol, labetalol, metoprolol, and timolol are metabolised in the liver, and their metabolites are excreted in urine. Atenolol and nadolol aren't metabolised and are excreted unchanged in urine and faeces. Betaxolol is metabolised in the liver and is primarily excreted in urine. Bisoprolol is partially eliminated by renal pathways. Approximately 50% of the drug is excreted in the urine and about 2% in faeces. Pindolol is metabolised in the liver (about 65% of the dose), and 35% to 50% of the dose is excreted unchanged in urine.

Pharmacodynamics
Beta-adrenergic blockers decrease blood pressure and block beta-adrenergic receptor sites in the heart muscle and conduction system. This decreases heart rate and reduces the force of the heart's contractions, resulting in a lower demand for oxygen by the myocardium.

Pharmacotherapeutics
Beta-adrenergic blockers are indicated for the long-term prevention of angina. Metaprolol may be given I.V. in acute coronary syndrome, followed by an oral dose. Bisprolol, carvedilol and nevbivol are indicated for heart failure. Beta-andrenergic blockers are also first-line therapy for treating hypertension and for improving symptoms and prognosis in heart failure.

Drug interactions
Several drugs interact with beta-adrenergic blockers:
* Antacids delay absorption of beta-adrenergic blockers.
* NSAIDs can decrease the hypotensive effects of beta-adrenergic blockers.
* Lidocaine toxicity may occur when the drug is taken with beta-adrenergic blockers.
* The requirements for insulin and oral antidiabetic drugs can be altered by beta-adrenergic blockers.
* The ability of theophylline to produce bronchodilation is impaired by nonselective beta-adrenergic blockers.
* Hypotensive effects may be increased when beta-adrenergic blockers are administered with diuretics.

Adverse reactions
Adverse reactions to beta-adrenergic blockers include:
* bradycardia, angina, heart failure, and arrhythmias, especially AV block
* fainting
* fluid retention

- peripheral oedema
- shock
- nausea and vomiting
- diarrhoea
- significant constriction of the bronchioles.

Slow to a halt

Suddenly stopping a beta-adrenergic blocker may trigger angina, hypertension, arrhythmias, and acute MI.

Nursing process

These nursing process steps are appropriate for patients undergoing treatment with beta-adrenergic blockers.

Assessment
- Obtain a baseline blood pressure and pulse rate and rhythm; recheck regularly.
- Monitor the ECG when therapy starts, when dosage is adjusted, and particularly during I.V. therapy.
- Monitor the patient's vital signs frequently; assess for signs of toxicity and adverse reactions.
- Measure the apical pulse rate and blood pressure before giving the drug.
- Monitor blood studies, such as liver function tests, as indicated.
- Be alert for adverse reactions and drug interactions.
- Evaluate the patient's and family's knowledge of drug therapy.

Key nursing diagnoses
- Risk for injury related to orthostatic hypotension.
- Risk for injury related to presence of hypertension.
- Deficient knowledge related to drug therapy.

Planning outcome goals
- Blood pressure will be maintained within acceptable limits.
- Risk for injury will be minimised.
- The patient will demonstrate correct drug administration.

Implementation
- Don't crush sustained-release tablets.
- Be aware that sustained-released and extended-release medications aren't interchangeable.
- Take safety precautions if adverse CNS reactions occur.
- Notify the prescriber about adverse reactions.
- Know that the dosage is usually adjusted to the patient's blood pressure and tolerance.

- Prevent or minimise orthostatic hypotension by assisting the patient to get up slowly, and by telling the patient not to make sudden movements.
- Use I.V. forms of the drug for treating severe hypertension. I.V. forms may be given as a loading dose I.V. or may be diluted with normal saline solution and given by intermittent infusion.
- If systolic blood pressure is below 90 mm Hg or heart rate is below 60 beats/minute, withhold the dose and notify the prescriber or follow the prescriber's parameters for withholding the medication.
- Know that the drug may be given with meals as indicated.
- Before any surgical procedure, notify the anaesthetist that the patient is receiving this drug.
- Don't discontinue I.V. administration abruptly.
- Provide patient teaching.

Evaluation
- Patient sustains no injury from orthostatic hypotension.
- Patient and family understand drug therapy.

Calcium channel blockers

Calcium channel blockers are commonly used to treat hypertension. Several are also used to treat arrhythmias and to prevent angina that doesn't respond to other antianginal drugs.

Calcium channel blockers used to treat hypertension include:
- amlodipine besylate (mesylate or maleate salts may also be used)
- diltiazem
- felodipine
- isradipine
- nicardipine
- nifedipine
- nisoldipine
- verapamil.

Pharmacokinetics

When administered orally, calcium channel blockers are absorbed quickly and almost completely. Because of the first-pass effect, however, the bioavailability of these drugs is much lower. Food decreases amlodipine absorption by 30%, and high-fat foods increase the peak concentration of nisoldipine. Calcium channel blockers are highly bound to plasma proteins.

All calcium channel blockers are metabolised rapidly and almost completely in the liver and are primarily excreted in urine.

Pharmacodynamics

Calcium channel blockers prevent the passage of calcium ions across the myocardial cell membrane and vascular smooth-muscle cells. This causes dilation of the coronary and peripheral arteries, which decreases the force of the heart's contractions and reduces the workload of the heart and decreases blood pressure. By preventing arterioles from constricting, calcium channel blockers also reduce afterload, resulting in a decreased oxygen demand of the heart.

Some calcium channel blockers (diltiazem and verapamil) also reduce the heart rate by slowing conduction through the SA and AV nodes. A slower heart rate reduces the heart's need for additional oxygen.

Pharmacotherapeutics

Calcium channel blockers are used to treat hypertension and for long-term prevention of angina. They shouldn't be used for short-term relief of chest pain. Calcium channel blockers are particularly effective for preventing Prinzmetal's angina.

Drug interactions

These drug interactions can occur with calcium channel blockers:
• Calcium salts and vitamin D reduce the effectiveness of calcium channel blockers.
• Nondepolarising blocking drugs may enhance the muscle-relaxant effect when taken with calcium channel blockers.
• Verapamil and diltiazem increase the risk of digoxin toxicity, enhance the action of carbamazepine, and can produce myocardial depression.

Adverse reactions

Possible adverse reactions include headache, dizziness, weakness, orthostatic hypotension, heart failure, hypotension, peripheral oedema, palpitations, and arrhythmias such as tachycardia. Bradycardia and AV block also occur with diltiazem and verapamil.

Nursing process

These nursing process steps are appropriate for patients undergoing treatment with calcium channel blockers.

Assessment
• Obtain a history of the patient's underlying condition before therapy, and reassess regularly thereafter.

Calcium channel blockers are particularly effective for preventing Prinzmetal's angina.

- Obtain a baseline blood pressure and pulse rate and rhythm; recheck regularly.
- Monitor the ECG when therapy starts and when the dosage is adjusted.
- Monitor the patient's vital signs frequently, and assess for signs of toxicity and adverse reactions.
- Measure the apical pulse rate and blood pressure before giving the drug.
- Assist the patient with ambulation during the start of therapy because dizziness may occur.
- Advise the patient that fluid and sodium intake may need to be restricted to minimise oedema.
- Monitor serum drug levels as indicated.
- Monitor blood studies, such as liver function tests, as indicated.
- Be alert for adverse reactions and drug interactions.
- Evaluate the patient's and family's knowledge of drug therapy.

Key nursing diagnoses
- Risk for injury related to orthostatic hypotension.
- Risk for injury related to adverse reactions.
- Deficient knowledge related to drug therapy.

Planning outcome goals
- Blood pressure will be maintained within acceptable limits.
- Risk for injury will be minimised.
- Complications from adverse reactions will be diminished.
- The patient will demonstrate correct drug administration.

Implementation
- Don't crush sustained-release tablets.
- Be aware that sustained-released and extended-release medications aren't interchangeable.
- Take safety precautions if adverse CNS reactions occur.
- Notify the prescriber about adverse reactions.
- If systolic pressure is below 90 mm Hg or heart rate is below 60 beats/minute, withhold the dose and notify the prescriber or follow the prescribed parameters for withholding the medication.
- Assist the patient with walking because dizziness can occur.

Evaluation
- Patient sustains no injury from orthostatic hypotension.
- Patient has no serious adverse reactions.
- Patient states the importance of compliance with therapy.

Sympatholytic drugs

Sympatholytic drugs include several different types of drugs that reduce blood pressure by inhibiting or blocking the sympathetic nervous system. They're classified by their site or mechanism of action and include:

• central-acting sympathetic nervous system inhibitors (clonidine hydrochloride, and methyldopa) (See *Centrally acting sympatholytics: Clonidine.*)

• alpha-adrenergic blockers (doxazosin, phentolamine, prazosin, and terazosin) (See *Alpha-adrenergic blockers: Doxazosin.*)

• mixed alpha- and beta-adrenergic blockers (carvedilol and labetalol)

• noradrenaline (norepinephrine) depletors (guanethidine monosulphate). However, these drugs are rarely used.

Pharmacokinetics

Most sympatholytic drugs are absorbed well from the GI tract, distributed widely, metabolised in the liver, and excreted primarily in urine.

Pharmacodynamics

All sympatholytic drugs inhibit stimulation of the sympathetic nervous system. This causes dilation of the peripheral blood vessels or decreased cardiac output, thereby reducing blood pressure.

Prototype pro

Centrally acting sympatholytics: Clonidine

Actions

• Inhibits central vasomotor centres, decreasing sympathetic outflow to the heart, kidneys, and peripheral vasculature
• Decreases peripheral vascular resistance
• Decreases systolic and diastolic blood pressure
• Decreases heart rate

Indications

• Blood pressure reduction

Nursing considerations

• The drug is adjusted to the patient's blood pressure and tolerance.
• When stopping therapy in a patient receiving both clonidine and a beta-adrenergic blocker, gradually withdraw the beta-adrenergic blocker first to minimise adverse reactions.
• Discontinuing clonidine for surgery isn't recommended.

Pharmacotherapeutics

If blood pressure can't be controlled by beta-adrenergic blockers and diuretics, an alpha-adrenergic blocker (such as prazosin) or an alpha-beta blocker (such as labetalol) may be used.

Try and try again

If the patient still fails to achieve the desired blood pressure, the prescriber may add a drug from a different class, substitute a drug in the same class, or increase the drug dosage.

Drug interactions

Sympatholytic drugs can create the following drug interactions:
* Clonidine plus tricyclic antidepressants may increase blood pressure.
* Clonidine taken with CNS depressants may worsen CNS depression.
* Carvedilol taken with antidiabetic agents may result in an increased hypoglycaemic effect.
* Carvedilol taken with calcium channel blockers may result in increased digoxin levels.
* Carvedilol taken with rifampicin decreases levels of carvedilol.
* Sympatholytic drugs can also produce significant adverse reactions.

Adverse reactions

Possible adverse reactions to sympatholytic drugs vary by type. For example, alpha-adrenergic blockers may cause hypotension.

Central problems

Adverse reactions to central-acting drugs include:
* depression
* drowsiness
* oedema
* liver dysfunction
* numbness and tingling
* vertigo.

"G" whiz

Adverse reactions to guanethidine include:
* decreased heart contractility
* diarrhoea
* fluid retention
* orthostatic hypotension.

Prototype pro

Alpha-adrenergic blockers: Doxazosin

Actions

* Acts on peripheral vasculature to produce vasodilation

Indications

* Blood pressure reduction

Nursing considerations

* The dosage must be increased gradually, with adjustments every 2 weeks for hypertension.
* Monitor blood pressure.
* Monitor the electrocardiogram for arrhythmias.

Nursing process

These nursing process steps are appropriate for patients undergoing treatment with sympatholytics.

Assessment

- Obtain a baseline blood pressure and pulse rate and rhythm; recheck regularly.
- Monitor the patient for adverse reactions.
- Monitor the patient's weight and fluid and electrolyte status.
- Monitor the patient's compliance with treatment.
- Observe the patient's tolerance of the drug, and monitor for the drug's therapeutic effects. The patient may require a dosage adjustment.

Key nursing diagnoses

- Risk for injury related to orthostatic hypotension.
- Risk for injury related to presence of hypertension.
- Deficient knowledge related to drug therapy.

Planning outcome goals

- Blood pressure will be maintained within acceptable limits.
- Risk for injury to the patient will be minimised.
- The patient will demonstrate correct drug administration.

Implementation

- If giving orally, administer the drug with food or at bedtime, as indicated.
- Follow the manufacturer's guidelines when mixing and administering parenteral drugs.
- Prevent or minimise orthostatic hypotension by assisting the patient to get up slowly, and by telling the patient not to make sudden movements.
- Maintain the patient's nonpharmacologic therapies, such as sodium restriction, calorie reduction, stress management, and exercise program.
- Keep in mind that drug therapy may be given to lower blood pressure rapidly in some hypertensive emergency situations.
- The dosage is usually adjusted to the patient's blood pressure and tolerance.
- Periodic eye examinations are recommended.

Education edge

Teaching about antihypertensives

If antihypertensives are prescribed, review these points with the patient and caregivers:

- Take the drug exactly as prescribed. Don't stop the drug abruptly. Abrupt discontinuation may cause severe rebound hypertension.
- The last oral dose is usually administered at bedtime.
- The drug can cause drowsiness, but tolerance to this adverse effect will develop.
- Be aware of the adverse reactions caused by this drug, and notify your prescriber of serious or persistent reactions.

- Avoid sudden changes in position to prevent dizziness, light-headedness, or fainting, which are signs of orthostatic hypotension.
- Avoid hazardous activities until the full effects of the drug are known. Also avoid physical exertion, especially in hot weather.
- Consult with your prescriber before taking any over-the-counter medications or herbal remedies; serious drug interactions can occur.
- Comply with therapy.

Evaluation
- Patient sustains no trauma from orthostatic hypotension.
- Patient sustains no injury.
- Patient and family understand drug therapy. (See *Teaching about antihypertensives.*)

Direct vasodilators

Direct vasodilators decrease systolic and diastolic blood pressure. They act on arteries, veins, or both. Examples of these drugs include:
- diazoxide
- hydralazine
- minoxidil
- sodium nitroprusside.

Hydralazine and minoxidil are usually used to treat resistant or refractory hypertension. Diazoxide and nitroprusside are reserved for use in hypertensive crisis. (See *Vasodilators: Nitroprusside.*)

Pharmacokinetics

Most vasodilating drugs are absorbed rapidly and distributed well. They're all metabolised in the liver, and most are excreted by the kidneys.

Prototype pro

Vasodilators: Nitroprusside

Actions

- Relaxes arteriolar and venous smooth muscle

Indications

- Blood pressure reduction; preload and afterload reduction

Nursing considerations

- Monitor thiocyanate levels every 72 hours; excessive doses or rapid infusion (more than 15 mcg/kg/minute) can cause cyanide toxicity.
- Monitor for adverse effects and signs of cyanide toxicity, including profound hypotension, metabolic acidosis, dyspnea, headache, loss of consciousness, ataxia, and vomiting.
- Monitor blood pressure every 5 minutes at start of infusion and every 15 minutes thereafter.
- An I.V. infusion must be wrapped in foil because it's sensitive to light.

Pharmacodynamics

The direct vasodilators relax peripheral vascular smooth muscles, causing the blood vessels to dilate. This lowers blood pressure by increasing the diameter of the blood vessels, reducing total peripheral resistance.

Pharmacotherapeutics

Vasodilating drugs are rarely used alone to treat hypertension. Rather, they're usually used in combination with other drugs to treat the patient with moderate to severe hypertension (hypertensive crisis).

Drug interactions

Few drug interactions occur with vasodilating drugs. Some that may occur, however, include the following:
- The antihypertensive effects of hydralazine and minoxidil are increased when they're given with other antihypertensive drugs such as methyldopa.
- Vasodilating drugs may produce additive effects when given with nitrates, such as isosorbide dinitrate or glyceryl trinitrate.

Successful treatment of hypertension usually requires a team approach.

Adverse reactions

Direct vasodilators commonly produce adverse reactions related to reflex activation of the sympathetic nervous system. As blood pressure falls, the sympathetic nervous system is stimulated, producing such compensatory measures as vasoconstriction and tachycardia.

Other reactions to sympathetic stimulation include:
- palpitations
- angina
- oedema
- breast tenderness
- fatigue
- headache
- rash
- severe pericardial effusion.

Nursing process

These nursing process steps are appropriate for patients undergoing treatment with direct vasodilating drugs.

Assessment

- Obtain a baseline blood pressure and pulse rate and rhythm; recheck regularly.
- Because excessive doses or rapid infusion of more than 15 mcg/kg/minute of nitroprusside can cause cyanide toxicity, check thiocyanate levels every 72 hours. Levels above 100 mcg/ml may cause toxicity. Watch for profound hypotension, metabolic acidosis, dyspnea, headache, loss of consciousness, ataxia, and vomiting.
- Monitor the patient for adverse reactions and drug interactions.
- Monitor the patient's weight and fluid and electrolyte status.
- Observe the patient's compliance with the treatment.
- Observe the patient's tolerance of the drug, and monitor the drug's therapeutic effects. The dosage may need to be adjusted.

Key nursing diagnoses

- Risk for injury related to orthostatic hypotension.
- Ineffective tissue perfusion related to hypotension.
- Risk for injury related to presence of hypertension.
- Deficient knowledge related to drug therapy.

Planning outcome goals
- Blood pressure will be maintained within acceptable limits.
- Risk for injury will be minimised.
- The patient will demonstrate correct drug administration.

Implementation
- If giving orally, administer the drug with food or at bedtime, as indicated.
- Follow the manufacturer's guidelines when mixing and administering parenteral drugs.
- Prevent or minimise orthostatic hypotension by assisting the patient to get up slowly, and by telling the patient not to make sudden movements.
- Keep in mind that nitroprusside is sensitive to light; wrap I.V. solutions of this drug in foil. A fresh solution should have a faint brownish tint. Discard the drug after 24 hours.
- Infuse the I.V. forms with an infusion pump, usually piggybacked through a peripheral line with no other medications.
- If administering I.V., check blood pressure every 5 minutes at the start of the infusion and every 15 minutes thereafter with nitroprusside and titrate dosage according to blood pressure parameters prescribed. If severe hypotension occurs, stop the infusion and notify the prescriber. Effects of the drug quickly reverse.
- If cyanide toxicity occurs, stop the drug immediately and notify the prescriber.
- Maintain the patient's nonpharmacologic therapies, such as sodium restriction, calorie reduction, stress management, and exercise program.
- Keep in mind that drug therapy may be given to lower blood pressure rapidly in some hypertensive emergency situations.
- Know that the dosage is usually adjusted to the patient's blood pressure and tolerance.
- Periodic eye examinations are recommended.

Evaluation
- Patient sustains no injury from orthostatic hypotension.
- Patient maintains adequate tissue perfusion.
- Patient sustains no injury.
- Patient and family understand drug therapy.

Selective aldosterone-receptor antagonist

Eplerenone, the only selective aldosterone-receptor antagonist, produces sustained increases in plasma renin and serum aldosterone. This inhibits the negative feedback mechanism of aldosterone on renin secretion. It selectively binds to mineralocorticoids receptors. The result is an antihypertensive effect.

Eplerenone is in a class of its own!

Pharmacokinetics

Eplerenone has a plasma protein binding of 50% and is primarily bound to alpha-1-acid glycoproteins after oral administration. Its metabolism is controlled by CYP3A4, and less than 5% of the dose is excreted unchanged in urine and faeces.

Pharmacodynamics

Eplerenone blocks the binding of aldosterone, an important part of the RAAS. Aldosterone causes increases in blood pressure through sodium reabsorption.

Pharmacotherapeutics

Eplerenone is used to lower blood pressure.

Drug interactions

Eplerenone levels may be increased when the drug is taken with inhibitors of CYP3A4 (erythromycin, saquinavir, verapamil, and fluconazole).

Adverse reactions

Eplerenone may cause hyperkalaemia, which may result in arrhythmias.

Nursing process

These nursing process steps are appropriate for patients undergoing treatment with a selective aldosterone-receptor antagonist.

Assessment
- Obtain a baseline blood pressure and pulse rate and rhythm; recheck regularly.
- Monitor the patient for adverse reactions.
- Monitor the patient's weight and fluid and electrolyte status.
- Monitor the patient's compliance with treatment.

Key nursing diagnoses
- Risk for injury related to orthostatic hypotension.
- Risk for injury related to presence of hypertension.
- Deficient knowledge related to drug therapy.

Planning outcome goals
- Blood pressure will be maintained within acceptable limits.
- Risk for injury will be minimised.
- The patient will demonstrate correct drug administration.

Implementation
- If giving orally, administer the drug with food or at bedtime, as indicated.
- Prevent or minimise orthostatic hypotension by assisting the patient to get up slowly, and by telling the patient not to make sudden movements.
- Maintain the patient's nonpharmacologic therapies, such as sodium restriction, calorie reduction, stress management, and exercise program.
- Know that the dosage is usually adjusted to the patient's blood pressure and tolerance.
- Periodic eye examinations are recommended.

Evaluation
- Patient sustains no trauma from orthostatic hypotension.
- Patient sustains no injury.
- Patient and family understand drug therapy.

Diuretics

Diuretics are used to promote the excretion of water and electrolytes by the kidneys. By doing so, these drugs play a major role in the treatment of hypertension as well as other cardiovascular conditions.

The players

The major diuretics used as cardiovascular drugs include thiazide and thiazide-like diuretics, loop diuretics, and potassium-sparing diuretics.

Thiazide and thiazide-like diuretics

Thiazide and thiazide-like diuretics are sulphonamide derivatives.

Prototype pro

Thiazide diuretics: Hydrochlorothiazide

Actions

- Interferes with sodium transport across tubules of the cortical diluting segment of the nephron
- Increases renal excretion of sodium, chloride, water, potassium, and calcium
- Increases bicarbonate, magnesium, phosphate, bromide, and iodide excretion
- Decreases excretion of ammonia, causing increased serum ammonia levels

Indications

- Oedema
- Hypertension

Nursing considerations

- Monitor for adverse effects, such as pancreatitis, haematologic disorders, and electrolyte imbalances, especially hypokalaemia (signs of hypokalaemia include leg cramps and muscle aches).
- Frequently monitor weight and blood pressure.

Thiazide diuretics include:
- bendroflumethiazide
- benzthiazide
- hydrochlorothiazide
- hydroflumethiazide.

Thiazide-like diuretics include:
- chlortalidone
- indapamide
- metolazone.

Pharmacokinetics

Thiazide diuretics are absorbed rapidly but incompletely from the GI tract after oral administration. They cross the placenta and are secreted in breast milk. These drugs differ in how well they're metabolised and are excreted primarily in urine. (See *Thiazide diuretics: Hydrochlorothiazide.*)

Making a move

Thiazide-like diuretics are absorbed from the GI tract. Indapamide is distributed widely into body tissues and metabolised in the liver.

Prototype pro

Thiazide-like diuretics: Indapamide

Actions

- Interferes with sodium transport across the tubules of the cortical diluting segment in the nephron, thereby increasing renal excretion of sodium, chloride, water, potassium, and calcium

Indications

- Oedema from right-sided heart failure
- Mild to moderate left-sided heart failure
- Nephrotic syndrome
- Oedema and ascites caused by hepatic cirrhosis
- Hypertension
- Diabetes insipidus, especially nephrogenic diabetes insipidus

Nursing considerations

- Give the drug in the morning to prevent nocturia.
- The drug may be used with a potassium-sparing diuretic to prevent potassium loss.

Chlortalidone is 90% bound to erythrocytes. Little is known about chlortalidone metabolism. These drugs are excreted primarily in urine. (See *Thiazide-like diuretics: Indapamide.*)

Pharmacodynamics

Thiazide and thiazide-like diuretics prevent sodium from being reabsorbed in the kidney. As sodium is excreted, it pulls water along with it. Thiazide and thiazide-like diuretics also increase the excretion of chloride, potassium, and bicarbonate, which can result in electrolyte imbalances. With long-term use, thiazide diuretics also lower blood pressure by arteriolar vasodilation.

Up and down

Initially, these drugs decrease circulating blood volume, leading to reduced cardiac output. However, if the therapy is maintained, cardiac output stabilises but plasma fluid volume decreases.

Pharmacotherapeutics

Thiazides are used for the long-term treatment of hypertension and are also used to treat oedema caused by mild or moderate heart failure, liver disease, kidney disease, and corticosteroid and oestrogen therapy.

Stopping stones

Because these drugs decrease the level of calcium in the urine, they're also used alone or with other drugs to prevent the development and recurrence of renal calculi.

A paradoxical effect

In patients with diabetes insipidus (a disorder characterised by excessively large amounts of urine production and excessive thirst, caused by reduced secretion of antidiuretic hormone), thiazides paradoxically decrease urine volume, possibly through sodium depletion and plasma volume reduction.

That's strange. Thiazide diuretics help treat oedema and hypertension by causing the body to shed water...but with diabetes insipidus, these drugs *reduce* urine volume—a beneficial effect.

Drug interactions

Drug interactions related to thiazide and thiazide-like diuretics result in altered fluid volume, blood pressure, and serum electrolyte levels:
• Thiazide and thiazide-like diuretics may increase blood glucose levels, requiring higher doses of insulin and oral antidiabetic drugs.
• Hyponatraemia (low levels of sodium in the blood) and thiazide resistance may also occur.
• Taking corticosteroids, corticotropin, and amphotericin with these diuretics may cause hypokalaemia.
• Lithium levels may be increased by thiazide and thiazide-like diuretics.
• Thiazide and thiazide-like diuretics may increase the response to skeletal muscle relaxants.
• NSAIDs, including COX 2 inhibitors, may reduce the antihypertensive effect of these diuretics.

Adverse reactions

The most common adverse reactions to thiazide and thiazide-like diuretics are reduced blood volume, orthostatic hypotension, hyponatraemia (low blood sodium levels), and hypokalaemia.

Nursing process

These nursing process steps are appropriate for patients undergoing treatment with thiazide and thiazide-like diuretics.

Assessment

• Monitor the patient's intake, output, and serum electrolyte levels regularly.

Weighing in

- Weigh the patient each morning immediately after voiding and before breakfast, in the same type of clothing, and on the same scale. Weight provides a reliable indicator of the patient's response to diuretic therapy.
- Monitor blood glucose level in a diabetic patient. Diuretics may cause hyperglycaemia.
- Monitor serum creatinine and BUN levels regularly. The drug isn't as effective if these levels are more than twice normal. Also monitor blood uric acid level.

Key nursing diagnoses
- Risk for deficient fluid volume related to excessive diuresis.
- Deficient knowledge related to diuretic therapy.

Planning outcome goals
- Normal fluid volume is maintained as evidenced by blood pressure and heart rate.
- Adverse effects of the diuretic will be minimised.
- The patient will demonstrate correct drug administration.

Implementation
- Give the drug in the morning to prevent nocturia.
- Consult a dietitian to provide a high-potassium diet.
- Administer potassium supplements as prescribed to maintain an acceptable serum potassium level.
- Keep a urinal or commode readily available to the patient.

Evaluation
- Patient maintains adequate hydration.
- Patient states the importance of taking diuretic early in the day to prevent nocturia.
- Patient and family understand diuretic therapy. (See *Teaching about diuretics*.)

Make sure patients taking diuretics weigh themselves daily, at the same time, in the same clothing, and on the same scale. It's an important indicator of their progress.

Loop diuretics

Loop (high-ceiling) diuretics are highly potent drugs. They include bumetanide, furosemide and torasemide.

Pharmacokinetics

Loop diuretics usually are absorbed well and distributed rapidly. These diuretics are highly protein bound. For the most part, they undergo partial or complete metabolism in the liver, except for

Education edge

Teaching about diuretics

If diuretics are prescribed, review these points with the patient and caregivers:

- It's essential to understand the rationale for therapy and the importance of following the prescribed regimen.
- Take the drug at the same time each day to prevent nocturia. The drug may be taken with food to minimise GI irritation.
- Seek your prescriber's approval before taking any other drug, including over-the-counter medications and herbal remedies.
- Record your weight each morning after voiding and before breakfast, in the same type of clothing, and on the same scale.
- Be aware of adverse effects and report symptoms promptly, especially chest, back,

or leg pain; shortness of breath; dyspnea; increased oedema or weight; or excess diuresis (weight loss of more than 1 kg daily). Be aware of photosensitivity reactions that usually occur 10 to 14 days after initial sun exposure.

- Avoid high-sodium foods (smoked meats, processed cheeses), and don't add table salt to foods.
- Potassium-rich foods (such as bananas, oranges, and potatoes) are needed if taking potassium-depleting diuretics. If taking potassium-sparing diuretics, potassium-rich foods shouldn't be consumed in great quantity.
- Keep follow-up appointments to monitor effectiveness of therapy.

---

furosemide, which is excreted primarily unchanged. Loop diuretics are excreted primarily by the kidneys.

Pharmacodynamics

Loop diuretics are the most potent diuretics available, producing the greatest volume of diuresis (urine production). They also have a high potential for causing severe adverse reactions. (See *Loop diuretics warning*.)

Bumetanide is the shortest-acting diuretic. It's 40 times more potent than furosemide.

The scoop on the loop

Loop diuretics receive their name because they act primarily on the thick, ascending loop of Henle (the part of the nephron responsible for concentrating urine) to increase the secretion of sodium, chloride, and water. These drugs may also inhibit sodium, chloride, and water reabsorption.

Pharmacotherapeutics

Loop diuretics are used to treat oedema associated with heart failure as well as to treat hypertension (usually with a potassium-sparing diuretic or a potassium supplement to prevent hypokalaemia).

Before you give that drug!

Loop diuretics warning

Loop diuretics contain sulfa. A patient who has an allergy to sulfa may experience an allergic reaction. Use with caution, and alert the patient to this possibility.

Prototype pro

Loop diuretics: Furosemide

Actions

- Inhibits sodium and chloride reabsorption in the ascending loop of Henle, thus increasing renal excretion of sodium, chloride, and water
- Increases excretion of potassium (like thiazide diuretics)
- Produces greater maximum diuresis and electrolyte loss than a thiazide diuretic

Indications

- Acute pulmonary oedema
- Oedema
- Hypertension

Nursing considerations

- Monitor for adverse effects, such as pancreatitis, haematologic disorders, and electrolyte imbalances (especially hypokalaemia).
- Monitor weight and blood pressure frequently.
- Signs of hypokalaemia may include leg cramps and muscle aches.

They're also used to treat oedema associated with liver disease or nephrotic syndrome (kidney disease). (See *Loop diuretics: Furosemide*.)

Drug interactions

Loop diuretics produce a variety of drug interactions:
- The risk of ototoxicity (damage to the organs of hearing) is increased when aminoglycosides and cisplatin are taken with loop diuretics (especially high doses of furosemide).
- Loop diuretics reduce the hypoglycaemic effect of oral antidiabetic drugs, possibly resulting in hyperglycaemia.
- Loop diuretics may increase the risk of lithium toxicity.
- An increased risk of electrolyte imbalances that can trigger arrhythmias is present when cardiac glycosides and loop diuretics are taken together.

Adverse reactions

Because of the potent effects of these drugs, adverse reactions to loop diuretics may be severe. The most severe reactions involve fluid and electrolyte imbalances.

All too common

Common adverse reactions include:
- excess fluid volume loss (especially in elderly patients)
- orthostatic hypotension

- hyperuricaemia
- electrolyte imbalances, including hypokalaemia, hypochloraemia, hyponatraemia, hypocalcaemia, and hypomagnesaemia.

Nursing process

These nursing process steps are appropriate for patients undergoing treatment with loop diuretics.

Assessment
- Monitor blood pressure and pulse rate (especially during rapid diuresis). Establish baseline values before therapy begins, and watch for significant changes.
- Establish a baseline complete blood count (including WBC count), liver function test results, and levels of serum electrolytes, carbon dioxide, magnesium, BUN, and creatinine. Review periodically.
- Assess the patient for evidence of excessive diuresis: hypotension, tachycardia, poor skin turgor, excessive thirst, or dry and cracked mucous membranes.
- Monitor the patient for oedema and ascites. Observe the legs of ambulatory patients and the sacral area of patients on bed rest.
- Monitor and record the patient's weight and intake and output carefully every 24 hours.

Key nursing diagnoses
- Risk for deficient fluid volume related to excessive diuresis.
- Risk for injury related to electrolyte imbalance.
- Deficient knowledge related to diuretic therapy.

Planning outcome goals
- Normal fluid volume is maintained as evidenced by blood pressure and pulse.
- The patient won't exhibit adverse effects of electrolyte imbalance.
- The patient will demonstrate correct diuretic therapy administration.

Implementation
- Give diuretics in the morning to ensure that major diuresis occurs before bedtime. To prevent nocturia, administer diuretics before 6 p.m.
- Give an I.V. dose slowly over 1 to 2 minutes.
- If prescribed, reduce the dosage for a patient with hepatic dysfunction and increase the dosage for a patient with renal impairment, oliguria, or decreased diuresis. (Inadequate urine output may result in circulatory overload, causing water intoxication, pulmonary oedema, and heart failure). If ordered, increase the

dosage of insulin or oral hypoglycaemic in a diabetic patient and reduce the dosage of other antihypertensive drugs.
• Weigh the patient each morning immediately after voiding and before breakfast, in the same type of clothing, and on the same scale. Weight provides a reliable indicator of the patient's response to diuretic therapy.

Play it safe

• Take safety measures for all ambulatory patients until the response to the diuretic is known.
• Consult a dietitian about the need for potassium supplements.
• Keep a urinal or commode readily available.

Evaluation
• Patient maintains adequate hydration.
• Electrolyte levels remain with normal limits.
• Patient and family understand diuretic therapy.

Potassium-sparing diuretics

Potassium-sparing diuretics have weaker diuretic and antihypertensive effects than other diuretics but provide the advantage of conserving potassium. These drugs include amiloride, spironolactone, and triamterene.

Pharmacokinetics

Potassium-sparing diuretics are only available orally and are absorbed in the GI tract. They're metabolised in the liver (except for amiloride, which isn't metabolised) and excreted primarily in urine and bile.

Pharmacodynamics

The direct action of potassium-sparing diuretics on the distal tubule of the kidneys produces the following effects:
• Urinary excretion of sodium and water increases, as does excretion of chloride and calcium ions.
• The excretion of potassium and hydrogen ions decreases.
    These effects lead to reduced blood pressure and increased serum potassium levels.

Head to head

Spironolactone, one of the main potassium-sparing diuretics, is structurally similar to aldosterone and acts as an aldosterone antagonist. Recall that aldosterone promotes the retention of sodium and water and the loss of potassium. Spironolactone counteracts these effects by competing with aldosterone for receptor sites. As a result, sodium, chloride, and water are excreted and potassium is retained.

Pharmacotherapeutics

Potassium-sparing diuretics are used to treat:

- oedema
- diuretic-induced hypokalaemia in patients with heart failure
- cirrhosis
- nephrotic syndrome (abnormal condition of the kidneys)
- heart failure
- hypertension.

Spironolactone is also used to treat hyperaldosteronism (excessive secretion of aldosterone) and hirsutism (excessive hair growth), including hirsutism associated with Stein-Leventhal (polycystic ovary) syndrome.

A balancing act

Potassium-sparing diuretics are commonly used with other diuretics to potentiate their action or counteract their potassium-wasting effects.

Drug interactions

Few drug interactions are associated with the use of amiloride, spironolactone, and triamterene. Those that do occur are related not directly to the drugs but to their potassium-sparing effects.

Adverse reactions

Few adverse drug reactions occur with potassium-sparing diuretics. However, their potassium-sparing effects can lead to hyperkalaemia, especially if given with a potassium supplement or a high-potassium diet.

Enhance diuretic action or offset potassium loss—either way, I can carry my weight.

Nursing process

These nursing process steps are appropriate for patients undergoing treatment with potassium-sparing diuretics.

Assessment

- Monitor blood pressure and pulse rate (especially during rapid diuresis). Establish baseline values before therapy begins, and watch for significant changes.
- Establish a baseline complete blood count (including WBC count), liver function test results, and levels of serum electrolytes, carbon dioxide, magnesium, BUN, and creatinine. Review periodically.
- Assess the patient for evidence of excessive diuresis: hypotension, tachycardia, poor skin turgor, excessive thirst, or dry and cracked mucous membranes.
- Monitor the patient for oedema and ascites. Observe the legs of ambulatory patients and the sacral area of patients on bed rest.
- Weigh the patient each morning immediately after voiding and before breakfast, in the same type of clothing, and on the same scale.

Weight provides a reliable indicator of the patient's response to diuretic therapy.
• Monitor and record the patient's intake and output carefully every 24 hours.

Key nursing diagnoses
• Risk for deficient fluid volume related to excessive diuresis.
• Risk for injury related to electrolyte imbalance.
• Deficient knowledge related to diuretic therapy.

Planning outcome goals
• Normal fluid volume will be maintained as evidenced by blood pressure and pulse.
• No adverse effects of electrolyte imbalance will be exhibited.
• The patient will demonstrate correct diuretic therapy administration.

Implementation
• Give diuretics in the morning to ensure that major diuresis occurs before bedtime. To prevent nocturia, administer diuretics before 6 p.m.
• If prescribed, reduce the dosage for a patient with hepatic dysfunction and increase the dosage for a patient with renal impairment, oliguria, or decreased diuresis. (Inadequate urine output may result in circulatory overload, causing water intoxication, pulmonary oedema, and heart failure). If prescribed, increase the dosage of insulin or oral hypoglycaemic in a diabetic patient and reduce the dosage of other antihypertensive drugs.
• Take safety measures for all ambulatory patients until the response to the diuretic is known.
• Consult a dietitian about the need for education regarding potassium.
• Keep a urinal or commode readily available to the patient.

Evaluation
• Patient maintains adequate hydration.
• Electrolyte levels remain with normal limits.
• Patient and family understand diuretic therapy.

Lipid-regulating drugs

Lipid-regulating drugs are used to lower abnormally high blood levels of lipids, such as cholesterol, triglycerides, and phospholipids. The risk of developing coronary artery disease increases when serum lipid levels are elevated. These drugs are used in combination with lifestyle changes, such as proper diet, weight loss, and exercise, and treatment of any underlying disorder.

Lipid-regulating drug classes include:
- bile-sequestering drugs
- fibric-acid derivatives
- HMG-CoA reductase inhibitors
- nicotinic acid
- cholesterol absorption inhibitors.

Bile-sequestering drugs

The bile-sequestering drugs include colestyramine and colestipol hydrochloride. These drugs are resins that remove excess bile acids from the fat deposits under the skin.

Pharmacokinetics

Bile-sequestering drugs aren't absorbed from the GI tract. Instead, they remain in the intestine, where they combine with bile acids for about 5 hours, and are eventually excreted in faeces.

Pharmacodynamics

The bile-sequestering drugs lower blood levels of low-density lipoproteins (LDLs). These drugs combine with bile acids in the intestines to form an insoluble compound that's then excreted in faeces. The decreasing level of bile acid in the gallbladder triggers the liver to synthesise more bile acids from their precursor, cholesterol.

Come to a halt

As cholesterol leaves the bloodstream and other storage areas to replace the lost bile acids, blood cholesterol levels decrease. Because the small intestine needs bile acids to emulsify lipids and form chylomicrons, absorption of all lipids and lipid-soluble drugs decreases until the bile acids are replaced.

Pharmacotherapeutics

Bile-sequestering drugs are the drugs of choice for treating type IIa hyperlipoproteinaemia (familial hypercholesterolaemia) in a patient who isn't able to lower LDL levels through dietary changes. A patient whose blood cholesterol levels indicate a severe risk of coronary artery disease is most likely to require one of these drugs as a supplement to his diet.

Drug interactions

Bile-sequestering drugs produce the following drug interactions:
- Bile acid binding resins of bile-sequestering drugs may interfere with the absorption of digoxin, oral phosphate supplements, and hydrocortisone.

Bile-sequestering drugs are used to lower LDL levels that don't respond to diet changes.

- Bile-sequestering drugs may decrease absorption of propranolol, tetracycline, furosemide, benzylpenicillin, hydrochlorothiazide, and gemfibrozil.
- Bile-sequestering drugs may reduce absorption of lipid-soluble vitamins, such as A, D, E, and K. Poor absorption of vitamin K can affect prothrombin time significantly, increasing the risk of bleeding.

Adverse reactions

Short-term adverse reactions to bile-sequestering drugs are relatively mild. More severe reactions can result from long-term use. Adverse GI effects with long-term therapy include severe faecal impaction, vomiting, diarrhoea, and haemorrhoid irritation.

Less likely

Rarely, peptic ulcers and bleeding, gallstones, and inflammation of the gallbladder may occur.

Nursing process

These nursing process steps are appropriate for patients undergoing treatment with lipid-regulating drugs.

Assessment
- Assess the patient's cholesterol level and pruritus before therapy, as appropriate.
- Monitor blood cholesterol and lipid levels before and periodically during therapy. Monitor the drug's effectiveness by checking cholesterol and triglyceride levels every 4 weeks or asking the patient whether pruritus has diminished or abated, as appropriate.
- Monitor CK levels when therapy begins and every 6 months thereafter. Also check CK levels if a patient who takes a cholesterol synthesis inhibitor complains of muscle pain.
- Monitor the patient for adverse reactions and drug interactions.
- Monitor the patient for fat-soluble vitamin deficiency because long-term use may be linked to deficiency of vitamins A, D, E, and K and folic acid.
- Evaluate the patient's and family's knowledge of drug therapy.

Key nursing diagnoses
- Risk for injury related to elevated cholesterol levels.
- Risk for injury related to underlying condition.
- Deficient knowledge related to drug therapy.

Planning outcome goals
- Cholesterol levels will be lowered to acceptable levels.
- Risk for injury will be minimised.
- The patient will demonstrate correct drug administration.

Implementation
- If severe constipation develops, decrease the dosage, add a stool softener, or discontinue the drug.
- Give all other drugs at least 1 hour before or 4 to 6 hours after colestyramine to avoid blocking their absorption.

Mixing it up

- Mix powder forms of bile-sequestering drugs with 120 to 180 ml of liquid. Never administer dry powder alone because the patient may accidentally inhale it.
- To mix the powder, sprinkle it on the surface of a preferred drink or a wet food such as soup or custard. Let it stand for a few minutes, and then stir it to obtain uniform suspension. Know that mixing with fizzy drinks may result in excess foaming. Use a large glass and mix slowly.

Evaluation
- Patient maintains adequate cholesterol levels.
- Patient won't incur injury while taking medication.
- Patient and family understand drug therapy. (See *Teaching about lipid-regulating drugs.*)

Education edge
Teaching about lipid-regulating drugs

If lipid-regulating drugs are prescribed, review these points with the patient and caregivers:

- Take the drug exactly as prescribed. If you take a bile-sequestering drug, never take the dry form. Oesophageal irritation or severe constipation may result.
- Use a large glass and sprinkle the powder on the surface of a preferred drink. Let the mixture stand a few minutes; then stir thoroughly. The best diluents are water, milk, and juice (especially pulpy fruit juice). Mixing with fizzy drinks may result in excess foaming. After drinking this preparation, swirl a small additional amount of liquid in the same glass and then drink it to ensure ingestion of the entire dose.
- Diet is very important in controlling serum lipid levels. Maintain proper dietary management of serum lipids (restricting total fat and cholesterol intake) as well as control of other cardiac disease risk factors.
- Drink 2 to 3 L of fluid daily, and report persistent or severe constipation.
- Weight control, exercise, and smoking cessation programs may be appropriate.
- If you also take bile acid resin, take fenofibrate 1 hour before or 4 to 6 hours after bile acid resin.
- When taking fenofibrate, promptly report symptoms of unexplained muscle weakness, pain, or tenderness, especially if accompanied by malaise or fever.
- Have periodic eye examinations.
- Don't crush or chew extended-release tablets.

Fibric acid derivatives

Fibric acid is produced by several fungi. Two derivatives of this acid are fenofibrate and gemfibrozil. These drugs are used to reduce high triglyceride levels and, to a lesser extent, high LDL levels.

Pharmacokinetics

Fenofibrate and gemfibrozil are absorbed readily from the GI tract and are highly protein bound. Fenofibrate undergoes rapid hydrolysis, and gemfibrozil undergoes extensive metabolism in the liver. Both drugs are excreted in urine.

Pharmacodynamics

Although the exact mechanism of action for these drugs isn't known, researchers believe that fibric acid derivatives may:
- reduce cholesterol production early in its formation
- mobilise cholesterol from the tissues
- increase cholesterol excretion
- decrease synthesis and secretion of lipoproteins
- decrease synthesis of triglycerides.

A silver lining

Gemfibrozil produces two other effects:
- It increases high-density lipoprotein (HDL) levels in the blood (remember, this is "good" cholesterol).
- It increases the serum's capacity to dissolve additional cholesterol.

Pharmacotherapeutics

Fibric acid drugs are used primarily to reduce triglyceride levels, especially very-low-density triglycerides, and secondarily to reduce blood cholesterol levels.

Because of their ability to reduce triglyceride levels, fibric acid derivatives are useful in treating patients with types II, III, IV, and mild-type V hyperlipoproteinaemia.

Drug interactions

These drug interactions may occur:
- Fibric acid drugs may displace acidic drugs, such as barbiturates, phenytoin, thyroid derivatives, and cardiac glycosides.
- The risk of bleeding increases when fibric acid derivatives are taken with oral anticoagulants.
- Fibric acid derivatives can lead to adverse GI effects.

Adverse reactions

Adverse reactions to fibric acid drugs include headache, dizziness, blurred vision, arrhythmias, thrombocytopenia, and rash. GI effects include epigastric pain, dyspepsia, nausea, vomiting, and diarrhoea or constipation.

Nursing process

These nursing process steps are appropriate for patients undergoing treatment with fibric acid derivatives.

Assessment
- Assess the patient's cholesterol level and pruritus before therapy, as appropriate.
- Monitor blood cholesterol and lipid levels before and periodically during therapy. Monitor the drug's effectiveness by checking cholesterol and triglyceride levels every 4 weeks or asking the patient whether pruritus has diminished or abated, as appropriate.
- Assess liver function tests before starting therapy and periodically thereafter.
- Monitor CK levels when therapy begins and every 6 months thereafter. Also check CK levels if a patient who takes a cholesterol synthesis inhibitor complains of muscle pain.
- Monitor the patient for adverse reactions and drug interactions.
- Monitor the patient for fat-soluble vitamin deficiency because long-term use may be linked to deficiency of vitamins A, D, E, and K and folic acid.
- Evaluate the patient's and family's knowledge of drug therapy.

Key nursing diagnoses
- Risk for injury related to elevated cholesterol levels.
- Risk for injury related to underlying condition.
- Deficient knowledge related to drug therapy.

Planning outcome goals
- Cholesterol levels will be lowered to acceptable levels.
- Risk for injury will be minimised.
- The patient will demonstrate correct drug administration.

Implementation
- If severe constipation develops, decrease the dosage, add a stool softener, or discontinue the drug.
- Administer a daily fibric acid derivative at prescribed times.
- Withdraw therapy in a patient who doesn't have an adequate response after 2 months of treatment with the maximum dose.
- Give tablets with meals to increase bioavailability.

- Evaluate renal function and triglyceride levels of a patient with severe renal impairment before dosage increases.
- Reinforce the importance of adhering to a triglyceride-lowering diet.
- Instruct patient who also takes bile acid resin to take fenofibrate 1 hour before or 4 to 6 hours after bile acid resin.

Evaluation

- Patient maintains adequate cholesterol levels.
- Patient won't incur injury while taking medication.
- Patient and family understand drug therapy.

HMG-CoA reductase inhibitors

As their name implies, 3-hydroxy-3-methylglutaryl coenzyme A (HMG-CoA) reductase inhibitors (also known as the *statins*) lower lipid levels by interfering with cholesterol synthesis. These drugs include atorvastatin calcium, fluvastatin sodium, lovastatin, pravastatin sodium, and simvastatin. (See *Lipid-regulating drugs: Atorvastatin*.)

Prototype pro

Lipid-regulating drugs: Atorvastatin

Actions

- Inhibits HMG-CoA reductase

Indications

- Plasma cholesterol and lipoprotein level reduction

Nursing considerations

- Use the drug only after diet and other nonpharmacological treatments prove ineffective.
- Restrict the patient to a standard low-cholesterol diet before and during therapy.

- Before starting treatment, perform a baseline lipid profile to exclude secondary causes of hypercholesterolaemia. Liver function test results and lipid levels should be obtained before therapy, after 6 and 12 weeks, or following a dosage increase and periodically thereafter.
- Before starting treatment, a baseline creatine kinase may be performed and the patient should be routinely monitored for myopathy, which may be an indication of rhabdomyolysis.

Pharmacokinetics

With the exception of pravastatin, HMG-CoA reductase inhibitors are highly bound to plasma proteins. All undergo extensive first-pass metabolism. Their specific pharmacokinetic properties vary slightly.

Pharmacodynamics

HMG-CoA reductase inhibitors inhibit the enzyme that's responsible for the conversion of HMG-CoA to mevalonate, an early rate-limiting step in the biosynthesis of cholesterol.

Pharmacotherapeutics

Statin drugs are used primarily to reduce low-density lipoproteins (LDLs) and also to reduce total blood cholesterol levels. These agents also produce a mild increase in HDLs.

Because of their ability to lower cholesterol levels, statins are indicated for the treatment of primary hypercholesterolaemia (types IIa and IIb).

Heart to heart

As a result of their effect on LDL and total cholesterol, these drugs are indicated for primary and secondary prevention of cardiovascular events.

Drug interactions

These drug interactions may occur:
• Atorvastatin or simvastatin when combined with nicotinic acid, erythromycin, clarithromycin, immunosuppressant drugs (especially ciclosporine), gemfibrozil, itraconazole, ketoconazole, or fluconazole may increase the risk of myopathy (muscle wasting and weakness) or rhabdomyolysis (potentially fatal breakdown of skeletal muscle, causing renal failure).
• All HMG-CoA reductase inhibitors should be administered 1 hour before or 4 hours after bile acid sequestrants (colestyramine, colestipol).
• Simvastatin may increase the risk of bleeding when administered with warfarin.

Adverse reactions

HMG-CoA reductase inhibitors may alter liver function studies, increasing aspartate aminotransferase, alanine aminotransferase, alkaline phosphatase, and bilirubin levels. Other hepatic effects may include pancreatitis, hepatitis, and cirrhosis.

Myalgia is the most common musculoskeletal effect, although arthralgia and muscle cramps may also occur. Myopathy and rhabdomyolysis are rare but potentially severe reactions that may occur with these drugs.

Possible adverse GI reactions include nausea, vomiting, diarrhoea, abdominal pain, flatulence, and constipation.

Nursing process

These nursing process steps are appropriate for patients undergoing treatment with HMG-CoA reductase inhibitors.

Assessment
- Assess the patient's cholesterol level and pruritus before therapy, as appropriate.
- Monitor blood cholesterol and lipid levels before and periodically during therapy. Monitor the drug's effectiveness by checking cholesterol and triglyceride levels every 4 weeks or asking the patient whether pruritus has diminished or abated, as appropriate.
- Monitor CK levels when therapy begins and every 6 months thereafter. Also check CK levels if a patient who takes a cholesterol synthesis inhibitor complains of muscle pain.
- Liver function tests should be performed at the start of therapy and periodically thereafter. A liver biopsy may be performed if enzyme level elevations persist.
- Monitor the patient for adverse reactions and drug interactions.
- Monitor the patient for fat-soluble-vitamin deficiency because long-term use may be linked to deficiency of vitamins A, D, E, and K and folic acid.
- Evaluate the patient's and family's knowledge of drug therapy.

Key nursing diagnoses
- Risk for injury related to elevated cholesterol levels.
- Risk for imbalanced fluid volume related to adverse drug effects on the GI system.
- Deficient knowledge related to drug therapy.

Planning outcome goals
- Cholesterol levels will be lowered to acceptable levels.
- Risk for adverse GI effects will be minimised.
- The patient will demonstrate correct drug administration.

Implementation
- If severe constipation develops, decrease the dosage, add a stool softener, or discontinue the drug.
- Give the drug before meals and at bedtime, as applicable. Give simvastatin in the evening, and fluvastatin and pravastatin at bedtime.

Evaluation
- Patient maintains adequate cholesterol levels.
- Patient won't incur injury while taking medication.
- Patient and family understand drug therapy.

Nicotinic acid

Also known as *niacin*, nicotinic acid is a water-soluble vitamin that decreases triglyceride and apolipoprotein B-100 levels and increases HDL levels. The drug is available in immediate-release and extended-release tablets.

Pharmacokinetics

Nicotinic acid is moderately bound to plasma proteins; its overall binding ranges from 60% to 70%. The drug undergoes rapid metabolism by the liver to active and inactive metabolites. About 75% of the drug is excreted in urine.

Pharmacodynamics

The way that nicotinic acid lowers triglyceride and apolipoprotein levels is unknown. However, it may work by inhibiting hepatic synthesis of lipoproteins that contain apolipoprotein B-100, promoting lipoprotein lipase activity, reducing free fatty acid mobilisation from adipose tissue, and increasing faecal elimination of sterols.

Pharmacotherapeutics

Nicotinic acid is used primarily as an adjunct to lower triglyceride levels in patients with type IV or V hyperlipidaemia who are at high risk for pancreatitis. The drug also may be used to lower cholesterol and LDL levels in patients with hypercholesterolaemia. It's commonly used with other lipid-regulating drugs to meet LDL goals and to increase the HDL level for patients in whom it's below the desired level.

This lipid-regulating drug is contraindicated in patients who are hypersensitive to nicotinic acid and in those with hepatic dysfunction, active peptic ulcer disease, or arterial bleeding.

Drug interactions

These drug interactions can occur with nicotinic acid:
- Together, nicotinic acid and an HMG-CoA reductase inhibitor may increase the risk of muscle wasting and weakness, myopathy, or life-threatening breakdown of skeletal muscle, causing renal failure or rhabdomyolysis.
- A bile-sequestering drug, such as colestyramine or colestipol, can bind with nicotinic acid and decrease its effectiveness.
- When given with nicotinic acid, kava may increase the risk of hepatotoxicity.

Adverse reactions

High doses of nicotinic acid may produce vasodilation and cause flushing. Extended-release forms tend to produce less severe vasodilation than immediate-release forms. To help minimise flushing, aspirin may be given 30 minutes before nicotinic acid, or the extended-release form may be given at night.

Nicotinic acid can cause hepatotoxicity; the risk of this adverse reaction is greater with extended-release forms. Other adverse effects include nausea, vomiting, diarrhoea, and epigastric or substernal pain.

Nursing process

These nursing process steps are appropriate for patients undergoing treatment with nicotinic acid.

Assessment

- Assess the patient's cholesterol level and pruritus before therapy, as appropriate.
- Monitor blood cholesterol and lipid levels before and periodically during therapy. Monitor the drug's effectiveness by checking cholesterol and triglyceride levels every 4 weeks or asking the patient whether pruritus has diminished or abated, as appropriate.
- Monitor CK levels when therapy begins and every 6 months thereafter. Also check CK levels if a patient who takes a cholesterol synthesis inhibitor complains of muscle pain.
- Monitor the patient for adverse reactions and drug interactions.
- Monitor the patient for fat-soluble vitamin deficiency because long-term use may be linked to deficiency of vitamins A, D, E, and K and folic acid.
- Evaluate the patient's and family's knowledge of drug therapy.

Key nursing diagnoses

- Risk for injury related to elevated cholesterol levels.
- Risk for injury related to underlying condition.
- Deficient knowledge related to drug therapy.

Planning outcome goals

- Cholesterol levels will be lowered to acceptable levels.
- Risk for injury to the patient will be minimised.
- The patient will demonstrate correct drug administration.

Implementation

- If severe constipation develops, decrease the dosage, add a stool softener, or discontinue the drug.
- Administer aspirin, as appropriate, to help reduce flushing.
- Know that timed-released nicotinic acid or nicotinamide may prevent excessive flushing that occurs with large doses. However, timed-release nicotinic acid has been linked to hepatic dysfunction, even at doses as low as 1 g daily.

- Give the drug with meals to minimise GI adverse effects.
- To decrease flushing, advise the patient to take the drug with a low-fat snack and to avoid taking it after alcohol, hot beverages, hot or spicy foods, a hot shower, or exercise.

Evaluation
- Patient maintains adequate cholesterol levels.
- Patient won't incur injury while taking medication.
- Patient and family understand drug therapy.

Cholesterol absorption inhibitors

As their name implies, cholesterol absorption inhibitors inhibit the absorption of cholesterol and related phytosterols from the intestine. Ezetimibe is the drug that falls under this class.

Pharmacokinetics
Ezetimibe is absorbed and extensively conjugated to an active form and is highly bound to plasma proteins. The drug is primarily metabolised in the small intestine and is excreted by biliary and renal routes.

Pharmacodynamics
Ezetimibe reduces blood cholesterol levels by inhibiting the absorption of cholesterol by the small intestine.

On the edge

The drug works at the brush border of the small intestine to inhibit cholesterol absorption. This leads to a decrease in delivery of intestinal cholesterol to the liver, causing a reduction in hepatic cholesterol stores and an increase in clearance from the blood.

Pharmacotherapeutics
Ezetimibe may be administered alone as adjunctive therapy to diet for treatment of primary hypercholesterolaemia and homozygous sitosterolaemia. The drug is also indicated as adjunctive therapy, administered in addition to HMG-CoA reductase inhibitors, for the treatment of primary hypercholesterolaemia and homozygous familial hypercholesterolaemia. Ezetimibe provides additional lowering of total cholesterol, LDL, and an additional increase HDL cholesterol in patients unable to achieve their desired goals following maximum-dose HMG-CoA reductase inhibitor therapy.

Drug interactions
Colestyramine may decrease the effectiveness of ezetimibe. Fenofibrate, gemfibrozil, and ciclosporine lead to an increased level of ezetimibe.

Ezetimibe reduces blood cholesterol levels by inhibiting the absorption of cholesterol by the small intestine.

Adverse reactions

The most common adverse reactions to ezetimibe include:

- fatigue
- abdominal pain
- diarrhoea
- pharyngitis
- sinusitis
- arthralgia and back pain
- cough.

When ezetimibe is given with an HMG-CoA reductase inhibitor, the most common adverse reactions are:

- chest or abdominal pain
- dizziness
- headache
- diarrhoea
- pharyngitis
- sinusitis
- upper respiratory infection
- arthralgia, myalgia, and back pain.

Nursing process

These nursing process steps are appropriate for patients undergoing treatment with cholesterol absorption inhibitors.

Assessment

- Assess the patient's cholesterol level and pruritus before therapy, as appropriate.
- Monitor blood cholesterol and lipid levels before and periodically during therapy. Monitor the drug's effectiveness by checking cholesterol and triglyceride levels every 4 weeks or asking the patient whether pruritus has diminished or abated, as appropriate.
- Monitor CK levels when therapy begins and every 6 months thereafter. Also check CK levels if a patient who takes a cholesterol synthesis inhibitor complains of muscle pain.
- Be alert for adverse reactions and drug interactions.
- Monitor the patient for fat-soluble-vitamin deficiency because long-term use may be linked to deficiency of vitamins A, D, E, and K and folic acid.
- Evaluate the patient's and family's knowledge of drug therapy.

Key nursing diagnoses

- Risk for injury related to elevated cholesterol levels.
- Risk for injury related to underlying condition.
- Deficient knowledge related to drug therapy.

Planning outcome goals
- Cholesterol levels will be lowered to acceptable levels.
- Risk for injury to the patient will be minimised.
- The patient will demonstrate correct drug administration.

Implementation
- If severe constipation develops, decrease the dosage, add a stool softener, or discontinue the drug.
- Instruct on a cholesterol-lowering diet as appropriate.

Evaluation
- Patient maintains adequate cholesterol levels.
- Patient won't incur injury while taking medication.
- Patient and family understand drug therapy.

Quick quiz

1. A patient is receiving digoxin for treatment of atrial fibrillation. When you enter the room to give the medication, you find the patient irritable and complaining of nausea and blurred vision. She's also disoriented to place and time. The most appropriate action at this time is to:
- A. attempt to reorient the patient while helping her take the digoxin.
- B. return to the room later and see whether the patient will take the medication.
- C. withhold the digoxin and notify the prescriber about your assessment findings.
- D. check the medication profile for possible drug interactions after giving the digoxin to the patient.

Answer: C. Irritability, nausea, blurred vision, and confusion are signs and symptoms of digoxin toxicity. The digoxin dose should be withheld, the prescriber notified, and the digoxin level checked. You should try to reorient the patient and prepare for possible emergency treatment pending the laboratory results.

2. A patient comes to the emergency department complaining of chest pains, which started 1 hour ago while he was mowing the lawn. Glyceryl trinitrate was given sublingually as prescribed. Which of the following adverse reactions would be most likely to occur?
- A. Hypotension
- B. Dizziness
- C. GI distress
- D. Headache

Answer: D. The most common reaction to nitrates is headache. Nitrates dilate the blood vessels in the meningeal layers between the brain and cranium. Hypotension, dizziness, and GI distress may occur, but likelihood varies with each patient.

3. Which adverse reaction associated with ACE inhibitors is the most common and usually leads to disruption of therapy?
    A. Constipation
    B. Cough
    C. Sexual dysfunction
    D. Tachycardia

Answer: B. Cough causes discontinuation of ACE inhibitor therapy in more than 10% of patients taking this class of antihypertensives because it disrupts the patient's sleep patterns.

4. A patient is taking an HMG-CoA reductase inhibitor. Which of the following tests should be performed at the start of therapy and periodically thereafter?
    A. Liver function
    B. Electrolyte levels
    C. Complete blood count
    D. ECG

Answer: A. Because increased liver enzyme levels may occur in patients receiving long-term HMG-CoA therapy, liver function test results should be monitored.

Scoring

☆☆☆   If you answered all four questions correctly, A1! You're aces with ACE inhibitors and all of the other cardiovascular drugs.

☆☆   If you answered three questions correctly, cool! Cardiovascular drugs aren't causing you any complications.

☆   If you answered fewer than three questions correctly, stay mellow! This is a complex chapter, and it might just require another dose.

Just the facts

In this chapter, you'll learn:

♦ classes of drugs used to treat respiratory disorders

♦ uses and varying actions of these drugs

♦ absorption, distribution, metabolism, and excretion of these drugs

♦ drug interactions and adverse reactions to these drugs.

Drugs and the respiratory system

The respiratory system, which extends from the nose to the pulmonary capillaries, performs the essential function of gas exchange between the body and its environment. In other words, it takes in oxygen and expels carbon dioxide.

Drugs used to improve respiratory symptoms are available in inhalation and systemic formulations. These include:

- beta$_2$-adrenergic agonists
- anticholinergics
- corticosteroids
- leukotriene modifiers
- mast cell stabilisers
- methylxanthines
- expectorants
- antitussives
- mucolytics
- decongestants.

Are you ready to learn about respiratory system drugs? Then take a deep breath and let's get started.

Beta₂-adrenergic agonists

Beta₂-adrenergic agonists are used for the treatment of symptoms associated with asthma and chronic obstructive pulmonary disease (COPD). These drugs are analogous to the endogenous ligand noradrenaline (norepinephrine). Agents in this class can be divided into two categories:
* short-acting
* long-acting.

Beta-adrenergic agonists can be short- or long-acting.

The short...

Short-acting beta₂-adrenergic agonists include:
* salbutamol (systemic, inhalation)
* terbutaline (systemic).

...and long of it

Long-acting beta₂-adrenergic agonists include:
* salmeterol (inhalation)
* formoterol (inhalation).

Pharmacokinetics

Beta₂-adrenergic agonists are minimally absorbed from the GI tract. Inhaled formulations generally exert their effects locally. After inhalation, beta₂-adrenergic agonists appear to be absorbed over several hours from the respiratory tract. These drugs don't cross the blood-brain barrier. They're extensively metabolised in the liver to inactive compounds and are rapidly excreted in urine and faeces.

Pharmacodynamics

Beta₂-adrenergic agonists increase levels of cyclic adenosine monophosphate through the stimulation of beta₂-adrenergic receptors in the smooth muscle, resulting in bronchodilation. Beta₂-adrenergic agonists may lose their selectivity at higher doses, which can increase the risk of toxicity. Inhaled agents are preferred because they act locally in the lungs, resulting in fewer adverse effects than systemically absorbed formulations.

Pharmacotherapeutics

Short-acting inhaled beta$_2$-adrenergic agonists are the drugs of choice for fast relief of symptoms in asthmatic patients. They're primarily used on an as needed basis for asthma and chronic obstructive pulmonary disease (COPD) and are also effective for exercise-induced asthma.

From morning till night

Some patients with COPD use short-acting inhaled beta$_2$-adrenergic agonists around the clock on a specified schedule. However, excessive use of these agents may indicate poor asthma control, requiring reassessment of the therapeutic regimen.

Strictly regimented

Long-acting agents are more appropriately used with anti-inflammatory agents, specifically inhaled corticosteroids, to help control asthma. They must be administered on schedule in order to be most effective. They're especially useful when a patient exhibits nocturnal asthmatic symptoms. Because of their delayed onset, long-acting beta$_2$-adrenergic agonists aren't used for acute symptoms. They're also ineffective against the chronic inflammation associated with asthma.

Drug interactions

Interactions with beta$_2$-adrenergic agonists aren't as common when using inhaled formulations. Beta-adrenergic blockers decrease the bronchodilating effects of the beta$_2$-adrenergic agonists and, therefore, these drugs should be used together cautiously.

Adverse reactions

Adverse reactions to short-acting beta$_2$-adrenergic agonists include paradoxical bronchospasm, tachycardia, palpitations, tremors, and dry mouth.

Adverse reactions to long-acting beta$_2$-adrenergic agonists include bronchospasm, tachycardia, palpitations, hypertension, and tremors.

Nursing process

These nursing process steps are appropriate for patients undergoing treatment with beta$_2$-adrenergic agonists.

Assessment
• Assess the patient's respiratory condition before therapy and regularly thereafter.
• Assess peak flow readings before starting treatment and periodically thereafter.

- Be alert for adverse reactions and drug interactions.
- Evaluate the patient's and family's knowledge of drug therapy.

Key nursing diagnoses
- Ineffective breathing pattern related to respiratory condition.
- Impaired gas exchange related to underlying condition.
- Deficient knowledge related to drug therapy.

Planning outcome goals
- Breathing pattern will improve as evidenced by regular and even respiratory rate and rhythm.
- Gas exchange will be adequate as evidenced by improved peak flow rates, oxygen saturation, and arterial blood gas (ABG) levels.
- The patient will demonstrate correct drug administration.

Implementation
- Report insufficient relief or worsening condition.
- Obtain a prescription for a mild analgesic if a drug-induced headache occurs.
- Don't use long-acting beta$_2$-adrenergic agonists for reversing bronchospasm during an acute asthma attack.

Evaluation
- Patient exhibits normal breathing pattern.
- Patient exhibits improved gas exchange.
- Patient and family understand drug therapy. (See *Teaching about bronchodilators*.)

Anticholinergics

Anticholinergics competitively antagonise the actions of acetylcholine and other cholinergic agonists at receptors. Generally, oral anticholinergics aren't used to treat asthma and other COPDs because of their tendency to thicken secretions and form mucus plugs in the airways.

Ipratropium

Inhaled ipratropium bromide is a bronchodilator used primarily in patients suffering from COPD. It may also be used as an adjunct to beta$_2$-adrenergic agonists.

Pharmacokinetics
Ipratropium is minimally absorbed from the GI tract. It exerts its effects locally.

Education edge

Teaching about bronchodilators

If bronchodilators are prescribed, review these points with the patient and caregivers:

- Take the drug as directed. Note that some medications should be taken every 12 hours, even if you're feeling better, and other drugs, such as salbutamol, should only be used in an acute attack.
- Take the drug 30 to 60 minutes before exercise, as directed, to prevent exercise-induced bronchospasm.
- Contact your prescriber if the medication no longer provides sufficient relief or if you need more than four inhalations per day. This may be a sign that asthma symptoms are worsening. Don't increase the dosage of the drug.
- If you're taking an inhaled corticosteroid, continue to use it as directed by the prescriber.
- Don't take bronchodilators with other drugs, over-the-counter preparations, or herbal remedies without your prescriber's consent.
- Follow these instructions for using a metered-dose inhaler as appropriate:
  – Clear your nasal passages and throat.

  – Breathe out, expelling as much air from lungs as possible.
  – Place the mouthpiece well into mouth, and inhale deeply as you release the dose from the inhaler.
  – Hold your breath for several seconds, remove the mouthpiece, and exhale slowly.
- Avoid accidentally spraying the medication into your eyes. Temporary blurring of vision may result.
- If more than one inhalation is prescribed, wait at least 2 minutes between each subsequent inhalation.
- If you use a corticosteroid inhaler, use ipratropium first, and then wait about 5 minutes before using the corticosteroid. This process allows the bronchodilator to open air passages for maximum effectiveness of the corticosteroid.
- Take a missed dose as soon as you remember, unless it's almost time for the next dose; in that case, skip the missed dose. Don't double the dose.

Pharmacodynamics

Ipratropium blocks the parasympathetic nervous system rather than stimulating the sympathetic nervous system. To exert its anticholinergic effects, this drug inhibits muscarinic receptors, which results in bronchodilation.

Pharmacotherapeutics

Ipratropium is used in patients with COPD. It may also be used as an adjunctive therapy for the treatment of asthma; however, it's less effective as a form of long-term management. It's commonly used in combination with a short-acting beta$_2$-adrenergic agonist on a scheduled basis.

Drug interactions

Drug interactions aren't as likely when using an inhaled formulation of ipratropium. Use antimuscarinic and anticholinergic agents cautiously with ipratropium.

Adverse reactions

The most common adverse reactions to anticholinergics include:
* nervousness
* tachycardia
* nausea and vomiting
* paradoxical bronchospasm with excessive use.

Nursing process

These nursing process steps are appropriate for patients undergoing treatment with anticholinergics.

Assessment
* Assess the patient's respiratory condition before therapy and regularly thereafter.
* Assess peak flow readings before starting treatment and periodically thereafter.
* Be alert for adverse reactions and drug interactions.
* Evaluate the patient's and family's knowledge of drug therapy.

Key nursing diagnoses
* Ineffective breathing pattern related to respiratory condition.
* Impaired gas exchange related to underlying condition.
* Deficient knowledge related to drug therapy.

Planning outcome goals
* Breathing pattern improves as evidenced by regular and even respiratory rate and rhythm.
* Gas exchange will be adequate as evidenced by improved peak flow rates, oxygen saturation, and ABG levels.
* The patient will demonstrate correct drug administration.

Implementation
* Report insufficient relief or a worsening condition.
* Obtain a prescription for a mild analgesic if a drug-induced headache occurs.
* Be aware that the drug isn't effective for treating acute episodes of bronchospasm when rapid response is needed.
* Monitor the medication regimen. Total inhalations shouldn't exceed 12 in 24 hours, and total nasal sprays shouldn't exceed 8 in each nostril in 24 hours.

- If more than one inhalation is prescribed, 2 minutes should elapse between inhalations. If more than one type of inhalant is prescribed, always give the bronchodilator first and wait 5 minutes before administering the other.
- Give the drug on time to ensure maximal effect.
- Notify the prescriber if the drug fails to relieve bronchospasms.
- Provide patient teaching.

Evaluation
- Patient exhibits normal breathing pattern.
- Patient exhibits improved gas exchange.
- Patient and family understand drug therapy.

Corticosteroids

Corticosteroids are anti-inflammatory agents available in both inhaled and systemic formulations for the short- and long-term control of asthma symptoms. This class consists of many drugs with differing potencies.

Via nose

Inhaled corticosteroids include:
- beclometasone dipropionate
- budesonide
- flunisolide
- fluticasone propionate
- triamcinolone acetonide.

Via mouth

Oral corticosteroids include:
- prednisolone.

Via vein

I.V. corticosteroids include:
- methylprednisolone sodium succinate
- hydrocortisone sodium succinate.

Pharmacokinetics
Inhaled corticosteroids are minimally absorbed, although absorption increases as the dose is increased. Oral prednisolone is readily absorbed and I.V. forms have a rapid onset.

Before you give that drug!

Corticosteroid warning

Consider these points about special populations before administering corticosteroids:

- Growth should be monitored in children, especially when taking systemic agents or higher doses of inhaled agents.
- Older patients may benefit from specific medications, diet, and exercise intended to prevent osteoporosis while on these agents, especially when receiving higher doses of inhaled steroids or systemic agents.

- Patients with diabetes may require closer monitoring of blood glucose while on steroids.
- Corticosteroid levels are negligible in the breast milk of mothers who are receiving less than 20 mg/day of oral drug.
- To reduce the risk of adverse effects occurring with the inhaled agents, use the lowest possible doses to maintain control. Spacers should be used to administer doses, and patients should rinse their mouths out following administration.

Pharmacodynamics

Corticosteroids inhibit the production of cytokines, leukotrienes, and prostaglandins, the recruitment of eosinophils, and the release of other inflammatory mediators. These drugs typically inhibit the enzyme phospholipase A2 which is an essential component of the inflammatory cascade. They also have various effects elsewhere in the body that cause many of the long-term adverse effects associated with these agents. (See *Corticosteroid warning*.)

Pharmacotherapeutics

Corticosteroids are the most effective agents available for the long-term treatment and prevention of asthma exacerbations. Systemic formulations are commonly reserved for moderate to severe acute exacerbations but are also used in those with severe asthma that's refractory to other measures. Systemic corticosteroids should be used at the lowest effective dose and for the shortest possible period to avoid adverse effects.

Inhaled corticosteroids remain the mainstay of therapy to prevent future exacerbations for most asthmatics with mild to severe disease. Use of inhaled corticosteroids reduces the need for systemic steroids in many patients, thus reducing the risk of serious long-term adverse effects. Inhaled corticosteroids shouldn't be used for acute symptoms; rather, short-acting inhaled beta$_2$-adrenergic agonists should be used.

Prolonged use of systemic corticosteriods can result in serious adverse effects.

CAUTION!

Drug interactions

Interactions aren't likely when using inhaled formulations. Hormonal contraceptives, ketoconazole, and macrolide antibiotics can increase the activity of corticosteroids in general and may require a dosage decrease of the steroid. Barbiturates, colestyramine, and phenytoin can decrease the effectiveness of corticosteroids and may require a dosage increase of the steroid.

Adverse reactions

Possible adverse reactions to inhaled corticosteroids include:
* mouth irritation
* oral candidiasis
* upper respiratory tract infection.

Nursing process

These nursing process steps are appropriate for patients undergoing treatment with corticosteroids.

Assessment
* Assess the patient's respiratory condition before therapy and regularly thereafter.
* Assess peak flow readings before starting treatment and periodically thereafter.
* Assess smoking history and estimate lung deterioration.
* Be alert for adverse reactions and drug interactions.
* Evaluate the patient's and family's knowledge of drug therapy.

Key nursing diagnoses
* Ineffective breathing pattern related to respiratory condition.
* Impaired gas exchange related to underlying condition.
* Deficient knowledge related to drug therapy.

Planning outcome goals
* Breathing pattern will improve as evidenced by regular and even respiratory rate and rhythm.
* Gas exchange will be adequate as evidenced by improved peak flow rates, oxygen saturation, and ABG levels.
* The patient will demonstrate correct drug administration.

Implementation
* Report insufficient relief or worsening of condition.
* Give oral doses with food to prevent GI irritation.
* Take precautions to avoid exposing the patient to infection.
* Don't stop the drug abruptly.

- Notify the prescriber of severe or persistent adverse reactions.
- Avoid prolonged use of corticosteroids, especially in children.

Evaluation
- Patient exhibits normal breathing pattern.
- Patient exhibits improved gas exchange.
- Patient and family understand drug therapy.

Leukotriene modifiers

Leukotriene modifiers are used for the prevention and long-term control of mild asthma and include the *Leukotriene receptor antagonists* zafirlukast and montelukast. (See *Leukotriene modifiers: Zafirlukast*.)

Pharmacokinetics
All leukotriene modifiers are extensively metabolised, have a rapid absorption, and are highly protein bound (> 90%). Zafirlukast's absorption is decreased by food. Montelukast has a rapid absorption from the GI tract and may be given with food. Patients with hepatic impairment may require a dosage adjustment.

Prototype pro

Leukotriene modifiers: Zafirlukast

Actions

- Selectively competes for leukotriene receptor sites, blocking inflammatory action

Indications

- Prophylaxis and long-term management of asthma

Nursing considerations

- This drug isn't indicated for reversing bronchospasm in acute asthma attacks.

- Give cautiously to elderly patients and those with hepatic impairment.
- Drug absorption is decreased by food; the drug should be given 1 hour before or 2 hours after meals.
- Monitor liver function studies in patients with suspected hepatic dysfunction. The drug may need to be discontinued if hepatic dysfunction is confirmed.

Pharmacodynamics

Leukotrienes are substances that are released from mast cells, eosinophils, and basophils. They can result in smooth-muscle contraction of the airways, increased permeability of the vasculature, increased secretions, and activation of other inflammatory mediators. The leukotriene receptor antagonists zafirlukast and montelukast are competitive inhibitors of the leukotriene D4 and E4 receptors that inhibit leukotriene from interacting with its receptor and blocking its action.

Pharmacotherapeutics

Leukotriene modifiers are primarily used to prevent and control asthma exacerbations in patients with mild to moderate disease. They may also be used as steroid-sparing agents in some patients.

Drug interactions

• Because zafirlukast inhibits CYP 2C9, increased toxicity can result when the drug is used with phenytoin or warfarin.
• Zafirlukast inhibits CYP 3A4 which can result in increased toxicity if used with amlodipine, atorvastatin, carbamazepine, clarithromycin, ciclosporine, erythromycin, hormonal contraceptives, itraconazole, ketoconazole, lovastatin, nelfinavir, nifedipine, ritonavir, sertraline, simvastatin, or warfarin.
• Zafirlukast and montelukast are metabolised by CYP 2C9. Increased toxicity can result if these drugs are administered with amiodarone, cimetidine, fluconazole, fluoxetine, fluvoxamine, isoniazid, metronidazole, or voriconazole.
• Leukotrienes have a decreased effectiveness when given with carbamazepine, phenobarbital, phenytoin, primidone, or rifampicin.
• Montelukast is metabolised by CYP 3A4. Increased toxicity can result if this drug is given with amiodarone, cimetidine, clarithromycin, ciclosporine, erythromycin, fluoxetine, fluvoxamine, itraconazole, ketoconazole, metronidazole, or voriconazole.
• Decreased effectiveness of montelukast can result if administered with carbamazepine, efavirenz, garlic supplements, modafinil, nevirapine, oxcarbazepine, phenobarbital, phenytoin, rifabutin, or St. John's wort.

Adverse reactions

Adverse reactions to leukotriene modifiers include:
• headache
• dizziness
• nausea and vomiting
• myalgia.

Nursing process

These nursing process steps are appropriate for patients undergoing treatment with leukotriene modifiers.

Assessment
• Assess the patient's respiratory condition before therapy and regularly thereafter.
• Assess peak flow readings before starting treatment and periodically thereafter.
• Use cautiously in patients with hepatic impairment.
• Be alert for adverse reactions and drug interactions.
• Evaluate the patient's and family's knowledge of drug therapy.

Key nursing diagnoses
• Ineffective breathing pattern related to respiratory condition.
• Impaired gas exchange related to underlying condition.
• Deficient knowledge related to drug therapy.

Planning outcome goals
• Breathing pattern will improve as evidenced by regular and even respiratory rate and rhythm.
• Gas exchange will be adequate as evidenced by improved peak flow rates, oxygen saturation, and ABG levels.
• The patient will demonstrate correct drug administration.

Implementation
• Report insufficient relief or worsening of condition.
• Don't use these drugs for reversing bronchospasm during an acute asthma attack.
• Administer zafirlukast 1 hour before or 2 hours after meals.

Evaluation
• Patient exhibits normal breathing pattern.
• Patient exhibits improved gas exchange.
• Patient and family understand drug therapy.

Mast cell stabilisers

Mast cell stabilisers are used for the prevention and long-term control of asthma, especially in paediatric patients and patients with mild disease. These drugs aren't effective in the management of an acute asthma attack.

One of the most commonly used medications in this class is nedocromil.

Pharmacokinetics

Mast cell stabilisers are minimally absorbed from the GI tract. Inhaled formulations exert effects locally.

Pharmacodynamics

The mechanism of action of mast cell stabilisers is poorly understood, but these agents seem to inhibit the release of inflammatory mediators by stabilising the mast cell membrane, possibly through the inhibition of chloride channels.

Pharmacotherapeutics

Mast cell stabilisers control the inflammatory process and are used for the prevention and long-term control of asthma symptoms. They're the agents of choice for children and patients with exercise-induced asthma.

Drug interactions

There are no known drug interactions for nedocromil.

With the proper medication, exercise-induced asthma doesn't have to stop you in your tracks.

Adverse reactions

Adverse reactions to inhaled mast cell stabilisers may include:
- pharyngeal and tracheal irritation
- cough
- wheezing
- bronchospasm
- headache.

Nursing process

These nursing process steps are appropriate for patients undergoing treatment with mast cell stabilisers.

Assessment
- Assess the patient's respiratory condition before therapy and regularly thereafter.
- Assess peak flow readings before starting treatment and periodically thereafter.
- Be alert for adverse reactions and drug interactions.
- Evaluate the patient's and family's knowledge of drug therapy.

Key nursing diagnoses
- Ineffective breathing pattern related to respiratory condition.
- Impaired gas exchange related to underlying condition.
- Deficient knowledge related to drug therapy.

Planning outcome goals
- Breathing pattern will improve as evidenced by regular and even respiratory rate and rhythm.
- Gas exchange will be adequate as evidenced by improved peak flow rates, oxygen saturation, and ABG levels.
- The patient will demonstrate correct drug administration.

Implementation
- Report insufficient relief or worsening of condition.
- Don't use these drugs for reversing bronchospasm during an acute asthma attack.
- Obtain a prescription for a mild analgesic if a drug-induced headache occurs.
- Monitor for adverse effects of therapy.

Evaluation
- Patient exhibits normal breathing pattern.
- Patient exhibits improved gas exchange.
- Patient and family understand drug therapy.

Methylxanthines

Methylxanthines, also called *xanthines*, are used to treat breathing disorders. Examples of methylxanthines include:
- anhydrous theophylline
- aminophylline.

Aminophylline is a theophylline derivative. Theophylline is the most commonly used oral methylxanthine. Aminophylline is preferred when I.V. methylxanthine treatment is required.

Pharmacokinetics
When methylxanthines are given as an oral solution or a rapid-release tablet, they're absorbed rapidly and completely. They're converted in the body to an active form, which is principally theophylline. High-fat meals can increase theophylline concentrations and increase the risk of toxicity.

pH scale weighs in

Absorption of slow-release forms of theophylline depends on the patient's gastric pH. Food can also alter absorption. When converting patient dosages from I.V. aminophylline to theophylline by mouth, the dosage is decreased by 20%.

Theophylline is approximately 56% protein bound in adults and 36% protein bound in a neonate. It readily crosses the placental barrier and is secreted in breast milk. Smokers and patients on dialysis may need higher doses.

Theophylline is metabolised primarily in the liver by the cytochrome P450 IA2 (CYPIA2) enzyme. In adults and children, about 10% of a dose is excreted unchanged in urine. Therefore, no dosage adjustment is required in a patient with renal insufficiency. Elderly patients and patients with liver dysfunction may require lower doses. Because infants have immature livers with reduced metabolic functioning, as much as one-half of a dose may be excreted unchanged in their urine. Theophylline levels need to be collected to evaluate efficacy and avoid toxicity. The therapeutic serum concentration is 44 to 111 µmol/L. Levels need to be assessed when a dose is initiated or changed, and when drugs are added or removed from a patient's medication regimen.

Pharmacodynamics

Methylxanthines work in several ways.

Taking it easy

Methylxanthines decrease airway reactivity and relieve bronchospasm by relaxing bronchial smooth muscle. It's thought that theophylline inhibits phosphodiesterase (PDE), resulting in smooth-muscle relaxation in addition to bronchodilation and decreased inflammatory mediators (namely mast cells, T cells, and eosinophils). Much of theophylline's toxicity may be due to increased catecholamine release.

In nonreversible obstructive airway disease (chronic bronchitis, emphysema, and apnea), methylxanthines appear to increase the sensitivity of the brain's respiratory centre to carbon dioxide and stimulate the respiratory drive.

Pumped up

In chronic bronchitis and emphysema, these drugs reduce fatigue of the diaphragm, the respiratory muscle that separates the abdomen from the thoracic cavity. They also improve ventricular function and, therefore, the heart's pumping action.

Pharmacotherapeutics

Methylxanthines are used as second- or third-line agents for the long-term control of and presentation of symptoms related to:

- asthma
- chronic bronchitis
- emphysema.

Oh baby

Theophylline has been used to treat neonatal apnea (periods of not breathing in a neonate) and has been effective in reducing severe bronchospasm in infants with cystic fibrosis.

Drug interactions

Theophylline drug interactions occur with those substances that inhibit or induce the CYPIA2 enzyme system:

- Inhibitors of CYPIA2 decrease the metabolism of theophylline, thus increasing the serum concentrations. This results in increased adverse reactions or toxicity. The dose of theophylline may need to be reduced. Examples of CYPIA2 inhibitors include ketoconazole, erythromycin, clarithromycin, cimetidine, isoniazid, fluvoxamine, hormonal contraceptives, and ciprofloxacin.
- Inducers of CYPIA2 increase the metabolism of theophylline, decreasing the serum concentrations. This results in possible therapeutic failure. The dose of theophylline may need to be increased. Examples of CYPIA2 inducers include carbamazepine, phenobarbital, phenytoin, rifampacin and St. John's wort.
- Smoking cigarettes or marijuana increases theophylline elimination, decreasing its serum concentrations and effectiveness.
- Taking adrenergic stimulants or drinking beverages that contain caffeine or caffeine-like substances may result in additive adverse reactions to theophylline or signs and symptoms of methylxanthine toxicity.
- Activated charcoal may decrease theophylline levels.
- Receiving isoflurane with theophylline and theophylline derivatives increases the risk of cardiac toxicity.
- Theophylline and its derivatives may reduce the effects of lithium by increasing its rate of excretion.
- Thyroid hormones may reduce theophylline levels; antithyroid drugs may increase theophylline levels.

Memory jogger

How can you remember what theophylline and its salts are used to treat? Simple: Just remember to "ACE" this one! It's used for long-term control and prevention of symptoms related to:

Asthma

Chronic bronchitis

Emphysema.

Sleep tight, little one. Theophylline is used to treat neonatal apnea.

Adverse reactions

Adverse reactions to methylxanthines may be transient or symptomatic of toxicity.

Gut reactions

Adverse GI system reactions include:
- nausea and vomiting
- abdominal cramping
- epigastric pain
- anorexia
- diarrhoea.

Nerve racking

Adverse central nervous system (CNS) reactions include:
- headache
- irritability, restlessness, and anxiety
- insomnia
- dizziness.

Heart of the matter

Adverse cardiovascular reactions include:
- tachycardia
- palpitations
- arrhythmias.

Nursing process

These nursing process steps are appropriate for patients undergoing treatment with methylxanthines.

Assessment
- Assess the patient's respiratory condition before therapy and regularly thereafter.
- Assess peak flow readings before starting treatment and periodically thereafter.
- Be alert for adverse reactions and drug interactions.
- Monitor vital signs; measure fluid intake and output. Expected clinical effects include improvement in quality of pulse and respirations.
- Xanthine metabolism rate varies among individuals; dosage is determined by monitoring response, tolerance, pulmonary function, and serum theophylline level.
- Evaluate the patient's and family's knowledge of drug therapy.

Key nursing diagnoses
- Ineffective breathing pattern related to respiratory condition.
- Impaired gas exchange related to underlying condition.
- Deficient knowledge related to drug therapy.

Planning outcome goals
- Breathing pattern will improve as evidenced by regular and even respiratory rate and rhythm.
- Gas exchange will be adequate as evidenced by improved peak flow rates, oxygen saturation, and ABG levels.
- The patient will demonstrate correct drug administration.

Implementation
- Report insufficient relief or worsening of condition.
- Give oral doses around the clock, using a sustained-release product at bedtime.
- Use commercially available infusion solution for I.V. use, or mix the drug in 5% glucose, in water. Use an infusion pump for continuous infusion.
- Know that the dosage may need to be increased in cigarette smokers and in habitual marijuana smokers because smoking causes the drug to be metabolised faster.
- Know that the daily dose may need to be decreased in patients with heart failure or hepatic disease and in elderly patients because metabolism and excretion may be decreased.

Evaluation
- Patient exhibits normal breathing pattern.
- Patient exhibits improved gas exchange.
- Patient and family understand drug therapy. (See *Teaching about methylxanthines*.)

Expectorants

Expectorants thin mucus so it's cleared more easily out of airways.

Guaifenesin

The most commonly used expectorant is guaifenesin which is the active ingredient in many OTC products.

Pharmacokinetics
Guaifenesin is absorbed through the GI tract, metabolised by the liver, and excreted primarily by the kidneys.

Education edge

Teaching about methylxanthines

If methylxanthines are prescribed, review these points with the patient and caregivers:

- Don't dissolve, crush, or chew sustained-release products.
- For a child who can't swallow capsules, sprinkle the contents of capsules over soft food and instruct the child to swallow without chewing.
- Follow instructions for drug administration and dosage schedule.
- Relieve GI symptoms by taking an oral drug with a full glass of water after meals.
- Take the drug regularly as directed. Don't take extra medication.

- Dizziness may occur at start of therapy, especially in an elderly patient.
- Change position slowly and avoid hazardous activities during drug therapy.
- Check with your prescriber before using other drugs.
- If you're a smoker while on drug therapy and then you quit, notify your prescriber; your dosage may need to be reduced.
- Report signs of toxicity to your prescriber, including tachycardia, anorexia, nausea, vomiting, diarrhoea, restlessness, irritability, and headache.
- Have blood levels monitored periodically.

Pharmacodynamics

By increasing the production of respiratory tract fluids, guaifenesin reduces the thickness, adhesiveness, and surface tension of mucus, making it easier to clear from the airways. It also provides a soothing effect on mucosal membranes of the respiratory tract. The result is a more productive cough.

Pharmacotherapeutics

Guaifenesin helps make mucus easier to cough up and is used for the relief of symptoms caused by productive coughs from many disorders, such as:

- colds
- minor bronchial irritation
- bronchitis
- influenza
- sinusitis
- bronchial asthma
- emphysema.

Drug interactions

Guaifenesin isn't known to have specific drug interactions.

Adverse reactions

Adverse reactions to guaifenesin include:
- vomiting (if taken in large doses)
- diarrhoea
- drowsiness
- nausea
- abdominal pain
- headache
- hives or skin rash.

Nursing process

These nursing process steps are appropriate for patients undergoing treatment with guaifenesin.

Assessment
- Assess the patient's sputum production before and after giving the drug.
- Be alert for adverse reactions and drug interactions.
- Monitor the patient's hydration level if adverse GI reactions occur.
- Evaluate the patient's and family's knowledge of drug therapy.

Key nursing diagnoses
- Ineffective airway clearance related to underlying condition.
- Risk for deficient fluid volume related to adverse GI reactions.
- Deficient knowledge related to drug therapy.

Planning outcome goals
- The patient will have a patent airway.
- Fluid volume will be adequate as exhibited by blood pressure, pulse, and urine output.
- The patient will demonstrate correct drug administration.

Implementation
- Administer the medication as directed; give with a full glass of water as appropriate.
- Be aware that the drug may interfere with laboratory tests for 5-hydroxyindoleacetic acid and vanillylmandelic acid.
- Report ineffectiveness of the drug to the prescriber; also report if cough persists or if symptoms worsen.
- Encourage the patient to perform deep-breathing exercises.
- Advise the patient not to take other medications, over-the-counter products, or herbal remedies unless approved by the prescriber or a pharmacist.

Evaluation
• Patient's lungs are clear, and respiratory secretions are normal.
• Patient maintains adequate hydration.
• Patient and family understand drug therapy.

Antitussives

Antitussive drugs suppress or inhibit coughing. They're typically used to treat dry, nonproductive coughs. The major antitussives include:
• benzonatate
• codeine
• dextromethorphan hydrobromide
• diamorphine
• methadone

Pharmacokinetics
Antitussives are absorbed well through the GI tract, metabolised in the liver, and excreted in urine. Opioid antitussives are excreted in breast milk and should be used during pregnancy only if the benefits outweigh the risks.

Pharmacodynamics
Antitussives act in slightly different ways:
• Benzonatate acts by anaesthetising stretch receptors throughout the bronchi, alveoli, and pleura.
• Codeine, dextromethorphan, and diamorphine suppress the cough reflex by direct action on the cough centre in the medulla of the brain, thus lowering the cough threshold.

Pharmacotherapeutics
The uses of these drugs vary slightly, but each treats a serious, nonproductive cough that interferes with a patient's ability to rest or carry out activities of daily living.

Antitussives are used to relieve a dry, nonproductive cough, allowing for a good night's sleep.

Testing 1, 2, 3

Benzonatate relieves cough caused by pneumonia, bronchitis, the common cold, and chronic pulmonary diseases such as emphysema. It can also be used during bronchial diagnostic tests, such as bronchoscopy, when the patient must avoid coughing.

And the winner is...

Dextromethorphan one of the most widely used cough suppressants and may provide better antitussive activity than codeine. Its popularity may stem from the fact that it isn't associated with sedation, respiratory depression, or addiction at usual doses.

When the going gets tough

The opioid antitussives (typically codeine and diamorphine) are reserved for treating intractable cough, usually associated with lung cancer.

Drug interactions

Antitussives may interact with other drugs in the following ways:
- Codeine and diamorphine may cause excitation, an extremely elevated temperature, hypertension or hypotension, and coma when taken with monoamine oxidase (MAO) inhibitors.
- Dextromethorphan use with MAO inhibitors may produce excitation, an elevated body temperature, hypotension, and coma.
- Codeine may cause increased CNS depression, such as drowsiness, lethargy, stupor, respiratory depression, coma, and death, when taken with other CNS depressants, including alcohol, barbiturates, sedative-hypnotics, and phenothiazines.

Adverse reactions

Adverse reactions to antitussives vary by drug.

Benzonatate

Benzonatate needs to be swallowed whole; chewing or crushing can produce a local anaesthetic effect on the mouth and throat, which can compromise the airway. The following reactions can also occur when taking benzonatate:
- dizziness
- sedation
- headache
- nasal congestion
- burning in the eyes
- GI upset or nausea
- constipation
- skin rash, eruptions, or itching
- chills
- chest numbness.

Opioid antitussives

Common adverse reactions include nausea, vomiting, sedation, dizziness, and constipation. Other reactions include:
- pupil constriction
- bradycardia or tachycardia

Adverse reactions to antitussives are different for each drug.

- hypotension
- stupor
- seizures
- circulatory collapse
- respiratory arrest.

Nursing process

These nursing process steps are appropriate for patients undergoing treatment with antitussives.

Assessment
- Obtain a history of the patient's cough.
- Be alert for adverse reactions and drug interactions.
- Monitor the patient's hydration level if adverse GI reactions occur.
- Evaluate the patient's and family's knowledge of drug therapy.

Key nursing diagnoses
- Ineffective airway clearance related to underlying condition.
- Fatigue related to presence of nonproductive cough.
- Deficient knowledge related to drug therapy.

Planning outcome goals
- The patient will have a patent airway.
- The patient will state that fatigue is lessened.
- The patient will demonstrate correct drug administration.

Implementation
- Report ineffectiveness of the drug to the prescriber; also report if cough persists or if symptoms worsen.
- Encourage the patient to perform deep-breathing exercises.
- Use the drug with chest percussion and vibration.
- Advise the patient not to take other medications, over-the-counter products, or herbal remedies until talking with the prescriber or a pharmacist.

Evaluation
- Patient's lungs are clear, and respiratory secretions are normal.
- Patient's cough is relieved.
- Patient and family understand drug therapy.

Mucolytics

Mucolytics act directly on mucus, breaking down sticky, thick secretions and thus allowing easier elimination. The major mucolytics include:
- carbocisteine
- erdosteine
- mecysteine hydrochloride

Carbocisteine

Carbocisteine is the most common mucolytic used clinically for patients with abnormal or thick mucus.

Pharmacokinetics

Inhaled carbocisteine is absorbed from the pulmonary epithelium. The drug is metabolised in the liver, and its excretion is unknown.

Pharmacodynamics

Carbocisteine decreases the thickness of respiratory tract secretions by altering the molecular composition of mucus. It also irritates the mucosa to stimulate clearance and restores glutathione, a substance that plays an important role in oxidation-reduction processes.

Pharmacotherapeutics

Carbocisteine is used with other therapies to treat patients with abnormal or thick mucus secretions and may benefit patients with:
- bronchitis
- pulmonary complications related to cystic fibrosis
- atelectasis caused by mucus obstruction, as may occur in pneumonia, bronchiectasis, or chronic bronchitis.

Adverse reactions

With prolonged or persistent use, carbocisteine may produce:
- bronchospasm
- drowsiness
- nausea and vomiting
- severe runny nose
- stomatitis.

Carbocisteine isn't recommended in asthmatics because it may cause bronchospasm.

Nursing process

These nursing process steps are appropriate for patients undergoing treatment with mucolytics.

Assessment
- Assess the patient's sputum production before and after giving the drug.
- Be alert for adverse reactions and drug interactions.
- Monitor the patient's hydration if adverse GI reactions occur.
- Evaluate the patient's and family's knowledge of drug therapy.

Key nursing diagnoses
- Ineffective airway clearance related to underlying condition.
- Risk for deficient fluid volume related to adverse GI reactions.
- Deficient knowledge related to drug therapy.

Planning outcome goals
- The patient will have a patent airway.
- Fluid volume will be adequate as exhibited by blood pressure, pulse, and urine output.
- The patient will demonstrate correct drug administration.

Implementation
- As appropriate, dilute oral doses with cola, fruit juice, or water.
- Perform nebuliser treatments after the patient clears his airway. Use suction to clear air passages.
- Report ineffectiveness of the drug to the prescriber; also report if cough persists or if symptoms worsen.
- Encourage the patient to perform deep-breathing exercises.
- Advise the patient not to take other medications, over-the-counter products, or herbal remedies until talking with the prescriber or a pharmacist.

Evaluation
- Patient's lungs are clear, and respiratory secretions are normal.
- Adequate hydration is maintained.
- Patient and family understand drug therapy.

Decongestants

Decongestants may be classified as systemic or topical, depending on how they're administered.

How swell!

As sympathomimetic drugs, systemic decongestants stimulate the sympathetic nervous system to reduce swelling of the respiratory tract's vascular network. Systemic decongestants include:
*   ephedrine
*   phenylephrine
*   pseudoephedrine.

In the clear

Topical decongestants are also powerful vasoconstrictors. When applied directly to swollen mucosal membranes of the nose, they provide immediate relief from nasal congestion. Topical decongestants include:
*   ephedrine, adrenaline (epinephrine), and phenylephrine (sympathomimetic amines)
*   oxymetazoline and xylometazoline (imidazoline derivatives of sympathomimetic amines).

Pharmacokinetics

The pharmacokinetic properties of decongestants vary. When taken orally, the systemic decongestants are absorbed readily from the GI tract and widely distributed throughout the body into various tissues and fluids, including the cerebrospinal fluid, placenta, and breast milk.

All in a day's work

Systemic decongestants are slowly and incompletely metabolised by the liver and excreted largely unchanged in the urine within 24 hours of oral administration.

In the neighbourhood

Topical decongestants act locally on the alpha-adrenergic receptors of the vascular smooth muscle in the nose, causing the arterioles to constrict. As a result of this local action, absorption of the drug becomes negligible.

Pharmacodynamics

The properties of systemic and topical decongestants vary slightly.

Direct and to the point

The systemic decongestants cause vasoconstriction by directly stimulating alpha-adrenergic receptors in the blood vessels of the body. They also cause contraction of urinary and GI sphincters, dilation of the pupils of the eyes, and decreased secretion of insulin.

Indirect hit

These drugs may also act indirectly, resulting in the release of noradrenaline (norepinephrine) from storage sites in the body, which leads to peripheral vasoconstriction.

On a clear day...

Like systemic decongestants, topical decongestants stimulate alpha-adrenergic receptors in the smooth muscle of the blood vessels in the nose, resulting in vasoconstriction. The combination of reduced blood flow to the nasal mucosal membranes and decreased capillary permeability reduces swelling. This action improves respiration by helping to drain sinuses, clear nasal passages, and open eustachian tubes.

Pharmacotherapeutics

Systemic and topical decongestants are used to relieve the symptoms of swollen nasal membranes resulting from:
- allergic rhinitis (hay fever)
- vasomotor rhinitis
- acute coryza (profuse discharge from the nose)
- sinusitis
- the common cold.

It's a group effort

Systemic decongestants are usually given with other drugs, such as antihistamines, antimuscarinics, antipyretic-analgesics, and antitussives.

Advantage, topical

Topical decongestants provide two major advantages over systemics: minimal adverse reactions and rapid symptom relief.

when it comes to beating respiratory congestion, we're a winning team!

Drug interactions

Because they produce vasoconstriction, which reduces drug absorption, drug interactions involving topical decongestants seldom occur. However, systemic decongestants may interact with other drugs:
• Increased CNS stimulation may occur when systemic decongestants are taken with other sympathomimetic drugs, including adrenaline (epinephrine), noradrenaline (norepinephrine), dopamine, dobutamine, isoprenaline, and terbutaline.
• When taken with MAO inhibitors, systemic decongestants may cause severe hypertension or a hypertensive crisis, which can be life-threatening. These drugs shouldn't be used together.
• Alkalinising drugs may increase the effects of pseudoephedrine by reducing its urinary excretion.

Adverse reactions

Most adverse reactions to decongestants result from CNS stimulation and include:
• nervousness
• restlessness and insomnia
• nausea
• palpitations and tachycardia
• difficulty urinating
• elevated blood pressure.

Systemic decongestants

Systemic decongestants also exacerbate hypertension, hyperthyroidism, diabetes, benign prostatic hyperplasia, glaucoma, and heart disease.

Topical decongestants

The most common adverse reaction associated with prolonged use (more than 5 days) of topical decongestants is rebound nasal congestion. Other reactions include burning and stinging of the nasal mucosa, sneezing, and mucosal dryness or ulceration.

Nursing process

These nursing process steps are appropriate for patients undergoing treatment with decongestants.

Assessment

• Assess the patient's condition before and after giving the drug.
• Be alert for adverse reactions and drug interactions.
• Monitor the patient's hydration level if adverse GI reactions occur.
• Evaluate the patient's and family's knowledge of drug therapy.

Key nursing diagnoses

- Ineffective airway clearance related to underlying condition.
- Risk for deficient fluid volume related to adverse GI reactions.
- Deficient knowledge related to drug therapy.

Planning outcome goals

- The patient will have a patent airway.
- Fluid volume will be adequate as exhibited by blood pressure, pulse, and urine output.
- The patient will demonstrate correct drug administration.

Implementation

- Report ineffectiveness of the drug to the prescriber; also report if cough persists or if symptoms worsen.
- Encourage the patient to perform deep-breathing exercises.
- Advise the patient not to take other medications, over-the-counter products, or herbal remedies until talking with the prescriber or a pharmacist.
- Identify and correct hypoxia, hypercapnia, and acidosis, which may reduce drug effectiveness or increase adverse reactions, before or during ephedrine administration.
- Don't crush or break extended-release forms of the drug.
- Give the last dose at least 2 hours before bedtime to minimise insomnia.

Evaluation

- Patient's lungs are clear, and respiratory secretions are normal.
- Patient maintains adequate hydration.
- Patient and family understand drug therapy.

Quick quiz

1. You're instructing a patient with asthma about the use of bronchodilators. You should teach the patient:
    - A. to take the medication 4 hours before exercise to prevent exercise-induced bronchospasm.
    - B. to take only the specific drugs prescribed for acute bronchospasm, usually a short-acting beta$_2$-adrenergic agonist such as albuterol.
    - C. to double the dose of the medication in the event of a missed dose.
    - D. that long-acting beta$_2$ agonists, such as salmeterol, are effective in the treatment of acute asthma attacks.

Answer: B. Short-acting beta$_2$-adrenergic agonists are used in the treatment of acute bronchospasm. Long-acting agents aren't effective in acute attacks. To prevent exercise-induced asthma, medication should be taken 30 to 60 minutes before exercise.

2.   Which drug is an anticholinergic agent used to treat patients with COPD?
   A.   Atropine
   B.   Salbutamol
   C.   Budesonide
   D.   Ipratropium bromide

Answer: D. Inhaled ipratropium bromide is an anticholinergic agent used as a bronchodilator in patients with COPD.

3.   Which drug is a leukotriene modifier, the absorption of which is decreased by food and should be given 1 hour before or 2 hours after meals?
   A.   Aminophylline
   B.   Montelukast
   C.   Zafirlukast
   D.   Nedocromil

Answer: C. Absorption of zafirlukast is decreased by food, and it must be given 1 hour before meals or 2 hours after meals.

Scoring

☆☆☆   If you answered all three questions correctly, good job. You're slicker than a mucolytic in action!

☆☆   If you answered two questions correctly, you're as relaxed as bronchial smooth muscle on xanthines.

☆   If you answered fewer than two questions correctly, you may need another dose of the chapter to clear your head about respiratory drugs.

7 Gastrointestinal drugs

Just the facts

In this chapter, you'll learn:
- classes of drugs used to improve GI function
- uses and varying actions of these drugs
- absorption, distribution, metabolism, and excretion of these drugs
- drug interactions and adverse reactions to these drugs

Drugs and the GI system

The GI tract is basically a hollow, muscular tube that begins at the mouth and ends at the anus; it encompasses the pharynx, oesophagus, stomach, and the small and large intestines. Its primary functions are to digest and absorb foods and fluids and excrete metabolic waste.

Roll call

Classes of drugs used to improve GI function include:
- antiulcer drugs
- adsorbent, antiflatulent, and digestive drugs
- antidiarrhoeal and laxative drugs
- antiemetic and emetic drugs. (See *Where drugs affect GI secretions.*)

Antiulcer drugs

A peptic ulcer is a circumscribed lesion in the mucosal membrane, developing in the lower oesophagus, stomach, duodenum, or jejunum.

Pharm function

Where drugs affect GI secretions

Antiulcer drugs and digestive drugs that affect GI secretions can decrease secretory activity, block the action of secretions, form a protective coating on the lining, or replace missing enzymes. The illustration below depicts where these types of GI drugs act.

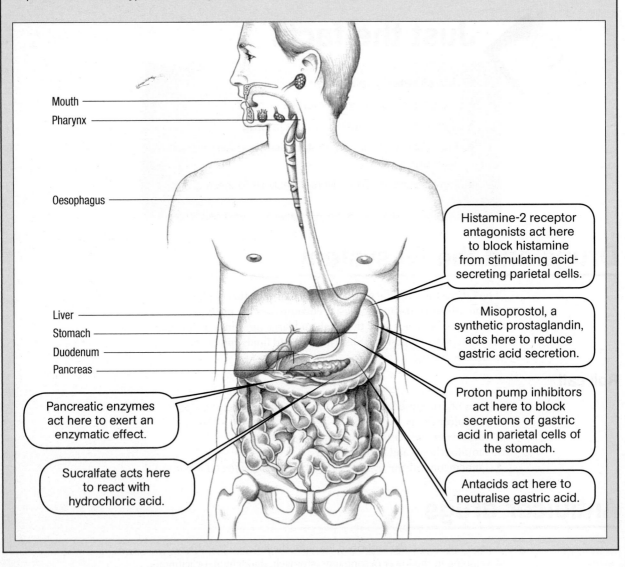

Mouth

Pharynx

Oesophagus

Liver

Stomach

Duodenum

Pancreas

Histamine-2 receptor antagonists act here to block histamine from stimulating acid-secreting parietal cells.

Misoprostol, a synthetic prostaglandin, acts here to reduce gastric acid secretion.

Proton pump inhibitors act here to block secretions of gastric acid in parietal cells of the stomach.

Pancreatic enzymes act here to exert an enzymatic effect.

Sucralfate acts here to react with hydrochloric acid.

Antacids act here to neutralise gastric acid.

Common culprits

The major causes of peptic ulcers include:
- bacterial infection with *Helicobacter pylori*
- the use of nonsteroidal anti-inflammatory drugs (NSAIDs)
- hypersecretory states such as Zollinger-Ellison syndrome
(a condition in which excessive gastric acid secretion causes peptic ulcers)
- cigarette smoking, which causes hypersecretion and impairs ulcer healing
- a genetic predisposition, which accounts for 20% to 50% of patients with peptic ulcers.

Busting bacteria or bolstering balance

Antiulcer drugs are formulated to eradicate *H. pylori* or restore the balance between acid and pepsin secretions and the GI mucosal defense. These drugs include:
- systemic antibiotics
- antacids
- histamine-2 (H_2) receptor antagonists
- proton pump inhibitors
- other antiulcer drugs, such as misoprostol and sucralfate.

One aim of antiulcer drugs is to restore the balance between acid and pepsin secretions and the GI mucosal defense.

Systemic antibiotics

H. pylori is a gram-negative bacteria that's thought to be a major causative factor in peptic ulcer formation and gastritis (inflammation of the stomach lining). Eradicating the bacteria promotes ulcer healing and decreases recurrence.

It takes two

Successful treatment involves the use of two or more antibiotics in combination with other drugs. Systemic antibiotics used to treat *H. pylori* include:
- amoxicillin
- clarithromycin
- metronidazole
- tetracycline.

Pharmacokinetics
Systemic antibiotics are variably absorbed from the GI tract.

Got milk?

Food, especially dairy products, decreases the absorption of tetracycline but doesn't significantly delay the absorption of the other antibiotics.

All of these antibiotics are distributed widely and are excreted primarily in urine.

Pharmacodynamics

Antibiotics act by treating the *H. pylori* infection. They're usually combined with an H_2-receptor antagonist or a proton pump inhibitor to decrease stomach acid and further promote healing.

Pharmacotherapeutics

Systemic antibiotics are indicated for *H. pylori* eradication to reduce the risk of a duodenal ulcer.

Sounds like a plan

Treatment plans that use at least two antimicrobial drugs and a proton pump inhibitor for 14 days, and then continue the proton pump inhibitor for 6 more weeks, help reduce acid in the patient with peptic ulcers.

Drug interactions

Tetracycline and metronidazole can interact with many other drugs. For example, tetracycline increases digoxin levels and, when combined with methoxyflurane, increases the risk of nephrotoxicity. Metronidazole and tetracycline increase the risk of bleeding when taken with oral anticoagulants.

Adverse reactions

Antibiotics used to improve GI tract function may lead to adverse reactions, such as those listed here:
• Metronidazole, clarithromycin, and tetracycline commonly cause mild GI disturbances.
• Clarithromycin and metronidazole may produce abnormal tastes.
• Metronidazole may cause a disulfiram-like reaction (nausea, vomiting, headache, cramps, flushing) when combined with alcohol. Discourage concomitant use.
• Amoxicillin may cause diarrhoea.
• Some antibiotics can cause contraceptive failure in oestrogen based preparations.

Dairy products and other foods decrease the absorption of the antibiotic tetracycline.

Don't combine metronidazole with alcohol. A severe reaction may occur.

Nursing process

These nursing process steps are appropriate for patients undergoing treatment with systemic antibiotics.

Assessment
- Assess the patient's infection before therapy and regularly thereafter.
- Assess signs and symptoms of the patient's ulcer.
- Watch for oedema, especially in the patient who's also receiving corticosteroids; antibiotics, such as metronidazole, may cause sodium retention.
- Assess for adverse reactions and drug interactions.
- Identify risk factors for peptic ulcer disease, such as cigarette smoking, stress, and drug therapy with irritating medications (aspirin, other NSAIDs, corticosteroids, or antineoplastics).
- Assess the patient's and family's understanding of drug therapy.

Key nursing diagnoses
- Ineffective health maintenance related to presence of susceptible organisms.
- Risk for deficient fluid volume related to drug-induced adverse GI reactions.
- Deficient knowledge related to drug therapy.

Planning outcome goals
- The patient's overall health status will improve.
- Stable vital signs and the patient's urine output will indicate improved fluid volume status.
- The patient and family will demonstrate an understanding of drug therapy.

Implementation
- Administer drugs as appropriate for the patient's condition and diagnosis.
- Use measures to prevent or minimise peptic ulcer disease and gastric acid-induced oesophageal disorders.
- Observe the patient for improvement in symptoms.

Evaluation
- Patient is free from infection.
- Patient maintains adequate hydration throughout therapy.
- Patient and family demonstrate an understanding of drug therapy. (See *Teaching about antiulcer drugs.*)

Make sure to evaluate for adequate hydration in the patient taking systemic antibiotics.

Education edge

Teaching about antiulcer drugs

If antiulcer drugs are prescribed, review these points with the patient and caregivers:

- Elevate the head of the bed.
- Avoid abdominal distention by eating small meals.
- Don't lie down for 1 to 2 hours after eating.
- Decrease intake of fats, chocolate, citric juices, coffee, and alcohol.
- Avoid smoking.
- Avoid obesity, constipation, and other conditions that increase intra-abdominal pressure.
- Take medications with enough water to avoid irritating the oesophagus.
- Take antiulcer drugs as directed; underuse decreases their effectiveness and overuse increases adverse effects.

- Swallow capsules whole unless otherwise instructed; some medications can be sprinkled on semi-solid food if they're difficult to swallow.
- Take medications as prescribed for maximum effectiveness.
- Take medications with or without food, as prescribed, when applicable.
- Eat a well-balanced diet.
- Get adequate rest.
- Exercise regularly.
- Avoid gastric irritants as well as nonsteroidal anti-inflammatory drugs.
- Reduce psychological stress; employ stress management techniques, as needed.
- Don't take other medications, over-the-counter preparations, or herbal remedies without first consulting with the prescriber.

Antacids

Antacids are over-the-counter (OTC) medications used in combination with other drugs to treat peptic ulcers. Types of antacids include:
- aluminium carbonate gel
- magnesium carbonate
- hydrotalcite (aluminium-magnesium complex)
- co-magaldrox (mixture of magnesium hydroxide and aluminium hydroxide)
- simeticone.

Pharmacokinetics

Antacids work locally in the stomach by neutralising gastric acid. They don't need to be absorbed to treat peptic ulcers. Antacids are distributed throughout the GI tract and are eliminated primarily in faeces.

Pharmacodynamics

The acid-neutralising action of antacids reduces the total amount of acid in the GI tract, allowing peptic ulcers time to heal.

> By reducing the amount of acid in the GI tract, antacids allow peptic ulcers time to heal.

Pepsin, a digestive enzyme, acts more effectively when the stomach is highly acidic; therefore, as acidity drops, pepsin action is also reduced.

Myth buster

Contrary to popular belief, antacids don't work by coating peptic ulcers or the lining of the GI tract.

Pharmacotherapeutics

Antacids are primarily prescribed to relieve pain and are used adjunctively in peptic ulcer disease.

Churn, churn, churn

Antacids also relieve symptoms of acid indigestion, heartburn, dyspepsia (burning or indigestion), or gastroesophageal reflux disease (GORD), where the contents of the stomach and duodenum flow back into the oesophagus.

Foiling phosphate absorption

Antacids may be used to control hyperphosphataemia (elevated blood phosphate levels) in kidney failure. Because calcium binds with phosphate in the GI tract, calcium carbonate antacids prevent phosphate absorption. (See *Antacids: Aluminium hydroxide*.)

Prototype pro

Antacids: Aluminium hydroxide

Actions

- Reduces total acid load in the GI tract
- Elevates gastric pH to reduce pepsin activity
- Strengthens the gastric mucosal barrier
- Increases oesophageal sphincter tone

Indications

- Relief of GI discomfort

Nursing considerations

- Shake suspensions well.
- When administering through a nasogastric tube, make sure that the tube is patent and placed correctly; after instilling, flush the tube with water to ensure passage to the stomach and to clear the tube.
- Don't give other oral drugs within 2 hours of antacid administration. This may cause premature release of enteric-coated drugs in the stomach.

Drug interactions

All antacids can interfere with the absorption of oral drugs if given at the same time. Absorption of digoxin, phenytoin, ketoconazole, iron salts, isoniazid, quinolones, and tetracycline may be reduced if taken within 2 hours of antacids. If a patient is taking an antacid in addition to other drugs, separate the drugs' administration times.

Adverse reactions

All adverse reactions to antacids are dose related and include:
- diarrhoea
- constipation
- electrolyte imbalances
- aluminium accumulation in serum.

Nursing process

These nursing process steps are appropriate for patients undergoing treatment with antacids.

Assessment
- Assess the patient's condition before therapy and regularly thereafter.
- Record the number and consistency of stools.
- Assess the patient for adverse reactions.
- Monitor the patient receiving long-term, high-dose aluminium carbonate and aluminium hydroxide for fluid and electrolyte imbalance, especially if he's on a sodium-restricted diet.
- Monitor phosphate levels in the patient receiving aluminium carbonate or aluminium hydroxide.
- Watch for signs of hypercalcaemia in the patient receiving calcium carbonate.
- Monitor magnesium levels in the patient with mild renal impairment who takes co-magaldrox.

Key nursing diagnoses
- Constipation related to adverse effects of antacids containing aluminium.
- Ineffective protection related to drug-induced electrolyte imbalance.
- Deficient knowledge related to drug therapy.

Planning outcome goals
- The patient's underlying symptoms will improve.
- Laboratory studies will show normal electrolyte balance.
- The patient and family will demonstrate an understanding of antacid therapy.

Education edge

Teaching about antacids

If antacids are prescribed, review these points with the patient and caregivers:

- Don't take antacids indiscriminately or switch antacids without the prescriber's consent.
- Don't take calcium carbonate with milk or other foods high in vitamin D.
- Don't take sodium bicarbonate with milk; doing so could cause hypercalcaemia.

- Don't use sodium bicarbonate regularly as an antacid. Use a nonabsorbable antacid if antacids are needed often.
- Shake the suspension form well before taking it.
- Some antacids, such as aluminium hydroxide, may colour stools white or cause white streaks.
- To prevent constipation, increase fluid and roughage intake and increase activity level.

Implementation

- Manage constipation with laxatives or stool softeners, or ask the prescriber about switching the patient to a magnesium preparation.
- If the patient suffers from diarrhoea, obtain a prescription for an antidiarrhoeal, as needed, and ask the prescriber about switching the patient to an antacid containing aluminium.
- Shake the container of a liquid form well.
- When giving the drug through a nasogastric (NG) tube, make sure that the tube is patent and placed correctly. After instilling the drug, flush the tube with water to ensure passage to the stomach and to clear the tube.

Evaluation

- Patient regains a normal bowel pattern.
- Patient maintains a normal electrolyte balance.
- Patient and family demonstrate an understanding of drug therapy. (See *Teaching about antacids*.)

Laxatives, stool softeners, or antidiarrhoeals may be prescribed to counteract the effects of antacids.

H$_2$-receptor antagonists

H$_2$-receptor antagonists are commonly prescribed as antiulcer drugs, although their use is declining in favour of proton pump inhibitors. Drugs in the H$_2$-receptor antagonist category include:

- cimetidine
- famotidine
- nizatidine
- ranitidine.

Pharmacokinetics

Cimetidine, nizatidine, and ranitidine are absorbed rapidly and completely from the GI tract. Famotidine isn't completely absorbed. Food and antacids may reduce the absorption of H_2-receptor antagonists.

H_2-receptor antagonists are distributed widely throughout the body, metabolised by the liver, and excreted primarily in urine.

Pharmacodynamics

H_2-receptor antagonists block histamine from stimulating the acid-secreting parietal cells of the stomach.

Really in a bind

Acid secretion in the stomach depends on the binding of gastrin, acetylcholine, and histamine to receptors on the parietal cells. If the binding of any one of these substances is blocked, acid secretion is reduced. The H_2-receptor antagonists, by binding with H_2 receptors, block the action of histamine in the stomach and reduce acid secretion. (See *H_2-receptor antagonists: Famotidine.*)

Pharmacotherapeutics

H_2-receptor antagonists are used therapeutically to:
* promote healing of duodenal and gastric ulcers
* provide long-term treatment of pathologic GI hypersecretory conditions such as Zollinger-Ellison syndrome
* reduce gastric acid production and prevent stress ulcers in severely ill patients and in those with reflux oesophagitis or upper GI bleeding.

Drug interactions

H_2-receptor antagonists may interact with antacids and other drugs:
* Antacids reduce the absorption of cimetidine, nizatidine, ranitidine, and famotidine.
* Cimetidine may increase the blood levels of oral anticoagulants, propranolol (and possibly other beta-adrenergic blockers), benzodiazepines, tricyclic antidepressants, theophylline, procainamide, lidocaine, phenytoin, calcium channel blockers, ciclosporine, carbamazepine, and opioid analgesics by reducing their metabolism in the liver and their subsequent excretion.
* Cimetidine taken with carmustine increases the risk of bone marrow toxicity.
* Cimetidine inhibits ethyl alcohol metabolism in the stomach, resulting in higher blood alcohol levels.

Adverse reactions

Using H_2-receptor antagonists may lead to adverse reactions, especially in elderly patients or in patients with altered hepatic or renal function:

- Cimetidine and ranitidine may produce headache, dizziness, malaise, muscle pain, nausea, diarrhoea or constipation, rashes, itching, loss of sexual desire, gynecomastia (cimetidine), and impotence.
- Famotidine and nizatidine produce few adverse reactions, with headache being the most common, followed by constipation or diarrhoea and rash.

Nursing process

These nursing process steps are appropriate for patients undergoing treatment with H_2-receptor antagonists.

Assessment
- Assess for adverse reactions, especially hypotension and arrhythmias.
- Periodically monitor laboratory tests, such as complete blood count and renal and hepatic studies.

Key nursing diagnoses
- Impaired tissue integrity related to the patient's underlying condition.
- Decreased cardiac output related to adverse cardiovascular effects (cimetidine).
- Deficient knowledge related to drug therapy.

Planning outcome goals
- The patient's tissue integrity will improve as evidenced by a reduction in underlying symptoms.
- Stable vital signs and the patient's urine output will indicate adequate cardiac output.
- The patient and family will demonstrate an understanding of drug therapy.

Implementation
- Administer a once-daily dose at bedtime to promote compliance. Twice-daily doses should be administered in the morning and evening; multiple doses, with meals and at bedtime.
- Don't exceed the recommended infusion rates when administering H_2-receptor antagonists I.V.; doing so increases the

Prototype pro

H_2-receptor antagonists: Famotidine

Actions

- Inhibits histamine's action at H_2 receptors in gastric parietal cells
- Reduces gastric acid output and concentration regardless of the stimulating agent (histamine, food, insulin, or caffeine) or basal conditions

Indications

- Gastroesophageal reflux disease
- Zollinger-Ellison syndrome
- Duodenal ulcer
- Gastric ulcer
- Heartburn

Nursing considerations

- Monitor for adverse effects such as headache.
- Monitor for signs of GI bleeding such as blood in the patient's faeces.

Education edge

Teaching about H₂-receptor antagonists

If histamine-2 (H₂) receptor antagonists are prescribed, review these points with the patient and caregivers:

- Take the drug with a snack if desired.
- Take the drug as prescribed; don't stop taking the drug suddenly.
- If taking the drug once daily, take it at bedtime for best results.
- Continue to take the drug, even after pain subsides, to allow for adequate healing.
- If the prescriber approves, antacids may also be taken, especially at the beginning of therapy, when pain is severe.
- Don't take antacids within 1 hour of taking an H₂-receptor antagonist.

- Don't take the drug for more than 8 weeks unless specifically requested by the prescriber.
- Don't self-medicate for heartburn longer than 2 weeks without consulting the prescriber.
- Be aware of possible adverse reactions, and report unusual effects.
- Avoid smoking during therapy; smoking stimulates gastric acid secretion and worsens the disease.
- Immediately report black tarry stools, diarrhoea, confusion, or rash.
- Don't take other drugs, over-the-counter products, or herbal remedies without first consulting with the prescriber or a pharmacist.

---

risk of adverse cardiovascular effects. Continuous I.V. infusion may suppress acid secretion more effectively.

- Administer antacids at least 1 hour before or after H₂-receptor antagonists. Antacids can decrease drug absorption.
- Anticipate dosage adjustments for the patient with renal disease.
- Avoid stopping the drug abruptly.

Evaluation

- Patient experiences decrease in or relief from upper GI symptoms with drug therapy.
- Patient maintains a normal heart rhythm.
- Patient and family demonstrate an understanding of drug therapy. (See *Teaching about H₂-receptor antagonists*.)

Proton pump inhibitors

Proton pump inhibitors disrupt chemical binding in stomach cells to reduce acid production, lessening irritation and allowing peptic ulcers to better heal. They include:

- esomeprazole
- lansoprazole
- omeprazole

> Be aware! Exceeding the recommended infusion rates when administering H₂-receptor antagonists I.V. increases the risk of adverse cardiovascular effects.

- pantoprazole
- rabeprazole.

Pharmacokinetics
Proton pump inhibitors are given orally in enteric-coated formulas to bypass the stomach because they're highly unstable in acid. They dissolve in the small intestine and are rapidly absorbed.

We just want to be-eee-eee-ee-eeee protein bound!

Highly protein bound

These drugs are highly protein bound and extensively metabolised by the liver to inactive compounds and then eliminated in urine.

Pharmacodynamics
Proton pump inhibitors block the last step in gastric acid secretion by combining with hydrogen, potassium, and adenosine triphosphate in the parietal cells of the stomach. (See *Proton pump inhibitors: Omeprazole.*)

Pharmacotherapeutics
Proton pump inhibitors are indicated for:
- short-term treatment of active gastric ulcers
- active duodenal ulcers
- erosive oesophagitis

Prototype pro

Proton pump inhibitors: Omeprazole

Actions

- Inhibits activity of acid (proton) pump and binds to hydrogen-potassium-adenosine triphosphate, located at the secretory surface of the gastric parietal cells, to block gastric acid formation

Indications

- Gastroesophageal reflux disease
- Zollinger-Ellison syndrome
- Duodenal ulcer
- Gastric ulcer
- *Helicobacter pylori* infection

Nursing considerations

- Monitor the patient for adverse effects, such as headache, dizziness, and nausea.
- Administer the drug 30 minutes before meals.

- symptomatic GORD that isn't responsive to other therapies
- active peptic ulcers associated with *H. pylori* infection (in combination with antibiotics)
- long-term treatment of hypersecretory states such as Zollinger-Ellison syndrome.

Drug interactions

Proton pump inhibitors may interfere with the metabolism of diazepam, phenytoin, and warfarin, causing increased half-lives and elevated plasma concentrations of these drugs. Proton pump inhibitors may also interfere with the absorption of drugs that depend on gastric pH for absorption, such as ketoconazole, digoxin, ampicillin, and iron salts.

Adverse reactions

Adverse reactions to proton pump inhibitors include:
- abdominal pain
- diarrhoea
- nausea and vomiting.

Nursing process

These nursing process steps are appropriate for patients undergoing treatment with proton pump inhibitors.

Assessment
- Assess the patient's condition before therapy and regularly thereafter.
- Assess the patient for adverse reactions and drug interactions.
- Monitor the patient's hydration status if adverse GI reactions occur.
- Assess the patient's and family's knowledge of drug therapy.

Key nursing diagnoses
- Impaired tissue integrity related to upper gastric disorder.
- Risk for deficient fluid volume related to drug-induced adverse GI reactions.
- Deficient knowledge related to drug therapy.

Planning outcome goals
- The patient's tissue integrity will improve as evidenced by a reduction in presenting symptoms.
- Adequate fluid volume, as evidenced by the patient's vital signs and urine output, will be maintained.
- The patient and family will demonstrate an understanding of drug therapy.

Education edge

Teaching about proton pump inhibitors

If proton pump inhibitors are prescribed, review these points with the patient and caregivers:

- Take the drug before eating; however, oral pantoprazole may be taken with or without food.
- Swallow the tablets or capsules whole; don't crush or chew them. These formulations are delayed-release and long-acting; opening, crushing, or chewing them destroys the drug's effects.
- If swallowing capsules is difficult, lansoprazole capsules can be opened and mixed with 60 ml of apple, orange, vegetable, or tomato juice.

Capsule contents can also be sprinkled on a small amount of semi-solid food. Swallow the mixture immediately without chewing the granules.
- Observe for the drug's effects; if symptoms persist or adverse reactions (such as headache, diarrhoea, abdominal pain, and nausea or vomiting) occur, notify the prescriber.
- Don't take over-the-counter preparations, other prescription drugs, or herbal remedies without first consulting with the prescriber.

Implementation

- Administer the drug 30 minutes before meals.
- Dosage adjustments aren't needed for patients with renal or hepatic impairment.
- Tell the patient to swallow capsules whole and not to open or crush them.

Evaluation

- Patient responds well to therapy.
- Patient maintains adequate hydration throughout therapy.
- Patient and family demonstrate an understanding of drug therapy. (See *Teaching about proton pump inhibitors*.)

Other antiulcer drugs

Research on the usefulness of other drugs in treating peptic ulcer disease continues. Two other antiulcer drugs currently in use are:
- misoprostol (a synthetic prostaglandin E_1)
- sucralfate.

Pharmacokinetics

Each of these drugs has slightly different pharmacokinetic properties.

After an oral dose, misoprostol is absorbed extensively and rapidly. It's metabolised to misoprostol acid, which is clinically

Remember: Give proton pump inhibitors 30 minutes before meals.

active, meaning it can produce a pharmacologic effect. Misoprostol acid is highly protein bound and is excreted primarily in urine.

Sucralfate is minimally absorbed from the GI tract. It's excreted in faeces.

Pharmacodynamics
The actions of these drugs vary.

Reduce and boost

Misoprostol protects against peptic ulcers caused by NSAIDs by reducing the secretion of gastric acid and by boosting the production of gastric mucus, a natural defense against peptic ulcers.

A sticky situation

Sucralfate works locally in the stomach, rapidly reacting with hydrochloric acid to form a thick, pastelike substance that adheres to the gastric mucosa and, especially, to ulcers. By binding to the ulcer site, sucralfate actually protects the ulcer from the damaging effects of acid and pepsin to promote healing. This binding usually lasts for 6 hours.

Once I get into the stomach, I stick like glue to ulcers like you!

Pharmacotherapeutics
Each of these drugs has its own therapeutic use.

Attention to prevention

Misoprostol prevents peptic ulcers caused by NSAIDs in patients at high risk for complications resulting from gastric ulcers.

To treat and prevent

Sucralfate is used for short-term treatment (up to 8 weeks) of duodenal or gastric ulcers and prevention of recurrent ulcers or stress ulcers.

Drug interactions
Misoprostol and sucralfate may interact with other drugs:
• Antacids may bind with misoprostol or decrease its absorption. However, this effect doesn't appear to be clinically significant.
• Cimetidine, digoxin, norfloxacin, phenytoin, ranitidine, tetracycline, and theophylline decrease the absorption of sucralfate.
• Antacids may reduce the binding of sucralfate to the gastric and duodenal mucosa, reducing its effectiveness.

Adverse reactions

Adverse reactions to misoprostol include:
- diarrhoea (common and usually dose-related)
- abdominal pain
- gas
- indigestion
- nausea and vomiting
- spontaneous abortion (women of childbearing age shouldn't become pregnant while taking misoprostol).
  Adverse reactions to sucralfate include:
- constipation
- nausea and vomiting
- metallic taste.

Nursing process

These nursing process steps are appropriate for patients undergoing treatment with the antiulcer drugs misoprostol and sucralfate.

Make sure you discuss contraceptive methods or alternative treatment with women who are taking misoprostol. This drug can harm the foetus if pregnancy occurs.

Assessment
- Assess the patient's condition before therapy and regularlv thereafter.
- Assess for adverse reactions and drug interactions.
- If the patient is taking misoprostol and is female, the drug can cause danger to the foetus if pregnancy occurs; discuss contraceptive methods or alternative treatment.
- Monitor the patient's hydration status if adverse GI reactions occur.
- Assess the patient's and family's understanding of drug therapy.

Key nursing diagnoses
- Impaired tissue integrity related to upper gastric disorder.
- Risk for deficient fluid volume related to drug-induced adverse GI reactions.
- Deficient knowledge related to drug therapy.

Planning outcome goals
- The patient's tissue integrity will improve as evidenced by a reduction in presenting symptoms.
- Adequate fluid volume will be maintained as evidenced by stable vital signs and urine output.
- The patient and family will demonstrate an understanding of drug therapy.

Implementation

- Administer sucralfate 1 hour before meals and at bedtime.
- Administer misoprostol with food.
- Tell the patient to continue the prescribed regimen at home to ensure complete healing. Pain and ulcerative symptoms may subside within the first few weeks of therapy.
- Urge the patient to avoid cigarette smoking because it may increase gastric acid secretion and worsen disease.
- Tell the patient to avoid alcohol, chocolate, spicy foods, or anything that irritates their stomach.
- Elevate the head of the bed for comfort.
- Tell the patient to avoid large meals within 2 hours before bedtime.
- In women, start misoprostol therapy on the second or third day of the next normal menses to ensure that the patient isn't pregnant.

Evaluation

- Patient responds well to therapy.
- Patient maintains adequate hydration throughout therapy.
- Patient and family demonstrate an understanding of drug therapy.

No butts about it! Cigarette smoking may increase gastric acid secretions and worsen ulcers.

Adsorbent, antiflatulent, and digestive drugs

Adsorbent, antiflatulent, and digestive drugs aid healthy GI function. They're used to fight undesirable toxins, acids, and gases in the GI tract.

Adsorbent drugs

Natural and synthetic adsorbent drugs, or adsorbents, are prescribed as antidotes for the ingestion of toxins, substances that can lead to poisoning or overdose.

It's no picnic

The most commonly used clinical adsorbent is activated charcoal, a black powder residue obtained from the distillation of various organic materials.

Adsorbent drugs are used as antidotes to toxins.

Pharmacokinetics

Quick action required

Activated charcoal must be administered soon after toxic ingestion because activated charcoal can only bind with drugs or poisons that haven't yet been absorbed from the GI tract. Activated charcoal, which isn't absorbed or metabolised by the body, is excreted unchanged in faeces.

A vicious cycle

After initial absorption, some poisons move back into the intestines, where they're reabsorbed. Activated charcoal may be administered repeatedly to break this cycle.

Pharmacodynamics

Because adsorbent drugs attract and bind toxins in the intestine, they inhibit toxins from being absorbed from the GI tract. However, this binding doesn't change toxic effects caused by earlier absorption of the poison.

Pharmacotherapeutics

Activated charcoal is a general-purpose antidote used for many types of acute oral poisoning. It isn't indicated in acute poisoning from mineral acids, alkalines, cyanide, ethanol, methanol, iron, sodium chloride alkali, inorganic acids, or organic solvents. It also shouldn't be used in children younger than aged 1. It shouldn't be used if the patient has a risk of GI obstruction, perforation, or haemorrhage; decreased or absent bowel sounds; or a history of recent GI surgery.

> Children younger than aged 1 shouldn't be given activated charcoal.

Drug interactions

Activated charcoal can decrease the absorption of oral medications; therefore, these medications (other than those used to treat the ingested toxin) shouldn't be taken orally within 2 hours of taking activated charcoal. Drugs used to induce vomiting, such as ipecac syrup, may decrease the effectiveness of activated charcoal. Generally, the use of such agents is not advised as there is little evidence to suggest that they affect absorption rates. However, if these drugs are used together to treat oral poisoning, activated charcoal should be used only after vomiting has stopped.

Adverse reactions

Activated charcoal turns stool black and may cause constipation.
A laxative, such as sorbitol, is usually given with activated charcoal to prevent constipation and improve taste.

Nursing process

These nursing process steps are appropriate for patients undergoing treatment with adsorbent drugs.

Assessment

• Obtain a history of the substance reportedly ingested, including time of ingestion, if possible. Activated charcoal isn't effective for all drugs and toxic substances.
• Assess for adverse reactions and drug interactions.
• Assess the patient's and family's knowledge of drug therapy.

Key nursing diagnoses

• Risk for injury related to ingestion of toxic substance or overdose.
• Risk for deficient fluid volume related to drug-induced vomiting.
• Deficient knowledge related to drug therapy.

Planning outcome goals

• The patient's risk of injury will be minimised.
• Fluid volume status will remain adequate as evidenced by vital signs and urine output.
• The patient and family will demonstrate an understanding of drug therapy.

Implementation

• Don't give the drug to a semiconscious or unconscious patient unless the airway is protected and an NG tube is in place for instillation.
• Mix the powdered form with tap water to form the consistency of thick syrup. Add a small amount of fruit juice or flavouring to make it more palatable.
• Give by NG tube after lavage, if needed.
• Don't give the drug in ice cream or milk, which may reduce absorption.
• Repeat the dose if the patient vomits shortly after administration.
• Keep airway, oxygen, and suction equipment nearby.
• Follow treatment with a stool softener or laxative to prevent constipation.
• Tell the patient that their stools will be black.

Here's a good tip: Mix powdered forms of adsorbents with a small amount of fruit juice to make them more palatable.

Evaluation
- Patient doesn't experience injury from ingesting toxic substance or from overdose.
- Patient exhibits no signs of deficient fluid volume.
- Patient and family demonstrate an understanding of drug therapy.

Antiflatulent drugs

Antiflatulent drugs, or antiflatulents, disperse gas pockets in the GI tract. They're available alone or in combination with antacids. The major antiflatulent drug currently in use is simeticone.

Pharmacokinetics

Simeticone isn't absorbed from the GI tract. It's distributed only in the intestinal lumen and is eliminated intact in faeces.

Pharmacodynamics

Simeticone creates foaming action in the GI tract. It produces a film in the intestines that disperses mucus-enclosed gas pockets and helps prevent their formation.

Pharmacotherapeutics

Simeticone is prescribed to treat conditions in which excess gas is a problem, such as:
- functional gastric bloating
- postoperative gaseous bloating
- diverticular disease
- spastic or irritable colon
- the swallowing of air.

Drug interactions

Simeticone doesn't interact significantly with other drugs.

Adverse reactions

Simeticone doesn't cause any known adverse reactions. It has, however, been associated with excessive belching or flatus.

We spell relief! Antiflatulent drugs treat conditions involving excessive amounts of air or gas in the stomach or intestine.

Nursing process

These nursing process steps are appropriate for patients undergoing treatment with antiflatulent drugs such as simeticone.

Assessment
• Assess the patient's condition before therapy and regularly thereafter.
• Assess for adverse GI reactions.
• Assess the patient's and family's knowledge of drug therapy.

Key nursing diagnoses
• Acute pain related to gas in the GI tract.
• Deficient knowledge related to drug therapy.

Planning outcome goals
• The patient's pain will decrease.
• The patient and family will demonstrate an understanding of drug therapy.

Implementation
• Make sure that the patient chews the tablet form before swallowing.
• If giving the suspension form, make sure to shake the bottle or container thoroughly to distribute the solution.
• Inform the patient that the drug doesn't prevent gas formation.
• Encourage the patient to change position frequently and to ambulate to help pass flatus.

Evaluation
• Patient's gas pain is relieved.
• Patient and family demonstrate an understanding of drug therapy.

Digestants (pancreatin and similar drugs)

Digestants aid digestion in patients who are missing enzymes or other substances needed to digest food. Digestive drugs that function in the GI tract, liver, and pancreas include:
• pancreatin, pancrelipase, lipase, protease, and amylase (pancreatic enzymes).

Shake shake shake. Shake shake shake. Shake your suspensions! Shake your suspensions!

Pharmacokinetics

Digestive drugs aren't absorbed; they act locally in the GI tract and are excreted in faeces.

Pharmacodynamics

The action of digestive drugs resembles the action of the body substances they replace. Dehydrocholic acid, a bile acid, increases the output of bile in the liver. The pancreatic enzymes replace normal pancreatic enzymes. They exert their effect in the duodenum and upper jejunum of the upper GI tract.

Key ingredients

These drugs contain trypsin to digest proteins, amylase to digest carbohydrates, and lipase to digest fats.

Pharmacotherapeutics

Because their action resembles the action of the body substances they replace, each digestive drug has its own indication.

For the enzyme impaired

Pancreatic enzymes are administered to patients with insufficient levels of pancreatic enzymes, such as those with pancreatitis or cystic fibrosis. They may also be used to treat steatorrhoea (a disorder of fat metabolism characterised by fatty, foul-smelling stools). (See *Pancreatic enzymes warning*.)

Drug interactions

Antacids reduce the effects of pancreatic enzymes and shouldn't be given at the same time. Pancreatic enzymes may also decrease the absorption of folic acid and iron.

Adverse reactions

Adverse reactions to pancreatic enzymes include:
- diarrhoea
- nausea
- abdominal cramping.

Nursing process

These nursing process steps are appropriate for patients undergoing treatment with digestive drugs.

Before you give that drug!

Pancreatic enzymes warning

Pancreatic enzymes should be given before meals. This ensures that the drug is available in the small intestine to help digestion. Giving pancreatic enzymes at another time, such as 1 hour or more after eating or during a meal, decreases the drug's effectiveness.

Patients with pancreatitis or cystic fibrosis may require pancreatic enzyme administration because their bodies may not produce enough on their own.

Assessment
• Assess the patient's condition before therapy and regularly thereafter. A decrease in the number of bowel movements and improved stool consistency indicate effective therapy.
• Monitor the patient's diet to ensure proper balance of fat, protein, and starch intake. This helps avoid indigestion. The dosage varies according to the degree of maldigestion and malabsorption, the amount of fat in the diet, and the enzyme activity of the drug.
• Assess the patient's and family's knowledge of drug therapy.
• Assess the patient's and family's knowledge and attitudes about nutrition.

Key nursing diagnoses
• Imbalanced nutrition: Less than body requirements related to the condition.
• Noncompliance related to long-term therapy.
• Deficient knowledge related to drug therapy.

Planning outcome goals
• The patient's nutritional status will improve as evidenced by laboratory tests and weight.
• The patient will comply with the prescribed drug regimen.
• The patient and family will demonstrate an understanding of drug therapy.

Implementation
• Administer the drug before or with each meal, as applicable.
• For infants, the powdered form may be mixed with a small amount of soft food and given before meals.
• Avoid contact with or inhalation of the powder form; it may be irritating.
• Older children may take capsules with food.
• Tell the patient not to crush or chew enteric-coated dosage forms. Capsules containing enteric-coated microspheres may be opened and their contents sprinkled on a small amount of soft food. Follow administration with a glass of water or juice.
• Review food preferences and diet with the patient and family.

A balanced diet, including adequate fat, protein, and starch intake, will prevent indigestion.

- Provide food and fluids that the patient enjoys at preferred times, if possible.
- Treat symptoms or disorders that may interfere with nutrition, such as pain, nausea, vomiting, or diarrhoea.
- Consult with a dietitian if special diets are required. Provide foods the patient likes that are nutritionally better choices but are within the prescribed diet.

Evaluation

- Patient maintains normal digestion of fats, carbohydrates, and proteins.
- Patient complies with prescribed drug regimen.
- Patient and family demonstrate an understanding of drug therapy. (See *Teaching about digestive drugs.*)

Antidiarrhoeal and laxative drugs

Diarrhoea and constipation represent the two major symptoms related to disturbances of the large intestine.

Antidiarrhoeals act systemically or locally and include:
- opioid-related drugs
- kaolin and morphine (a locally acting combination drug).

Laxatives stimulate defaecation and include:
- hyperosmolar drugs
- dietary fibre and related bulk-forming substances
- emollients
- stimulants
- lubricants.

Opioid-related drugs

Opioid-related drugs decrease peristalsis (involuntary, progressive wavelike intestinal movement that pushes faecal matter along) in the intestines and include:
- co-phenotrope (diphenoxylate with atropine)
- loperamide.

Education edge

Teaching about digestive drugs

If digestive drugs are prescribed, review these points with the patient and caregivers:

- Exercise and stay active to aid in digestion and improve appetite.
- Minimise the use of strong pain medications and sedatives because these drugs may cause drowsiness and deter eating and drinking.
- Have routine checkups to monitor weight, fluid intake, urine output, and laboratory study results and to assess nutritional outcome.

Opioid-related drugs decrease the wavelike movement of peristalsis.

Pharmacokinetics

Co-phenotrope is readily absorbed from the GI tract. However, loperamide isn't absorbed well after oral administration.

Both drugs are distributed in serum, metabolised in the liver, and excreted primarily in faeces. Co-phenotrope is metabolised to difenoxin, its biologically active major metabolite.

Pharmacodynamics

Co-phenotrope and loperamide slow GI motility by depressing the circular and longitudinal muscle action (peristalsis) in the large and small intestines. These drugs also decrease expulsive contractions throughout the colon.

Pharmacotherapeutics

Co-phenotrope and loperamide are used to treat acute, nonspecific diarrhoea. Loperamide is also used to treat chronic diarrhoea. (See *Antidiarrhoeals: Loperamide.*)

Drug interactions

Both co-phenotrope, and loperamide may enhance the depressant effects of barbiturates, alcohol, opioids, tranquilisers, and sedatives.

Adverse reactions

Adverse reactions to co-phenotrope and loperamide include:
- nausea
- vomiting
- abdominal discomfort or distention
- drowsiness
- fatigue
- central nervous system (CNS) depression
- tachycardia (fast heart rate)
- paralytic ileus (reduced or absent peristalsis in the intestines).

Nursing process

These nursing process steps are appropriate for patients undergoing treatment with opioid-related drugs.

Prototype pro

Anti-diarrhoeals: Loperamide

Actions

- Inhibits peristaltic activity, prolonging transit of intestinal contents

Indications

- Diarrhoea

Nursing considerations

- Monitor the drug's effect on bowel movements.
- If giving by nasogastric tube, flush the tube to clear it and to ensure the drug's passage to the stomach.
- Oral liquids are available in different concentrations. Check the dosage carefully.
- For children, consider an oral liquid that doesn't contain alcohol.

Assessment

- Assess the patient's condition before therapy and regularly thereafter.
- Assess the patient's diarrhoea before therapy and regularly thereafter.
- Monitor fluid and electrolyte balance.
- Monitor hydration status if adverse GI reactions occur.
- Evaluate the patient for adverse reactions.
- Assess the patient's and family's knowledge of drug therapy.

Key nursing diagnoses

- Diarrhoea related to the underlying condition.
- Risk for deficient fluid volume related to GI upset.
- Deficient knowledge related to drug therapy.

Planning outcome goals

- The patient will have normal bowel movements.
- Adequate fluid balance will be maintained as evidenced by the patient's intake and output.
- The patient and family will demonstrate an understanding of drug therapy.

Implementation

- Administer the drug exactly as prescribed.
- Correct fluid and electrolyte disturbances before starting the drug; dehydration may increase the risk of delayed toxicity in some cases.
- Use naloxone to treat respiratory depression caused by overdose.
- Take safety precautions if the patient experiences adverse CNS reactions.
- Notify the prescriber about serious or persistent adverse reactions.

Before giving antidiarrhoeals, make sure you correct fluid and electrolyte disturbances, which may cause dehydration.

Evaluation

- Patient's diarrhoea is relieved.
- Patient maintains adequate hydration.
- Patient and family demonstrate an understanding of drug therapy. (See *Teaching about antidiarrhoeals.*)

Education edge

Teaching about antidiarrhoeals

If antidiarrhoeals are prescribed, review these points with the patient and caregivers:

- Take the drug exactly as prescribed; be aware that excessive use of opium preparations can lead to dependence.
- Notify your prescriber if diarrhoea lasts for more than 2 days, if acute abdominal signs and symptoms occur, or if the drug is ineffective.
- Report adverse reactions.
- Avoid hazardous activities that require alertness if central nervous system depression occurs.
- Maintain intake of fluids and electrolytes, up to 2 to 3 L per day. Water, clear soup, weak tea, gelatin, and noncarbonated, caffeine-free drinks are well tolerated.
- Avoid food and fluids that can irritate the GI tract while diarrhoea is present, such as raw fruits and vegetables and spicy foods.

- Schedule rest periods and decrease activity while diarrhoea persists to reduce peristalsis.

Prevention tips

To help prevent diarrhoea:

- Prepare and store food properly and avoid products that have been prepared under unsanitary conditions.
- Wash hands before handling any food, after handling raw meat and poultry, and before eating.
- Chew food well.
- Avoid overuse of laxatives or over-the-counter products that contain senna or other stimulant laxatives.

Kaolin mixtures

Kaolin mixtures are locally acting over-the-counter antidiarrhoeals. They work by adsorbing irritants and soothing the intestinal mucosa.

Pharmacokinetics
Kaolin mixtures aren't absorbed and, therefore, aren't distributed throughout the body. They're excreted in faeces.

Pharmacodynamics
Kaolin mixtures act as adsorbents, binding with bacteria, toxins, and other irritants on the intestinal mucosa.

Pharmacotherapeutics
Kaolin mixtures are used to relieve mild to moderate acute diarrhoea.

Just a stop-gap

They also may be used to temporarily relieve chronic diarrhoea until the cause is determined and definitive treatment starts.

Drug interactions

These antidiarrhoeals can interfere with the absorption of digoxin or other drugs from the intestinal mucosa if administered at the same time.

Adverse reactions

Kaolin mixtures cause few adverse reactions. However, constipation may occur, especially in elderly or debilitated patients or in cases of overdose or prolonged use.

Nursing process

These nursing process steps are appropriate for patients undergoing treatment with kaolin mixtures.

Kaolin mixtures may cause constipation, especially in elderly or debilitated patients.

Assessment

- Assess the patient's condition before therapy and regularly thereafter.
- Assess the patient's diarrhoea before therapy and regularly thereafter.
- Monitor fluid and electrolyte balance.
- Monitor hydration status if adverse GI reactions occur.
- Assess the patient for adverse reactions.
- Assess the patient's and family's knowledge of drug therapy.

Key nursing diagnoses

- Diarrhoea related to the underlying condition.
- Risk for deficient fluid volume related to GI upset.
- Deficient knowledge related to drug therapy.

Planning outcome goals

- The patient will have normal bowel movements.
- Adequate fluid balance will be maintained as evidenced by the patient's intake and output.
- The patient and family will demonstrate an understanding of drug therapy.

Implementation
- Administer the drug exactly as prescribed.
- Correct fluid and electrolyte disturbances before starting the drug; dehydration may increase the risk of delayed toxicity in some cases.
- Take safety precautions if the patient experiences adverse CNS reactions.
- Notify the prescriber about serious or persistent adverse reactions.

Evaluation
- Patient's diarrhoea is relieved.
- Patient maintains adequate hydration.
- Patient and family demonstrate an understanding of drug therapy.

Hyperosmolar laxatives

Hyperosmolar laxatives work by drawing water into the intestine, thereby promoting bowel distention and peristalsis. They include:
- glycerin
- lactulose
- saline compounds, such as magnesium salts, sodium biphosphate, sodium phosphate, polyethylene glycol (PEG), and electrolytes.

Pharmacokinetics
The pharmacokinetic properties of hyperosmolar laxatives vary.

Enter from the rear

Glycerin is placed directly into the colon by enema or suppository and isn't absorbed systemically.

Intestine marks the spot

Lactulose enters the GI tract orally and is minimally absorbed. As a result, the drug is distributed only in the intestine. It's metabolised by bacteria in the colon and excreted in faeces.

Saline away

After saline compounds are introduced into the GI tract orally or as an enema, some of their ions are absorbed. Absorbed ions are excreted in urine, the unabsorbed drug in faeces.

And then there's PEG

PEG is a nonabsorbable solution that acts as an osmotic drug but doesn't alter electrolyte balance.

Pharmacodynamics

Hyperosmolar laxatives produce a bowel movement by drawing water into the intestine. Fluid accumulation distends the bowel and promotes peristalsis and a bowel movement. (See *Hyperosmolar laxatives: Magnesium hydroxide.*)

Pharmacotherapeutics

The uses of hyperosmolar laxatives vary:
• Glycerin is helpful in bowel retraining.
• Lactulose is used to treat constipation and help reduce ammonia production and absorption from the intestines in liver disease.
• Saline compounds are used when prompt and complete bowel evacuation is required.

Drug interactions

Hyperosmolar laxatives don't interact significantly with other drugs. However, the absorption of oral drugs administered 1 hour before PEG is significantly decreased.

I come bearing water to help promote peristalsis!

Prototype pro

Hyperosmolar laxatives: Magnesium hydroxide

Actions

• Reduces total acid in the GI tract
• Elevates gastric pH to reduce pepsin activity
• Strengthens the gastric mucosal barrier
• Increases oesophageal sphincter tone

Indications

• Upset stomach
• Constipation
• To increase the magnesium level

Nursing considerations

• Monitor the drug's effect on bowel movements.
• Shake the suspension well. Give the drug with a large amount of water when used as a laxative.
• When used with a nasogastric tube, make sure the tube is placed properly and is patent. After instilling the drug, flush the tube with water to ensure passage to the stomach and to maintain tube patency.

Adverse reactions

Adverse reactions to hyperosmolar laxatives involve fluid and electrolyte imbalances.

Adverse reactions to glycerin include:

- weakness
- fatigue.

Lactulose may cause these adverse reactions:

- abdominal distention, gas, and abdominal cramps
- nausea and vomiting
- diarrhoea
- hypokalaemia
- hypovolaemia
- increased blood glucose level.

Adverse reactions to saline compounds include:

- weakness
- lethargy
- dehydration
- hypernatraemia
- hypermagnesaemia
- hyperphosphataemia
- hypocalcaemia
- cardiac arrhythmias
- shock.

These adverse reactions may occur with PEG:

- nausea
- abdominal fullness
- explosive diarrhoea
- bloating.

Nursing process

These nursing process steps are appropriate for patients undergoing treatment with hyperosmolar laxatives.

Assessment

- Obtain a baseline assessment of the patient's bowel patterns and GI history before giving a laxative.
- Determine whether the patient maintains adequate fluid intake and diet and whether he exercises.
- Assess the patient's bowel pattern throughout therapy. Assess bowel sounds and colour and consistency of stools.
- Monitor fluid and electrolyte status during administration.
- Assess for adverse reactions and drug interactions.
- Assess the patient's and family's knowledge of drug therapy.

Key nursing diagnoses
- Diarrhoea related to adverse GI effects.
- Acute pain related to abdominal discomfort.
- Deficient knowledge related to drug therapy.

Planning outcome goals
- Regular bowel movements will be maintained. The patient's pain will decrease.
- The patient and family will demonstrate an understanding of drug therapy.

Implementation
- Time drug administration so that bowel evacuation doesn't interfere with scheduled activities or sleep.
- Shake suspensions well; give with a large amount of water, as applicable.
- If administering the drug through an NG tube, make sure that the tube is placed properly and is patent. After instilling the drug, flush the tube with water to ensure passage to the stomach and to maintain tube patency.
- Don't crush enteric-coated tablets.
- Make sure that the patient has easy access to a bedpan or bathroom.
- Institute measures to prevent constipation.

Evaluation
- Patient regains normal bowel pattern.
- Patient states that pain is relieved with stool evacuation.
- Patient and family demonstrate an understanding of drug therapy.

Schedule laxative administration so that the drug's effects don't interfere with the patient's activities or sleep.

Dietary fibre and related bulk-forming laxatives

A high-fibre diet is the most natural way to prevent or treat constipation. Dietary fibre is the part of plants not digested in the small intestine.

Close resemblance

Bulk-forming laxatives, which resemble dietary fibre, contain natural and semisynthetic polysaccharides and cellulose. These laxatives include:
- Ispaghula husk
- methylcellulose
- psyllium hydrophilic mucilloid
- sterculia.

A high-fibre diet is the most natural way to prevent or treat constipation, but bulk-forming laxatives can offer a little help if nature isn't cooperating!

Prototype pro

Bulk-forming laxatives: Sterculia

Actions

- Absorbs water and expands to increase bulk and moisture content of stool, thus encouraging peristalsis and bowel movements

Indications

- Constipation

Nursing considerations

- Mix the drug with at least 240 ml of cold, pleasant-tasting liquid, such as orange juice, to mask grittiness. Stir only a few seconds. Have the patient drink the mixture immediately, before it congeals.

Follow administration with another glass of liquid.

- Sterculia may reduce the patient's appetite if taken before meals.
- This drug isn't absorbed systemically and is nontoxic.
- Stercula is useful in debilitated patients and in patients with postpartum constipation, irritable bowel syndrome, or diverticular disease. It's also used to treat chronic laxative abuse and combined with other laxatives to empty the colon before barium enema examination.
- Advise patients with diabetes to check the drug's label and to use a brand that doesn't contain sugar.

Pharmacokinetics

Dietary fibre and bulk-forming laxatives aren't absorbed systemically. The polysaccharides in these drugs are converted by intestinal bacterial flora into osmotically active metabolites that draw water into the intestine. Dietary fibre and bulk-forming laxatives are excreted in faeces.

Pharmacodynamics

Dietary fibre and bulk-forming laxatives increase stool mass and water content, promoting peristalsis. (See *Bulk-forming laxatives: Sterculia*.)

Pharmacotherapeutics

Bulk-forming laxatives are used to:
- treat simple cases of constipation, especially constipation resulting from a low-fibre or low-fluid diet
- aid patients recovering from acute myocardial infarction (MI) or cerebral aneurysms who need to avoid Valsalva's manoeuvre (forced expiration against a closed airway) and maintain soft stool
- manage patients with IBS and diverticulosis.

Drug interactions

Decreased absorption of digoxin, warfarin, and salicylates occurs if these drugs are taken within 2 hours of fibre or bulk-forming laxatives.

Adverse reactions

Adverse reactions to dietary fibre and related bulk-forming laxatives include:
*   flatulence
*   a sensation of abdominal fullness
*   intestinal obstruction
*   faecal impaction (hard faeces that can't be removed from the rectum)
*   oesophageal obstruction (if sufficient liquid hasn't been administered with the drug)
*   severe diarrhoea.

Nursing process

These nursing process steps are appropriate for patients undergoing treatment with dietary fibre and bulk-forming laxatives.

Assessment
*   Obtain a baseline assessment of the patient's bowel patterns and GI history before giving a laxative.
*   Assess the patient for adverse reactions and drug interactions.
*   Monitor the patient's bowel pattern throughout therapy. Assess bowel sounds and colour and consistency of stools.
*   Assess the patient's fluid and electrolyte status during administration.
*   Determine whether the patient maintains adequate fluid intake and diet and whether he exercises regularly.
*   Assess the patient's and family's knowledge of drug therapy.

Key nursing diagnoses
*   Diarrhoea related to adverse GI effects.
*   Acute pain related to abdominal discomfort.
*   Deficient knowledge related to drug therapy.

Planning outcome goals
*   Regular bowel movements will be maintained.
*   The patient's pain will decrease.
*   The patient and family will demonstrate an understanding of drug therapy.

Implementation

- Time drug administration so that the drug's effects don't interfere with scheduled activities or sleep.
- Mix drugs as directed and give with a large amount of water, as applicable.
- Don't crush enteric-coated tablets.
- The laxative effect usually occurs in 12 to 24 hours but may be delayed for up to 3 days.
- Make sure that the patient has easy access to a bedpan or bathroom.
- Institute measures to prevent constipation.

Evaluation

- Patient regains normal bowel pattern.
- Patient states that pain is relieved with stool evacuation.
- Patient and family demonstrate an understanding of drug therapy.

Emollient laxatives

Emollient laxatives—also known as *stool softeners*—primarily include the sodium salts of docusate.

Pharmacokinetics

Administered orally, emollient laxatives are absorbed and excreted through bile in faeces.

Pharmacodynamics

Emollient laxatives emulsify the fat and water components of faeces in the small and large intestines. This detergent action allows water and fats to penetrate the stool, making it softer and easier to eliminate. Emollients also stimulate electrolyte and fluid secretion from intestinal mucosal cells. (See *Emollient laxatives: Docusate.*)

Pharmacotherapeutics

Emollient laxatives are the drugs of choice for softening stools in patients who should avoid straining during a bowel movement, including those with:

- recent MI or surgery
- disease of the anus or rectum
- increased intracranial pressure (ICP)
- hernias.

Prepare to emulsify

Prototype pro

Emollient laxatives: Docusate

Actions

- Reduces surface tension of interfacing liquid contents of the bowel, promoting incorporation of additional liquid into stool, thus forming a softer mass

Indications

- Stool softener for patients who should avoid straining during a bowel movement

Nursing considerations

- Monitor the drug's effect on bowel movements.

- Be alert for adverse reactions and drug interactions.
- This drug is the laxative of choice for patients who shouldn't strain during defaecation (including those recovering from myocardial infarction or rectal surgery), for patients with rectal or anal disease that makes passage of firm stool difficult, and for patients with postpartum constipation.
- Discontinue the drug if abdominal cramping occurs and notify the prescriber.
- Docusate doesn't stimulate intestinal peristaltic movements.

Drug interactions

Taking oral doses of mineral oil with oral emollient laxatives increases the systemic absorption of mineral oil. This increased absorption may result in tissue deposits of the oil.

Proceed with caution

Because emollient laxatives may enhance the absorption of many oral drugs, drugs with low margins of safety (narrow therapeutic index) should be administered cautiously.

Adverse reactions

Although adverse reactions to emollient laxatives seldom occur, they may include:
- a bitter taste
- diarrhoea
- throat irritation
- mild, transient abdominal cramping.

Nursing process

These nursing process steps are appropriate for patients undergoing treatment with emollient laxatives.

Assessment

- Obtain a baseline assessment of the patient's bowel patterns and GI history before giving a laxative.
- Assess the patient for adverse reactions and drug interactions.
- Monitor the patient's bowel pattern throughout therapy. Assess bowel sounds and colour and consistency of stools.
- Assess the patient's fluid and electrolyte status during administration.
- Determine whether the patient maintains adequate fluid intake and diet and whether he exercises.
- Assess the patient's and family's knowledge of drug therapy.

Key nursing diagnoses

- Diarrhoea related to adverse GI effects.
- Acute pain related to abdominal discomfort.
- Deficient knowledge related to drug therapy.

Planning

- Regular bowel movements will be maintained.
- The patient's pain will decrease.
- The patient and family will demonstrate an understanding of drug therapy.

Implementation

- Time drug administration so that bowel evacuation doesn't interfere with scheduled activities or sleep.
- Shake suspensions well; give with a large amount of water, as applicable.
- If administering the drug through an NG tube, make sure that the tube is placed properly and is patent. After instilling the drug, flush the tube with water to ensure passage to the stomach and to maintain tube patency.
- Don't crush enteric-coated tablets.
- Make sure that the patient has easy access to a bedpan or bathroom.
- Institute measures to prevent constipation.

Evaluation

- Patient regains normal bowel pattern.
- Patient states that pain is relieved with stool evacuation.
- Patient and family demonstrate an understanding of drug therapy.

Stimulant laxatives

Stimulant laxatives, also known as *irritant cathartics*, include:
* bisacodyl
* cascara
* dantron
* senna
* sodium picosulfate

Pharmacokinetics

Stimulant laxatives are minimally absorbed and are metabolised in the liver. The metabolites are excreted in urine and faeces.

Pharmacodynamics

Stimulant laxatives stimulate peristalsis and produce a bowel movement by irritating the intestinal mucosa or stimulating nerve endings of the intestinal smooth muscle. (See *Stimulant laxatives: Bisacodyl*.)

Powering up peristalsis

Castor oil and cascara (an anthriquinone) also increase peristalsis in the small intestine, although these two powerful stimulant laxatives are now considered obsolete.

Prototype pro

Stimulant laxatives: Bisacodyl

Actions

* Increases peristalsis, probably by acting directly on the smooth muscle of the intestine
* Thought to irritate musculature or stimulate colonic intramural plexus
* Promotes fluid accumulation in the colon and small intestine

Indications

* Constipation
* Emptying of the bowel before general surgery, sigmoidoscopic, and radiologic procedures

Nursing considerations

* Monitor the drug's effect on bowel movements.
* Be alert for adverse reactions and drug interactions.
* Don't give tablets within 60 minutes of milk or antacids.
* Insert a suppository as high as possible into the rectum and try to position it against the rectal wall. Avoid embedding the drug within faecal material because this may delay onset of action.
* Soft-formed stool is usually produced 15 to 60 minutes after rectal administration.

Pharmacotherapeutics

Stimulant laxatives are the preferred drugs for emptying the bowel before general surgery, sigmoidoscopic, and radiologic procedures such as barium studies of the GI tract. Stimulant laxatives are also used to treat constipation caused by prolonged bed rest, neurologic dysfunction of the colon, and constipating drugs such as opioids.

Drug interactions

No significant drug interactions occur with stimulant laxatives. However, because stimulant laxatives produce increased intestinal motility, they reduce the absorption of other oral drugs administered at the same time, especially sustained-release forms.

Adverse reactions

Adverse reactions to stimulant laxatives include:
- weakness
- nausea
- abdominal cramps
- mild inflammation of the rectum and anus
- urine discolouration (especially with senna use).

> Stimulant laxatives are used to empty the bowel before general surgery, sigmoidoscopic and radiologic procedures.

Nursing process

These nursing process steps are appropriate for patients undergoing treatment with stimulant laxatives.

Assessment
- Obtain a baseline assessment of the patient's bowel patterns and GI history before giving a laxative.
- Assess the patient for adverse reactions and drug interactions.
- Monitor the patient's bowel pattern throughout therapy. Assess bowel sounds and colour and consistency of stools.
- Assess the patient's fluid and electrolyte status during administration.
- Determine whether the patient maintains adequate fluid intake and diet and whether he exercises.
- Assess the patient's and family's knowledge of drug therapy.

Key nursing diagnoses
- Diarrhoea related to adverse GI effects.
- Acute pain related to abdominal discomfort.
- Deficient knowledge related to drug therapy.

Planning outcome goals
- Regular bowel movements will be maintained.
- The patient's pain will decrease.
- The patient and family will demonstrate an understanding of drug therapy.

Implementation
- Time drug administration so that bowel evacuation doesn't interfere with scheduled activities or sleep.
- Shake suspensions well; give with a large amount of water, as indicated.
- If administering the drug through an NG tube, make sure that the tube is placed properly and is patent. After instilling the drug, flush the tube with water to ensure passage to the stomach and to maintain tube patency.
- Don't crush enteric-coated tablets.
- Make sure that the patient has easy access to a bedpan or bathroom.
- Institute measures to prevent constipation.

Evaluation
- Patient regains normal bowel pattern.
- Patient states that pain is relieved with stool evacuation.
- Patient and family demonstrate an understanding of drug therapy.

Lubricant laxatives

Mineral oil is the main lubricant laxative in current clinical use.

Pharmacokinetics
In its nonemulsified form, mineral oil is minimally absorbed; the emulsified form is about half absorbed. Absorbed mineral oil is distributed to the mesenteric lymph nodes, intestinal mucosa, liver, and spleen. Mineral oil is metabolised by the liver and excreted in faeces. (See *Lubricant laxatives: Mineral oil.*)

Pharmacodynamics
Mineral oil lubricates the stool and the intestinal mucosa and prevents water reabsorption from the bowel lumen. The increased fluid content of faeces increases peristalsis. Rectal administration by enema also produces distention.

Prototype pro

Lubricant laxatives: Mineral oil

Actions
- Increases water retention in stool by creating a barrier between the colon wall and faeces that prevents colonic reabsorption of faecal water.

Indications
- Constipation.

Nursing considerations
- Monitor the drug's effect on bowel movements.
- Be alert for adverse reactions and drug interactions.
- Give the drug on an empty stomach.
- Give the drug with fruit juice or a carbonated drink to disguise its taste.

Pharmacotherapeutics

Mineral oil is used to treat constipation and maintain soft stools when straining is contraindicated, such as after a recent MI (to avoid Valsalva's manoeuvre), eye surgery (to prevent increased pressure in the eye), or cerebral aneurysm repair (to avoid increased ICP). Administered orally or by enema, mineral oil is also used to treat patients with faecal impaction.

Drug interactions

To minimise drug interactions, administer mineral oil at least 2 hours before other drugs. These drug interactions may occur:
• Mineral oil may impair the absorption of many oral drugs, including fat-soluble vitamins, hormonal contraceptives, and anticoagulants.
• Mineral oil may interfere with the antibacterial activity of nonabsorbable sulphonamides.

Adverse reactions

Adverse reactions to mineral oil include:
• nausea
• vomiting
• diarrhoea
• abdominal cramping.

You can minimise drug interactions by giving mineral oil at least 2 hours before other drugs.

Nursing process

These nursing process steps are appropriate for patients undergoing treatment with lubricant laxatives.

Assessment

• Obtain a baseline assessment of the patient's bowel patterns and GI history before giving a laxative.
• Assess the patient for adverse reactions and drug interactions.
• Monitor the patient's bowel pattern throughout therapy. Assess bowel sounds and colour and consistency of stools.
• Assess the patient's fluid and electrolyte status during administration.
• Determine whether the patient maintains adequate fluid intake and diet and whether he exercises.
• Assess the patient's and family's knowledge of drug therapy.

Key nursing diagnoses

• Diarrhoea related to adverse GI effects.
• Acute pain related to abdominal discomfort.
• Deficient knowledge related to drug therapy.

Planning outcome goals
- Regular bowel movements will be maintained.
- The patient's pain will decrease.
- The patient and family will demonstrate an understanding of drug therapy.

Implementation
- Time drug administration so that bowel evacuation doesn't interfere with scheduled activities or sleep.
- When giving mineral oil by mouth, give it on an empty stomach.
- Perform rectal administration according to facility protocol.
- Make sure that the patient has easy access to a bedpan or bathroom.
- Institute measures to prevent constipation.

Evaluation
- Patient regains normal bowel pattern.
- Patient states that pain is relieved with stool evacuation.
- Patient and family demonstrate an understanding of drug therapy. (See *Teaching about laxatives*.)

Education edge

Teaching about laxatives

If laxatives are prescribed, review these points with the patient and caregivers:

- Therapy should be short term. Abuse or prolonged use can result in nutritional imbalances.
- Diet, exercise, and fluid intake are important in maintaining normal bowel function and preventing or treating constipation.
- Drink at least 6 to 10 glasses (240 ml each) of fluid daily, unless contraindicated.
- Exercise regularly to help with bowel elimination.
- Stool softeners and bulk-forming laxatives may take several days to achieve results.

- If using a bulk-forming laxative, remain active and drink plenty of fluids.
- Stimulant laxatives may cause harmless urine discolouration.
- Include foods high in fibre, such as bran and other cereals, fresh fruit, and vegetables, in diet.
- Frequent or prolonged use of some laxatives can result in dependence.
- Never take laxatives when acute abdominal pain, nausea, or vomiting is present. A ruptured appendix or other serious complication may result.
- Notify the prescriber if symptoms persist or if the laxative doesn't work.

Antiemetic and emetic drugs

Antiemetics and emetics represent two groups of drugs with opposing actions. Emetic drugs, which are derived from plants, produce vomiting. Antiemetic drugs decrease nausea, reducing the urge to vomit.

Antiemetics

The major antiemetics include:
• antihistamines, including cinnarzine, dimenhydrinate, buclizine hydrochloride, cyclizine hydrochloride, and hydroxyzine hydrochloride
• phenothiazines, including chlorpromazine hydrochloride, perphenazine, prochlorperazine maleate, promethazine hydrochloride, and trifluoperazine
• serotonin receptor (5-HT$_3$) antagonists, including ondansetron, dolasetron, and granisetron.

No.1 nausea fighter

Ondansetron is one of the most commonly used antiemetics.

Pharmacokinetics

The pharmacokinetic properties of antiemetics may slightly vary. Oral antihistamine antiemetics are absorbed well from the GI tract and are metabolised primarily by the liver. Their inactive metabolites are excreted in urine.

Phenothiazines and serotonin receptor antagonists are absorbed well and extensively metabolised by the liver. They are excreted in urine and faeces.

Pharmacodynamics

The action of antiemetics may vary.

Mechanism unknown

The mechanism of action that produces the antiemetic effect of antihistamines is unclear.

The trigger zone

Phenothiazines produce their antiemetic effect by blocking the dopaminergic receptors in the chemoreceptor trigger zone in the brain. (This area of the brain, near the medulla, stimulates the vomiting centre in the medulla, causing vomiting). These drugs may also directly depress the vomiting centre.

Two spots to block

The serotonin receptor antagonists block serotonin stimulation centrally in the chemoreceptor trigger zone and peripherally in the vagal nerve terminals, both of which stimulate vomiting.

Pharmacotherapeutics
The uses of antiemetics may vary.

Motion potion

With the exception of trimethobenzamide, the antihistamines are specifically used for nausea and vomiting caused by inner ear stimulation. As a consequence, these drugs prevent or treat motion sickness. They usually prove most effective when given before activities that produce motion sickness and are much less effective when nausea or vomiting has already begun.

Much more severe

Phenothiazines and serotonin receptor antagonists control severe nausea and vomiting from various causes. They're used when vomiting becomes severe and potentially hazardous, such as postsurgical or viral nausea and vomiting. Both types of drugs are also prescribed to control the nausea and vomiting resulting from cancer chemotherapy and radiotherapy. (See *Other antiemetics*.)

Other antiemetics

Here are other antiemetics currently in use.

Hyoscine

Hyoscine prevents motion sickness, but its use is limited because of its sedative and anticholinergic effects. A number of transdermal preparations are highly effective without producing the usual adverse effects.

Metoclopramide

Metoclopramide hydrochloride is principally used to treat GI motility disorders, including gastroparesis in diabetic patients. It's also used to prevent chemotherapy-induced nausea and vomiting.

Drug interactions

Antiemetics may have many significant interactions:

- Antihistamines and phenothiazines can produce additive CNS depression and sedation when taken with CNS depressants, such as barbiturates, tranquilisers, antidepressants, alcohol, and opioids.
- Antihistamines can cause additive anticholinergic effects, such as constipation, dry mouth, vision problems, and urine retention, when taken with anticholinergic drugs, including tricyclic antidepressants, phenothiazines, and antiparkinsonian drugs.
- Phenothiazine antiemetics taken with anticholinergic drugs increase the anticholinergic effect and decrease antiemetic effects.

Adverse reactions

The use of these antiemetic drugs may lead to adverse reactions:

- Antihistamine and phenothiazine antiemetics produce drowsiness; paradoxical CNS stimulation may also occur.
- CNS effects associated with phenothiazine and serotonin receptor antagonist antiemetics include confusion, anxiety, euphoria, agitation, depression, headache, insomnia, restlessness, and weakness.
- The anticholinergic effect of antiemetics may cause constipation, dry mouth and throat, painful or difficult urination, urine retention, impotence, and visual and auditory disturbances.
- Hypotension and orthostatic hypotension with an increased heart rate, fainting, and dizziness are common adverse reactions to phenothiazines.

Nursing process

These nursing process steps are appropriate for patients undergoing treatment with antiemetics.

Assessment

- Assess the patient's condition before therapy and regularly thereafter.
- Assess for adverse reactions and drug interactions.
- Assess the patient's and family's knowledge of drug therapy.

Key nursing diagnoses

- Ineffective health maintenance related to the underlying condition.
- Risk for deficient fluid volume related to the underlying condition.
- Deficient knowledge related to drug therapy.

> Antihistamines and phenothiazines can produce additive CNS depression and sedation when taken with CNS depressants.

Planning outcome goals
- The patient will exhibit improved health as evidenced by decreased vomiting.
- Fluid volume balance will remain adequate as evidenced by the patient's intake and output, vital signs, and electrolyte evaluations.
- The patient and family will demonstrate an understanding of drug therapy.

Implementation
- Monitor the patient for the drug's effect.
- Administer the drug as directed to promote GI effectiveness and relieve distress.
- Give I.M. injections deeply into large muscle mass. Rotate injection sites.
- Don't give antiemetics subcutaneously.
- If the drug is being used to prevent motion sickness, the patient should take the dose 30 to 60 minutes before travel.
- Warn the patient to avoid alcohol and hazardous activities until the drug's CNS effects are known.
- Stop the drug 4 days before allergy skin tests.

Evaluation
- Patient responds well to therapy.
- Patient maintains fluid volume.
- Patient and family demonstrate an understanding of drug therapy.

It isn't my job! Don't give antiemetics subcutaneously.

Emetics

Emetics are used to induce vomiting in a person who has ingested toxic substances. For example, ipecac syrup is used to induce vomiting in the early management of oral poisoning or drug overdose.

Current controversy

The use of ipecac syrup has become controversial because it delays the use of activated charcoal. In addition, there's a risk of potential abuse by individuals with eating disorders.

Pharmacokinetics
Little information exists concerning the absorption, distribution, and excretion of ipecac syrup. After administration, vomiting occurs within 10 to 30 minutes.

Measuring success

The success of treatment is directly linked to fluid intake with ipecac administration.

Pharmacodynamics

Ipecac syrup induces vomiting by stimulating the vomiting centre located in the brain's medulla.

Pharmacotherapeutics

Ipecac syrup is used to induce vomiting in the early management of oral poisoning and drug overdose in patients who are fully conscious.

Drug interactions

Because ipecac syrup is used only in acute situations, drug interactions rarely occur. If poisoning results from ingestion of a phenothiazine, the phenothiazine's antiemetic effect may decrease the emetic effect of ipecac syrup. If prescribed, give ipecac syrup before activated charcoal (when given together, the activated charcoal adsorbs and inactivates the ipecac syrup).

Adverse reactions

Ipecac syrup rarely produces adverse reactions when used in the recommended dosages. However, prolonged vomiting for more than 1 hour or repeated vomiting involving more than six episodes in 1 hour, lethargy, and diarrhoea may occur.

Nursing process

These nursing process steps are appropriate for patients undergoing treatment with emetics.

Assessment
- Assess the patient's condition before therapy and regularly thereafter.
- Assess for adverse reactions and drug interactions.
- Assess the patient's and family's knowledge of drug therapy.

Key nursing diagnoses
- Ineffective health maintenance related to the underlying condition.
- Risk for deficient fluid volume related to the underlying condition.
- Deficient knowledge related to drug therapy.

Emetics are used to induce vomiting when a patient has ingested a toxic substance.

EMERGENCY

Planning outcome goals
- The patient will exhibit improved health as evidenced by normal vital signs.
- Fluid volume balance will remain adequate as evidenced by the patient's intake and output, vital signs, and electrolyte evaluations.
- The patient and family will demonstrate an understanding of drug therapy.

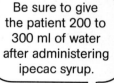

Be sure to give the patient 200 to 300 ml of water after administering ipecac syrup.

Implementation
- Monitor the patient for the drug's effect.
- Administer the drug as directed; don't administer if the patient ingested petroleum distillates or volatile oils. Retching and vomiting can cause aspiration and lead to bronchospasm, pulmonary oedema, or aspiration pneumonitis.
- Don't give ipecac syrup after the patient ingests caustic substances, such as lye; additional injury to the oesophagus and mediastinum may occur.
- Administer 200 to 300 ml of water after giving a dose.
- If two doses don't induce vomiting, be prepared to perform gastric lavage.
- Position the patient on their side to prevent aspiration of vomitus. Have airway and suction equipment nearby.
- Advise the parent or guardian to consult the prescriber or poison control centre before giving ipecac syrup to a child.

Evaluation
- Patient responds well to therapy.
- Patient maintains fluid volume.
- Patient and family demonstrate an understanding of drug therapy.

Quick quiz

1. A patient is taking calcium carbonate for peptic ulcer disease. You should monitor the patient for:
- A. hypercalcaemia.
- B. hypocalcaemia.
- C. hyperkalaemia.
- D. hypokalaemia.

Answer: A. Watch for signs of hypercalcaemia in the patient receiving calcium carbonate.

2. Which adverse reaction is common and usually dose related in patients taking misoprostol?
- A. Diarrhoea
- B. Nausea
- C. Vomiting
- D. Bloating

Answer: A. Misoprostol commonly causes diarrhoea. This reaction is usually dose related.

3. Which drug or drug type may interact with the H$_2$-receptor antagonist cimetidine?
   A. Hormonal contraceptives
   B. Lipid-regulating agents
   C. Digoxin
   D. Oral anticoagulants

Answer: D. Cimetidine may increase the blood levels of oral anticoagulants by reducing their metabolism in the liver and excretion.

4. A patient is admitted to the emergency department with salicylate poisoning. Which drug should the nurse anticipate giving the patient?
   A. Chlorpromazine
   B. Activated charcoal
   C. Magnesium citrate
   D. Docusate

Answer: B. Activated charcoal is a general-purpose antidote that's used for various types of acute oral poisoning.

Scoring

☆☆☆   If you answered all four questions correctly, thumbs up! Your knowledge of GI drugs is gastronomical.

   ☆☆   If you answered three questions correctly, nice work! You certainly aren't lacking learning in the laxative department.

      ☆   If you answered fewer than three questions correctly, don't panic. You may need some more time to digest the material.

Are you ready to roll into the next chapter?

(8) Haematologic drugs

Just the facts

In this chapter, you'll learn:

♦ classes of drugs used to treat haematologic disorders

♦ uses and varying actions of these drugs

♦ absorption, distribution, metabolism, and excretion of these drugs

♦ drug interactions and adverse reactions to these drugs.

Drugs and the haematologic system

The haematologic system includes plasma (the liquid component of blood) and blood cells, such as red blood cells (RBCs), white blood cells, and platelets. Types of drugs used to treat disorders of the haematologic system include:
• haematinic drugs
• anticoagulant drugs
• thrombolytic drugs.

Haematinic drugs

Haematinic drugs provide essential building blocks for RBC production. They do so by increasing haemoglobin, the necessary element for oxygen transportation.

Taking aim at anaemia

This section discusses haematinic drugs used to treat microcytic and macrocytic anaemia—iron, vitamin B_{12}, and folic acid—as well as

I'm really popular here! You'll find me as plasma, blood cells, and platelets in the haematologic system.

epoetin alfa and darbepoetin alfa, which are used to treat normocytic anaemia.

Iron

Iron preparations are used to treat the most common form of anaemia—iron deficiency anaemia. Iron preparations discussed in this section include ferrous fumarate, ferrous gluconate, ferrous sulphate, iron dextran, and polysaccharide iron complex.

Pharmacokinetics

Iron is absorbed primarily from the duodenum and upper jejunum of the intestine. The formulations don't vary in their rate of absorption, but they do vary in the amount of elemental iron supplied.

What's in store?

The amount of iron absorbed depends partially on the body's stores of iron. When body stores are low or RBC production is accelerated, iron absorption may increase by 20% to 30%. On the other hand, when total iron stores are large, only about 5% to 10% of iron is absorbed.

Form and function

Enteric-coated preparations decrease iron absorption because, in that form, iron isn't released until after it leaves the duodenum. The lymphatic system absorbs the parenteral form after I.M. injections.

Iron is transported by the blood and bound to transferrin, it's carrier plasma protein. About 30% of the iron is stored primarily as haemosiderin or ferritin in the reticuloendothelial cells of the liver, spleen, and bone marrow. About 66% of the total body iron is contained in haemoglobin. Excess iron is excreted in urine, stool, sweat, and through intestinal cell sloughing. Excess iron is also secreted in breast milk.

Pharmacodynamics

Although iron has other roles, its most important role is the production of haemoglobin. About 80% of iron in the plasma goes to the bone marrow, where it's used for erythropoiesis (production of RBCs).

Pharmacotherapeutics

Oral iron therapy is used to prevent or treat iron deficiency anaemia. It's also used to prevent anaemia in children aged 6 months to 2 years because this is a period of rapid growth and development.

Iron's most important role is to produce haemoglobin.

Baby makes two

A pregnant woman may need iron supplements to replace the iron used by the developing foetus. Oral iron therapy should be used unless she's unable to take iron.

An alternate route

Parenteral iron therapy is used for patients who can't absorb oral preparations, aren't compliant with oral therapy, or have bowel disorders (such as ulcerative colitis or Crohn's disease). Patients with end-stage renal disease who receive haemodialysis may also receive parenteral iron therapy at the end of their dialysis session. Parenteral iron therapy corrects the iron store deficiency quickly; however, the anaemia isn't corrected any faster than it would be with oral preparations.

Two of a kind

There are two parenteral iron products available. Iron dextran is given by either I.M. injection or slow continuous I.V. infusion. Iron sucrose is indicated for use in the haemodialysis patient and is administered by I.V. infusion.

Drug interactions

Iron absorption is reduced by antacids as well as by such foods as coffee, tea, eggs, and milk. Other drug interactions involving iron include:
- Tetracycline, demeclocycline, minocycline, oxytetracycline, doxycycline, methyldopa, quinolones, levofloxacin, norfloxacin, ofloxacin, moxifloxacin, ciprofloxacin, levothyroxine, and penicillamine absorption may be reduced when taken with oral iron preparations.
- Colestyramine, cimetidine, magnesium trisilicate, and colestipol may reduce iron absorption in the GI tract.
- Cimetidine and other histamine-2 receptor antagonists may decrease GI absorption of iron.

Adverse reactions

The most common adverse reaction to iron therapy is gastric irritation and constipation. Iron preparations also darken the stool. The liquid form can stain the teeth. Parenteral iron has been associated with an anaphylactoid reaction. (See *Parenteral iron.*)

Nursing process

These nursing process steps are appropriate for patients undergoing treatment with iron.

Before you give that drug!

Parenteral iron

Before administering parenteral iron, be aware that it has been associated with an anaphylactoid reaction. Administer initial test doses before full dose infusion to evaluate for potential reactions. Continue to monitor the patient closely because delayed reactions can occur up to 1 to 2 days later.

Symptoms of an anaphylactoid reaction to parenteral iron include:
- arthralgia
- backache
- chills
- dizziness
- headache
- malaise
- fever
- myalgia
- nausea
- vomiting
- hypotension
- respiratory distress.

Assessment
- Assess the patient's iron deficiency before starting therapy.
- Monitor iron's effectiveness by evaluating haemoglobin level, haematocrit, and reticulocyte count.
- Monitor the patient's health status.
- Assess for adverse reactions and drug interactions.
- Observe the patient for delayed reactions from therapy.
- Assess the patient's and family's knowledge of drug therapy.

Key nursing diagnoses
- Ineffective health maintenance related to iron deficiency.
- Risk for injury related to the underlying condition.
- Deficient knowledge related to drug therapy.

Planning outcome goals
- The patient's iron deficiency will improve as evidenced by laboratory studies.
- The risk of injury to the patient will be minimised.
- The patient and family will demonstrate an understanding of drug therapy.

Implementation
- Don't give iron dextran with oral iron preparations.
- If I.M. or I.V. injections of iron are recommended, a test dose may be required in the facility.
- If administering iron I.M., give with a 19G or 20G needle that's 29 to 39mm long. Inject into the upper outer quadrant of the buttock. Use the Z-track method to avoid leakage into subcutaneous tissue and staining of the skin.
- Minimise skin staining with I.M. injections of iron by using a separate needle to withdraw the drug from it's container.
- I.V. iron is given if the patient has insufficient muscle mass for deep I.M. injection, impaired absorption from muscle as a result of stasis or oedema, the potential for uncontrolled I.M. bleeding from trauma (as in patients with haemophilia), or the need for massive and prolonged parenteral therapy (as in patients with chronic substantial blood loss).
- Promote a varied diet that's adequate in protein, calories, minerals, and electrolytes.
- Encourage foods high in iron, as applicable, to help the delay onset of iron deficiency anaemia.
- Administer I.V. fluids and electrolytes as necessary to provide nutrients. Oral food intake or tube feedings are preferable to I.V. therapy.
- Correct underlying disorders that contribute to mineral and electrolyte deficiency or excess.

To give iron I.M., use a 19G or 20G needle that's 29 to 39mm long.

Education edge

Teaching about haematinic drugs

If haematinic drugs are prescribed, review these points with the patient and caregivers:

- The best source of minerals and electrolytes is a well-balanced diet that includes a variety of foods.
- Don't take over-the-counter preparations, other drugs, or herbal remedies without first talking to the prescriber or a pharmacist. Adverse interactions can occur with haematinic drugs. For example, herbal preparations of chamomile, feverfew, and St. John's wort may inhibit iron absorption.
- Keep all mineral and electrolyte substances out of the reach of children; accidental overdose can occur.

- Keep follow-up appointments for periodic blood tests and procedures to make sure treatment is appropriate.
- Take the drug as prescribed. Iron supplements should be taken with or after meals with 240 ml of fluid.
- Don't crush or chew slow-release tablets or capsules. Liquid preparations can be diluted with water and sipped through a straw.
- Rinse the mouth after taking liquid preparations to prevent staining of the teeth.
- Iron preparations may cause dark green or black stools.
- Get plenty of rest and rise slowly to avoid dizziness. Take rest periods during the day to conserve energy.

- Promote measures to relieve anorexia, nausea, vomiting, diarrhoea, pain, and other symptoms.
- Arrange for a nutritional consult, as needed.

Evaluation
- Patient's haemoglobin level, haematocrit, and reticulocyte counts are normal.
- Patient doesn't experience anaphylaxis.
- Patient and family demonstrate an understanding of drug therapy. (See *Teaching about haematinic drugs*.)

Vitamin B$_{12}$

Vitamin B$_{12}$ preparations are used to treat pernicious anaemia. Common vitamin B$_{12}$ preparations include cyanocobalamin and hydroxocobalamin.

Pharmacokinetics
Vitamin B$_{12}$ is available in parenteral, oral, and intranasal forms.

It's fundamental

A substance called *intrinsic factor*, secreted by the gastric mucosa, is needed for vitamin B$_{12}$ absorption. People who have a deficiency of intrinsic factor develop a special type of anaemia known as *vitamin B₁₂-deficiency pernicious anaemia*. Because individuals with this disorder can't absorb vitamin B₁₂, an injectable or intranasal form of the drug is used to treat it.

Final destination: Liver

When cyanocobalamin is injected by the I.M. or subcutaneous route, it's absorbed and binds to transcobalamin II for transport to the tissues. It's then transported in the bloodstream to the liver, where 90% of the body's vitamin B₁₂ supply is stored. Although hydroxocobalamin is absorbed more slowly from the injection site, its uptake in the liver may be greater than that of cyanocobalamin.

Slow release

With either drug, the liver slowly releases vitamin B₁₂ as needed. It's secreted in breast milk during lactation. About 3 to 8 mcg of vitamin B₁₂ are excreted in bile each day and then reabsorbed in the ileum. Within 48 hours after a vitamin B₁₂ injection, 50% to 95% of the dose is excreted unchanged in urine.

Pharmacodynamics

When vitamin B₁₂ is administered, it replaces vitamin B₁₂ that the body normally would absorb from the diet.

A burst of B₁₂

This vitamin is essential for cell growth and replication and for the maintenance of myelin (nerve coverings) throughout the nervous system. Vitamin B₁₂ also may be involved in lipid and carbohydrate metabolism.

Pharmacotherapeutics

Cyanocobalamin and hydroxocobalamin are used to treat pernicious anaemia, a megaloblastic anaemia characterised by decreased gastric production of hydrochloric acid and the deficiency of intrinsic factor, a substance normally secreted by the parietal cells of the gastric mucosa that's essential for vitamin B₁₂ absorption.

Common ground

Intrinsic factor deficiencies are common in patients who have undergone total or partial gastrectomies or total ileal resection. Oral vitamin B₁₂ preparations are used to supplement nutritional deficiencies of the vitamin.

Why is vitamin B₁₂ so important?

Because it's essential for cell growth and replication and for maintaining myelin throughout the nervous system.

Drug interactions
Alcohol, aspirin, aminosalicylic acid, neomycin, chloramphenicol, and colchicine may decrease the absorption of oral cyanocobalamin.

Adverse reactions
No dose-related adverse reactions occur with vitamin B_{12} therapy. However, some rare reactions may occur when vitamin B_{12} is administered parenterally.

Don't be so (hyper)sensitive
Adverse reactions to parenteral administration can include hypersensitivity reactions that could result in anaphylaxis and death, pulmonary oedema, heart failure, peripheral vascular thrombosis, polycythaemia vera, hypokalaemia, itching, transient rash, hives, and mild diarrhoea.

Adverse reactions can get dicey when vitamin B_{12} is given parenterally.

Nursing process
These nursing process steps are appropriate for patients undergoing treatment with vitamin B_{12}.

Assessment
- Assess the patient's vitamin B_{12} deficiency before therapy.
- Monitor the drug's effectiveness by evaluating haemoglobin level, haematocrit, and reticulocyte count.
- Monitor the patient's health status.
- Assess for adverse reactions and drug interactions.
- Observe the patient for delayed reactions to therapy.
- Assess the patient's and family's knowledge of drug therapy.

Key nursing diagnoses
- Ineffective health maintenance related to vitamin B_{12} deficiency.
- Risk for injury related to the underlying condition.
- Deficient knowledge related to drug therapy.

Planning outcome goals
- The patient's vitamin B_{12} deficiency will improve as evidenced by laboratory studies.
- The risk of injury to the patient will be minimised.
- The patient and family will demonstrate an understanding of drug therapy.

Implementation
- Promote a varied diet that's adequate in protein, calories, minerals, and electrolytes.
- Encourage foods high in iron, as applicable, to help delay the onset of iron deficiency anaemia.
- Administer I.V. fluids and electrolytes as necessary to provide nutrients. Oral food intake or tube feedings are preferable to I.V. therapy.
- Correct underlying disorders that contribute to mineral and electrolyte deficiency or excess.
- Promote measures to relieve anorexia, nausea, vomiting, diarrhoea, pain, and other symptoms.

Evaluation
- Patient's haemoglobin level, haematocrit, and reticulocyte counts are normal.
- Patient's underlying condition improves.
- Patient and family demonstrate an understanding of drug therapy.

Folic acid

Folic acid is given to treat megaloblastic anaemia caused by folic acid deficiency. This type of anaemia usually occurs in infants, adolescents, pregnant and lactating women, the elderly, alcoholics, and in those with intestinal or malignant diseases. Folic acid is also used as a nutritional supplement.

Pharmacokinetics
Folic acid is absorbed rapidly in the first third of the small intestine and distributed into all body tissues. Synthetic folic acid is readily absorbed even in malabsorption syndromes.

Folic acid is metabolised in the liver. Excess folate is excreted unchanged in urine, and small amounts of folic acid are excreted in faeces. Folic acid is also secreted in breast milk.

Pharmacodynamics
Folic acid is an essential component for normal RBC production and growth. A deficiency in folic acid results in megaloblastic anaemia and low serum and RBC folate levels.

Pharmacotherapeutics
Folic acid is used to treat folic acid deficiency. Patients who are pregnant or undergoing treatment for liver disease, haemolytic

> Good news! Synthetic folic acid is readily absorbed even in patients with malabsorption syndromes.

anaemia, alcohol abuse, skin disorders, or renal disorders typically need folic acid supplementation. Serum folic acid levels less than 5 mg indicate folic acid deficiency.

Drug interactions
These drug interactions may occur with folic acid:
- Methotrexate, sulfasalazine, hormonal contraceptives, aspirin, triamterene, pentamidine, and trimethoprim reduce the effectiveness of folic acid.
- In large doses, folic acid may counteract the effects of anticonvulsants, such as phenytoin, potentially leading to seizures.

Seize this warning! Large doses of folic acid may counteract the effects of anticonvulsants.

Adverse reactions
Adverse reactions to folic acid include:
- erythema
- itching
- rash
- anorexia
- nausea
- altered sleep patterns
- difficulty concentrating
- irritability
- overactivity.

Nursing process
These nursing process steps are appropriate for patients undergoing treatment with folic acid.

Assessment
- Assess the patient's folic acid deficiency before therapy.
- Monitor the therapy's effectiveness by evaluating haemoglobin level, haematocrit, and reticulocyte count.
- Monitor the patient's health status.
- Assess for adverse reactions and drug interactions.
- Observe the patient for delayed reactions to therapy.
- Assess the patient's and family's knowledge of drug therapy.

Key nursing diagnoses
- Ineffective health maintenance related to folic acid deficiency.
- Risk for injury related to the underlying condition.
- Deficient knowledge related to drug therapy.

Planning outcome goals
- The patient's folic acid deficiency will improve as evidenced by laboratory studies.
- The risk of injury to the patient will be minimised.
- The patient and family will demonstrate an understanding of drug therapy.

Implementation
- Promote a varied diet that's adequate in protein, calories, minerals, and electrolytes.
- Administer I.V. fluids and electrolytes as necessary to provide nutrients. Oral food intake or tube feedings are preferable to I.V. therapy.
- Correct underlying disorders that contribute to mineral and electrolyte deficiency or excess.
- Promote measures to relieve anorexia, nausea, vomiting, diarrhoea, pain, and other symptoms.
- If using the I.M. route, don't mix folic acid and other drugs in the same syringe.

Evaluation
- Patient's haemoglobin level, haematocrit, and reticulocyte counts are normal.
- Patient's underlying condition improves.
- Patient and family demonstrate an understanding of drug therapy.

If you're using the I.M. route, don't mix folic acid and other drugs in the same syringe. You'll need both of us for proper administration.

Epoetin alfa and darbepoetin alfa

Erythropoietin is a substance that forms in the kidneys in response to hypoxia (reduced oxygen) and anaemia. It stimulates RBC production (erythropoiesis) in the bone marrow. For the patient experiencing decreased erythropoietin production, epoetin alfa and darbepoetin alfa are glycoproteins that are used to stimulate RBC production.

Pharmacokinetics
Epoetin alfa and darbepoetin alfa may be given by the subcutaneous or I.V. route.

Their own agenda
After subcutaneous administration, peak serum levels of epoetin alfa occur in 5 to 24 hours. The peak level of darbepoetin alfa occurs within 24 to 72 hours. The circulating half-life is 4 to 13 hours for epoetin alfa and 49 hours for darbepoetin alfa. The therapeutic effect of these drugs lasts for several days after administration.

I'm SO stimulating! Epoetin alfa and darbepoetin alfa are used to stimulate RBC production.

Pharmacodynamics

Patients with conditions that decrease erythropoietin production (such as chronic renal failure) typically develop normocytic anaemia. Epoetin alfa and darbepoetin alfa are structurally similar to erythropoietin. Therapy with these drugs corrects normocytic anaemia within 5 to 6 weeks.

Pharmacotherapeutics

Epoetin alfa is used to:
• treat patients with anaemia associated with chronic renal failure
• treat anaemia associated with zidovudine therapy in patients with human immunodeficiency virus infection
• treat anaemia in cancer patients receiving chemotherapy
• reduce the need for allogenic blood transfusions in patients undergoing surgery.

Darbepoetin alfa is indicated for anaemia associated with chronic renal failure.

Drug interactions

No known drug interactions exist.

Adverse reactions

Hypertension is the most common adverse reaction to epoetin alfa and darbepoetin alfa. Other adverse reactions may include:
• headache
• joint pain
• nausea
• oedema
• fatigue
• diarrhoea
• vomiting
• chest pain
• skin reactions at the injection site
• weakness
• dizziness.

Nursing process

These nursing process steps are appropriate for patients undergoing treatment with epoetin alfa or darbepoetin alfa.

Assessment
• Assess the patient's iron deficiency before starting therapy.

Hip hip hooray! Epoetin alfa and darbepoetin alfa have no known drug interactions!

- Monitor the drug's effectiveness by evaluating haemoglobin level, haematocrit, and reticulocyte count.
- Monitor the patient's health status.
- Assess vital signs, especially blood pressure.
- Assess for adverse reactions and drug interactions.
- Observe the patient for delayed reactions to therapy.
- Assess the patient's and family's knowledge of drug therapy.

Key nursing diagnoses
- Ineffective health maintenance related to iron deficiency.
- Risk for injury related to the underlying condition.
- Deficient knowledge related to drug therapy.

Planning outcome goals
- The patient's iron deficiency will improve as evidenced by laboratory studies.
- The risk of injury to the patient will be minimised.
- The patient and family will demonstrate an understanding of drug therapy.

Implementation
- Give I.V. drug by direct injections.
- Additional heparin may be needed to prevent blood clotting if the patient is on dialysis.
- Promote a varied diet that's adequate in protein, calories, minerals, and electrolytes.
- Encourage foods high in iron, as applicable, to help delay the onset of iron deficiency anaemia.
- Administer I.V. fluids and electrolytes as necessary to provide nutrients. Oral food intake or tube feedings are preferable to I.V. therapy.
- Correct underlying disorders that contribute to mineral and electrolyte deficiency or excess.
- Promote measures to relieve anorexia, nausea, vomiting, diarrhoea, pain, and other symptoms.
- Administer supplementation, as necessary.

Evaluation
- Patient's haemoglobin level, haematocrit, and reticulocyte counts are normal.
- Patient's underlying condition improves.
- Patient and family demonstrate an understanding of drug therapy.

Anticoagulant drugs

Anticoagulant drugs are used to reduce the ability of the blood to clot. Major categories of anticoagulant drugs include:
- heparin
- oral anticoagulants
- antiplatelet drugs
- direct thrombin inhibitors
- factor Xa inhibitors.

Blood trying to clot? I think not! Anticoagulant drugs reduce the blood's ability to clot.

Heparin and heparin derivatives

Heparin, prepared commercially from animal tissue, is an antithrombolytic agent used to prevent clot formation. Because it doesn't affect the synthesis of clotting factors, heparin can't dissolve already formed clots.

The lightweights

Low-molecular-weight heparins, such as dalteparin sodium and enoxaparin sodium, are derived by decomposing unfractionated heparin into simpler compounds. They were developed to prevent deep vein thrombosis (DVT), a blood clot in the deep veins (usually of the legs), in surgical patients. Their use is preferred because they can be given subcutaneously and don't require as much monitoring as unfractionated heparin.

Pharmacokinetics

Because heparin and its derivatives aren't absorbed well from the GI tract, they must be administered parenterally. Unfractionated heparin is administered by continuous I.V. infusion. Low-molecular-weight heparins have the advantage of a prolonged circulating half-life. They can be administered subcutaneously once or twice daily. Distribution is immediate after I.V. administration, but it isn't as predictable with subcutaneous injection.

I.M. is out

Heparin and its' derivatives aren't given I.M. because of the risk of local bleeding. These drugs metabolise in the liver. Their metabolites are excreted in urine. (See *Anticoagulant drugs: Heparin and heparin derivatives.*)

Listen up! Don't give heparin or its' derivatives I.M.

Pharmacodynamics

Heparin and heparin derivatives prevent the formation of new thrombi. Here's how heparin works:
- Heparin inhibits the formation of thrombin and fibrin by activating antithrombin III.

Prototype pro

Anticoagulant drugs: Heparin and heparin derivatives

Actions

- Accelerates formation of an antithrombin III-thrombin complex
- Inactivates thrombin and prevents the conversion of fibrinogen to fibrin

Indications

- Deep vein thrombosis
- Pulmonary embolism
- Open-heart surgery
- Disseminated intravascular coagulation
- Maintaining patency of I.V. indwelling catheters
- Unstable angina
- Post-myocardial infarction
- Cerebral thrombosis in evolving stroke
- Left ventricular thrombi
- Heart failure
- History of embolism and atrial fibrillation.

Nursing considerations

- Monitor the patient for adverse effects, such as haemorrhage, prolonged clotting time, thrombocytopenia, and hypersensitivity reactions.
- Regularly inspect the patient for bleeding gums, bruises, petechiae, epistaxis, tarry stools, haematuria, and haematemesis.
- Effects can be neutralised by protamine sulphate.
- Monitor partial thromboplastin time regularly.

- Antithrombin III then inactivates factors IXa, Xa, XIa, and XIIa in the intrinsic and common pathways. The end result is the prevention of a stable fibrin clot.
- In low doses, heparin increases the activity of antithrombin III against factor Xa and thrombin and inhibits clot formation.
- Much larger doses are necessary to inhibit fibrin formation after a clot has been formed. This relationship between dose and effect is the rationale for using low-dose heparin to prevent clotting.
- Whole blood clotting time, thrombin time, and partial thromboplastin time (PTT) are prolonged during heparin therapy. However, these times may be only slightly prolonged with low or ultra-low preventive doses.

Pharmacotherapeutics

Heparin may be used in many clinical situations to prevent the formation of new clots or the extension of existing clots. These situations include:

• preventing or treating venous thromboemboli, characterised by inappropriate or excessive intravascular activation of blood clotting as well as extending embolisms
• treating disseminated intravascular coagulation, a complication of other diseases, resulting in accelerated clotting
• treating arterial clotting and preventing embolus formation in patients with atrial fibrillation, an arrhythmia in which ineffective atrial contractions cause blood to pool in the atria, increasing the risk of clot formation
• preventing thrombus formation and promoting cardiac circulation in an acute myocardial infarction (MI) by preventing further clot formation at the site of the already formed clot.

An out-of-body experience

Heparin can be used to prevent clotting whenever the patient's blood must circulate outside the body through a machine, such as the cardiopulmonary bypass machine and haemodialysis machine, as well as during extracorporeal circulation and blood transfusions.

No bones about it

Heparin is also useful for preventing clotting during intra-abdominal or orthopaedic surgery. (These types of surgery, in many cases, activate the coagulation mechanisms excessively.) In fact, heparin is the drug of choice for orthopaedic surgery. (See *Monitoring heparin therapy*.)

Pulling the plug on DVT

Low-molecular-weight heparins are used to prevent DVT.

Drug interactions

Watch for these drug interactions in patients taking heparin or heparin derivatives:
• Because heparin and heparin derivatives act synergistically with all the oral anticoagulants, the risk of bleeding increases when the patient takes both drugs together. The prothrombin time (PT) and International Normalised Ratio (INR), used to monitor the effects of oral anticoagulants, may also be prolonged.
• The risk of bleeding increases when the patient takes nonsteroidal anti-inflammatory drugs (NSAIDs), iron dextran, clopidogrel, cilostazol, or an antiplatelet drug, such as aspirin, and dipyridamole, while also receiving heparin or its derivatives.
• Drugs that antagonise or inactivate heparin and heparin derivatives include antihistamines, digoxin, penicillins,

---

Monitoring heparin therapy

Therapy with unfractionated heparin requires close monitoring. Dosage adjustments may be needed to ensure therapeutic effectiveness without increasing the risk of bleeding. Monitor partial thromboplastin time to measure the effectiveness of unfractionated heparin therapy.

When to switch

Heparin therapy is associated with thrombocytopenia. If heparin-induced thrombocytopenia develops, use thrombin inhibitors, such as lepirudin or bivalirudin, instead of heparin.

cephalosporins, glyceryl trinitrate, nicotine, phenothiazines, tetracycline hydrochloride, neomycin sulphate, and I.V. penicillin.
• Nicotine may inactivate heparin and heparin derivatives.
• Glyceryl trinitrate may inhibit the effects of heparin and heparin derivatives.
• Protamine sulphate and administration of fresh frozen plasma counteract the effects of heparin and heparin derivatives.

Adverse reactions

One advantage of heparin and its derivatives is that they produce relatively few adverse reactions. These reactions can usually be prevented if the patient's PTT is maintained within the therapeutic range (1.5 to 2.5 times the control).

Reversal of fortune

Bleeding, the most common adverse effect, can be reversed easily by administering protamine sulphate, which binds to heparin and forms a stable salt with it. Other effects include bruising, haematoma formation, necrosis of the skin or other tissue, and thrombocytopenia.

Nursing process

These nursing process steps are appropriate for patients undergoing treatment with heparin or heparin derivatives.

Assessment
• Assess the patient for bleeding and other adverse reactions.
• Assess the patient's underlying condition before therapy.
• Monitor the patient's vital signs, haemoglobin level, haematocrit, platelet count, PT, INR, and PTT.
• Assess the patient's urine, stool, and emesis for blood.

Key nursing diagnoses
• Ineffective protection related to the drug's effects on the body's normal clotting and bleeding mechanisms.
• Risk for deficient fluid volume related to bleeding.
• Deficient knowledge related to drug therapy.

Planning outcome goals
• The patient will have clotting times appropriate for drug therapy.
• Adequate fluid volume will be maintained as evidenced by the patient's vital signs and laboratory studies.
• The patient and family will demonstrate an understanding of drug therapy.

Hmmmm. The potential for bleeding with heparin use is a clue that leads me to believe that there's a risk for deficient fluid volume.

Implementation
- Carefully and regularly monitor PTT. Anticoagulation is present when PTT values are 1.5 to 2.5 times the control values.
- Don't administer heparin I.M.; avoid I.M. injections of any anticoagulant, if possible.
- Keep protamine sulphate available to treat severe bleeding caused by the drug.
- Notify the prescriber about serious or persistent adverse reactions.
- Maintain bleeding precautions throughout therapy.
- Administer I.V. solutions using an infusion pump, as appropriate.
- Avoid excessive I.M. injection of other drugs to minimise the risk of haematoma.

Evaluation
- Patient's health status improves.
- Patient has no evidence of bleeding or haemorrhaging.
- Patient and family demonstrate an understanding of drug therapy.

Maintain bleeding precautions throughout anticoagulant therapy.

Oral anticoagulants

One of the major oral anticoagulants in use is the coumarin compound warfarin sodium.

Pharmacokinetics
Warfarin is absorbed rapidly and almost completely when it's taken orally.

Why the delay?

Despite its rapid absorption, warfarin's effects aren't seen for about 48 hours, and it may take 3 to 4 days for the full effect to occur. This is because warfarin antagonises the production of vitamin K-dependent clotting factors. Before warfarin can exhibit its full effect, the circulating vitamin K clotting factors must be exhausted.

Warfarin is bound extensively to plasma albumin, metabolised in the liver, and excreted in urine. Because warfarin is highly protein bound and metabolised in the liver, using other drugs at the same time may alter the amount of warfarin in the body. This may increase the risk of bleeding and clotting, depending on which drugs are used.

Pharmacodynamics

Oral anticoagulants alter the ability of the liver to synthesise vitamin K-dependent clotting factors, including prothrombin and factors VII, IX, and X. However, clotting factors already in the bloodstream continue to coagulate blood until they become depleted, so anticoagulation doesn't begin immediately. (See *Monitoring warfarin therapy*.)

Pharmacotherapeutics

Oral anticoagulants are prescribed to treat thromboembolism and, in this situation, are started while the patient is still receiving heparin. Warfarin, however, may be started without heparin in outpatients at high risk for thromboembolism. (See *Anticoagulant drugs: Warfarin*.)

The chosen one

Oral anticoagulants also are the drugs of choice to prevent DVT and treat patients with prosthetic heart valves or diseased mitral valves. They sometimes are combined with an antiplatelet drug, such as aspirin, clopidogrel, or dipyridamole, to decrease the risk of arterial clotting.

Drug interactions

Many patients who take oral anticoagulants also receive other drugs, placing them at risk for serious drug interactions:

Monitoring warfarin therapy

Warfarin therapy requires close monitoring to ensure that the patient maintains therapeutic levels of the drug. Frequent assessment of the prothrombin time and International Normalised Ratio is necessary. Dosage adjustments should be made in cases that fall outside the therapeutic range.

I'm having trouble making vitamin K-dependent clotting factors. It must be the warfarin!

Prototype pro

Anticoagulant drugs: Warfarin

Actions

- Inhibits vitamin K-dependent activation of clotting factors II, VII, IX, and X formed in the liver

Indications

- Prevention of pulmonary embolism caused by deep vein thrombosis, myocardial infarction, rheumatic fever, prosthetic heart valves, or chronic atrial fibrillation

Nursing considerations

- Monitor the patient for adverse effects, such as haemorrhage, prolonged clotting time, rash, fever, diarrhoea, and hepatitis.
- Regularly inspect the patient for bleeding gums, bruises, petechiae, epistaxis, tarry stools, haematuria, and haematemesis.
- The drug's effects can be neutralised by vitamin K.
- Monitor prothrombin time regularly.

- Many drugs, such as highly protein-bound medications, increase the effects of warfarin, resulting in an increased risk of bleeding. Examples include paracetamol, allopurinol, amiodarone, cephalosporins, cimetidine, ciprofloxacin, danazol, diazoxide, disulfiram, erythromycin, glucagon, heparin, ibuprofen, isoniazid, ketoprofen, metronidazole, miconazole, neomycin, propafenone, propylthiouracil, streptokinase, sulphonamides, tamoxifen, tetracyclines, thiazides, thyroid drugs, tricyclic antidepressants, urokinase, and vitamin E.
- Drugs metabolised by the liver may increase or decrease the effectiveness of warfarin. Examples include barbiturates, carbamazepine, corticosteroids, corticotropin, mercaptopurine, hormonal contraceptives containing oestrogen, rifampicin, spironolactone, sucralfate, and trazodone.
- A diet high in vitamin K reduces the effectiveness of oral anticoagulants.
- The risk of phenytoin toxicity increases when phenytoin is taken with warfarin. Phenytoin may increase or decrease the effects of warfarin.
- Chronic alcohol abuse increases the risk of clotting in patients taking warfarin. Patients with acute alcohol intoxication have an increased risk of bleeding.
- Vitamin K and fresh frozen plasma reduce the effects of warfarin.

Adverse reactions

The primary adverse reaction to oral anticoagulant therapy is minor bleeding. Severe bleeding can occur, however, with the most common site being the GI tract. Bleeding into the brain may be fatal. Bruises and haematomas may form at arterial puncture sites (for example, after a blood gas sample is drawn). Neurosis or gangrene of the skin and other tissue can occur.

In reverse

The effects of oral anticoagulants can be reversed with phytomenadione (vitamin K).

Nursing process

These nursing process steps are appropriate for patients undergoing treatment with oral anticoagulants.

Assessment

- Assess the patient's underlying condition before starting therapy.

> Keep an eye on your patient's diet if he's taking oral anticoagulants. A diet high in vitamin K reduces the effectiveness of these drugs.

- Monitor the patient closely for bleeding and other adverse reactions.
- Monitor the patient's vital signs, haemoglobin level, haematocrit, platelet count, PT, INR, and PTT.
- Assess the patient's urine, stool, and emesis for blood.

Key nursing diagnoses
- Ineffective protection related to the drug's effects on the body's normal clotting and bleeding mechanisms.
- Risk for deficient fluid volume related to bleeding.
- Deficient knowledge related to drug therapy.

Planning outcome goals
- The patient's clotting times will respond appropriately to drug therapy.
- Adequate fluid volume will be maintained as evidenced by the patient's vital signs and laboratory studies.
- The patient and family will demonstrate an understanding of drug therapy.

Implementation
- Carefully and regularly monitor PT and INR values.
- Keep vitamin K available to treat frank bleeding caused by warfarin.
- Notify the prescriber about serious or persistent adverse reactions.
- Maintain bleeding precautions throughout therapy.
- Administer the drug at the same time each day.

Evaluation
- Patient has no adverse change in health status.
- Patient has no evidence of bleeding or haemorrhaging.
- Patient and family demonstrate an understanding of drug therapy. (See *Teaching about anticoagulant drugs*.)

Antiplatelet drugs

Antiplatelet drugs are used to prevent arterial thromboembolism, particularly in patients at risk for MI, stroke, and arteriosclerosis (hardening of the arteries). Antiplatelet drugs include:
- aspirin
- clopidogrel
- dipyridamole
- sulfinpyrazone.

Education edge

Teaching about anticoagulant drugs

If anticoagulant drugs are prescribed, review these points with the patient and caregivers:

- Take the drug exactly as prescribed. If taking warfarin, take it at night.
- If taking warfarin, have blood drawn for prothrombin time or International Normalised Ratio tests in the morning to ensure accurate results.
- Consult the prescriber before taking other drugs, including over-the-counter medications and herbal remedies.

- Institute ways to prevent bleeding during daily activities. For example, remove safety hazards from the home to reduce the risk of injury.
- Don't increase intake of green, leafy vegetables because vitamin K in these foods may antagonise the anticoagulant effects of the drug.
- Report bleeding or other adverse reactions promptly.
- Keep appointments for blood tests and follow-up examinations.
- Report planned or known pregnancy

I.V. instances

I.V. antiplatelet drugs are used in the treatment of acute coronary syndromes and include the medications eptifibatide, tirofiban, and abciximab.

Pharmacokinetics

Antiplatelet drugs that are taken orally are absorbed very quickly and reach peak concentration between 1 and 2 hours after administration. Aspirin maintains its antiplatelet effect for approximately 10 days, or as long as platelets normally survive. The effects of clopidogrel last about 5 days. Sulfinpyrazone may require several days of administration before its antiplatelet effects are seen.

Within minutes

Antiplatelet drugs administered I.V. are quickly distributed throughout the body. They're minimally metabolised and excreted unchanged in urine. The effects of the drugs are seen within 15 to 20 minutes of administration and last approximately 6 to 8 hours. Elderly patients and patients with renal failure may have decreased clearance of these drugs, prolonging their antiplatelet effect.

Pharmacodynamics

Antiplatelet drugs interfere with platelet activity in different drug-specific and dose-related ways.

> Elderly patients and patients with renal failure may have decreased clearance of antiplatelet drugs, which can prolong their antiplatelet effects.

Block that clot

Low dosages of aspirin appear to inhibit clot formation by blocking the synthesis of prostaglandin, which in turn prevents formation of the platelet-aggregating substance thromboxane A_2. Clopidogrel inhibits platelet aggregation by inhibiting platelet-fibrinogen binding.

Prevent that platelet

I.V. antiplatelet drugs block platelet function by inhibiting the glycoprotein IIa-IIIb receptor, which is the major receptor involved in platelet aggregation.

Dipyridamole may inhibit platelet aggregation by its ability to increase adenosine, which is a coronary vasodilator and platelet aggregation inhibitor.

Multifunctional

Sulfinpyrazone inhibits several platelet functions; it lengthens platelet survival and prolongs the patency of arteriovenous shunts used for haemodialysis. A single dose rapidly inhibits platelet aggregation.

Pharmacotherapeutics

Antiplatelet drugs have many different uses.

A familiar face

Aspirin is used in patients with a previous MI or unstable angina to reduce the risk of death, and in men to reduce the risk of transient ischaemic attacks (TIAs) (temporary reduction in circulation to the brain).

After an MI, sulfinpyrazone may be used to decrease the risk of sudden cardiac death. In patients with mitral stenosis (a narrowed mitral valve) caused by rheumatic fever, it may decrease the risk of systemic embolism.

Risky business

Clopidogrel is used to reduce the risk of an ischaemic stroke or vascular death in patients with a history of a recent MI, stroke, or established peripheral artery disease. This drug is also used to treat acute coronary syndromes, especially in patients who undergo percutaneous transluminal coronary angioplasty (PTCA) or coronary artery bypass grafting.

Dynamic duos

Dipyridamole is used with a coumarin compound to prevent thrombus formation after cardiac valve replacement. Dipyridamole with aspirin has been used to prevent thromboembolic disorders in patients with aortocoronary bypass grafts (bypass surgery) or prosthetic (artificial) heart valves.

The list goes on

Eptifibatide is indicated in the treatment of acute coronary syndrome and in those patients undergoing percutaneous coronary intervention (PCI). Tirofiban is indicated in the treatment of acute coronary syndrome. Abciximab is indicated as an adjunct to PCI.

Drug interactions

Several drug interactions can occur in patients taking antiplatelet drugs:
- Antiplatelet drugs taken in combination with NSAIDs, heparin, or oral anticoagulants increase the risk of bleeding.
- Sulfinpyrazone taken with aspirin and oral anticoagulants increases the risk of bleeding.
- Aspirin increases the risk of toxicity of methotrexate and valproic acid.
- Aspirin may reduce the effectiveness of sulfinpyrazone to relieve signs and symptoms of gout.
- Cimetidine increases the risk of ticlopidine toxicity and bleeding.

Adverse reactions

Hypersensitivity reactions, particularly anaphylaxis, can occur. Bleeding is the most common adverse effect of I.V. antiplatelet drugs.

Adverse reactions to aspirin include:
- stomach pain
- heartburn
- nausea
- constipation
- blood in the stool
- slight gastric blood loss.

Patients taking sulfinpyrazone may experience abdominal discomfort.

Clopidogrel may cause these adverse reactions:
- headache
- skin ulceration
- joint pain
- flu-like symptoms
- upper respiratory tract infection.

Drugs that interact with antiplatelet drugs include NSAIDs, heparin, oral anticoagulants, methotrexate, valproic acid, antacids, and cimetidine.

Dipyridamole may cause:
- headache
- dizziness
- nausea
- flushing
- weakness and fainting
- mild GI distress.

Nursing process

These nursing process steps are appropriate for patients undergoing treatment with antiplatelet drugs.

Assessment
- Assess the patient's underlying condition before starting therapy.
- Monitor the patient closely for bleeding and other adverse reactions.
- During long-term therapy with aspirin, monitor the patient's serum salicylate level.
- Monitor the patient's vital signs, haemoglobin level, haematocrit, and platelet count.
- Assess the patient's urine, stool, and emesis for blood.

Key nursing diagnoses
- Ineffective protection related to the drug's effects on the body's normal clotting and bleeding mechanisms.
- Risk for deficient fluid volume related to bleeding.
- Deficient knowledge related to drug therapy.

Planning outcome goals
- The patient's clotting times will respond appropriately to drug therapy.
- Adequate fluid volume will be maintained as evidenced by the patient's vital signs and laboratory studies.
- The patient and family will demonstrate an understanding of drug therapy.

Implementation
- Notify the prescriber about serious or persistent adverse reactions.
- Maintain bleeding precautions throughout therapy.
- Avoid excessive I.V., I.M., or subcutaneous injection of other drugs to minimise the risk of haematoma.
- Give aspirin with food, milk, an antacid, or a large glass of water to reduce adverse GI reactions.
- If the patient has trouble swallowing, crush aspirin, combine it with soft food, or dissolve it in liquid. Give the drug immediately after mixing it with liquid because the drug doesn't stay in solution.
- Don't crush enteric-coated products.

Patients receiving long-term aspirin therapy need to have their serum salicylate level monitored.

Here's a bright idea: If the patient can't swallow aspirin, crush it and combine it with soft food or dissolve it in liquid.

- Withhold the dose and notify the prescriber if bleeding, salicylism (tinnitus, hearing loss), or adverse GI reactions develop.
- Stop antiplatelet drugs 5 to 7 days before elective surgery, as appropriate.

Evaluation
- Patient has no adverse change in health status.
- Patient has no evidence of bleeding or haemorrhaging.
- Patient and family demonstrate an understanding of drug therapy.

Direct thrombin inhibitors

Direct thrombin inhibitors are anticoagulant drugs used to prevent the formation of harmful blood clots in the body. Bivalirudin and lepirudin are examples of direct thrombin inhibitors.

Pharmacokinetics
Direct thrombin inhibitors are usually administered I.V., typically by continuous infusion. They're metabolised by the liver. Reduced dosages may be necessary in individuals with hepatic impairment. Effects on PTT become apparent within 4 to 5 hours of administration. Platelet count recovery becomes apparent within 3 days.

When you'll reach the peak

Direct thrombin inhibitors have a rapid onset after I.V. bolus administration. Bivalirudin reaches peak response in 15 minutes and has a duration of 2 hours. Peak levels of lepirudin occur in 10 minutes, and its duration also lasts until the infusion stops. Both of these drugs are excreted renally.

Pharmacodynamics
Direct thrombin inhibitors interfere with the blood clotting mechanism by blocking the direct activity of soluble and clot-bound thrombin. When these drugs bind to thrombin, they inhibit:
- platelet activation, granule release, and aggregation
- fibrinogen cleavage
- fibrin formation and further activation of the clotting cascade.

Creating a complex

Lepirudin binds rapidly with thrombin to form tight complexes, but it doesn't inhibit other proteases.

But don't crush enteric-coated drugs!

Hipper than heparin

Compared with heparin, direct thrombin inhibitors have three advantages:

They have activity against clot-bound thrombin.

They have more predictable anticoagulant effects.

They aren't inhibited by the platelet release reaction.

Pharmacotherapeutics

Lepirudin is used to treat heparin-induced thrombocytopenia (HIT). Bivalirudin has been approved for use in patients with unstable angina who are undergoing PTCA. It should be used in conjunction with aspirin therapy.

Keep track of contraindications

Bivalirudin is contraindicated in patients with cerebral aneurysm, intracranial haemorrhage, or general uncontrolled haemorrhage. In addition, the dose may need to be reduced in those with impaired renal function because 20% of the drug is excreted unchanged in urine. Bivalirudin also increases the risk of haemorrhage in those with GI ulceration or hepatic disease. Hypertension may increase the risk of cerebral haemorrhage. Use bivalirudin with caution after recent surgery or trauma and during lactation.

Drug interactions

Don't give direct thrombin inhibitors with drugs that may enhance the risk of bleeding. Haemorrhage may occur. Patients at greatest risk for haemorrhage include those with severe hypertension, lumbar puncture, or spinal anaesthesia; those undergoing major surgery, especially involving the brain, spinal cord, or eye; those with haematologic conditions associated with increased bleeding tendencies; or those with GI lesions. Use direct thrombin inhibitors cautiously in these patients.

Adverse reactions

The major adverse effect of direct thrombin inhibitors is bleeding with the possibility of major haemorrhage; this rarely occurs. Other adverse reactions include:
- intracranial haemorrhage
- retroperitoneal haemorrhage
- nausea, vomiting, abdominal cramps, and diarrhoea
- headache
- haematoma at the I.V. infusion site.

> Don't give direct thrombin inhibitors with drugs that may enhance the risk of bleeding. Haemorrhage may occur.

Nursing process

These nursing process steps are appropriate for patients undergoing treatment with direct thrombin inhibitors.

Assessment
- Assess the patient's underlying condition before starting therapy.
- Monitor the patient closely for bleeding and other adverse reactions.
- Check PT, INR, and PTT.
- Monitor the patient's vital signs, haemoglobin level, haematocrit, and platelet count.
- Assess the patient's urine, stool, and emesis for blood.

Key nursing diagnoses
- Ineffective protection related to the drug's effects on the body's normal clotting and bleeding mechanisms.
- Risk for deficient fluid volume related to bleeding.
- Deficient knowledge related to drug therapy.

Planning outcome goals
- The patient's clotting times will respond appropriately to drug therapy.
- Adequate fluid volume will be maintained as evidenced by the patient's vital signs and laboratory studies.
- The patient and family will demonstrate an understanding of drug therapy.

Implementation
- Notify the prescriber about serious or persistent adverse reactions.
- Maintain bleeding precautions throughout therapy.
- Administer I.V. solutions using an infusion pump as appropriate; dilute solutions according to the manufacturer's recommendations.
- Avoid excessive I.M., I.V., or subcutaneous administration of other drugs to minimise the risk of haematoma.

Evaluation
- Patient has no adverse change in health status.
- Patient has no evidence of bleeding or haemorrhaging.
- Patient and family demonstrate an understanding of drug therapy.

Factor Xa inhibitor drugs

Factor Xa inhibitor drugs are used to prevent DVT in patients undergoing total hip and knee replacement surgery or hip fracture surgery. The only factor Xa inhibitor drug available in the United Kingdom is fondaparinux.

Phew! There's only one factor Xa inhibitor drug to keep track of: fondaparinux.

Pharmacokinetics

Fondaparinux is administered subcutaneously and absorbed rapidly and completely. It's excreted primarily unchanged in urine. The peak effect is seen within 2 hours of administration and lasts for approximately 17 to 24 hours.

Pharmacodynamics

Fondaparinux binds to antithrombin III and potentiates by about 300 times the natural neutralisation of factor Xa by antithrombin III. Factor Xa neutralization interrupts the coagulation cascade, which inhibits thrombin and thrombus formation.

Pharmacotherapeutics

Currently, fondaparinux is only indicated for preventing DVT in patients undergoing total hip and knee replacement surgery and fractured hip surgery.

Drug interactions

Avoid giving factor Xa inhibitors with drugs that may enhance the risk of bleeding.

Adverse effects

Adverse effects that can occur with factor Xa inhibitor therapy include:
- bleeding
- nausea
- anaemia
- fever
- rash
- constipation
- oedema.

Nursing process

These nursing process steps are appropriate for patients undergoing treatment with fondaparinux.

Assessment
- Assess the patient's underlying condition before starting therapy.
- Monitor the patient closely for bleeding and other adverse reactions.
- Check PT, INR, and PTT.
- Monitor the patient's vital signs, haemoglobin level, haematocrit, and platelet count.
- Assess the patient's urine, stool, and emesis for blood.

Key nursing diagnoses
- Ineffective protection related to the drug's effects on the body's normal clotting and bleeding mechanisms.
- Risk for deficient fluid volume related to bleeding.
- Deficient knowledge related to drug therapy.

Planning outcome goals
- The patient's clotting times will respond appropriately to drug therapy.
- Adequate fluid volume will be maintained as evidenced by the patient's vital signs and laboratory studies.
- The patient and family will demonstrate an understanding of drug therapy.

Implementation
- Administer the drug by subcutaneous injection into fatty tissue only; rotate injection sites.
- Don't mix the drug with other injections or infusions.
- Notify the prescriber about serious or persistent adverse reactions.
- Maintain bleeding precautions throughout therapy.
- Avoid excessive I.V., I.M., or subcutaneous administration of other drugs to minimise the risk of haematoma.

Evaluation
- Patient has no adverse change in health status.
- Patient has no evidence of bleeding or haemorrhaging.
- Patient and family demonstrate an understanding of drug therapy.

Fondaparinux affects the body's normal clotting and bleeding mechanisms. That means I should include "ineffective protection related to the drug's effects" in my key nursing diagnoses.

Thrombolytic drugs

Thrombolytic drugs are used to dissolve a preexisting clot or thrombus, commonly in an acute or emergency situation. Some of the thrombolytic drugs currently used include alteplase, reteplase, tenecteplase, urokinase, and streptokinase.

Pharmacokinetics
After I.V. or intracoronary administration, thrombolytic drugs are distributed immediately throughout the circulation, quickly activating plasminogen (a precursor to plasmin, which dissolves fibrin clots).

In the blink of an eye

Alteplase, tenecteplase, reteplase, and urokinase are cleared rapidly from circulating plasma, primarily by the liver. Streptokinase is removed rapidly from the circulation by antibodies and the reticuloendothelial system (a body system involved in defending

Thrombolytic drugs are commonly used in acute or emergency situations.

EMERGENCY

against infection and disposing products of cell breakdown). These drugs don't appear to cross the placental barrier.

Pharmacodynamics

Thrombolytic drugs convert plasminogen to plasmin, which lyses (dissolves) thrombi, fibrinogen, and other plasma proteins. (See *How alteplase helps restore circulation*.)

Pharm function

How alteplase helps restore circulation

When a thrombus forms in an artery, it obstructs the blood supply, causing ischaemia and necrosis. Alteplase can dissolve a thrombus in either the coronary or pulmonary artery, restoring the blood supply to the area beyond the blockage.

Obstructed artery

A thrombus blocks blood flow through the artery, causing distal ischaemia.

Inside the thrombus

Alteplase enters the thrombus, which consists of plasminogen bound to fibrin. Alteplase binds to the fibrin-plasminogen complex, converting the inactive plasminogen into active plasmin. This active plasmin digests the fibrin, dissolving the thrombus. As the thrombus dissolves, blood flow resumes.

Prototype pro

Thrombolytic drugs: Streptokinase

Actions

- Dissolves clots by converting plasminogen to plasmin

Indications

- Deep vein thrombosis
- Pulmonary embolism
- Arterial thrombosis and embolism
- Acute myocardial infarction.

Nursing considerations

- Monitor the patient for adverse effects, such as arrhythmias, bleeding, pulmonary oedema, and hypersensitivity reactions.
- Monitor the patient's vital signs frequently.
- Monitor the patient for bleeding frequently.

Pharmacotherapeutics

Thrombolytic drugs have several uses. They're used to treat certain thromboembolic disorders (such as acute MI, acute ischaemic stroke, and peripheral artery occlusion) and have also been used to dissolve thrombi in arteriovenous cannulas (used in dialysis) and I.V. catheters to reestablish blood flow. (See *Thrombolytic drugs: Streptokinase.*)

Here's the breakdown

Thrombolytic drugs are the drugs of choice to break down newly formed thrombi. They seem most effective when administered within 6 hours after the onset of symptoms.

To be more specific…

In addition, each drug has specific uses:
- Alteplase is used to treat acute MI, pulmonary embolism, acute ischaemic stroke, and peripheral artery occlusion and to restore patency to clotted grafts and I.V. access devices.
- Streptokinase is used to treat acute MI, pulmonary embolism, and DVT.
- Reteplase and tenecteplase are used to treat acute MI.
- Urokinase is used to treat pulmonary embolism, coronary artery thrombosis, and catheter clearance.

Drug interactions

These drug interactions can occur with thrombolytic drugs:
- Thrombolytic drugs interact with heparin, oral anticoagulants, antiplatelet drugs, and NSAIDs to increase the patient's risk of bleeding.

Thrombolytic drug precautions

Before administering thrombolytic drugs, familiarize yourself with their contraindications and precautions.

Contraindications

Thrombolytic drugs are contraindicated in patients with:

- active internal bleeding
- intracranial neoplasm
- arteriovenous malformation
- aneurysm
- severe uncontrolled hypertension
- history of recent stroke (within 2 months)
- subarachnoid haemorrhage
- known bleeding diathesis
- intraspinal or intracranial trauma
- surgery within the past 2 months.

Precautions

Thrombolytic drugs are used cautiously in patients who have:

- undergone major surgery within the past 10 days

- undergone organ biopsy
- traumatic injury (including cardiopulmonary resuscitation)
- GI or genitourinary bleeding
- cerebrovascular disease
- hypertension
- mitral stenosis, atrial fibrillation, or other condition that may lead to left-sided heart thrombus
- acute pericarditis
- subacute bacterial endocarditis
- septic thrombophlebitis
- diabetic haemorrhagic retinopathy.

Thrombolytic drugs are also used cautiously in patients who are:

- receiving anticoagulants
- pregnant
- 10 days or fewer postpartum
- lactating.

Adverse reactions

The major reactions associated with the thrombolytic drugs are bleeding and allergic responses, especially with streptokinase. Streptokinase from bacterial sources is antigenic and may only be administered on one occasion. (See *Thrombolytic drug precautions*.)

Nursing process

These nursing process steps are appropriate for patients undergoing treatment with thrombolytic drugs.

Assessment
- Assess the patient's underlying condition before starting therapy.
- Monitor the patient closely for bleeding and other adverse reactions.
- Check PT, INR, and PTT.
- Monitor the patient's vital signs, haemoglobin level, haematocrit, and platelet count.
- Assess the patient's urine, stool, and emesis for blood.
- Assess the patient's cardiopulmonary status, including electrocardiogram and vital signs, before and during therapy.
- Monitor the patient for internal bleeding and check puncture sites frequently.

Key nursing diagnoses
- Ineffective cardiopulmonary tissue perfusion related to the patient's underlying condition.
- Risk for deficient fluid volume related to adverse effects of drug therapy.
- Deficient knowledge related to drug therapy.

Planning outcome goals
- The patient's cardiopulmonary assessment findings will improve.
- Adequate fluid volume will be maintained as evidenced by the patient's vital signs and laboratory studies.
- The patient and family will demonstrate an understanding of drug therapy.

Implementation
- Notify the prescriber about serious or persistent adverse reactions.
- Maintain bleeding precautions throughout therapy.
- Administer I.V. solutions using an infusion pump, as appropriate; reconstitute solutions per facility protocol.
- Avoid excessive I.M., I.V., or subcutaneous administration of other drugs to minimise the risk of haematoma.
- Administer heparin with thrombolytics according to facility protocol.
- Have antiarrhythmics available; monitor cardiac status closely.
- Avoid invasive procedures during thrombolytic therapy.

Evaluation
- Patient's cardiopulmonary assessment findings demonstrate improved perfusion.
- Patient has no evidence of bleeding or haemorrhaging.
- Patient and family demonstrate an understanding of drug therapy.

Quick quiz

1. Which administration method for parenteral iron helps avoid leakage into subcutaneous tissue?

    A. Z-track method
    B. I.M. into the deltoid
    C. Subcutaneous injection
    D. Intradermal injection

Answer: A. The Z-track method helps to avoid leakage into subcutaneous tissue and staining of the skin.

2. Which test should the nurse check in her assessment of a patient receiving heparin?

    A. Complete blood count
    B. PTT
    C. Arterial blood gas
    D. Haemoglobin level

Answer: B. PTT should be monitored to measure the effectiveness of heparin therapy.

3. What's the most common adverse reaction experienced with antiplatelet drugs?

    A. Nausea
    B. Joint pain
    C. Headache
    D. Bleeding

Answer: D. Bleeding is the most common adverse effect of I.V. antiplatelet drugs.

Scoring

✩✩✩ If you answered all three questions correctly, magnificent! You're on top when it comes to managing clots.

✩✩ If you answered two questions correctly, way to go! You're in the know about drugs and blood flow.

✩ If you answered fewer than two questions correctly, stay calm. Another look at this chapter with efficiency should reverse any deficiencies.

⑨ Endocrine drugs

Just the facts

In this chapter, you'll learn:

♦ classes of drugs that affect the endocrine system

♦ uses and varying actions of these drugs

♦ absorption, distribution, metabolism, and excretion of these drugs

♦ drug interactions and adverse reactions to these drugs.

Drugs and the endocrine system

The endocrine system consists of glands, which are specialised cell clusters, and hormones, the chemical transmitters secreted by the glands in response to stimulation.

A delicate balance

Together with the central nervous system, the endocrine system regulates and integrates the body's metabolic activities and maintains homeostasis (the body's internal equilibrium). The drug types that treat endocrine system disorders include:
- natural hormones and their synthetic analogues, such as insulin and glucagon
- hormonelike substances
- drugs that stimulate or suppress hormone secretion.

Antidiabetic drugs and glucagon

Insulin, a pancreatic hormone, and oral antidiabetic drugs are classified as *hypoglycaemic drugs* because they lower blood glucose levels. Glucagon, another pancreatic hormone, is classified as a *hyperglycaemic drug* because it raises blood glucose levels.

Aaaaoooooooooooom. The endocrine system, made up of glands and hormones, helps maintain the body's internal equilibrium.

Low insulin = high glucose

Diabetes mellitus, known simply as *diabetes*, is a chronic disease of insulin deficiency or resistance. It's characterised by disturbances in carbohydrate, protein, and fat metabolism. This leads to elevated levels of the sugar glucose in the body. The disease comes in two primary forms:

type 1, previously referred to as insulin-dependent diabetes mellitus

type 2, previously referred to as non–insulin-dependent diabetes mellitus.

Downward spiral

Situations that can decrease glucose levels in patients with diabetes include:
- an antidiabetic drug dosage that's too high
- an increase in activity (such as exercise)
- noncompliance with drug therapy (for example, taking an antidiabetic drug but not eating afterward).

Insulin

Patients with type 1 diabetes require an external source of insulin to control blood glucose levels. Insulin may also be given to patients with type 2 diabetes in certain situations.

Pick a rate, any rate

Types of insulin include:
- rapid-acting, such as insulin lispro
- short-acting, such as insulin apart (regular)
- intermediate-acting, such as isophane insulin
- long-acting, such as insulin detemir.

Pharmacokinetics

Insulin isn't effective when taken orally because the GI tract breaks down the protein molecule before it reaches the bloodstream.

Skin deep

All insulins, however, may be given by subcutaneous injection. Absorption of subcutaneous insulin varies according to the injection site, the blood supply, and degree of tissue hypertrophy at the injection site.

The amount of insulin absorbed depends on the injection site, the patient's blood supply, and the degree of tissue hypertrophy at the injection site.

In the I.V. league

Insulin apart may also be given I.V. as well as in dialysate fluid infused into the peritoneal cavity for patients on peritoneal dialysis therapy.

Far and wide

After absorption into the bloodstream, insulin is distributed throughout the body. Insulin-responsive tissues are located in the liver, adipose tissue, and muscle. Insulin is metabolised primarily in the liver and, to a lesser extent, in the kidneys and muscle. It's excreted in faeces and urine.

Pharmacodynamics

Insulin is an anabolic or building hormone that promotes:
- storage of glucose as glycogen (see *How insulin aids glucose uptake*)
- increase in protein and fat synthesis
- deceleration of the breakdown of glycogen, protein, and fat
- balance of fluids and electrolytes.

Extracurricular activity

Although it has no antidiuretic effect, insulin can correct the polyuria (excessive urination) and polydipsia (excessive thirst) associated with the osmotic diuresis that can occur with hyperglycaemia by decreasing the blood glucose level. Insulin also facilitates the movement of potassium from the extracellular fluid into the cell.

Okay, Team Insulin. Let's show this body what we building hormones can do!

Pharmacotherapeutics

Insulin is indicated for:
- type 1 diabetes
- type 2 diabetes when other methods of controlling blood glucose levels have failed or are contraindicated
- type 2 diabetes when blood glucose levels are elevated during periods of emotional or physical stress (such as infection and surgery)
- type 2 diabetes when oral antidiabetic drugs are contraindicated because of pregnancy or hypersensitivity.

Calming complications

Insulin is also used to treat two complications of diabetes: diabetic ketoacidosis (DKA), which is more common with type 1 diabetes, and hyperosmolar hyperglycaemic nonketotic syndrome, which is more common with type 2 diabetes.

Pharm function

How insulin aids glucose uptake

These illustrations show how insulin allows a cell to use glucose for energy.

☝ Glucose can't enter the cell without the aid of insulin.

✌ Normally produced by the beta cells of the pancreas, insulin binds to the receptors on the surface of the target cell. Insulin and its receptor first move to the inside of the cell, which activates glucose transporter channels to move to the surface of the cell.

✌ These channels allow glucose to enter the cell. The cell can then use the glucose for metabolism.

Insulin receptor ○— Glucose Glucose transport channel

Insulin

Glucose available for metabolism

Nondiabetic duty

Insulin is also used to treat severe hyperkalaemia (elevated serum potassium levels) in patients without diabetes. Potassium moves with glucose from the bloodstream into the cell, lowering serum potassium levels. (See *Hypoglycaemic drugs: Insulin*.)

Drug interactions

Some drugs interact with insulin, altering its ability to decrease the blood glucose level; other drugs directly affect glucose levels:

• Anabolic steroids, salicylates, alcohol, and monoamine oxidase (MAO) inhibitors may increase the hypoglycaemic effect of insulin.

Did you hear? Insulin can be used in patients without diabetes to treat severe hyperkalaemia!

Prototype pro

Hypoglycaemic drugs: Insulin

Actions

- Increases glucose transport across muscle and fat cell membranes to reduce blood glucose levels
- Promotes conversion of glucose to its storage form, glycogen
- Triggers amino acid uptake and conversion to protein in muscle cells and inhibits protein degradation
- Stimulates triglyceride formation and inhibits the release of free fatty acids from adipose tissue
- Stimulates lipoprotein lipase activity, which converts circulating lipoproteins to fatty acids

Indications

- Type 1 diabetes
- Adjunct treatment in type 2 diabetes
- Diabetic ketoacidosis

Nursing considerations

- Monitor the patient for adverse effects, such as hypoglycaemia and hypersensitivity reactions.

- Corticosteroids, sympathomimetic drugs, and thiazide diuretics may reduce the effects of insulin, resulting in hyperglycaemia.
- Beta-adrenergic blockers may prolong the hypoglycaemic effect of insulin and may mask signs and symptoms of hypoglycaemia.

Adverse reactions

Adverse reactions to insulin include:
- hypoglycaemia (below-normal blood glucose levels)
- Somogyi effect (hypoglycaemia followed by rebound hyperglycaemia)
- hypersensitivity reactions
- lipodystrophy (disturbance in fat deposition)
- insulin resistance.

Nursing process

These nursing process steps are appropriate for patients undergoing treatment with insulin.

Assessment

- Assess the patient's glucose level before therapy and regularly thereafter. Monitor level more frequently if he's under stress or if the patient is unstable, pregnant, recently diagnosed with diabetes, or taking drugs that can interact with insulin.

- Monitor the patient's glycosylated haemoglobin level regularly.
- Monitor the patient's urine ketone level when the glucose level is elevated.
- Assess for adverse reactions and drug interactions.
- Monitor injection sites for local reactions.
- Assess the patient's and family's knowledge of drug therapy.

Key nursing diagnoses
- Ineffective health maintenance related to hyperglycaemia.
- Risk for injury related to drug-induced hypoglycaemia.
- Deficient knowledge related to drug therapy.

Planning outcome goals
- Blood glucose levels will be maintained within normal limits.
- The risk of injury to the patient will be minimised.
- The patient and family will demonstrate an understanding of drug therapy.

Implementation
- Use regular insulin in patients with circulatory collapse, DKA, or hyperkalaemia. Don't use regular insulin concentration (500 units/ ml) I.V. Don't use intermediate- or long-acting insulins for coma or other emergencies that needs rapid drug action.
- Insulin resistance may develop; large insulin doses are needed to control symptoms of diabetes in these cases. U-500 insulin is available in concentrated form for such patients. Give the facility pharmacy sufficient notice before you need to refill an in-house prescription because every pharmacy may not stock it. Never store U-500 insulin in the same area as other insulin preparations because of the danger of severe overdose if given accidentally to other patients.

> Don't shake vials containing insulin suspension. Doing so causes bubbling and creates air in the syringe.

In the mix

- To mix the insulin suspension, swirl the vial gently, or rotate it between your palms or between your palm and thigh. Don't shake the vial vigorously; doing so causes bubbling and creates air in the syringe.
- Insulin lispro has a rapid onset of action and should be given within 15 minutes before meals.
- Some types of insulin can be mixed in any proportion but remember that switching from separate injections to a prepared mixture may alter the patient's response.

- Don't use insulin that has changed colour or become clumped or granular.
- Check the expiration date on the vial before using.
- Use only regular insulin if administering by the I.V. route. Inject directly at the prescribed rate into the vein, through an intermittent infusion device, or into a port close to the I.V. access site. If given by continuous infusion, infuse the drug diluted in normal saline solution at the prescribed rate.
- If administering subcutaneously, pinch a fold of skin with the fingers starting at least 7.5 cm apart, and insert the needle at a 45- to 90-degree angle. Press but don't rub the site after injection. Rotate and chart injection sites to avoid overuse of one area. A patient with diabetes may achieve better control if injection sites are rotated within the same anatomic region.

Only regular insulin should be given I.V.

Highs and lows

- Ketosis-prone type 1, severely ill, and newly diagnosed diabetic patients with very high glucose levels may require hospitalisation and I.V. treatment with fast-acting insulins.
- Notify the prescriber of sudden changes in glucose levels, dangerously high or low levels, or ketosis.
- Be prepared to provide supportive measures if the patient develops DKA or hyperglycaemic nonketotic coma.
- Treat hypoglycaemic reactions with an oral form of rapid-acting glucose (if the patient can swallow) or with glucagon or I.V. glucose (if the patient can't be roused). Follow administration with a complex carbohydrate snack when the patient is awake, and then determine the cause of the reaction.
- Make sure that the patient is following appropriate diet and exercise programs. Expect to adjust the insulin dosage when other aspects of the regimen are altered.
- Discuss with the prescriber how to handle noncompliance.
- Teach the patient and family how to monitor glucose level and administer insulin. (See *Teaching about insulin*.)

Evaluation
- Patient's glucose level is normal.
- Patient sustains no injury from drug-induced hypoglycaemia.
- Patient and family demonstrate an understanding of drug therapy.

Education edge

Teaching about insulin

If insulin therapy is prescribed, review these points with the patient and caregivers:

- Insulin relieves symptoms but doesn't cure the disease; therapy is lifelong.
- Glucose monitoring is an essential guide to determining dosage and success of therapy; know the proper use of equipment for monitoring glucose level.
- Follow the prescribed therapeutic regimen; adhere to specific diet, weight reduction, exercise, and personal hygiene programs— including daily foot inspection—and consult with the prescriber about ways to avoid infection.
- Review the timing of injections and eating with the prescriber; don't skip meals.
- Accuracy of drug measurement is very important, especially with concentrated regular insulin. Aids, such as a magnifying sleeve or dose magnifier, may improve accuracy. Review with the prescriber and your family how to measure and give insulin.
- Don't alter the order in which insulin types are mixed or change the model or brand of the syringe or needle used.
- Learn to recognise signs and symptoms of hyperglycaemia and hypoglycaemia and what to do if they occur.
- Avoid consuming alcohol during drug therapy.
- Don't smoke within 30 minutes after an insulin injection. Smoking decreases the drug's absorption.
- Wear or carry medical identification at all times.
- Carry an ample supply of insulin and syringes on trips. Note time-zone changes for dose schedules when travelling.
- Have carbohydrates (glucose tablets) on hand for emergencies.

Oral antidiabetic drugs

Types of oral antidiabetic drugs available include:
- first-generation sulphonylureas (such as chlorpropamide and tolbutamide)
- second-generation sulphonylureas (such as glimepiride, glibenclamide and gliclazide)
- thiazolidinedione drugs (pioglitazone and rosiglitazone)
- metformin (a biguanide drug)
- alpha-glucosidase inhibitors (acarbose)
- meglitinides (such as repaglinide)

- nateglinide (an amino acid derivative)
- combination therapies (such as glipizide and metformin, glyburide and metformin, and rosiglitazone and metformin).

Pharmacokinetics

Oral antidiabetic drugs are absorbed well from the GI tract and distributed via the bloodstream throughout the body. They're metabolised primarily in the liver and are excreted mostly in urine, with some excreted in bile. Glyburide is excreted equally in urine and faeces; rosiglitazone and pioglitazone are largely excreted in both. (See *Oral hypoglycaemic drugs: Gliclazide*.)

Pharmacodynamics

It's believed that oral antidiabetic drugs produce actions within and outside the pancreas (extrapancreatic) to regulate blood glucose.

If the pancreas isn't functioning properly, it's believed that oral antidiabetic drugs can temporarily stimulate it to release insulin.

To the pancreas...

Oral antidiabetic drugs probably stimulate pancreatic beta cells to release insulin in a patient with a minimally functioning pancreas. Within a few weeks to a few months of starting sulphonylureas, pancreatic insulin secretion drops to pretreatment levels, but blood glucose levels remain normal or near normal. Most likely, it's the actions of the oral antidiabetic drugs outside of the pancreas that maintain this glucose control.

...and beyond!

Oral antidiabetic drugs provide several extrapancreatic actions to decrease and control blood glucose. They can go to work in the liver and decrease glucose production (gluconeogenesis) there. Also, by increasing the number of insulin receptors in the peripheral tissues, they provide more opportunities for the cells to bind sufficiently with insulin, initiating the process of glucose metabolism. Meglitinides have a short duration and are given preprandially for this reason.

Oral antidiabetic drugs also work in the liver to decrease glucose production.

Let's get specific

These oral antidiabetic drugs produce specific actions:
- Pioglitazone and rosiglitazone improve insulin sensitivity.
- Metformin decreases liver production of glucose and intestinal absorption of glucose and improves insulin sensitivity.
- Acarbose inhibits enzymes, delaying glucose absorption.

Pharmacotherapeutics

Oral antidiabetic drugs are indicated for patients with type 2 diabetes if diet and exercise can't control blood glucose levels. These drugs aren't effective in patients with type 1 diabetes because the pancreatic beta cells aren't functioning at a minimal level.

Calling all combos

Combinations or an oral antidiabetic drug and insulin therapy may be indicated for some patients who don't respond to either drug alone.

Drug interactions

Hypoglycaemia and hyperglycaemia are the main risks when oral antidiabetic drugs interact with other drugs.

Low blow

Hypoglycaemia may occur when sulphonylureas are combined with alcohol, anabolic steroids, chloramphenicol, gemfibrozil, MAO inhibitors, salicylates, sulphonamides, fluconazole, cimetidine, warfarin, and ranitidine. It may also occur when metformin is combined with cimetidine, nifedipine, procainamide, ranitidine, and vancomycin. Hypoglycaemia is less likely to occur when metformin is used as a single agent.

High fly

Hyperglycaemia may occur when sulphonylureas are taken with corticosteroids, rifampicin, sympathomimetics, and thiazide diuretics. Metformin administration with iodinated contrast dyes can result in acute renal failure. Doses should be withheld in patients undergoing procedures that require I.V. contrast dyes.

Adverse reactions

Hypoglycaemia is a major adverse reaction of oral antidiabetic drugs, especially when combination therapy is used.

Adverse reactions specific to sulphonylureas include:
- nausea
- epigastric fullness
- blood abnormalities
- water retention
- rash
- hyponatraemia
- photosensitivity.

Adverse reactions to metformin include:
- metallic taste
- nausea and vomiting
- abdominal discomfort.

Prototype pro

Oral hypogly-caemic drugs: Gliclazide

Actions

- Augments insulin release from the pancreatic beta cells and reduces glucose output by the liver
- Extrapancreatic effect increases peripheral sensitivity to insulin and causes mild diuretic effect

Indications

- Type 2 diabetes

Nursing considerations

- Monitor the patient for adverse effects, such as nausea, vomiting, diarrhoea and constipation, although these are normally mild and infrequent.
- During times of stress, the patient may need insulin; monitor for hypoglycaemia.

Acarbose may cause these reactions:
* abdominal pain
* diarrhoea
* gas.

Thiazolidinediones may cause:
* weight gain
* swelling.

Sun may not be fun for patients using sulphonylureas. Photosensitivity may occur.

Nursing process

These nursing process steps are appropriate for patients undergoing treatment with oral antidiabetic drugs.

Assessment
* Assess the patient's blood glucose level regularly.
* The patient transferring from insulin therapy to oral antidiabetics needs glucose monitoring at least three times daily before meals.
* Assess for adverse reactions and drug interactions.
* Assess the patient's compliance with drug therapy and other aspects of treatment.
* Assess the patient's and family's knowledge of drug therapy.

Key nursing diagnoses
* Ineffective health maintenance related to hyperglycaemia.
* Risk for injury related to hypoglycaemia.
* Deficient knowledge related to drug therapy.

Planning outcome goals
* Blood glucose level will be maintained within normal limits.
* The risk of injury to the patient will be minimised.
* The patient and family will demonstrate an understanding of drug therapy.

Implementation
* Give sulphonylureas 30 minutes before the morning meal (once-daily dosing) or 30 minutes before morning and evening meals (twice-daily dosing). Give metformin with morning and evening meals. Alpha-glucosidase inhibitors should be taken with the first bite of each main meal three times daily.
* A patient who takes a thiazolidinedione should have liver enzyme levels measured at the start of therapy, every 2 months for the first year of therapy, and periodically thereafter.
* A patient transferring from one oral hypoglycaemic to another (except chlorpropamide) usually doesn't need a transition period.
* Although most patients take oral hypoglycaemics once daily, patients taking increased doses may achieve better results with twice-daily dosage.

• Treat hypoglycaemic reactions with an oral form of rapid-acting carbohydrates (if the patient can swallow) or with glucagon or I.V. glucose (if the patient can't swallow or is comatose). Follow up treatment with a complex carbohydrate snack when the patient is awake, and determine the cause of the reaction.

• Anticipate that the patient may need insulin therapy during periods of increased stress, such as with infection, fever, surgery, or trauma. Increase monitoring, especially for hyperglycaemia, during these situations.

• Make sure that adjunct therapy, such as diet and exercise, is being used appropriately.

• Teach the patient how and when to monitor glucose levels and to recognise signs and symptoms of hyperglycaemia and hypoglycaemia. (See *Teaching about antidiabetic drugs.*)

Patients using oral antidiabetics may need insulin therapy during times of stress, such as when they have surgery.

Evaluation

- Patient sustains no injury.
- Patient maintains adequate hydration.
- Patient complies with therapy, as evidenced by normal or near-normal glucose level.
- Patient and family demonstrate an understanding of drug therapy.

Glucagon

Glucagon, a hyperglycaemic drug that raises blood glucose levels, is a hormone normally produced by the alpha cells of the islets of Langerhans in the pancreas. (See *How glucagon raises glucose levels.*)

Pharm function

How glucagon raises glucose levels

When adequate stores of glycogen are present, glucagon can raise glucose levels in patients with severe hypoglycaemia. What happens is easy to follow:

- Initially, glucagon stimulates the formation of adenylate cyclase in the liver cell.
- Adenylate cyclase then converts adenosine triphosphate (ATP) to cyclic adenosine monophosphate (cAMP).

- This product initiates a series of reactions that result in an active phosphorylated glucose molecule.
- In this phosphorylated form, the large glucose molecule can't pass through the cell membrane.
- Through glycogenolysis (the breakdown of glycogen, the stored form of glucose), the liver removes the phosphate group and allows the glucose to enter the bloodstream, raising blood glucose levels for short-term energy needs.

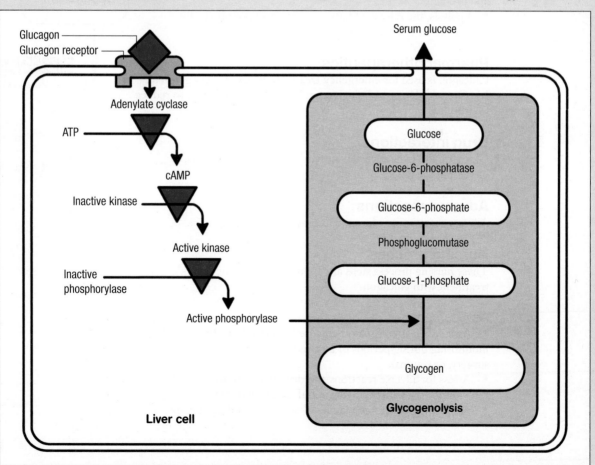

Pharmacokinetics

After subcutaneous, I.M., or I.V. injection, glucagon is absorbed rapidly. It's distributed throughout the body, although its effect occurs primarily in the liver.

Here, there, and (almost) everywhere

Glucagon is degraded extensively by the liver, kidneys, and plasma and at its tissue receptor sites in plasma membranes. It's removed from the body by the liver and kidneys.

Pharmacodynamics

Glucagon regulates the rate of glucose production through:
- glycogenolysis, the conversion of glycogen back into glucose by the liver
- gluconeogenesis, the formation of glucose from free fatty acids and proteins
- lipolysis, the release of fatty acids from adipose tissue for conversion to glucose.

Pharmacotherapeutics

Glucagon is used for emergency treatment of severe hypoglycaemia. It's also used during radiologic examination of the GI tract to reduce GI motility.

Drug interactions

Glucagon interacts adversely only with oral anticoagulants, increasing the tendency to bleed.

Adverse reactions

Adverse reactions to glucagon are rare.

Nursing process

These nursing process steps are appropriate for patients undergoing treatment with glucagon.

Assessment
- Assess the patient's blood glucose level regularly. Increase monitoring during periods of increased stress (infection, fever, surgery, or trauma).
- Assess for adverse reactions and drug interactions.
- Monitor the patient's hydration if vomiting occurs.
- Assess the patient's and family's knowledge of drug therapy.

Glucagon is used for emergency treatment of severe hypoglycaemia.

EMERGENCY

Key nursing diagnoses
- Ineffective health maintenance related to hyperglycaemia.
- Risk for injury related to hypoglycaemia.
- Deficient knowledge related to drug therapy.

Planning outcome goals
- Blood glucose will remain within normal limits.
- The risk of injury to the patient will be reduced.
- The patient and family will demonstrate an understanding of drug therapy.

Implementation
- For I.M. and subcutaneous use, reconstitute the drug in a 1-unit vial with 1 ml of diluent; reconstitute the drug in a 10-unit vial with 10 ml of diluent.
- For I.V. administration, a drip infusion, such as gluose solution, may be used, which is compatible with glucagon; the drug forms precipitate in chloride solutions. Inject the drug directly into the vein or into I.V. tubing over 2 to 5 minutes.
- Arouse the lethargic patient as quickly as possible. Give additional carbohydrates orally to prevent a secondary hypoglycaemic episode, and then determine the cause of the reaction.
- Notify the prescriber that the patient's hypoglycaemic episode required glucagon use.
- Be prepared to provide emergency intervention if the patient doesn't respond to glucagon administration. An unstable, hypoglycaemic patient with diabetes may not respond to glucagon; give I.V. glucose 50% instead.
- Notify the prescriber if the patient can't retain some form of sugar for 1 hour because of nausea or vomiting.

Evaluation
- Patient sustains no injury.
- Patient maintains adequate hydration.
- Patient and family demonstrate an understanding of drug therapy.

> If a patient doesn't respond to glucagon, give I.V. glucose 50% instead.

Thyroid and antithyroid drugs

Thyroid and antithyroid drugs function to correct thyroid hormone deficiency (hypothyroidism) and thyroid hormone excess (hyperthyroidism).

Thyroid drugs

Thyroid drugs can be natural or synthetic hormones and may contain triiodothyronine (T_3), thyroxine (T_4), or both.

Synthesise from sodium

Synthetic thyroid drugs actually are the sodium salts of the L-isomers of the hormones. These synthetic hormones include:
- levothyroxine sodium, which contains T_4
- liothyronine sodium, which contains T_3.

Pharmacokinetics

Thyroid hormones are absorbed variably from the GI tract, distributed in plasma, and bound to serum proteins. They're metabolised through deiodination, primarily in the liver, and excreted unchanged in faeces.

Pharmacodynamics

The principal pharmacologic effect is an increased metabolic rate in body tissues. Thyroid hormones affect protein and carbohydrate metabolism and stimulate protein synthesis. They promote gluconeogenesis and increase the use of glycogen stores.

Taken to heart

Thyroid hormones increase heart rate and cardiac output (the amount of blood pumped by the heart each minute). They may even increase the heart's sensitivity to catecholamines and increase the number of beta-adrenergic receptors in the heart (stimulation of beta receptors in the heart increases heart rate and contractility).

More flow

Thyroid hormones may increase blood flow to the kidneys and increase the glomerular filtration rate (the amount of plasma filtered through the kidney each minute) in patients with hypothyroidism, producing diuresis. (See *Thyroid hormones: Levothyroxine*.)

Talk about increasing productivity! Thyroid hormones increase my rate and output in addition to increasing the metabolic rate of body tissues.

Pharmacotherapeutics

Thyroid drugs act as replacement or substitute hormones in these situations:

- to treat the many forms of hypothyroidism
- with antithyroid drugs to prevent goitre formation (an enlarged thyroid gland) and hypothyroidism
- to differentiate between primary and secondary hypothyroidism during diagnostic testing
- to treat papillary or follicular thyroid carcinoma.

A winning choice

Levothyroxine is the drug of choice for thyroid hormone replacement and thyroid-stimulating hormone (TSH) suppression therapy.

Drug interactions

Thyroid drugs interact with several common drugs:

- They increase the effects of oral anticoagulants, increasing the tendency to bleed.
- Colestyramine and colestipol reduce the absorption of thyroid hormones.
- Phenytoin may displace T_4 from plasma binding sites, temporarily increasing levels of free thyroxine.
- Taking thyroid drugs with digoxin may reduce serum digoxin levels, increasing the risk of arrhythmias or heart failure.
- Carbamazepine, phenytoin, phenobarbital, and rifampicin increase thyroid hormone metabolism, reducing the effectiveness.
- Serum theophylline levels may increase when theophylline is administered with thyroid drugs.

Adverse reactions

Most adverse reactions to thyroid drugs result from toxicity.

Gut reactions

Adverse reactions in the GI system include diarrhoea, abdominal cramps, weight loss, and increased appetite.

Cardiac concerns

Adverse reactions in the cardiovascular system include palpitations, sweating, rapid heart rate, increased blood pressure, angina, and arrhythmias.

Prototype pro

Thyroid hormones: Levothyroxine

Actions

- Stimulates metabolism of all body tissues by accelerating the rate of cellular oxidation

Indications

- Cretinism
- Myxoedema coma
- Thyroid hormone replacement

Nursing considerations

- Monitor the patient for adverse effects, such as nervousness, insomnia, tremor, tachycardia, palpitations, angina, arrhythmias, and cardiac arrest.
- Use with extreme caution in elderly patients and in patients with cardiovascular disorders.

Effects all around

General manifestations of toxic doses include:
- headache
- tremor
- insomnia
- nervousness
- fever
- heat intolerance
- menstrual irregularities.

Nursing process

These nursing process steps are appropriate for patients undergoing treatment with thyroid drugs.

Assessment
- Assess the patient's thyroid function test results regularly.
- Assess the patient's condition before therapy and regularly thereafter. Normal levels of T_4 should occur within 24 hours, followed by a threefold increase in the T_3 level in 3 days.
- Assess for adverse reactions and drug interactions.
- In a patient with coronary artery disease receiving thyroid hormone, watch for possible coronary insufficiency.
- Monitor the patient's pulse rate and blood pressure.
- Monitor the patient for signs of thyrotoxicosis or inadequate dosage, including diarrhoea, fever, irritability, listlessness, rapid heartbeat, vomiting, and weakness.
- Monitor prothrombin time (PT) and International Normalised Ratio; a patient taking anticoagulants usually needs lower doses.
- Assess the patient's and family's knowledge of drug therapy.

Key nursing diagnoses
- Ineffective health maintenance related to the presence of hypothyroidism.
- Risk for injury related to drug-induced adverse reactions.
- Deficient knowledge related to drug therapy.

Planning outcome goals
- Thyroid levels will be within normal limits.
- The risk of injury to the patient will be minimised.
- The patient and family will demonstrate an understanding of drug therapy.

Remember: Patients are at risk for injury related to adverse reactions to thyroid drugs.

Implementation
- Thyroid hormone dosages vary widely. Begin treatment at the lowest level, adjusting to higher doses according to the patient's symptoms and laboratory data, until a euthyroid state is reached.
- When changing from levothyroxine to liothyronine, stop levothyroxine and then start liothyronine. Dosage is increased in small increments after residual effects of levothyroxine disappear. When changing from liothyronine to levothyroxine, start levothyroxine several days before withdrawing liothyronine to avoid relapse.
- Give thyroid hormones at the same time each day, preferably in the morning, to prevent insomnia.
- Thyroid drugs may be supplied either in micrograms (mcg) or in milligrams (mg). Don't confuse these dose measurements.
- Thyroid hormones alter thyroid function test results. A patient taking levothyroxine who needs radioactive iodine uptake studies must discontinue the drug 4 weeks before the test.
- A patient taking a prescribed anticoagulant with thyroid hormones usually needs a reduced anticoagulant dosage.

Give thyroid hormones at the same time each day, preferably in the morning, to prevent insomnia.

Evaluation
- Patient's thyroid hormone levels are normal.
- Patient sustains no injury from adverse reactions.
- Patient complies with therapy as evidenced by normal thyroid hormone levels and resolution of the underlying disorder.

Antithyroid drugs

A number of drugs act as antithyroid drugs, or *thyroid antagonists*. Used for patients with hyperthyroidism (thyrotoxicosis), these drugs include:
- thioamides, which include propylthiouracil and carbimazole
- iodides, which include stable iodine and radioactive iodine.

Pharmacokinetics
Thioamides and iodides are absorbed through the GI tract, concentrated in the thyroid, and metabolised by conjugation. They are excreted in urine.

Pharmacodynamics
Drugs used to treat hyperthyroidism work in different ways.

Stopping synthesis

Thioamides block iodine's ability to combine with tyrosine, thereby preventing thyroid hormone synthesis.

Inhibited by iodine

Stable iodine inhibits hormone synthesis through the Wolff-Chaikoff effect, in which excess iodine decreases the formation and release of thyroid hormone.

Reduced by radiation

Radioactive iodine reduces hormone secretion by destroying thyroid tissue through induction of acute radiation thyroiditis (inflammation of the thyroid gland) and chronic gradual thyroid atrophy. Acute radiation thyroiditis usually occurs 3 to 10 days after administering radioactive iodine. Chronic thyroid atrophy may take several years to appear.

Pharmacotherapeutics

Antithyroid drugs commonly are used to treat hyperthyroidism, especially Graves' disease (hyperthyroidism caused by autoimmunity), which accounts for 85% of all cases.

Thioamides

Propylthiouracil, which lowers serum T_3 levels faster than carbimazole, is usually used for rapid improvement of severe hyperthyroidism.

Good for gravidas

Propylthiouracil is preferred over carbimazole in pregnant women because its rapid action reduces transfer across the placenta and because it doesn't cause aplasia cutis (a severe skin disorder) in the foetus.

Bad for breast-feeding

Propylthiouracil and carbimazole are distributed in breast milk. Patients receiving these drugs shouldn't breast-feed. If nursing is absolutely necessary, propylthiouracil is the preferred drug.

Once a day

Because carbimazole blocks thyroid hormone formation for a longer time, it's better suited for administration once per day to a patient with mild to moderate hyperthyroidism. Therapy may continue for 12 to 24 months before remission occurs.

Iodides

To treat hyperthyroidism, the thyroid gland may be removed by surgery or destroyed by radiation. Before surgery, stable iodine is used to prepare the gland for surgical removal by firming it and decreasing its vascularity. Stable iodine is also used after radioactive iodine therapy to control symptoms of hyperthyroidism while the radiation takes effect.

Drug interactions

Iodide preparations may react synergistically with lithium, causing hypothyroidism. Other interactions with antithyroid drugs aren't clinically significant.

Adverse reactions

The most serious adverse reaction to thioamide therapy is granulocytopenia. Hypersensitivity reactions may also occur.

(Not) a spoonful of sugar

The iodides can cause an unpleasant brassy taste and burning sensation in the mouth, increased salivation, and painful swelling of the parotid glands.

Rare, but be aware

Rarely, I.V. iodine administration can cause an acute hypersensitivity reaction. Radioactive iodine also can cause a rare—but acute—reaction 3 to 14 days after administration.

Nursing process

These nursing process steps are appropriate for patients undergoing treatment with antithyroid drugs.

Assessment

• Assess the patient's condition and thyroid function test before therapy and regularly thereafter. Normal levels of T_4 should occur within 24 hours, followed by a threefold increase in the T_3 level in 3 days.
• Assess for adverse reactions and drug interactions.
• Watch for signs of hypothyroidism (depression; cold intolerance; hard, nonpitting oedema); adjust the dosage, as directed.
• Monitor complete blood count, as directed, to detect impending leucopenia, thrombocytopenia, and agranulocytosis.
• Monitor the patient's hydration status if adverse GI reactions occur.
• Assess the patient's and family's knowledge of drug therapy.

Key nursing diagnoses
- Ineffective health maintenance related to the presence of a thyroid condition
- Risk for injury related to drug-induced adverse reactions
- Deficient knowledge related to drug therapy

Planning outcome goals
- Thyroid levels will be within normal limits.
- The risk of injury to the patient will be minimised.
- The patient and family will demonstrate an understanding of drug therapy.

Implementation
- Thyroid hormone dosages vary widely. Begin treatment at the lowest level, adjusting to higher doses according to the patient's symptoms and laboratory data until an euthyroid state is reached.
- Give thyroid hormones at the same time each day, preferably in the morning, to prevent insomnia.
- Give the drug with meals to reduce GI reactions.
- Discontinue the drug and notify the prescriber if the patient develops a severe rash or enlarged cervical lymph nodes.
- Thyroid drugs may be supplied either in micrograms (mcg) or in milligrams (mg). Don't confuse these dose measurements.

Evaluation
- Patient's thyroid hormone levels are normal.
- Patient sustains no injury from adverse reactions.
- Patient complies with therapy as evidenced by normal thyroid hormone levels and resolution of the underlying disorder. (See *Teaching about thyroid and antithyroid drugs*.)

> Start patients at the lowest thyroid hormone dose, and then adjust to higher doses as needed.

Pituitary drugs

Pituitary drugs are natural or synthetic hormones that mimic the hormones produced by the pituitary gland. The pituitary drugs consist of two groups:

Anterior pituitary drugs may be used diagnostically or therapeutically to control the function of other endocrine glands, such as the thyroid gland, adrenals, ovaries, and testes.

Posterior pituitary drugs may be used to regulate fluid volume and stimulate smooth-muscle contraction in selected clinical situations.

> Anterior pituitary drugs control the function of endocrine glands. Posterior pituitary drugs regulate fluid volume and stimulate smooth-muscle contraction.

Education edge

Teaching about thyroid and antithyroid drugs

If thyroid or antithyroid drugs are prescribed, review these points with the patient and caregivers:

- Take the drug exactly as prescribed. Take the dose at the same time each day, preferably in the morning before breakfast, to maintain constant hormone levels. Taking the drug in the morning prevents insomnia.
- Report signs and symptoms of thyroid hormone overdose (chest pain, palpitations, sweating, nervousness) or aggravated cardiovascular disease (chest pain, dyspnea, tachycardia).
- If taking antithyroid drugs, report skin eruptions (signs of hypersensitivity), fever, sore throat, or mouth sores (early signs of agranulocytosis).

- Ask the prescriber about using iodised salt and eating shellfish, especially if taking antithyroid medications, to avoid possible toxic levels of iodine.
- If a stable response has been achieved, don't change drug brands.
- Children may lose hair during the first months of therapy; this is a temporary reaction.
- Report unusual bleeding or bruising.
- Keep follow-up appointments and have thyroid levels tested regularly.
- Don't use other drugs, over-the-counter products, or herbal remedies without first consulting with the prescriber or a pharmacist.

Anterior pituitary drugs

The protein hormones produced in the anterior pituitary gland regulate growth, development, and sexual characteristics by stimulating the actions of other endocrine glands. Anterior pituitary drugs include:
- the adrenocorticotropic, corticotropin
- the growth hormone somatropin
- gonadotropics, which include chorionic gonadotropin and menotropins
- thyrotropics, which include TSH, thyrotropin alfa, and protirelin.

Pharmacokinetics
Anterior pituitary drugs aren't given orally because they're destroyed in the GI tract. Some of these hormones can be administered topically, but most require injection.

Sometimes slower than Mother Nature

Usually, natural hormones are absorbed, distributed, and metabolised rapidly. Some analogues, however, are absorbed and metabolised more slowly. Anterior pituitary hormone drugs are metabolised at the receptor site and in the liver and kidneys. The hormones are excreted primarily in urine.

Pharmacodynamics

Anterior pituitary drugs exert a profound effect on the body's growth and development. The hypothalamus controls secretions of the pituitary gland. In turn, the pituitary gland secretes hormones that regulate secretions or functions of other glands.

Production managers

The concentration of hormones in the blood helps determine hormone production rate. Increased hormone levels inhibit hormone production; decreased levels raise production and secretion. Anterior pituitary drugs, therefore, control hormone production by increasing or decreasing the body's hormone levels.

Anterior pituitary drugs are used for diagnostic *and* therapeutic purposes.

Pharmacotherapeutics

The clinical indications for anterior pituitary hormone drugs are diagnostic and therapeutic:
• Corticotropin is used diagnostically to differentiate between primary and secondary failure of the adrenal cortex.
• Corticotropin is also used to treat adrenal insufficiency.
• In males, chorionic gonadotropin is used to evaluate testosterone production, treat hypogonadism, and treat cryptorchidism (undescended testes).
• In women, chorionic gonadotropin and menotropins are used to help induce ovulation during infertility treatments.
• Thyrotropin is used diagnostically to help distinguish between primary hypothyroidism (caused by a thyroid disorder) and secondary hypothyroidism (pituitary malfunction).
• Thyrotropin alfa is a synthetic TSH used to treat thyroid cancer.

Drug interactions

Anterior pituitary drugs interact with several different types of drugs:
• Administering immunisations to a person receiving corticotropin increases the risk of neurologic complications and may reduce the antibody response.
• Corticotropin reduces salicylate levels.
• Enhanced potassium loss may occur when diuretics are taken with corticotropins.

- Barbiturates, phenytoin, and rifampicin increase the metabolism of corticotropin, reducing its effects.
- Oestrogen increases the effect of corticotropin.

Adverse reactions
The major adverse reactions to pituitary drugs are hypersensitivity reactions. Long-term corticotropin use can cause Cushing's syndrome.

Nursing process
These nursing process steps are appropriate for patients undergoing treatment with anterior pituitary drugs.

Children taking anterior pituitary drugs should have their growth assessed regularly.

Assessment
- Assess the patient's underlying condition before therapy and regularly during therapy.
- Assess the child's growth before therapy and regularly thereafter. Monitor the patient's height and blood with regular checkups; radiologic studies may also be needed.
- Assess for hypersensitivity and allergic reactions and have adrenal responsiveness verified before starting corticotropin treatment.
- Assess for adverse reactions and drug interactions.
- Note and record weight changes, fluid exchange, and resting blood pressures until the minimal effective dosage is achieved.
- Assess neonates of corticotropin-treated mothers for signs of hypoadrenalism.
- Monitor the patient for stress.
- Assess the patient's and family's knowledge about the diagnostic test or drug therapy prescribed.

Key nursing diagnoses
- Ineffective protection related to the underlying condition.
- Risk for injury related to drug-induced adverse reactions.
- Deficient knowledge related to drug test or therapy.

Planning outcome goals
- The patient's underlying condition will improve.
- The risk of injury to the patient will be minimised.
- The patient and family will demonstrate an understanding of the diagnostic test or prescribed drug therapy.

Implementation

- Administer the drug as prescribed and monitor for effects.
- Corticotropin should be adjunct, not sole, therapy. The oral form is preferred for long-term therapy.
- If administering corticotropin I.V., dilute it in 500 ml of 5% glucose in water and infuse over 8 hours.
- If administering corticotropin gel, warm it to room temperature and draw it into a large needle. Replace the needle with a 21G or 22G needle. Give slowly as a deep I.M. injection. Warn the patient that the injection is painful.
- Refrigerate reconstituted solution and use it within 24 hours.
- Counteract oedema with a low-sodium, high-potassium diet; nitrogen loss with a high-protein diet; and psychotic changes with a reduction in corticotropin dosage or use of sedatives.
- Stress to the patient the importance of informing healthcare team members about corticotropin. Unusual stress may require additional use of rapidly acting corticosteroids. When possible, gradually reduce corticotropin dosage to the smallest effective dose to minimise induced adrenocortical insufficiency. Therapy can be restarted if a stressful situation, such as trauma, surgery, or severe illness, occurs shortly after stopping the drug.

Evaluation

- Patient's underlying condition improves with drug therapy.
- Patient doesn't experience injury as a result of drug-induced adverse reactions.
- Patient and family demonstrate an understanding of the diagnostic test or drug therapy.

Posterior pituitary drugs

Posterior pituitary hormones are synthesised in the hypothalamus and stored in the posterior pituitary, which, in turn, secretes the hormones into the blood. Posterior pituitary drugs include:
- all forms of antidiuretic hormone (ADH), such as desmopressin acetate, and vasopressin
- the oxytocic drug, oxytocin.

Pharmacokinetics

Because enzymes in the GI tract can destroy all protein hormones, these drugs can't be given orally. Posterior pituitary drugs may be given by injection or intranasal spray.

Posterior pituitary drugs can't be given orally because enzymes in the GI tract destroy protein hormones.

ADH on the move

ADH is distributed throughout extracellular fluid and doesn't appear to bind with protein. Most of the drug is metabolised rapidly in the liver and kidneys. It's excreted in urine.

Slower (or maybe faster) by a nose

Like other natural hormones, oxytocin is absorbed, distributed, and metabolised rapidly. However, when oxytocin is administered intranasally, absorption is erratic.

Pharmacodynamics

Under neural control, posterior pituitary hormones affect:
- smooth-muscle contraction in the uterus, bladder, and GI tract
- fluid balance through kidney reabsorption of water
- blood pressure through stimulation of the arterial wall muscles.

On the rise

ADH increases cyclic adenosine monophosphate, which increases the permeability of the tubular epithelium in the kidneys, promoting reabsorption of water. High dosages of ADH stimulate contraction of blood vessels, increasing blood pressure.

Less…and more

Desmopressin reduces diuresis and promotes clotting by increasing the plasma level of factor VIII (antihaemophillic factor).

Mother's little helper

In a pregnant woman, oxytocin may stimulate uterine contractions by increasing the permeability of uterine cell membranes to sodium ions. It also can stimulate lactation through its effect on mammary glands.

Pharmacotherapeutics

ADH is prescribed for hormone replacement therapy in patients with neurogenic diabetes insipidus (an excessive loss of urine caused by a brain lesion or injury that interferes with ADH synthesis or release). However, it doesn't effectively treat nephrogenic diabetes insipidus (caused by renal tubular resistance to ADH).

The long and short of ADH therapy

Short-term ADH therapy is indicated for patients with transient diabetes insipidus after head injury or surgery; therapy may be lifelong for patients with idiopathic hormone deficiency.

The dirt on desmopressin

Desmopressin is the drug of choice for chronic ADH deficiency. It's also indicated for primary nocturnal enuresis. Desmopressin is administered intranasally. It has a long duration of action and a relative lack of adverse effects.

A lesson on vasopressin

Used for short-term therapy, vasopressin elevates blood pressure in patients with hypotension caused by lack of vascular tone. It also relieves postoperative gaseous distention. Additionally, vasopressin may be used for transient polyuria resulting from ADH deficiency related to neurosurgery or head injury.

Partum me, is this the delivery suite?

Oxytocin is used to:
- induce labour and complete incomplete abortions
- treat preeclampsia, eclampsia, and premature rupture of the membranes
- control bleeding and uterine relaxation after delivery
- hasten uterine shrinking after delivery
- stimulate lactation.

It's a chore

Oxytocin is used to induce or reinforce labour only when:
- the mother's pelvis is known to be adequate
- vaginal delivery is indicated
- the foetus is mature
- the foetal position is favourable
- critical care facilities and an experienced clinician are immediately available.

> Oxytocin may be used under certain conditions to induce or reinforce labour.

Drug interactions

Various drugs may interact with posterior pituitary drugs:
- Alcohol, demeclocycline, and lithium may decrease ADH activity of desmopressin and vasopressin.
- Chlorpropamide, carbamazepine, and cyclophosphamide increase ADH activity.
- Synergistic effects may occur when barbiturates are used concurrently with ADH, leading to coronary insufficiency or arrhythmias.
- Cyclophosphamide may increase the effect of oxytocin.
- Concurrent use of vasopressors and oxytocin increases the risk of hypertensive crisis and postpartum rupture of cerebral blood vessels.

Adverse reactions

Hypersensitivity reactions are the most common adverse reactions to posterior pituitary drugs. With natural ADH, anaphylaxis may occur after injection. Natural ADH can also cause:

- ringing in the ears
- anxiety
- hyponatraemia (low serum sodium levels)
- proteins in the urine
- eclamptic attacks
- pupil dilation
- transient oedema.
  Adverse reactions to synthetic ADH are rare.

"Expecting" some problems

Synthetic oxytocin can cause adverse reactions for pregnant women, including:

- bleeding after delivery
- GI disturbances
- sweating
- headache
- dizziness
- ringing in the ears
- severe water intoxication.

Watch for hypersensitivity reactions in patients receiving posterior pituitary drugs.

Nursing process

These nursing process steps are appropriate for patients undergoing treatment with posterior pituitary hormones.

Assessment

- Obtain a history of the patient's underlying condition before therapy.
- Assess for adverse reactions and drug interactions.
- Assess the patient's and family's knowledge of drug therapy.

Key nursing diagnoses

- Deficient fluid volume related to underlying condition.
- Risk for injury related to drug-induced adverse reactions.
- Deficient knowledge related to drug therapy.

Planning outcome goals

- Adequate fluid volume will be maintained as evidenced by the patient's vital signs and urine output.
- The risk of injury to the patient will be minimised.
- The patient and family will demonstrate an understanding of drug therapy.

Education edge

Teaching about ADH

If an antidiuretic hormone (ADH) is prescribed, review these points with the patient and caregivers:

- Clear the nasal passages before using the drug intranasally.
- Report such conditions as nasal congestion, allergic rhinitis, or upper respiratory tract infection; a dosage adjustment may be needed.

- If using subcutaneous desmopressin, rotate injection sites to avoid tissue damage.
- Drink only enough water to satisfy thirst.
- Monitor fluid intake and output.
- Wear or carry medical identification indicating that you're using ADH.

Implementation

- Administer the drug according to the prescriber's instructions and monitor for effect.
- Assess the effectiveness of ADH by checking the patient's fluid intake and output, serum and urine osmolality, and urine specific gravity.
- Monitor the patient carefully for hypertension and water intoxication when giving ADH drugs. Seizures, coma, and death can occur from water intoxication. Watch for excessively elevated blood pressure or lack of response to the drug, which may be indicated by hypotension. Weigh the patient daily.
- Use a rectal tube to facilitate gas expulsion after vasopressin injection.
- Desmopressin injection shouldn't be used to treat severe cases of von Willebrand's disease or haemophilia A with factor VIII levels of 0% to 5%.
- When desmopressin is used to treat diabetes insipidus, dosage or frequency of administration may be adjusted according to the patient's fluid output. Morning and evening doses are adjusted separately for adequate diurnal rhythm of water turnover.
- Oxytocin is administered only by I.V. infusion, not by I.V. bolus.
- When administering oxytocin, monitor and record uterine contractions, heart rate, blood pressure, intrauterine pressure, foetal heart rate, and blood loss every 15 minutes. Also monitor the patient's fluid intake and output. Antidiuretic effect may lead to fluid overload, seizures, and coma.
- Have magnesium sulphate (20% solution) available for relaxation of the myometrium when administering oxytocin.

Patients taking posterior pituitary drugs should be weighed daily.

• If contractions are less than 2 minutes apart, if they're above 50 mm Hg, or if they last 90 seconds or longer, stop oxytocin infusion, turn the patient on her left side, and notify the prescriber.
• Teach the patient and caregivers how to properly measure and inhale the intranasal form of ADH. (See *Teaching about ADH*.)

Evaluation
• Patient achieves normal fluid and electrolyte balance.
• Patient is free from injury.
• Patient and family demonstrate an understanding of drug therapy.

Oestrogens

Oestrogens mimic the physiologic effects of naturally occurring female sex hormones. They're used to correct oestrogen-deficient states and, along with hormonal contraceptives, prevent pregnancy.

Natural and synthetic oestrogens

Oestrogens that treat endocrine system disorders include:
• natural conjugated oestrogenic substances (estradiol and oestropipate)
• synthetic oestrogens (esterified oestrogens, estradiol valerate, and ethinyl estradiol).

Pharmacokinetics
Oestrogens are absorbed well and distributed throughout the body. Metabolism occurs in the liver, and the metabolites are excreted primarily by the kidneys.

Pharmacodynamics
The exact mechanism of action of oestrogen isn't clearly understood. It's believed to increase synthesis of deoxyribonucleic acid, ribonucleic acid, and protein in oestrogen-responsive tissues in the female breast, urinary tract, and genital organs. (See *Oestrogens: Conjugated oestrogenic substances*.)

Prototype pro

Oestrogens: Conjugated oestrogenic substances

Actions

- Increases synthesis of deoxyribonucleic acid, ribonucleic acid, and protein in responsive tissues
- Reduces release of follicle-stimulating hormone and luteinising hormone from the pituitary gland

Indications

- Abnormal uterine bleeding
- Palliative treatment of breast cancer at least 5 years after menopause
- Female castration
- Primary ovarian failure
- Osteoporosis
- Hypogonadism
- Vasomotor menopausal symptoms
- Atrophic vaginitis, kraurosis vulvae
- Palliative treatment of inoperable prostate cancer
- Vulvar and vaginal atrophy

Nursing considerations

- Monitor the patient for adverse reactions, such as seizures, thromboembolism and increased risk of stroke, pancreatitis, pulmonary embolism, myocardial infarction, endometrial cancer, hepatic adenoma, and breast cancer.
- Because of the risk of thromboembolism, therapy should be discontinued at least 1 month before procedures that may cause prolonged immobilisation or thromboembolism, such as knee or hip surgery.
- Give oral forms at mealtime or at bedtime (if only one daily dose is required) to minimise nausea.

Pharmacotherapeutics

Ostrogens are prescribed:
- primarily for hormone replacement therapy in postmenopausal women to relieve symptoms caused by loss of ovarian function (See *Hormone replacement therapy risks*.)
- less commonly for hormonal replacement therapy in women with primary ovarian failure or female hypogonadism (reduced hormonal secretion by the ovaries) and in patients who have undergone surgical castration
- palliatively to treat advanced, inoperable breast cancer in postmenopausal women and prostate cancer in men.

Drug interactions

Relatively few drugs interact with oestrogens:
- Oestrogens may decrease the effects of anticoagulants, increasing the risk of blood clots.

Want to provide some relief from those hot flushes? Try hormone replacement therapy with oestrogen.

- Carbamazepine, barbiturates, antibiotics, phenytoin, primidone and rifampicin reduce oestrogen's effectiveness.
- Oestrogens interfere with the absorption of dietary folic acid, which may result in a folic acid deficiency.

Adverse reactions

Adverse reactions to oestrogens include:
- hypertension
- thromboembolism (blood vessel blockage caused by a blood clot)
- thrombophlebitis (vein inflammation associated with clot formation).

Nursing process

These nursing process steps are appropriate for patients undergoing treatment with oestrogens.

Assessment
- Obtain a history of the patient's underlying condition before therapy, and reassess regularly thereafter.
- Make sure that the patient has a thorough physical examination before starting oestrogen therapy.
- A patient receiving long-term therapy should have yearly examinations. Periodically monitor lipid levels, blood pressure, body weight, and liver function.
- Monitor the patient regularly to detect improvement or worsening of symptoms.
- Assess for adverse reactions and drug interactions.
- If the patient has diabetes mellitus, watch closely for loss of diabetes control.
- If the patient is also receiving a warfarin-type anticoagulant, monitor PT. If prescribed, adjust the anticoagulant dosage.
- Assess the patient's and family's knowledge of drug therapy.

Key nursing diagnoses
- Ineffective health maintenance related to the underlying condition.
- Risk of injury related to adverse effects.
- Deficient knowledge related to drug therapy.

Planning outcome goals
- The patient's underlying condition will improve.
- The risk for injury to the patient will be minimised.
- The patient and her family will demonstrate an understanding of drug therapy.

Hormone replacement therapy risks

A number of recent studies have reported an increased risk of myocardial infarction, stroke, breast cancer, pulmonary emboli, and deep vein thrombosis in menopausal women who received combination therapy with conjugated oestrogens and progesterone for 5 years. Because of these risks, it is recommended that oestrogens (with or without progestins) be used at the lowest effective dose and for the shortest duration possible. Furthermore, the use oestrogen and progestin solely to prevent coronary artery disease has been restricted.

Implementation
- Notify the pathologist about the patient's oestrogen therapy when sending specimens for evaluation.
- Keep in mind that oestrogens usually are given cyclically (once daily for 3 weeks, followed by 1 week without drugs; repeated as needed).
- Administer the drug as prescribed and monitor for effects.
- Withhold the drug and notify the prescriber if a thromboembolic event is suspected; be prepared to provide supportive care, as indicated.
- Teach the patient how to apply oestrogen ointments or transdermal oestrogen, or how to insert an intravaginal oestrogen suppository. Also inform the patient of the symptoms that accompany a systemic reaction to ointments. (See *Teaching about oestrogens*.)

Evaluation
- Patient's condition improves.
- Patient doesn't develop serious complications of oestrogen therapy.
- Patient and her family understand drug therapy.

Stop oestrogen therapy if a thromboembolic event is suspected.

Education edge
Teaching about oestrogens

If oestrogens are prescribed, review these points with the patient and caregivers:

- Read the package insert describing the drug's adverse reactions and keep it for later reference.
- Take the drug with meals or at bedtime to relieve nausea. Nausea usually disappears with continued therapy.
- Review with the prescriber how to apply oestrogen ointments or transdermal oestrogen.
- Be aware of symptoms that accompany a systemic reaction to ointments.
- Use sanitary pads instead of tampons when using the suppository.
- Stop taking the drug immediately if pregnancy occurs because oestrogens can harm the foetus.
- Don't breast-feed during oestrogen therapy.
- If receiving cyclic therapy for postmenopausal symptoms, withdrawal bleeding may occur during the week off. However, fertility isn't restored and ovulation doesn't occur.

- Medical supervision is essential during prolonged therapy.
- Males on long-term therapy may experience temporary gynecomastia and impotence, which will disappear when therapy ends.
- Report abdominal pain; pain, numbness, or stiffness in the legs or buttocks; pressure or pain in the chest; shortness of breath; severe headaches; vision disturbances (such as blind spots, flashing lights, blurriness); vaginal bleeding or discharge; breast lumps; swelling of hands or feet; yellow skin and sclera; dark urine; or light-coloured stools to the prescriber immediately.
- If diabetic, report symptoms of hyperglycaemia or glycosuria.
- Keep follow-up appointments for gynecologic examinations, clinical breast examinations, and mammography. Perform breast self-examinations as instructed.

Quick quiz

1. Which type of insulin would the nurse expect to administer to a patient with DKA?

    A. Regular insulin

    B. Intermediate-acting insulin

    C. Long-acting insulin

    D. Rapid-acting insulin

Answer: A. Use regular insulin in a patient with circulatory collapse, DKA, or hyperkalaemia.

2. Which implementation step is appropriate for switching a patient from liothyronine therapy to levothyroxine therapy?

    A. Stop liothyronine before starting levothyroxine.

    B. Start levothyroxine several days before stopping liothyronine.

    C. Start levothyroxine several days after stopping liothyronine.

    D. Give a supplemental I.V. thyroid drug in between liothyronine therapy and levothyroxine therapy.

Answer: B. When changing from liothyronine to levothyroxine, levothyroxine is started several days before withdrawing liothyronine to avoid relapse.

3. Which drug is typically prescribed for a patient with diabetes insipidus?

    A. ADH

    B. Oxytocin

    C. Thyroxine

    D. Corticotropin

Answer: A. ADH is prescribed for hormone replacement therapy in a patient with neurogenic diabetes insipidus.

4. A patient who's taking oestrogen and anticoagulants together is at increased risk for which condition?

    A. Hypertension

    B. Hypotension

    C. Bleeding

    D. Blood clots

Answer: D. Oestrogens may decrease the effects of anticoagulants, increasing the risk of blood clots.

Scoring

☆☆☆ If you answered all four questions correctly, perfect! There's no end to your endocrine drug knowledge!

☆☆ If you answered three questions correctly, marvellous! You've done your homework on homeostasis and hormones.

☆ If you answered fewer than three questions correctly, don't sink too low. You can always give the chapter another go.

10 Psychotropic drugs

Just the facts

In this chapter, you'll learn:

♦ classes of drugs that alter psychogenic behaviour and promote sleep

♦ uses and varying actions of these drugs

♦ absorption, distribution, metabolism, and excretion of these drugs

♦ drug interactions and adverse reactions to these drugs.

Drugs and psychiatric disorders

This chapter discusses drugs that are used to treat various sleep and psychogenic disorders, such as anxiety, depression, attention deficit hyperactivity disorder (ADHD), and psychotic disorders.

Sedative and hypnotic drugs

Sedatives reduce activity, tension, or excitement. Some degree of drowsiness commonly accompanies sedative use.

You're getting very sleepy...

When given in large doses, sedatives are considered *hypnotic drugs*, which induce a state resembling natural sleep. The three main classes of synthetic drugs used as sedatives and hypnotics are:

 benzodiazepines

 barbiturates

 nonbenzodiazepine-nonbarbiturate drugs.

Excuse me! When given in large doses, sedatives induce a state resembling natural sleep.

Benzodiazepines

Benzodiazepines produce many therapeutic effects, including some that aren't classified as sedative or hypnotic. These drugs exert their effects by increasing intracellular levels of chloride ion, thus hyperpolarising neurones. A stronger stimulus is required to reach the threshold potential, making nerve impulses more likely.

"Chill" pills

Benzodiazepines used primarily for their primary or secondary sedative or hypnotic effects include:
- alprazolam
- flurazepam
- lorazepam
- lormetazopam
- nitrazepam
- temazepam.

Pharmacokinetics

Benzodiazepines are absorbed rapidly and completely from the GI tract and distributed widely in the body. Penetration into the brain is rapid. The rate of absorption determines how quickly the drug will work. Flurazepam has the fastest rate of onset.

Distribution determines duration

The duration of effect is determined by the extent of distribution. For example, lormetazepam is highly lipophilic and widely distributed; therefore, it has a short duration of effect.

The ins and outs

Benzodiazepines are usually given orally, but may be given parenterally in certain situations, such as when a highly anxious patient needs sedation. All benzodiazepines are metabolised in the liver and excreted primarily in urine. Some benzodiazepines have active metabolites, which may give them a longer action.

Pharmacodynamics

Researchers believe that benzodiazepines work by stimulating gamma-aminobutyric acid (GABA) receptors in the ascending reticular activating system (RAS) of the brain. This RAS is associated with wakefulness and attention and includes the cerebral cortex and limbic, thalamic, and hypothalamic levels of the central nervous system (CNS). (See *How benzodiazepines work*.)

Pharm function

How benzodiazepines work

These illustrations show how benzodiazepines work at the cellular level.

Speed and passage

The speed of impulses from a presynaptic neuron across a synapse is influenced by the amount of chloride ions in the postsynaptic neuron. The passage of chloride ions into the postsynaptic neuron depends on the inhibitory neurotransmitter called *gamma-aminobutyric acid,* or *GABA.*

It binds

When GABA is released from the presynaptic neuron, it travels across the synapse and binds to GABA receptors on the postsynaptic neuron. This binding opens the chloride channels, allowing chloride ions to flow into the postsynaptic neuron and causing the nerve impulses to slow down.

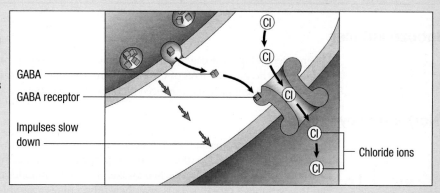

The result is another kind of depression

Benzodiazepines bind to receptors on or near the GABA receptor, enhancing the effect of GABA and allowing more chloride ions to flow into the postsynaptic neuron. This depresses the nerve impulses, causing them to slow down or stop.

Prototype pro

Benzodiazepines: Alprazolam

Actions

- Sites and mechanisms of action not known
- Enhances or facilitates the action of gamma-aminobutyric acid, an inhibitory neurotransmitter in the central nervous system (CNS)
- Acts at the limbic, thalamic, and hypothalamic levels of the CNS
- Produces anxiolytic, sedative, hypnotic, skeletal muscle relaxant, and anticonvulsant effects
- CNS-depressant activities

Indications

- Anxiety
- Panic disorders

Nursing considerations

- Monitor the patient for adverse reactions, such as drowsiness, light-headedness, depression, dry mouth, diarrhoea, and constipation.
- The drug isn't recommended for long-term use.
- Don't withdraw the drug abruptly; seizures may occur.

Snooze inducer

When given in higher dosages, benzodiazepines induce sleep, probably because they depress the RAS of the brain. Benzodiazepines increase total sleep time and produce a reduced number of awakenings.

(Not) a real eye opener

In most cases, benzodiazepines don't decrease the time spent in rapid eye movement sleep (the state of sleep in which brain activity resembles the activity it shows when awake; the body's muscles relax, and the eyes move rapidly). This gives benzodiazepines a significant advantage over barbiturates. (See *Benzodiazepines: Alprazolam*.)

Pharmacotherapeutics

Clinical indications for benzodiazepines include:
- relaxing the patient before surgery
- treating insomnia
- producing I.V. anaesthesia
- treating alcohol withdrawal symptoms
- treating anxiety and seizure disorders
- producing skeletal muscle relaxation.

Drug interactions

Except for other CNS depressants, such as alcohol, few drugs interact with benzodiazepines.

Benzodiazepines increase total sleep time and decrease the number of awakenings.

A lethal combination

When benzodiazepines are taken with other CNS depressants (including alcohol and anticonvulsants), the result is enhanced sedative and CNS depressant effects, including reduced level of consciousness (LOC), reduced muscle coordination, respiratory depression, and death.

Hormonal contraceptives may reduce the metabolism of flurazepam, increasing the risk of toxicity.

Be careful! Taking benzodiazepines with other CNS depressants, such as alcohol, enhances sedative and CNS depressant effects.

Adverse reactions

Benzodiazepines may cause:
- amnesia
- fatigue
- muscle weakness
- mouth dryness
- nausea and vomiting
- dizziness
- ataxia (impaired ability to coordinate movement).

Feeling a little out of it?

Unintentional daytime sedation, hangover effect (residual drowsiness and impaired reaction time on awakening), and rebound insomnia may also occur. Additionally, benzodiazepines have a potential for abuse, tolerance, and physical dependence.

Senior alert!

Benzodiazepines with a long half-life or active metabolites may accumulate and cause adverse effects in elderly patients and should be avoided. If they must be used, start the patient at a lower dosage and gradually increase it.

Nursing process

These nursing process steps are appropriate for patients undergoing treatment with benzodiazepines.

Assessment
- Assess the patient's anxiety before therapy and frequently thereafter.
- In the patient receiving repeated or prolonged therapy, monitor liver, renal, and haematopoietic function test results periodically.
- Assess for adverse reactions and drug interactions.
- Assess the patient's and family's knowledge of drug therapy.

Key nursing diagnoses
- Anxiety related to the patient's underlying condition.
- Risk for injury related to drug-induced reactions.
- Deficient knowledge related to drug therapy.

Planning outcome goals
- The patient will state that his anxiety is reduced.
- The risk of injury to the patient will be minimised.
- The patient and family will demonstrate an understanding of drug therapy.

Implementation
- Don't give benzodiazepines for everyday stress or use them for long-term therapy (more than 4 months).
- Check to see that the patient has swallowed tablets before leaving his room.
- Expect to give lower doses at longer intervals in an elderly or a debilitated patient.
- Don't withdraw benzodiazepines abruptly after long-term use; withdrawal symptoms may occur. Abuse or addiction is possible.

Evaluation
- Patient is less anxious.
- Patient doesn't experience injury from adverse CNS reactions.
- Patient and family demonstrate an understanding of drug therapy.

Benzodiazepines shouldn't be given for more than 4 months.

Barbiturates

The major pharmacologic action of barbiturates is to reduce overall CNS alertness. Barbiturates used primarily as sedatives and hypnotics include:
- amobarbital
- butabarbital
- phenobarbital
- secobarbital.

The highs and lows

Low doses of barbiturates depress the sensory and motor cortex in the brain, causing drowsiness. High doses may cause respiratory depression and death because of their ability to depress all levels of the CNS.

Are you paying attention? Barbiturates reduce overall CNS alertness.

Prototype pro

Barbiturates: Phenobarbital

Actions

- Induces an imbalance in central inhibitory and facilitatory mechanisms, which influence cerebral cortex and reticular formation
- Decreases presynaptic and postsynaptic membrane excitability
- Produces all levels of central nervous system (CNS) depression (mild sedation to coma to death)
- Facilitates the action of gamma-aminobutyric acid, an inhibitory neurotransmitter in the CNS
- Exerts a central effect, which depresses respiration and GI motility
- Reduces nerve transmission and decreases excitability of the nerve cell as its principal anticonvulsant mechanism of action
- Raises the seizure threshold

Indications

- Epilepsy
- Febrile seizures
- Sedation

Nursing considerations

- Monitor the patient for adverse reactions, such as drowsiness, lethargy, hangover, respiratory depression, apnea, Stevens-Johnson syndrome, and angioedema.
- Don't withdraw the drug abruptly; seizures may worsen.
- Watch for signs of toxicity: coma, asthmatic breathing, clammy skin, and cyanosis.
- Phenobarbital doesn't have an analgesic action and may increase the reaction to painful stimuli when given in subanaesthetic doses.

Pharmacokinetics

Barbiturates are absorbed well from the GI tract. They're distributed rapidly, metabolised by the liver, and excreted in urine.

Pharmacodynamics

As sedative and hypnotics, barbiturates depress the sensory cortex of the brain, decrease motor activity, alter cerebral function, and produce drowsiness, sedation, and hypnosis. These drugs appear to act throughout the CNS; however, the RAS of the brain, which is responsible for wakefulness, is a particularly sensitive site. (See *Barbiturates: Phenobarbital*.)

Pharmacotherapeutics

Barbiturates have many clinical indications, some of which go beyond sedative and hypnotic uses. They're used for:
- daytime sedation (for short periods only, typically less than 2 weeks)
- insomnia

- preoperative sedation and anaesthesia
- relief from anxiety
- anticonvulsant effects.

A little too good

Tolerance to barbiturates occurs more rapidly as compared to benzodiazepines. Physical dependence may be induced even with a small daily dosage. In comparison, benzodiazepines are relatively effective and safe and, for these reasons, have replaced barbiturates as the sedatives and hypnotics of choice.

Drug interactions

Barbiturates may interact with many other drugs:
- They may reduce the effects of beta-adrenergic blockers (such as metoprolol and propranolol), chloramphenicol, corticosteroids, doxycycline, oral anticoagulants, hormonal contraceptives, tricyclic antidepressants, metronidazole, theophylline, and ciclosporine.
- Hydantoins, such as phenytoin, reduce the metabolism of phenobarbital, resulting in increased toxic effects.
- Their use with other CNS depressants may cause excessive CNS depression.
- Valproic acid may increase barbiturate levels.
- Monoamine oxidase (MAO) inhibitors slow down barbiturate metabolism, increasing sedative effects.
- When taken with paracetamol, an increased risk of liver toxicity results.

Adverse reactions

Barbiturates may have widespread adverse effects.

Striking the wrong "chord"

CNS reactions include:
- drowsiness
- lethargy
- headache
- depression.

"Heart-y" responses

Cardiovascular effects include:
- mild bradycardia
- hypotension.

"Air" ways

Respiratory effects include:
- hypoventilation
- spasm of the larynx (voice box) and bronchi
- reduced rate of breathing
- severe respiratory depression.

And the rest of the story

Other reactions include:
- vertigo
- nausea and vomiting
- diarrhoea
- epigastric pain
- allergic reactions.

Nursing process

These nursing process steps are appropriate for patients undergoing treatment with barbiturates.

Assessment
- Assess the patient's condition before therapy and regularly thereafter.
- Assess the patient's LOC and sleeping patterns before and during therapy to evaluate the drug's effectiveness. Monitor his neurologic status for alteration or deterioration.
- Assess the patient's vital signs frequently, especially during I.V. administration.
- Assess for adverse reactions and drug interactions.

Key nursing diagnoses
- Risk for injury related to adverse drug reaction.
- Risk for trauma related to the underlying condition.
- Deficient knowledge related to drug therapy.

Planning outcome goals
- The risk of injury to the patient will be minimised.
- The risk of trauma to the patient will be minimised.
- The patient and family will demonstrate an understanding of drug therapy.

Implementation
- When giving parenteral forms, avoid extravasation, which may cause local tissue damage and tissue necrosis; inject I.V. or deep I.M. only. Don't exceed 5 ml for any I.M. injection site to avoid tissue damage.
- Be prepared to resuscitate. Too-rapid I.V. administration may cause respiratory depression, apnea, laryngospasm, or hypotension.

Keep an eye on the patient's loss of consciousness and sleeping patterns during barbiturate therapy.

• Take seizure precautions, as necessary. Monitor seizure character, frequency, and duration for changes, as indicated.
• Institute safety measures to prevent patient falls and injury. Raise side rails, assist the patient out of bed, and keep the call light within easy reach.
• Monitor blood level of the drug closely. Therapeutic levels range from 15 to 40 mcg/ml.
• Observe the patient to prevent hoarding or self-dosing, especially if they are depressed, suicidal, or drug dependent.
• Stop the drug slowly. Abrupt discontinuation may cause withdrawal symptoms or worsen seizures.

Evaluation
• Patient sustains no injury from sedation.
• Patient sustains no trauma during therapy.
• Patient and family demonstrate an understanding of drug therapy. (See *Teaching about barbiturates*.)

Nonbenzodiazepines-nonbarbiturates

Nonbenzodiazepines-nonbarbiturates act as hypnotics for short-term treatment of simple insomnia. These drugs, which offer no special advantages over other sedatives, include:
• chloral hydrate
• zaleplon
• zolpidem.

Education edge

Teaching about barbiturates

If barbiturates are prescribed, review these points with the patient and caregivers:

• Barbiturates can cause physical or psychological dependence.
• Take the drug exactly as prescribed. Don't change the dosage or take other drugs, including over-the-counter drugs or herbal remedies, without the prescriber's approval.
• A morning hangover is common after therapeutic use of barbiturates.

• Avoid hazardous tasks, driving, or operating machinery while taking the drug. Review other safety measures with your healthcare provider to prevent injury.
• The drug's full effects don't occur for 2 to 3 weeks, except when a loading dose is used.
• Don't stop taking the drug abruptly.
• If using hormonal contraceptives, consider using other birth control methods such as condoms.
• Report skin eruptions or other significant adverse effects.

Full on for only a fortnight

With the exception of zolpidem, which may be effective for up to 35 days, nonbenzodiazepines-nonbarbiturates lose their effectiveness by the end of the second week.

Pharmacokinetics

Nonbenzodiazepines-nonbarbiturates are absorbed rapidly from the GI tract. They're metabolised in the liver and excreted in urine.

Pharmacodynamics

The mechanism of action for nonbenzodiazepines-nonbarbiturates isn't fully known. They produce depressant effects similar to barbiturates.

Pharmacotherapeutics

Nonbenzodiazepines-nonbarbiturates are typically used for:
* short-term treatment of simple insomnia
* sedation before surgery
* sedation before EEG studies.

Drug interactions

Drug interactions involving nonbenzodiazepines-nonbarbiturates primarily occur when they're used with other CNS depressants, causing additive CNS depression resulting in drowsiness, respiratory depression, stupor, coma, and death.

> Nonbenzodiazepines-nonbarbiturates are used for short-term treatment of insomnia and sedation before surgery or EEG studies.

These mixes don't match

Chloral hydrate may increase the risk of bleeding in patients taking oral anticoagulants. Use with I.V. furosemide may produce sweating, flushing, variable blood pressure, and uneasiness.

Adverse reactions

The most common dose-related adverse reactions involving nonbenzodiazepines-nonbarbiturates include:
* nausea and vomiting
* gastric irritation
* hangover effects (possibly leading to respiratory depression or even respiratory failure).

Nursing process

These nursing process steps are appropriate for patients undergoing treatment with nonbenzodiazepines-nonbarbiturates.

Assessment
- Assess the patient's underlying condition.
- Evaluate the drug's effectiveness after administration.
- Assess for adverse reactions and drug interactions.
- Assess the patient's and family's knowledge of drug therapy.

Key nursing diagnoses
- Disturbed sleep pattern related to patient's underlying condition.
- Risk for injury related to adverse CNS reactions.
- Deficient knowledge related to drug therapy.

Planning outcome goals
- The patient's sleep pattern will improve.
- The risk of injury to the patient will be minimised.
- The patient and family will demonstrate an understanding of drug therapy.

When using nonbenzodiazepines-nonbarbiturates, I have to keep in mind that there's a risk of injury related to adverse CNS reactions.

Implementation
- Administer the drug as prescribed and monitor for its effects.
- To minimise the unpleasant taste of liquid forms, dilute or give the drug with liquid.
- Administer the drug after meals.
- Rectal suppositories should be refrigerated.
- Long-term use isn't recommended; nonbenzodiazepines-nonbarbiturates lose their efficacy in promoting sleep after 14 days of continued use. Long-term use may cause drug dependence. The patient may experience withdrawal symptoms if the drug is suddenly stopped.
- Caution the patient about performing activities that require mental alertness or physical coordination. For an inpatient, supervise walking and raise bed rails, particularly for an elderly patient.
- Tell the patient to report adverse effects, such as severe hangover or feelings of oversedation, so the prescriber can be consulted to adjust the dosage or change the drug.

Supervise patients taking nonbenzodiazepines-nonbarbiturates when they're walking.

Evaluation
- Patient states drug effectively induced sleep.
- Patient's safety is maintained.
- Patient and family demonstrate an understanding of drug therapy.

Antianxiety drugs

Antianxiety drugs, also called *anxiolytics*, include some of the most commonly prescribed drugs in the UK. They're used primarily to treat anxiety disorders. The three main types of antianxiety drugs are:
- benzodiazepines
- barbiturates
- buspirone.

Experiencing drug déjà vu?

Benzodiazepines and barbiturates were discussed earlier in this chapter in regard to their sedative and hypnotic use, but they're also used to treat anxiety.

Anxiety "it" list

Benzodiazepines used primarily to treat anxiety include:
- alprazolam
- chlordiazepoxide
- clonazepam
- diazepam
- lorazepam
- oxazepam.

Taking the edge off

When given in low dosages, these benzodiazepines decrease anxiety by acting on the limbic system and other areas of the brain that help regulate emotional activity. The drugs can usually calm the patient without causing drowsiness.

Back to the barbiturates

Barbiturates used to treat anxiety include:
- amobarbital
- secobarbital.

The difference is in the dosage

Benzodiazepines and barbiturates act the same way as when they're used as sedatives and hypnotics. However, the dosages may vary.

Addendum for anxiolytic use

When these drugs are used to treat anxiety, the nursing process steps are generally the same as when they're used as sedative hypnotics. However, keep these additional points in mind:

• Benzodiazepines and barbiturates are generally prescribed for short-term use. Patients undergoing long-term therapy should be referred to psychiatric counselling.

• The patient will need to identify and examine the source of his anxiety in order to reduce or eliminate it.

• Teach the patient various relaxation techniques, such as deep breathing and meditation, to help reduce anxiety. (See *Teaching about antianxiety drugs*.)

Buspirone

Buspirone is the first antianxiety drug in a class of drugs known as *azaspirodecanedione derivatives*. This drug's structure and mechanism of action differ from those of other antianxiety drugs.

Education edge
Teaching about antianxiety drugs

If antianxiety drugs are prescribed, review these points with the patient and caregivers:

• These drugs help relieve symptoms temporarily, but don't cure or solve the underlying problem. Counselling or psychotherapy can help find ways to decrease nervousness and assist with sleep.

• Use other methods to promote relaxation, such as physical exercise, reading, crafts, stress-management techniques, and relaxation techniques.

• Identify factors that cause symptoms. Avoiding such products as caffeine, cold medications, and appetite suppressants can help reduce symptoms of nervousness and insomnia.

• Tell other healthcare providers what drugs you're using to avoid being prescribed other drugs with similar effects. This reduces the chances of combined adverse effects.

• Avoid hazardous activities that require alertness and psychomotor coordination until the central nervous system effects of the drug are known.

• Avoid alcohol consumption and smoking while taking the drug.

• Don't take other drugs, over-the-counter products, or herbal remedies without first consulting the prescriber or a pharmacist.

• Take the drug as prescribed; don't stop taking it without the prescriber's approval.

• Dependence on the drug may occur if it's taken longer than directed.

• Increase fluid intake and fibre intake as well as activity levels to help avoid constipation.

• Take the drug later in the day or at night, as indicated, to help decrease daytime drowsiness.

• Keep all drugs out of the reach of children.

• Don't share drugs with anyone.

Advantage, buspirone

Buspirone has several advantages, including:
- less sedation
- no increase in CNS depressant effects when taken with alcohol or sedative-hypnotics
- lower abuse potential.

Pharmacokinetics
Buspirone is absorbed rapidly, undergoes extensive first-pass effect, and is metabolised in the liver to at least one active metabolite. The drug is eliminated in urine and faeces.

Pharmacodynamics
Although buspirone's mechanism of action remains unknown, it's clear that buspirone doesn't affect GABA receptors like benzodiazepines. Buspirone seems to produce various effects in the midbrain and acts as a midbrain modulator, possibly due to its high affinity for serotonin receptors. Recent evidence suggests that it may also act on dopamine-2 receptors

Pharmacotherapeutics
Buspirone is used to treat generalised anxiety states. Patients who haven't received benzodiazepines seem to respond better to buspirone.

Slow as a tortoise

Because of its slow onset of action, buspirone is ineffective when quick relief from anxiety is needed.

Not for simple stress

Although buspirone hasn't shown potential for abuse and hasn't been classified as a controlled substance, it isn't recommended for relief of everyday stress.

Drug interactions
Unlike other antianxiety drugs, buspirone doesn't interact with alcohol or other CNS depressants. However, when buspirone is given with MAO inhibitors, hypertensive reactions may occur.

> Buspirone has less sedation and a lower abuse potential. Now that's a winning combination!

> A toast to buspirone! Cheers to you for not interacting with alcohol or other CNS depressants.

Adverse reactions

The most common reactions to buspirone include:

- dizziness
- light-headedness
- insomnia
- rapid heart rate
- palpitations
- headache.

Nursing process

These nursing process steps are appropriate for patients undergoing treatment with buspirone.

Assessment

- Obtain a history of the patient's anxiety before therapy and reassess regularly thereafter.
- Assess for adverse reactions and drug interactions.
- Assess the patient's and family's understanding of drug therapy.

Key nursing diagnoses

- Anxiety related to the underlying condition.
- Fatigue related to drug-induced adverse reactions.
- Deficient knowledge related to drug therapy.

Planning outcome goals

- The patient will state his anxiety is reduced.
- The patient won't experience fatigue.
- The patient and family will demonstrate an understanding of drug therapy.

Implementation

- Before starting therapy in the patient already being treated with a benzodiazepine, make sure that they don't stop the benzodiazepine abruptly; a withdrawal reaction may occur.
- Give the drug with food or milk.
- The dosage may be increased in 2 to 4-day intervals, as ordered.
- Warn the patient to avoid hazardous activities that require alertness and psychomotor coordination until the CNS effects of the drug are known.
- Signs of improvement usually appear within 7 to 10 days; optimal results occur after 3 to 4 weeks of therapy.

Tell the patient to avoid activities that require alertness and psychomotor coordination until the CNS effects of buspirone are known.

Evaluation
- Patient's anxiety is relieved.
- Patient's fatigue is decreased.
- Patient and family demonstrate an understanding of drug therapy.

Antidepressant and mood stabiliser drugs

Antidepressant and mood stabiliser drugs are used to treat affective disorders—disturbances in mood, characterised by depression or elation.

One pole

Unipolar disorders, characterised by periods of clinical depression, are treated with:
- selective serotonin reuptake inhibitors (SSRIs)
- MAO inhibitors
- tricyclic antidepressants (TCAs)
- other antidepressants.

Two poles

Lithium is used to treat bipolar disorders, characterised by alternating periods of manic behavior and clinical depression.

Selective serotonin reuptake inhibitors

Developed to treat depression with fewer adverse effects, SSRIs are chemically different from TCAs and MAO inhibitors. Some of the SSRIs currently available are:
- citalopram
- escitalopram
- fluoxetine
- fluvoxamine
- paroxetine
- sertraline.

Good news! SSRIs treat depression with fewer adverse effects.

Pharmacokinetics
SSRIs are absorbed almost completely after oral administration and are highly protein bound. They're primarily metabolised in the liver and excreted in urine.

Prototype pro

Selective serotonin reuptake inhibitors: Fluoxetine

Actions

- Presumed to be linked to the inhibition of central nervous system (CNS) neuronal uptake of serotonin

Indications

- Depression
- Treatment of binge eating and vomiting behaviours in patients with moderate to severe bulimia nervosa
- Premenstrual dysphoric disorder
- Anorexia nervosa
- Panic disorder
- Alcohol dependence

Nursing considerations

- Monitor the patient for adverse reactions, such as anxiety, nervousness, insomnia, drowsiness, nausea, diarrhoea, dry mouth, and respiratory distress.
- Give the drug in the morning to prevent insomnia.
- Warn the patient to avoid hazardous activities that require alertness and psychomotor coordination until the CNS effects of the drug are known.

Pharmacodynamics

SSRIs inhibit the neuronal reuptake of the neurotransmitter serotonin. (See *Selective serotonin reuptake inhibitors: Fluoxetine.*)

Pharmacotherapeutics

SSRIs are used to treat major depressive episodes. They have the same degree of effectiveness as TCAs.

Here's the (SSRI) scope

SSRIs may also be useful in treating panic disorders, eating disorders, personality disorders, impulse control disorders, and anxiety disorders. For example, paroxetine is indicated for social anxiety disorder. Fluoxetine is approved for the treatment of bulimia. Fluoxetine and sertraline are approved for the treatment of premenstrual (dysphoric) disorder. Fluvoxamine, fluoxetine, sertraline, and paroxetine are also used to treat obsessive-compulsive disorder.

Drug interactions

Drug interactions with SSRIs are associated with their ability to competitively inhibit a liver enzyme that's responsible for oxidation of numerous drugs,

> Hey! You're getting in the way of my enzyme activity! I can't oxidise other drugs because of you!

including TCAs; antipsychotics, such as clozapine; carbamazepine; metoprolol; flecainide; and encainide.

Danger ahead!

Using SSRIs with MAO inhibitors can cause serious, potentially fatal reactions. Individual SSRIs also have their own particular interactions:
• Using citalopram and paroxetine with warfarin may lead to increased bleeding.
• Carbamazepine may increase the clearance of citalopram.
• Fluoxetine increases the half-life of diazepam and displaces highly protein-bound drugs, leading to toxicity.
• Fluvoxamine use with diltiazem may cause bradycardia.
• Paroxetine shouldn't be used with tryptophan because this combination can cause headache, nausea, sweating, and dizziness.
• Paroxetine may increase procyclidine levels, causing increased anticholinergic effects.
• Cimetidine, phenobarbital, and phenytoin may reduce paroxetine metabolism by the liver, increasing the risk of toxicity.
• Paroxetine and sertraline may interact with other highly protein-bound drugs, causing adverse reactions to either drug. (See *Prozac peril.*)

Adverse reactions

Anxiety, insomnia, somnolence, and palpitations may occur with the use of an SSRI. Sexual dysfunction (anorgasm and delayed ejaculation) as well as various skin rashes have been reported. Decreased glucose concentrations in plasma can occur with fluoxetine. Orthostatic hypotension may occur with citalopram and paroxetine use.

Stopping…may be starting

Other symptoms may develop when a patient stops taking an SSRI (See *SSRI discontinuation syndrome*).

Nursing process

These nursing process steps are appropriate for patients undergoing treatment with SSRIs.

Assessment
• Assess the patient's condition before therapy, and reassess regularly throughout therapy.
• Assess for adverse reactions and drug interactions.
• Assess the patient's and family's knowledge of drug therapy.

Prozac peril

In the late 1980s, a widely publicised report on fluoxetine (Prozac) suggested that akathisia, a movement disorder characterised by restlessness and extreme agitation (possible adverse reactions to fluoxetine), may lead to suicidal behaviour. However, many subsequent studies have failed to show a direct association between fluoxetine administration and suicidal ideation.

Keep in mind, however, that caution must be used in patients who are already suicidal and who develop extreme agitation while taking fluoxetine, because the severe discomfort associated with akathisia may exacerbate suicidal ideation.

SSRI discontinuation syndrome

Abrupt discontinuation of selective serotonin reuptake inhibitors (SSRIs) may result in a condition called *SSRI discontinuation syndrome*. This syndrome is characterised by symptoms of dizziness, vertigo, ataxia, nausea, vomiting, muscle pains, fatigue, tremor, and headache. The patient may also experience psychological symptoms, such as anxiety, crying spells, irritability, sad feelings, memory problems, and vivid dreams.

The half-life of it

SSRI discontinuation syndrome occurs in up to one-third of patients taking SSRIs. It's more common in patients who are stopping SSRIs with a short half-life, such as paroxetine. Fluoxetine is the least likely to cause this problem because of its extremely long half-life.

How to deal

This syndrome is self-limited. With treatment, it usually resolves within 2 to 3 weeks. Tapering the drug dosage slowly over several weeks can help prevent it.

Key nursing diagnoses
- Ineffective coping related to the underlying condition.
- Disturbed sleep pattern related to drug-induced insomnia.
- Deficient knowledge related to drug therapy.

Planning outcome goals
- The patient's ability to cope will improve.
- Improved sleep patterns will be exhibited.
- The patient and family will demonstrate an understanding of drug therapy.

Implementation
- Elderly or debilitated patients and patients with renal or hepatic dysfunction may need lower dosages or less frequent dosing.
- Give SSRIs in the morning to prevent insomnia.
- Give antihistamines or topical corticosteroids to treat rashes or pruritus.
- Lower-weight children may need several weeks between dosage increases.

Elderly or debilitated patients and patients with renal or hepatic dysfunction may need lower dosages of SSRIs or less frequent dosing.

Education edge

Teaching about SSRIs

If selective serotonin reuptake inhibitors (SSRIs) are prescribed, review these points with the patient and caregivers:

- Take the drug as directed; don't alter the dose, even when symptoms subside. SSRIs are usually given for several months—sometimes longer.
- Relief from symptoms may not occur for 2 to 4 weeks after the drug is started; don't stop taking the drug prematurely.
- Don't take other drugs, over-the-counter products, or herbal remedies without first consulting with the prescriber. Serious drug interactions may occur.
- Tell other healthcare providers that you're taking an SSRI to avoid drug interactions.

- Avoid activities that require alertness and psychomotor coordination until the drug's effects on the central nervous system are known.
- SSRIs may be taken without regard to food.
- Take the drug in the morning to help avoid insomnia or nervousness, unless otherwise directed.
- Report excessive drowsiness, dizziness, difficulty breathing, or other adverse effects to the prescriber.
- Don't stop taking the drug without first consulting with the prescriber.
- Counselling, support groups, stress management techniques, and relaxation techniques may be helpful in addition to drug therapy.

Evaluation
- Patient behavior and communication indicate an improvement of depression with drug therapy.
- Patient has no insomnia with drug use.
- Patient and family demonstrate an understanding of drug therapy. (See *Teaching about SSRIs*.)

Monoamine oxidase inhibitors

MAO inhibitors are divided into two classifications based on their chemical structure:

 hydrazines, which include phenelzine

 nonhydrazines, comprised of a single drug, tranylcypromine.

Pharmacokinetics
MAO inhibitors are absorbed rapidly and completely from the GI tract and are metabolised in the liver to inactive metabolites. These metabolites are excreted mainly by the GI tract and, to a lesser degree, by the kidneys.

Pharmacodynamics

MAO inhibitors appear to work by inhibiting monoamine oxidase, the widely distributed enzyme that normally metabolises many neurotransmitters, including noradrenaline (norepinephrine) and serotonin. This action makes more noradrenaline (norepinephrine), dopamine, and serotonin available to the receptors, thereby relieving the symptoms of depression.

Pharmacotherapeutics

Indications for MAO inhibitors are similar to those for other antidepressants. They're particularly effective in panic disorder with agoraphobia, eating disorders, posttraumatic stress syndrome, and pain disorder.

Not a typical depression

MAO inhibitors are also thought to be effective in atypical depression. Atypical depression produces signs opposite of those of typical depression. For example, the patient gains weight, sleeps more, and has a higher susceptibility to rejection.

Battling the blues

MAO inhibitors may be used to treat typical depression resistant to other therapies or when other therapies are contraindicated. Other uses include the treatment of:
- phobic anxieties
- neurodermatitis (an itchy skin disorder seen in anxious, nervous people)
- hypochondriasis (abnormal concern about health)
- refractory narcolepsy (sudden sleep attacks).

Drug interactions

MAO inhibitors interact with many drugs:
- Taking MAO inhibitors with amphetamines, methylphenidate, levodopa, sympathomimetics, or nonamphetamine appetite suppressants may increase catecholamine release, causing hypertensive crisis. (See *Stopping MAO inhibitors*.)
- Using MAO inhibitors with fluoxetine, tricyclic antidepressants, citalopram, clomipramine, trazodone, sertraline, paroxetine, and

MAO inhibitors increase the amount of noradrenaline (norepinephrine), dopamine, and serotonin that's available to receptors, which helps relieve symptoms of depression.

Stopping MAO inhibitors

Monoamine oxidase (MAO) inhibitors should be discontinued 2 weeks before starting an alternative antidepressant. If a patient is switching from another antidepressant to an MAO inhibitor, a waiting period of 2 weeks (5 weeks for fluoxetine) is recommended before starting the MAO inhibitor.

fluvoxamine may result in an elevated body temperature, excitation, and seizures.
- When taken with doxapram, MAO inhibitors may cause hypertension and arrhythmias and may increase the adverse reactions to doxapram.
- The hypoglycaemic effects of antidiabetic drugs may be enhanced.
- Administering MAO inhibitors with pethidine may result in excitation, hypertension or hypotension, extremely elevated body temperature, and coma.

Eat, drink and...be careful

Certain foods can interact with MAO inhibitors and produce severe reactions. The most serious reactions involve tyramine-rich foods, such as red wine, aged cheese, and fava beans. Foods with moderate tyramine contents—for example, yogurt and ripe bananas—may be eaten occasionally, but with care. Caffeine may also interact with MAO inhibitors, but the reactions aren't as serious as with tyramine-rich foods.

Patients taking MAO inhibitors need to watch what they eat. Tyramine-rich foods can interact with these drugs and produce hypertensive crisis.

Adverse reactions

Administering MAO inhibitors in small, divided doses may relieve some of the following adverse reactions:
- hypertensive crisis (when taken with tyramine-rich foods)
- orthostatic hypertension
- restlessness, drowsiness, dizziness, and insomnia
- headache
- constipation, anorexia, and nausea and vomiting
- weakness and joint pain
- dry mouth
- blurred vision
- peripheral oedema
- urine retention and transient impotence
- rash
- skin and mucous membrane haemorrhage.

Nursing process

These nursing process steps are appropriate for patients undergoing treatment with MAO inhibitors.

Assessment
- Assess the patient's condition before therapy and regularly thereafter.
- Assess the patient for risk of self-harm.
- Obtain baseline blood pressure, heart rate, complete blood count (CBC), and liver function test results before beginning therapy; monitor these throughout treatment.
- Assess for adverse reactions and drug interactions.
- Assess the patient's and family's knowledge of drug therapy.

You can relieve adverse reactions by giving MAO inhibitors in small divided doses.

Key nursing diagnoses
- Disturbed thought processes related to presence of depression.
- Risk for injury related to drug-induced adverse CNS reactions.
- Deficient knowledge related to drug therapy.

Planning outcome goals
- The patient will exhibit improved thought processes.
- The risk of injury to the patient will be minimised.
- The patient and family will demonstrate an understanding of drug therapy.

Implementation
- The dosage is usually reduced to a maintenance level as soon as possible.
- Don't withdraw the drug abruptly.
- Discontinue MAO inhibitors 14 days before elective surgery, as indicated, to avoid interaction with anaesthetics.
- If the patient develops symptoms of overdose (such as palpitations, severe hypotension, or frequent headaches), withhold dose and notify the prescriber.
- Have phentolamine available to combat severe hypertension.
- Continue precautions for 10 days after stopping drug because it has long-lasting effects.

Signs of MAO inhibitor overdose include palpitations, severe hypotension, and frequent headaches.

Evaluation
- Patient's behaviour and communication exhibit improved thought processes.
- Patient doesn't experience injury from adverse CNS reactions.
- Patient and family demonstrate an understanding of drug therapy. (See *Teaching about MAO inhibitors*.)

Tricyclic antidepressants

TCAs are used to treat depression. They include:
- amitriptyline hydrochloride
- clomipramine
- doxepin
- imipramine hydrochloride
- nortriptyline
- trimipramine.

Pharmacokinetics
All of the TCAs are active pharmacologically, and some of their metabolites are also active. They're absorbed completely when taken orally but undergo first-pass effect.

Education edge

Teaching about MAO inhibitors

If monoamine oxidase (MAO) inhibitors are prescribed, review these points with the patient and caregivers:

- Avoid foods high in tyramine (such as aged cheese, red wine, beer, avocados, chocolate, bananas, and meat tenderisers) as well as large amounts of caffeine. Tranylcypromine is the MAO inhibitor most commonly reported to cause hypertensive crisis with ingestion of foods high in tyramine.

- Sit up for 1 minute before getting out of bed to avoid dizziness.
- Avoid overexertion because MAO inhibitors may suppress angina.
- Consult the prescriber before taking other prescription or over-the-counter drugs. Severe adverse effects can occur if MAO inhibitors are taken with cold, hay fever, or diet aids.
- Don't stop taking the drug suddenly.

Passing it on

With first-pass effect, a drug passes from the GI tract to the liver, where it's partially metabolised before entering the circulation. TCAs are metabolised extensively in the liver and eventually excreted as inactive compounds (only small amounts of active drug are excreted) in urine.

Oh-so-soluble

The extreme fat solubility of these drugs accounts for their wide distribution throughout the body, slow excretion, and long half-lives.

Pharmacodynamics

Researchers believe that TCAs increase the amount of noradrenaline (norepinephrine), serotonin, or both in the CNS by preventing their reuptake (reentry) into the storage granules in the presynaptic nerves. Preventing reuptake results in increased levels of these neurotransmitters in the synapses, relieving depression. TCAs also block acetylcholine and histamine receptors.

Pharmacotherapeutics

TCAs are used to treat episodes of major depression. They're especially effective in treating depression of insidious onset accompanied by weight loss, anorexia, or insomnia. Physical signs and symptoms may respond after 1 to 2 weeks of therapy, psychological symptoms after 2 to 4 weeks.

TCAs prevent the reuptake of noradrenaline (norepinephrine) and serotonin. More noradrenaline (norepinephrine) and serotonin in the synapses provides relief from depression.

Working together

TCAs may be helpful when used with a mood stabiliser in treating acute episodes of depression in patients with type 1 bipolar disorder.

Prototype pro

Tricyclic antidepressants: Imipramine

Actions

- May inhibit the reuptake of noradrenaline (norepinephrine) and serotonin in central nervous system (CNS) nerve terminals (presynaptic neurons), thus enhancing the concentration and activity of neuro-transmitters in the synaptic cleft.
- Exerts antihistaminic, sedative, anticholinergic, vasodilatory, and quinidine-like effects

Indications

- Depression
- Enuresis in children older than aged 6

Nursing considerations

- Monitor the patient for adverse reactions, such as sedation, anticholinergic effects, and orthostatic hypotension.
- Don't withdraw the drug abruptly; gradually reduce the dosage over several weeks.
- Warn the patient to avoid hazardous activities that require alertness and psychomotor coordination until the CNS effects of the drug are known.

Additional assistance

TCAs are also used to prevent migraine headaches and treat:
- panic disorder with agoraphobia
- urinary incontinence
- ADHD
- obsessive-compulsive disorder
- diabetic neuropathy
- enuresis. (See *Tricyclic antidepressants: Imipramine*.)

Drug interactions

TCAs interact with several commonly used drugs:
- TCAs increase the catecholamine effects of amphetamines and sympathomimetics, leading to hypertension.
- Barbiturates increase the metabolism of TCAs and decrease their blood levels.
- Cimetidine impairs the metabolism of TCAs by the liver, increasing the risk of toxicity.
- Using TCAs concurrently with MAO inhibitors may cause an extremely elevated body temperature, excitation, and seizures.

- An increased anticholinergic effect, such as dry mouth, urine retention, and constipation, is seen when anticholinergic drugs are taken with TCAs.
- TCAs reduce the antihypertensive effects of clonidine and guanethidine.

Adverse reactions

Adverse reactions to TCAs include:
- orthostatic hypotension (a drop in blood pressure on standing)
- sedation
- jaundice
- rashes and photosensitivity reactions
- resting tremor
- decreased sexual desire and inhibited ejaculation
- transient eosinophilia
- reduced white blood cell (WBC) count
- manic episodes (in patients with or without bipolar disorder)
- exacerbation of psychotic symptoms in susceptible patients.

TCAs increase the effects of anticholinergic drugs, which can result in dry mouth, urine retention, and constipation.

On the rare side

Although rare, TCA therapy may also lead to:
- granulocytopenia
- palpitations
- conduction delays
- rapid heartbeat
- impaired cognition and cardiovascular effects.

Nursing process

These nursing process steps are appropriate for patients undergoing treatment with TCAs.

Assessment
- Check an ECG in patients older than aged 40 before starting therapy.
- Observe the patient for mood changes to monitor drug effectiveness; benefits may not appear for 3 to 6 weeks.
- Assess the patient's vital signs regularly for decreased blood pressure or tachycardia (fast heart rate); observe them carefully for other adverse reactions and report changes. In particular, assess for anticholinergic adverse reactions (urine retention or constipation), which may require a dosage reduction.

Key nursing diagnoses
- Disturbed thought processes related to adverse effects.
- Risk for injury related to sedation and orthostatic hypotension.
- Noncompliance related to long-term therapy.

Planning outcome goals
- The patient will exhibit improved thought processes.
- The risk of injury to the patient will be minimised.
- The patient will comply with therapy.

Implementation
- Make sure that the patient swallows each dose; a depressed patient may hoard pills for a suicide attempt, especially when symptoms begin to improve.
- Don't withdraw the drug abruptly; gradually reduce the dosage over several weeks to avoid a rebound effect or other adverse reactions.
- Follow the manufacturer's instructions for reconstitution, dilution, and storage of drugs.

Evaluation
- Patient regains normal thought processes.
- Patient sustains no injury from adverse reactions.
- Patient complies with therapy.
- Patient's depression is alleviated. (See *Teaching about TCAs*.)

Miscellaneous antidepressants

Other antidepressants in use today include:
- mirtazapine, a tetracyclic antidepressant
- bupropion, a dopamine reuptake blocking drug

Withdraw TCAs gradually to avoid a rebound effect or other adverse reactions.

- venlafaxine, a serotonin-noradrenaline (norepinephrine) reuptake inhibitor (SNRI)
- trazodone, a triazopyridine drug.

Pharmacokinetics

The paths these antidepressants take through the body may vary:
- Mirtazapine is absorbed from the GI tract, distributed widely in the body, metabolised by the liver, and excreted by the kidneys.
- Bupropion is well absorbed from the GI tract and metabolised by the liver. Its metabolites are excreted by the kidneys. It appears to be highly bound to plasma proteins.
- Venlafaxine is rapidly absorbed after oral administration, partially bound to plasma proteins, metabolised in the liver, and excreted in urine.
- Trazodone is well absorbed from the GI tract, distributed widely in the body, metabolised by the liver, and about 75% is excreted in urine. The rest is excreted in faeces.

Pharmacodynamics

Much about how these drugs work has yet to be fully understood:
- Maprotiline and mirtazapine probably increase the amount of noradrenaline (norepinephrine), serotonin, or both in the CNS by blocking their reuptake by presynaptic neurons (nerve terminals).
- Bupropion was once thought to inhibit the reuptake of the neurotransmitter dopamine; however, its action is more likely on nonadrenergic receptors.
- Venlafaxine is thought to potentiate neurotransmitter activity in the CNS by inhibiting the neural reuptake of serotonin and noradrenaline (norepinephrine).
- Trazodone, although its effect is unknown, is thought to exert antidepressant effects by inhibiting the reuptake of noradrenaline (norepinephrine) and serotonin in the presynaptic neurons.
- Nefazodone's action isn't precisely defined. It inhibits neuronal uptake of serotonin and noradrenaline (norepinephrine). It's also a serotonin antagonist, which explains its effectiveness in treating anxiety.

Pharmacotherapeutics

These miscellaneous drugs are all used to treat depression. Trazodone may also be effective in treating aggressive behavior and panic disorder.

Venafaxine is an SNRI that lacks the sedative and antimuscarinic effects of tricyclic antidepressants-so it can be used to treat general anxiety as well as depression.

Drug interactions

All of these antidepressants may have serious, potentially fatal, reactions when combined with MAO inhibitors. Each of these drugs also carries individual, specific risks when used with other drugs:

• Mirtazapine interacts with CNS depressants, resulting in additive effects.

• Bupropion, when combined with levodopa, phenothiazines, and TCAs, increases the risk of adverse reactions, including seizures.

• Trazodone may increase serum levels of digoxin and phenytoin. Its use with antihypertensive drugs may cause increased hypotensive effects. CNS depression may be enhanced if trazodone is administered with other CNS depressants.

Adverse reactions

Adverse reactions to venlaxafine include:

• headache
• somnolence
• dizziness
• nausea.

Combining MAO inhibitors with other antidepressants can cause serious reactions.

Mirtazapine maladies

Mirtazapine may cause:

• tremors
• confusion
• nausea
• constipation.

Bupropion blues

These adverse reactions may occur with bupropion:

• headache
• confusion
• tremor
• agitation
• tachycardia
• anorexia
• nausea and vomiting.

Trazodone trouble

Trazodone may cause:

• drowsiness
• dizziness.

Nursing process

These nursing process steps are appropriate for patients undergoing treatment with miscellaneous antidepressants.

Assessment
• Assess the patient's condition before therapy and regularly thereafter.
• Assess for adverse reactions and drug interactions.
• Assess the patient's and family's knowledge of drug therapy.

Key nursing diagnoses
• Ineffective coping related to the underlying condition.
• Disturbed sleep pattern related to drug-induced insomnia.
• Deficient knowledge related to drug therapy.

Planning outcome goals
• The patient's ability to cope will improve.
• The patient's sleep patterns will improve.
• The patient and family will demonstrate an understanding of drug therapy.

Implementation
• Elderly or debilitated patients and patients with renal or hepatic dysfunction may need lower dosages or less frequent dosing.
• Give these drugs in the morning to prevent insomnia, unless otherwise directed.
• Administer the drugs as prescribed.
• Monitor the patient for effects of drug therapy.

Evaluation
• Patient's behaviour and communication indicate improvement of depression with drug therapy.
• Patient has no insomnia with drug use.
• Patient and family demonstrate an understanding of drug therapy.

Antidepressants such as bupropion should be taken in the morning to prevent insomnia.

Lithium

Lithium carbonate and lithium citrate are mood stabilisers used to prevent or treat mania. The discovery of lithium was a milestone in treating mania and bipolar disorders.

Pharmacokinetics
When taken orally, lithium is absorbed rapidly and completely and is distributed to body tissues. An active drug, lithium isn't metabolised and is excreted from the body unchanged.

Pharmacodynamics

In mania, one theory is that the patient experiences excessive catecholamine stimulation. In bipolar disorder, the patient is affected by swings between the excessive catecholamine stimulation of mania and the diminished catecholamine stimulation of depression. Lithium is also thought to reduce dopamine levels in the CNS.

I hear excessive catecholamine stimulation results in mania, and diminished catecholamine stimulation causes depression.

Yes, but lithium (that's us) may regulate catecholamine release to treat mania and bipolar disorders. Aren't we great?!

Curbing catecholamines

Lithium's exact mechanism is unknown. A few of the ways it may regulate catecholamine release in the CNS are by:
• increasing noradrenaline (norepinephrine) and serotonin uptake
• reducing the release of noradrenaline (norepinephrine) from the synaptic vesicles (where neurotransmitters are stored) in the presynaptic neuron
• inhibiting noradrenaline's (norepinephrine's) action in the postsynaptic neuron.

Under study

Researchers are also examining lithium's effects on electrolyte and ion transport. It may also modify actions of second messengers, such as cyclic adenosine monophosphate.

Pharmacotherapeutics

Lithium is used primarily to treat acute episodes of mania and to prevent relapses of bipolar disorders. Other uses of lithium being researched include preventing unipolar depression and migraine headaches and treating depression, alcohol dependence, anorexia nervosa, syndrome of inappropriate antidiuretic hormone, and neutropenia.

Lithium has a narrow therapeutic margin. So watch out for serious drug interactions.

Drug interactions

Lithium has a narrow therapeutic margin of safety. A blood level that's even slightly higher than the therapeutic level can be dangerous. Serious interactions with other drugs can occur because of this narrow therapeutic range:
• The risk of lithium toxicity increases when lithium is taken with thiazide and loop diuretics and nonsteroidal anti-inflammatory drugs.
• Administration of lithium with haloperidol, phenothiazines, and carbamazepine may produce an increased risk of neurotoxicity.
• Lithium may increase the hypothyroid effects of potassium iodide.

- Sodium bicarbonate may increase lithium excretion, reducing its effects.
- Lithium's effects are reduced when taken with theophylline.

Salt at fault?

A patient on a severe salt-restricted diet is susceptible to lithium toxicity. On the other hand, an increased intake of sodium may reduce the therapeutic effects of lithium.

Adverse reactions

Common adverse reactions to lithium include:
- reversible ECG changes
- thirst
- polyuria
- elevated WBC count.

Toxic times

Toxic blood levels of lithium may produce:
- confusion
- lethargy
- slurred speech
- increased reflex reactions
- seizures.

Nursing process

These nursing process steps are appropriate for patients undergoing treatment with lithium.

Assessment

- Assess the patient's condition before therapy and regularly thereafter. Expect a delay of 1 to 3 weeks before the drug's beneficial effects are noticed.
- Obtain a baseline ECG, thyroid and kidney studies, and electrolyte levels. Monitor lithium blood levels 8 to 12 hours after the first dose, usually before morning dose, two or three times weekly in the first month, and then weekly to monthly during maintenance therapy.
- Perform outpatient follow-up of thyroid and kidney function every 6 to 12 months. Palpate the thyroid to check for enlargement.
- Assess for adverse reactions and drug interactions.

Key nursing diagnoses

- Disturbed thought processes related to manic disorder.
- Ineffective health maintenance related to drug-induced endocrine dysfunction.
- Deficient knowledge related to drug therapy.

Remember: It may take 1 to 3 weeks to notice lithium's beneficial effects.

Planning outcome goals
- The patient's behaviour will improve.
- The patient's health status will improve.
- The patient and family will demonstrate an understanding of drug therapy.

Implementation
- Determination of lithium blood levels is crucial to safe use of the drug. Lithium shouldn't be used in a patient who can't have his blood level checked regularly.
- Give the drug with plenty of water and after meals to minimise GI reactions.
- Before leaving the bedside, make sure that the patient has swallowed the drug.
- Notify the prescriber if the patient's behaviour hasn't improved in 3 weeks or if it worsens.
- Adverse reactions usually are mild when the blood level of lithium remains below 1.5 mmol/l.
- If the patient has diuresis, check his urine specific gravity and report a level below 1.005, which may indicate diabetes insipidus.
- Lithium may alter glucose tolerance in a patient with diabetes. Monitor his glucose level closely.

Evaluation
- Patient exhibits improved behaviour and thought processes.
- Patient maintains normal endocrine function throughout therapy.
- Patient and family demonstrate an understanding of drug therapy. (See *Teaching about lithium*.)

Education edge

Teaching about lithium

If lithium is prescribed, review these points with the patient and caregivers:

- Take the drug with plenty of water and after meals to minimise GI upset.
- Lithium has a narrow therapeutic margin of safety. A blood level that's even slightly high can be dangerous.
- Watch for signs of toxicity, such as diarrhoea, vomiting, tremor, drowsiness, muscle weakness, and ataxia. Withhold one dose of the drug and call the prescriber if toxic symptoms appear. Don't stop the drug abruptly.

- Expect transient nausea, polyuria, thirst, and discomfort during the first few days of therapy.
- Avoid activities that require alertness and good psychomotor coordination until the drug's central nervous system effects are known.
- Don't switch brands or take other prescription or over-the-counter drugs without the prescriber's approval.
- Wear or carry medical identification.

Antipsychotic drugs

Antipsychotic drugs can control psychotic symptoms (delusions, hallucinations, and thought disorders) that can occur with schizophrenia, mania, and other psychoses; these disorders are thought to arise through disturbance of normal dopamine receptor activity.

Antipsychotic drugs can control psychotic symptoms, such as delusions, hallucinations, and thought disorders.

The name game

Drugs used to treat psychoses have several different names, including:
- antipsychotic, because they can eliminate signs and symptoms of psychoses
- major tranquilliser, because they can calm an agitated patient
- neuroleptic, because they have an adverse neurobiologic effect that causes abnormal body movements.

One...or the other

Regardless of what they're called, all antipsychotic drugs belong to one of two major groups:

 atypical antipsychotics

 typical antipsychotics.

Atypical antipsychotics

Atypical antipsychotics are drugs designed to treat schizophrenia. They include:
- clozapine
- olanzapine
- risperidone
- quetiapine
- aripiprazole.

Pharmacokinetics

Atypical antipsychotics are absorbed after oral administration. They're metabolised by the liver. Metabolites of clozapine, quetiapine, and olanzapine are inactive, whereas risperidone has an active metabolite. They're highly plasma protein bound and eliminated in urine, with a small portion eliminated in faeces.

Pharmacodynamics

Atypical antipsychotics typically block the dopamine receptors, but to a lesser extent than the typical antipsychotics, resulting in far fewer extrapyramidal adverse effects. Additionally, atypical antipsychotics block serotonin receptor activity. These combined actions

I'm not your run-of-the-mill antipsychotic. I block the activity of two receptors, dopamine and serotonin, to treat schizophrenia.

account for the effectiveness of atypical antipsychotics against the positive and negative symptoms of schizophrenia.

Pharmacotherapeutics

Atypical antipsychotics are considered the first line of treatment for patients with schizophrenia because of equal or improved effectiveness and improved tolerability. They're commonly used to treat behavioural and psychotic symptoms in patients with dementia, but dosages are significantly lower.

Drug interactions

Drugs that alter the P-450 enzyme system will alter the metabolism of some atypical antipsychotics.

The straight "dopa"

Atypical antipsychotics counteract the effects of levodopa and other dopamine agonists.

Adverse reactions

Atypical antipsychotics have fewer extrapyramidal effects than typical antipsychotics and a minimal risk of seizures (except for clozapine). Clozapine is associated with agranulocytosis. Weight gain is also common. Seizures may also occur.

Extra! Extra!

Olanzapine places the patient at minimal risk for extrapyramidal effects, but weight gain is common. Risperidone has a higher risk for extrapyramidal effects than other atypical antipsychotics if it's prescribed at doses higher than 6 mg/day.

Quetiapine and aripiprazole (a newer atypical antipsychotic) are associated with sedation.

Nursing process

These nursing process steps are appropriate for patients undergoing treatment with atypical antipsychotics.

Assessment
• Assess the patient's disorder before therapy and regularly thereafter.
• Assess for adverse reactions and drug interactions.
• Monitor the patient for tardive dyskinesia (involuntary movements). It may occur after prolonged use. This sign may not appear until months or years later and it may disappear spontaneously or persist for life despite stopping the drug.
• Assess the patient's and family's knowledge of drug therapy.

Tardive dyskinesia can occur after prolonged use of atypical antipsychotics. It may persist even after the drug is stopped.

Key nursing diagnoses
- Disturbed thought processes related to the underlying condition.
- Impaired physical mobility related to extrapyramidal effects.
- Deficient knowledge related to drug therapy.

Planning outcome goals
- The patient will exhibit improved thought processes.
- Adequate physical mobility will be exhibited.
- The patient and family will demonstrate an understanding of drug therapy.

Implementation
- Administer the drug as prescribed and monitor for its effect.
- When changing forms of the drug, the dosage will change to meet the patient's needs.
- Protect the drug from light, as indicated. Discard the drug if it's markedly discoloured.
- Don't stop the drug abruptly unless severe adverse reactions occur.
- Acute dystonic reactions may be treated with diphenhydramine.
- Warn the patient to avoid activities that require alertness and psychomotor coordination until the drug's CNS effects are known.
- Advise the patient to avoid alcohol while taking atypical antipsychotics.
- Tell the patient to chew sugarless gum or suck ice cubes to help relieve dry mouth.

Evaluation
- Patient demonstrates decreased psychotic behaviour and agitation.
- Patient maintains physical mobility.
- Patient and family demonstrate an understanding of drug therapy.

Typical antipsychotics

Typical antipsychotics, which include phenothiazines and nonphenothiazines, can be broken down into smaller classifications.

A sorted affair

Many clinicians believe that the phenothiazines should be treated as three distinct groups of drug because of the differences in the adverse reactions they cause:

Group 1: chlorpromazine, levomepromazine and promazine, generally characterised by pronounced sedative effects and moderate antimuscarinic and extrapyramidal side-effects.

Group 2: pericyazine and pipotiazine, generally characterised by moderate sedative effects and marked extrapyramidal side-effects.

Group 3: fluphenazine, perphenazine, prochlorperazine and trifluoperazine, generally characterised by by fewer sedative and antimuscarinic effects, but more pronounced extrapyramidal side-effects than groups 1 and 2.

Pharmacokinetics

Although typical antipsychotics are absorbed erratically, they're very lipid-soluble and highly protein-bound. Therefore, they're distributed to many tissues and are highly concentrated in the brain. All typical antipsychotics are metabolised in the liver and excreted in urine and bile.

Effects keep going and going and going and going

Because fatty tissues slowly release accumulated phenothiazine metabolites into the plasma, phenothiazines may produce effects up to 3 months after they're stopped.

Pharmacodynamics

Although the mechanism of action of typical antipsychotics isn't understood fully, researchers believe that these drugs work by blocking postsynaptic dopaminergic receptors in the brain.

Blocking...

The antipsychotic effect of phenothiazines and nonphenothiazines comes about from a receptor blockade in the limbic system. Their antiemetic effects result from the receptor blockade in the chemoreceptor trigger zone located in the brain's medulla.

and stimulating

Phenothiazines also stimulate the extrapyramidal system (motor pathways that connect the cerebral cortex with the spinal nerve pathways). (See *Phenothiazines: Chlorpromazine*.)

Pharmacotherapeutics

Phenothiazines are used primarily to:
- treat schizophrenia
- calm anxious or agitated patients
- improve a patient's thought processes
- alleviate delusions and hallucinations.

Even more uses

Other therapeutic uses have been found for phenothiazines:
- They're administered to treat other psychiatric disorders, such as brief reactive psychosis, atypical psychosis, schizoaffective psychosis, autism, and major depression with psychosis.

Because they're lipid-soluble and highly protein-bound, typical antipsychotics are distributed to many tissues and are highly concentrated in the brain.

Access denied! Typical antipsychotics block postsynaptic dopaminergic receptors in the brain.

Prototype pro

Phenothiazines: Chlorpromazine

Actions

- Functions as a dopamine antagonist by blocking postsynaptic dopamine receptors in various parts of the central nervous system (CNS)
- Produces antiemetic effects by blocking the chemoreceptor trigger zone
- Produces varying degrees of anticholinergic and alpha-adrenergic receptor blocking actions

Indications

- Agitated psychotic state, hallucinations, manic-depressive illness, excessive motor and autonomic activity
- Severe nausea and vomiting induced by CNS disturbances
- Moderate anxiety
- Behavioural problems caused by chronic organic mental syndrome, tetanus, acute intermittent porphyria, intractable hiccups, itching, and symptomatic rhinitis

Nursing considerations

- Monitor the patient for adverse reactions and extrapyramidal symptoms (ranging from akathisia during early treatment to tardive dyskinesia after long-term use).
- A neuroleptic malignant syndrome resembling severe parkinsonism may occur.
- Elevated liver enzyme levels that progress to obstructive jaundice usually indicate an allergic reaction.
- Don't withdraw the drug abruptly; gradually reduce the dosage over several weeks.
- Warn the patient to avoid hazardous activities that require alertness and psychomotor coordination until the drug's CNS effects are known.

- In combination with lithium, they're used in the treatment of patients with bipolar disorder, until the slower-acting lithium produces its therapeutic effect.
- They're prescribed to quiet mentally challenged children and agitated elderly patients, particularly those with dementia.
- They may be given to boost the preoperative effects of analgesics.
- They're helpful in the management of pain, anxiety, and nausea in patients with cancer.

News on the nons

As a group, nonphenothiazines are used to treat psychotic disorders. In addition, haloperidol and pimozide may be used to treat Tourette syndrome.

Drug interactions

Phenothiazines interact with many different types of drugs and may have serious effects:

• Increased CNS depressant effects, such as stupor, may occur when they're taken with CNS depressants.

• CNS depressants may reduce phenothiazine effectiveness, resulting in increased psychotic behavior or agitation.

• Taking anticholinergic drugs with phenothiazines may result in increased anticholinergic effects, such as dry mouth and constipation. By increasing phenothiazine metabolism, anticholinergic drugs may also reduce the antipsychotic effects of phenothiazines.

• Phenothiazines may reduce the antiparkinsonian effects of levodopa.

• Concurrent use with lithium increases the risk of neurotoxicity.

• The threshold for seizures is lowered when phenothiazines are used with anticonvulsants.

• Phenothiazines may increase the serum levels of TCAs and beta-adrenergic blockers.

Voted less likely to interact

Nonphenothiazines interact with fewer drugs than phenothiazines. Their dopamine-blocking activity can inhibit levodopa and may cause disorientation in patients receiving both drugs. Haloperidol may boost the effects of lithium, producing encephalopathy (brain dysfunction).

Adverse reactions

Neurologic reactions are the most common and serious adverse reactions associated with phenothiazines. Extrapyramidal symptoms may appear after the first few days of therapy; tardive dyskinesia may occur after several years of treatment.

On a more serious note

Neuroleptic malignant syndrome is a potentially fatal condition that produces muscle rigidity, extreme extrapyramidal symptoms, severely elevated body temperature, hypertension, and rapid heart rate. If left untreated, it can result in respiratory failure and cardiovascular collapse.

Shared traits

Most nonphenothiazines cause the same adverse reactions as phenothiazines.

Nursing process

These nursing process steps are appropriate for patients undergoing treatment with typical antipsychotics.

Assessment

• Assess the patient's vital signs regularly for decreased blood pressure (especially before and after parenteral therapy) or tachycardia; observe him carefully for other adverse reactions.
• Assess intake and output, watching for urine retention or constipation, which may require a dosage reduction.
• Monitor bilirubin levels weekly for the first 4 weeks. Obtain baseline CBC, ECG, liver and renal function test results, electrolyte levels (especially potassium), and eye examination findings. Monitor these findings periodically thereafter, especially in the patient receiving long-term therapy.
• Assess the patient for mood changes and monitor his progress.
• Monitor the patient for involuntary movements. Check the patient receiving prolonged treatment at least once every 6 months.

Key nursing diagnoses

• Risk for injury related to adverse reactions.
• Impaired mobility related to extrapyramidal symptoms.
• Noncompliance related to long-term therapy.

Planning outcome goals

• The risk of injury to the patient will be minimised.
• The patient will maintain mobility.
• The patient will comply with drug therapy.

Implementation

• Don't withdraw the drug abruptly. Although physical dependence doesn't occur with antipsychotic drugs, rebound worsening of psychotic symptoms may occur, and many drug effects may persist.
• Follow the manufacturer's guidelines for reconstitution, dilution, administration, and storage of drugs; slightly discoloured liquids may or may not be acceptable for use. Check with the pharmacist.

Evaluation

• Patient remains free from injury.
• Extrapyramidal symptoms don't develop.
• Patient complies with therapy, as evidenced by improved thought processes. (See *Teaching about antipsychotic drugs*.)

Watch closely for extrapyramidal symptoms, which may appear after the first few days of phenothiazine therapy.

Education edge

Teaching about antipsychotic drugs

If antipsychotic drugs are prescribed, review these points with the patient and caregivers:

- Take the drug as prescribed. Don't increase the dosage or discontinue the drug without the prescriber's approval.
- Take the full dose at bedtime if daytime sedation occurs.
- The drug's full therapeutic effect may not occur for several weeks.
- Watch for adverse reactions and report unusual effects, especially involuntary movements.
- Avoid alcohol while taking this drug.

- Don't take other drugs, including over-the-counter or herbal products, without the prescriber's approval.
- Avoid hazardous tasks until the drug's full effects are established. Sedative effects will lessen after several weeks.
- Excessive exposure to sunlight, heat lamps, or tanning beds may cause photosensitivity reactions.
- Avoid exposure to extreme heat or cold.
- Phenothiazines may cause pink or brown discolouration of urine.

Other psychotropic drugs

Other commonly used psychotropic drugs include stimulants.

Stimulants

Stimulants are used to treat attention deficit hyperactivity disorder (ADHD), a condition characterised by inattention, impulsiveness, and hyperactivity. Examples of stimulants include:
- amoxetine
- dexamfetamine
- methylphenidate
- mixed amphetamine salts
- modafinil.

Pharmacokinetics
Stimulants are absorbed well from the GI tract and are distributed widely in the body. Methylphenidate, however, undergoes significant first-pass effect. Stimulants are metabolised in the liver and excreted primarily in urine.

Pharmacodynamics
Stimulants are believed to work by increasing levels of dopamine and noradrenaline (norepinephrine) either by blocking the reuptake of dopamine and noradrenaline (norepinephrine), enhancing the presynaptic release, or by inhibiting MAO.

My first-pass effect limits how much methyldopa is absorbed by the body.

Pharmacotherapeutics

Stimulants are the treatment of choice for ADHD. They're helpful in improving attention span, leading to improved school or work performance, and decreasing impulsiveness and hyperactivity.

Wake-up call

Dexamfetamine and methylphenidate are also used in the treatment of narcolepsy. Modafinil, similarly can be used in the treatment of narcolepsy.

Drug interactions

Stimulants shouldn't be used within 14 days of discontinuing an MAO inhibitor. Also, methylphenidate may decrease the effect of guanethidine and increase the effects of TCAs, warfarin, and some anticonvulsants.

Adverse reactions

Stimulants are highly abused substances. Close monitoring of the patient is required. Although controversial, some prescribers recommend stopping the drug for a brief period, such as when children are on summer break from school, to reassess the need for therapy. Stimulants may affect growth. Monitor children closely for height and weight changes.

Crossed out

Modafinil is not recommended for use in children.

Dexamfetamine downers

Adverse reactions specific to dexamfetamine include:
- restlessness
- tremor
- insomnia
- tachycardia
- palpitations
- arrhythmias
- dry mouth
- unpleasant taste
- diarrhoea.

Stimulants are highly abused drugs. Monitor the patient closely.

Methylphenidate misfortune

Methylphenidate may cause:
- dizziness
- insomnia
- seizures
- palpitations
- arrhythmias
- abdominal pain
- rash
- thrombocytopenia.

Modafinil muddle

Adverse reactions to modafinil include:
- abdominal pain
- appetite changes
- gasto-intestinal disturbances
- palpitation
- visual disturbances
- aplastic anemia.

Nursing process

These nursing process steps are appropriate for patients undergoing treatment with stimulants.

Assessment
- Obtain a history of the patient's underlying condition before therapy, and reassess regularly throughout therapy.
- Assess for adverse reactions and drug interactions.
- Monitor the patient's sleeping pattern and observe him for signs of excessive stimulation.
- Assess the patient's and family's knowledge of drug therapy.

Key nursing diagnoses
- Ineffective health maintenance related to underlying condition.
- Disturbed sleep pattern related to drug-induced insomnia.
- Deficient knowledge related to drug therapy.

Planning outcome goals
- The patient's underlying condition will improve.
- The patient will exhibit an adequate sleeping pattern.
- The patient and family will demonstrate an understanding of drug therapy.

Implementation
- Give the drug at least 6 hours before bedtime to avoid sleep interference.
- Prolonged use may cause psychological dependence or habituation, especially in patients with histories of drug addiction.
- After prolonged use, reduce the dosage gradually to prevent acute rebound depression.
- Advise the patient to avoid hazardous activities until the drug's CNS effects are known.
- Tell the patient to avoid drinks containing caffeine, which increases the effects of amphetamines and related amines.
- Report adverse effects, such as excess stimulation, tolerance to effect, or decreased effectiveness, to the prescriber.

Evaluation
- Patient maintains improvement in underlying condition.
- Patient experiences no insomnia with drug use.
- Patient and family demonstrate an understanding of drug therapy.

Hold the lattes for patients taking stimulants! Caffeine increases the effects of these drugs.

Quick quiz

1. Which benzodiazepine is used primarily to treat anxiety?
- A. Lorazepam
- B. Temazepam
- C. Nitrazepam
- D. Flurazepam

Answer: A. Benzodiazepines used to treat anxiety include lorazepam, alprazolam, chlordiazepoxide hydrochloride, clonazepam, diazepam, halazepam, and oxazepam.

2. Which adverse reaction is common in the patient taking buspirone?
- A. Nausea
- B. Diarrhoea
- C. Constipation
- D. Headache

Answer: D. Common reactions to buspirone include headache, dizziness, light-headedness, insomnia, rapid heart rate, and palpitations.

3. Which food should the patient taking an MAO inhibitor avoid?
- A. Cheese
- B. Apples
- C. Bananas
- D. Beer

Answer: A. Certain foods can interact with MAO inhibitors and produce severe reactions. The most serious reactions involve tyramine-rich foods, such as red wine, aged cheese, and fava beans. Foods with moderate tyramine contents, such as ripe bananas, may be eaten occasionally.

Scoring

☆☆☆ If you answered all three questions correctly, great job! You're solid with the psychotropics.

☆☆ If you answered two questions correctly, you did just fine! There's no reason for you to be depressed.

☆ If you answered only one question correctly, stay calm. A quick review of the chapter may help relieve your anxiety.

⑪ Anti-infective drugs

Just the facts

In this chapter, you'll learn:

♦ classes of drugs that act as anti-infectives

♦ uses and varying actions of these drugs

♦ absorption, distribution, metabolism, and excretion of these drugs

♦ drug interactions and adverse reactions to these drugs.

Selecting an anti-infective drug

Selecting an appropriate anti-infective drug to treat a specific infection involves several important factors:

First, the microorganism must be isolated and identified—generally through growing a culture.

Then its susceptibility to various drugs must be determined. Because culture and sensitivity results take 48 hours, treatment typically starts at assessment and is then reevaluated when test results are obtained.

The location of the infection must be considered. For therapy to be effective, an adequate concentration of the anti-infective drug must be delivered to the infection site.

Finally, the cost of the drug as well as its potential adverse effects and the possibility of patient allergies must be considered.

> Before therapy with anti-infective drugs can begin, the microorganism involved in the infection must be identified.

Preventing pathogen resistance

The usefulness of anti-infective drugs is limited by the pathogens that may develop resistance to a drug's action.

The mutants strike back

Resistance is the ability of a microorganism to live and grow in the presence of an anti-infective drug. Resistance usually results from genetic mutation of the microorganism. (See *The rise of the resistance movement*.)

Antibacterial drugs

Antibacterial drugs, also known as *antibiotics*, are drugs that either kill bacteria or inhibit the growth of bacteria. They're mainly used to treat systemic (involving the whole body rather than a localised area) bacterial infections. Antibacterial drugs include:

- aminoglycosides
- penicillins
- cephalosporins
- tetracyclines
- lincomycin derivatives
- macrolides
- vancomycin
- carbapenems
- monobactams

Antibacterial drugs treat systemic bacterial infections.

The rise of the resistance movement

Indiscriminate use of anti-infective drugs has serious consequences. Unnecessary exposure of organisms to these drugs encourages the emergence of resistant strains. These resistant strains are likely to do far more damage than their predecessors.

Make reservations

Use of anti-infective drugs should be reserved for patients with infections caused by susceptible organisms and should be used in high enough doses and for an appropriate period. New anti-infective drugs should be reserved for severely ill patients with serious infections that don't respond to conventional drugs.

- fluoroquinolones
- sulphonamides
- nitrofurantoin.

Aminoglycosides

Aminoglycosides are bactericidal (they destroy bacteria). They're effective against:
- gram-negative bacilli
- some aerobic gram-positive bacteria
- mycobacteria
- some protozoa.

Naming names

Aminoglycosides currently in use include:
- amikacin sulphate
- gentamicin sulphate
- neomycin sulphate
- paromomycin sulphate
- streptomycin sulphate
- tobramycin.

Pharmacokinetics

Because aminoglycosides are absorbed poorly from the GI tract, they're usually given parenterally. After I.V. or I.M. administration, aminoglycoside absorption is rapid and complete.

Flowing with extracellular fluid

Aminoglycosides are distributed widely in extracellular fluid. They readily cross the placental barrier but don't cross the blood-brain barrier.

You're kidney-ing me!

Aminoglycosides aren't metabolised. They're excreted primarily by the kidneys.

Pharmacodynamics

Aminoglycosides act as bactericidal drugs against susceptible organisms by binding to the bacteria's 30S subunit, a specific ribosome in the microorganism, thereby interrupting protein synthesis and causing the bacteria to die.

Reasons behind resistance

Bacterial resistance to aminoglycosides may be related to:
- failure of the drug to cross the cell membrane
- altered binding to ribosomes
- destruction of the drug by bacterial enzymes.

Aminoglycosides kill bacteria by binding to their 30S subunit ribosomes.

Prototype pro

Aminoglycosides: Gentamicin

Actions

- Inhibits protein synthesis by binding directly to the 30S ribosomal subunit; usually bactericidal

Indications

- Serious infections caused by susceptible organisms
- Prevention of endocarditis during GI and genitourinary procedures or surgery

Nursing considerations

- Monitor the patient for adverse effects, such as seizures, ototoxicity, nephrotoxicity, apnea, anaphylaxis, leucopenia, thrombocytopenia, and agranulocytosis.
- Peak gentamicin level occurs 1 hour after I.M. injection or 30 minutes after I.V. infusion; check trough levels before the next dose.

Penetration power provided by penicillin

Some gram-positive enterococci resist aminoglycoside transport across the cell membrane. When penicillin is used with aminoglycoside therapy, the cell wall is altered, allowing the aminoglycoside to penetrate the bacterial cell. (See *Aminoglycosides: Gentamicin.*)

Pharmacotherapeutics

Aminoglycosides are most useful in treating:
- infections caused by gram-negative bacilli
- serious nosocomial (hospital-acquired) infections, such as gram-negative bacteraemia (abnormal presence of microorganisms in the bloodstream), peritonitis (inflammation of the peritoneum, the membrane that lines the abdominal cavity), and pneumonia in critically ill patients
- urinary tract infections (UTIs) caused by enteric bacilli that are resistant to less-toxic antibacterial drugs, such as penicillins and cephalosporins
- infections of the central nervous system (CNS) and the eye (treated with local instillation).

Combo care

Aminoglycosides are used in combination with penicillins to treat infections caused by gram-positive organisms, such as staphylococci and enterococci. Combination therapy increases the drugs' effectiveness.

Taming strains

Individual aminoglycosides may have their own particular usefulness:
• Streptomycin is active against many strains of mycobacteria, including *Mycobacterium tuberculosis*, and against the gram-positive bacteria *Nocardia* and *Erysipelothrix*.
• Amikacin, gentamicin, and tobramycin are active against *Acinetobacter, Citrobacter, Enterobacter, Escherichia coli, Klebsiella, Proteus* (indole-positive and indole-negative), *Providencia, Pseudomonas aeruginosa*, and *Serratia*.

When the drug's a dud

Aminoglycosides are inactive against anaerobic bacteria.

Drug interactions

Carbenicillin and ticarcillin reduce the effects of amikacin, gentamicin, neomycin, streptomycin, and tobramycin. This is especially true if the penicillin and aminoglycoside are mixed in the same container or I.V. line.

Amplified effects

Amikacin, gentamicin, neomycin, streptomycin, and tobramycin administered with neuromuscular blockers increase neuromuscular blockade, resulting in increased muscle relaxation and respiratory distress.

Toxic mix

Toxicity to the kidneys may result in renal failure and toxicity to the neurologic system results in peripheral neuropathy with numbness and tingling of extremities. The risk of renal toxicity also increases when amikacin, gentamicin, or tobramycin is taken with ciclosporine, amphotericin B, or aciclovir.

Oh dear, those poor ears

The symptoms of ototoxicity (damage to the ear) caused by aminoglycosides may be masked by antiemetic drugs. Loop diuretics taken with aminoglycosides increase the risk of ototoxicity. Hearing loss may occur in varying degrees and may be irreversible.

Adverse reactions

Serious adverse reactions limit the use of aminoglycosides and include:
• neuromuscular reactions, ranging from peripheral nerve toxicity to neuromuscular blockade

- ototoxicity
- renal toxicity.

Oral report

Adverse reactions to oral aminoglycosides include:
- nausea
- vomiting
- diarrhoea.

Nursing process

These nursing process steps are appropriate for patients undergoing treatment with aminoglycosides.

Assessment
- Obtain the patient's allergy history.
- Obtain culture and sensitivity tests before giving the first dose; therapy may begin pending test results. Check these tests periodically to assess the drug's efficacy.
- Assess vital signs, electrolyte levels, hearing ability, and renal function studies before and during therapy.
- Weigh the patient and review baseline renal function studies before therapy and then regularly during therapy. Notify the prescriber of changes so that the dosage may be adjusted.
- Assess for drug interactions and adverse reactions.
- Assess the patient's and family's knowledge of drug therapy.

Key nursing diagnoses
- Risk for injury related to adverse effects of drug.
- Risk for infection related to drug-induced superinfection.
- Risk for deficient fluid volume related to adverse GI reactions.

Planning outcome goals
- The patient's risk of injury will be minimised.
- The patient's risk of superinfection will be minimised.
- Fluid volume will remain within normal limits as evidenced by vital signs and intake and output.

Implementation
- Keep the patient well hydrated to minimise chemical irritation of the renal tubules.
- Don't add or mix other drugs with I.V. infusions, particularly penicillins, which inactivate aminoglycosides. If other drugs must be given I.V., temporarily stop infusion of the primary drug.

Because of the potential for ototoxicity, make sure you assess the patient's hearing ability before and during therapy with aminoglycosides.

- Follow the manufacturer's instructions for reconstitution, dilution, and storage of drugs; check expiration dates.
- Shake oral suspensions well before administering.
- Administer an I.M. dose deep into a large muscle mass (gluteal or midlateral thigh); rotate injection sites to minimise tissue injury. Apply ice to the injection site to relieve pain.
- Because too-rapid I.V. administration may cause neuromuscular blockade, infuse an I.V. drug continuously or intermittently over 30 to 60 minutes for adults and over 1 to 2 hours for infants; dilution volume for children is determined individually.
- With gentamicin, draw blood to check for peak level 1 hour after I.M. injection (30 minutes to 1 hour after I.V. infusion); for trough level, draw a sample just before the next dose. Peak gentamicin levels above 12 mcg/ml and trough levels above 2 mcg/ml may increase the risk of toxicity. Time and date all blood samples. Don't use a heparinised tube to collect blood samples because it interferes with results.
- Be aware that haemodialysis (8 hours) removes up to 50% of gentamicin from blood. Scheduling of dosages may need to be adjusted accordingly.
- Notify the prescriber about signs of decreasing renal function or changes in hearing.
- Be aware that therapy usually continues for 7 to 10 days. If no response occurs in 3 to 5 days, therapy may be stopped and new specimens obtained for culture and sensitivity testing.
- Encourage adequate fluid intake; the patient should be well hydrated while taking the drug to minimise chemical irritation of the renal tubules.

Applying ice can help relieve pain at an I.M. injection site.

Evaluation
- Patient maintains pretreatment renal function and hearing levels.
- Patient is free from infection.
- Patient maintains adequate hydration.

Penicillins

Penicillins remain one of the most important and useful antibacterial drugs, despite the availability of numerous others. The penicillins can be divided into four groups:
- natural penicillins (benzylpenicillin, phenoxymethylpenicillin)
- penicillinase-resistant penicillins (flucoxacillin)
- aminopenicillins (amoxicillin, ampicillin)
- extended-spectrum penicillins (piperacillin, ticarcillin disodium).

Pharmacokinetics

After oral administration, penicillins are absorbed mainly in the duodenum and the upper jejunum of the small intestine.

Affecting absorption

Absorption of oral penicillin varies and depends on such factors as:
- particular penicillin used
- pH of the patient's stomach and intestine
- presence of food in the GI tract.

Food factors

Most penicillins should be given on an empty stomach (1 hour before or 2 hours after a meal) to enhance absorption. Penicillins that can be given without regard to meals include amoxicillin, phenoxymethylpenicillin, and amoxicillin-clavulanate potassium (co-amoxiclav).

Well travelled

Penicillins are distributed widely to most areas of the body, including the lungs, liver, kidneys, muscle, bone, and placenta. High concentrations also appear in urine, making penicillins useful in treating UTIs.

Exit route

Penicillins are metabolised to a limited extent in the liver to inactive metabolites. Most penicillins are excreted 60% unchanged by the kidneys.

Pharmacodynamics

Penicillins are usually bactericidal in action. They bind reversibly to several enzymes outside the bacterial cytoplasmic membrane. These enzymes, known as *penicillin-binding proteins (PBPs)*, are involved in cell-wall synthesis and cell division. Interference with these processes inhibits cell-wall synthesis, causing rapid destruction of the cell.

Pharmacotherapeutics

No other class of antibacterial drugs provides as wide a spectrum of antimicrobial activity as the penicillins. As a class, they cover gram-positive, gram-negative, and anaerobic organisms, although specific penicillins are more effective against specific organisms.

Can't build walls! Can't divide! Too many PBPs attacked by penicillins!

Prototype pro

Natural penicillins: Benzylpenicillin

Actions

- Inhibits cell wall synthesis during microorganism multiplication
- Resists penicillinase enzymes produced by bacteria that convert penicillins to inactive penicilloic acid

Indications

- Bacterial infection caused by non-penicillinase-producing strains of gram-positive and gram-negative aerobic cocci, spirochetes, or certain gram-positive aerobic and anaerobic bacilli

Nursing considerations

- Monitor the patient for adverse effects, such as seizures, anaphylaxis, leucopenia, and thrombocytopenia.
- Obtain a specimen for culture and sensitivity tests before giving the first dose. Therapy may begin pending results.

I.M. the way to go (sometimes)

Penicillin is given by I.M. injection when oral administration is inconvenient or a patient's compliance is questionable. Because long-acting preparations of benzylpenicillins are relatively insoluble, they must be administered by the I.M. route. (See *Natural penicillins: benzylpenicillin*.)

Drug interactions

Penicillins may interact with various drugs:
- Probenecid increases the plasma concentration of penicillins.
- Penicillins reduce tubular secretion of methotrexate in the kidney, increasing the risk of methotrexate toxicity.
- Tetracyclines and chloramphenicol reduce the bactericidal action of penicillins.
- Neomycin decreases the absorption of phenoxymethylpenicillin.
- The effectiveness of hormonal contraceptives is reduced when they're taken with phenoxymethylpenicillin or ampicillin. If applicable, advise the patient to use a reliable alternative method of contraception in addition to hormonal contraceptives during penicillin therapy.
- Large doses of I.V. penicillins can increase the bleeding risks of anticoagulants by prolonging bleeding time.

Taking phenoxymethyl-penicillin or ampicillin with hormonal contraceptives reduces the effectiveness of the contraceptives. Using alternative contraception methods is advised.

• High dosages of benzylpenicillin and extended-spectrum penicillins (pipericillin, ticarcillin) inactivate aminoglycosides.

Adverse reactions

Hypersensitivity reactions are the major adverse reactions to penicillins, including:
• anaphylactic reactions
• serum sickness (a hypersensitivity reaction occurring 1 to 2 weeks after injection of a foreign serum)
• drug fever
• various skin rashes.

GI didn't know this could happen

Adverse GI reactions are associated with oral penicillins and include:
• tongue inflammation
• nausea and vomiting
• diarrhoea.

Dangerous diarrhoea

The aminopenicillins and extended-spectrum penicillins can produce pseudomembranous colitis (diarrhoea caused by a change in the flora of the colon or an overgrowth of a toxin-producing strain of *Clostridium difficile*).

Nursing process

These nursing process steps are appropriate for patients undergoing treatment with penicillins.

Assessment

• Obtain a history of the patient's infection before therapy; reassess for improvement regularly thereafter.
• Assess the patient's allergy history. Try to find out whether previous reactions were true hypersensitivity reactions or adverse reactions (such as GI distress) that the patient interpreted as an allergy.
• Obtain culture and sensitivity tests before giving the first dose; therapy may begin pending test results. Repeat these tests periodically to assess the drug's effectiveness.
• Monitor vital signs, electrolytes, and renal function studies.
• Assess the patient's consciousness and neurologic status when giving high doses; CNS toxicity can occur.

- Because coagulation abnormalities and bleeding can follow high doses, especially of extended-spectrum penicillins, monitor prothrombin time (PT), International Normalised Ratio (INR), and platelet counts, and assess the patient for signs of bleeding.
- Assess for adverse reactions and drug interactions.
- Assess the patient's and family's knowledge of drug therapy.

Key nursing diagnoses
- Risk for infection related to altered immune status.
- Risk for deficient fluid volume related to adverse GI reactions.
- Deficient knowledge related to drug therapy.

Planning outcome goals
- The patient's infection will resolve as evidenced by negative cultures, normal temperature, and normal white blood cell (WBC) counts.
- The patient will maintain adequate fluid hydration.
- The patient and family will demonstrate an understanding of drug therapy.

Implementation
- Give penicillins at least 1 hour before bacteriostatic antibacterial drugs (tetracyclines, erythromycins, and chloramphenicol); these drugs inhibit bacterial cell growth and decrease the rate of penicillin uptake by bacterial cell walls.
- Follow the manufacturers' directions for reconstituting, diluting, and storing drugs; check expiration dates.
- Give oral penicillins at least 1 hour before or 2 hours after meals to enhance GI absorption.
- Refrigerate oral suspensions (stable for 14 days); shake well before administering to ensure correct dosage.
- Give an I.M. dose deep into large muscle mass (gluteal or midlateral thigh), rotate injection sites to minimise tissue injury, and apply ice to the injection site to relieve pain. Don't inject more than 2 g of drug per injection site.
- With I.V. infusions, don't add or mix another drug, especially an aminoglycoside, which becomes inactive if mixed with a penicillin. If other drugs must be given I.V., temporarily stop infusion of the primary drug.
- Infuse an I.V. drug continuously or intermittently (over 30 minutes). Rotate the infusion site every 48 hours. An intermittent I.V. infusion may be diluted in 50 to 100 ml sterile water, normal saline solution, glucose 5% in water, glucose 5% in water and half-normal saline, or lactated Ringer-Lactate solution.

> Oral penicillins should be given 1 hour before or 2 hours after meals to enhance GI absorption.

Education edge

Teaching about anti-infective therapy

If anti-infective therapy is prescribed, review these points with the patient and caregivers:

- Take this drug exactly as prescribed. Complete the entire prescribed regimen, comply with instructions for around-the-clock scheduling, and keep follow-up appointments.
- Report unusual reactions, such as a rash, fever, or chills. These may be signs and symptoms of hypersensitivity to the drug.
- Check the drug's expiration date before taking it. Discard unused drug after the prescribed therapeutic regimen is taken.
- Don't share the drug with family or friends.
- If using hormonal contraceptives, use an additional form of contraception during drug therapy.
- Dispose of tissues properly and use proper hand-washing techniques to avoid spreading infection.

- Eat a balanced diet and maintain adequate fluid intake, rest, and exercise to help fight infection.
- Don't stop taking the drug, even if symptoms are relieved. The symptoms of the current infection may recur or a new infection may develop.
- Don't take drugs leftover from a previous illness or take someone else's drugs.
- Don't take other drugs, over-the-counter products, or herbal remedies without first consulting with the prescriber.
- Take the drug on an empty stomach, 1 hour before or 2 hours after meals. Food may decrease drug absorption.
- Take the drug with a full glass of water.
- Store the drug appropriately; some drugs may need refrigeration.

- Monitor the patient continuously for possible allergic reactions. A patient who has never had a penicillin hypersensitivity reaction may still have future allergic reactions.
- Monitor patients (especially elderly patients, debilitated patients, and patients receiving immunosuppressants or radiation) receiving long-term therapy for possible superinfection.
- Monitor the patient's hydration status if adverse GI reactions occur.

Evaluation
- Patient is free from infection.
- Patient maintains adequate hydration.
- Patient and family demonstrate understanding of drug therapy. (See *Teaching about anti-infective therapy*.)

Cephalosporins

Many antibacterial drugs introduced for clinical use in recent years have been cephalosporins.

Just because a patient hasn't had an allergic reaction to penicillin before doesn't mean he won't have one in the future. Make sure you monitor for possible allergic reactions during penicillin therapy.

Prototype pro

First-generation cephalosporins: Cefradine

Actions

- Inhibits cell wall synthesis promoting osmotic instability
- Usually are bactericidal

Indications

- Infection caused by susceptible organisms

Nursing considerations

- Obtain a specimen for culture and sensitivity tests before giving the first dose. Therapy may begin pending results.
- Monitor the patient for adverse effects, such as diarrhoea, haematologic disorders, rash, and hypersensitivity reactions.
- With large doses or prolonged treatment, monitor the patient for superinfections.

Therapy that spans generations

Cephalosporins are grouped into generations according to their effectiveness against different organisms, their characteristics, and their development:
- First-generation cephalosporins include cephradine. (See *First-generation cephalosporins: Cephradine*.)
- Second-generation cephalosporins include cefaclor and cefuroxime sodium.
- Third-generation cephalosporins include cefotaxime sodium, cefpodoxime, ceftazidime, and ceftriaxone sodium.
- Fourth-generation cephalosporins include cefepime hydrochloride.

Similar components = similar reactions

Because penicillins and cephalosporins are chemically similar (they both have what's called a *beta-lactam* molecular structure), cross-sensitivity occurs in 3% to 16% of patients. This means that someone who has had a reaction to penicillin is also at risk for a reaction to cephalosporins.

I'm proud to be part of four generations of infection-fighting cephalosporins!

Pharmacokinetics

Many cephalosporins are administered parenterally because they aren't absorbed from the GI tract. Some cephalosporins are absorbed from the GI tract and can be administered orally, but food usually decreases their absorption rate, although not the amount absorbed. Two cephalosporins (oral cefuroxime and cefpodoxime) actually have increased absorption when given with food.

No service to the CNS

After absorption, cephalosporins are distributed widely, although most aren't distributed in the CNS.

Crossing the line

Cefuroxime (second-generation) and the third-generation drugs cefotaxime, ceftriaxone, and ceftazidime cross the blood-brain barrier. Cefepime (fourth-generation) also crosses the blood-brain barrier, but the extent to which it does isn't known.

Much ado about metabolism

Many cephalosporins aren't metabolised at all. Cefotaxime is metabolised to the nonacetyl forms, which provide less antibacterial activity than the parent compounds. To a small extent, ceftriaxone is metabolised in the intestines to inactive metabolites, which are excreted via the biliary system.

Making an exit

All cephalosporins are excreted primarily unchanged by the kidneys with the exception of ceftriaxone, which is excreted in faeces via bile.

Pharmacodynamics

Like penicillins, cephalosporins inhibit cell-wall synthesis by binding to the bacterial PBP enzymes located on the cell membrane. After the drug damages the cell wall by binding with the PBPs, the body's natural defense mechanisms destroy the bacteria. (See *How cephalosporins attack bacteria*.)

Pharmacotherapeutics

The four generations of cephalosporins have particular therapeutic uses:
• First-generation cephalosporins, which act primarily against gram-positive organisms, may be used as alternative therapy in patients allergic to penicillin, depending on how sensitive to

> There's always an exception to the rule! Although the absorption of oral cephalosporins usually decreases when given with food, the absorption of oral cefuroxime and cefpodoxime increases with food.

Pharm function

How cephalosporins attack bacteria

The antibacterial action of cephalosporins depends on their ability to penetrate the bacterial wall and bind with proteins on the cytoplasmic membrane, as shown below.

> Cephalosporins penetrate and bind. That's how they wipe me out!

Mature bacterial cell

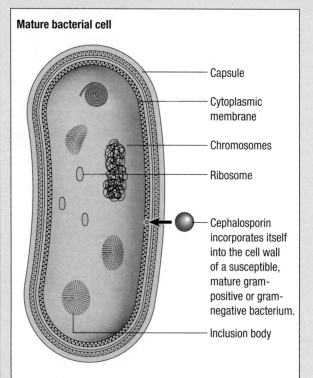

- Capsule
- Cytoplasmic membrane
- Chromosomes
- Ribosome
- Cephalosporin incorporates itself into the cell wall of a susceptible, mature gram-positive or gram-negative bacterium.
- Inclusion body

Daughter cells after division

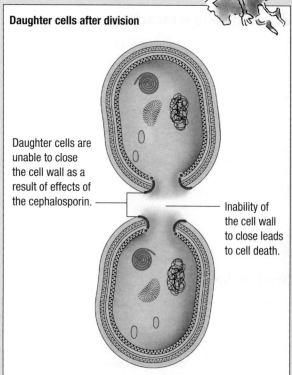

Daughter cells are unable to close the cell wall as a result of effects of the cephalosporin.

Inability of the cell wall to close leads to cell death.

penicillin the person is. They're also used to treat staphylococcal and streptococcal infections, including pneumonia, cellulitis (skin infection), and osteomyelitis (bone infection).

- Second-generation cephalosporins act against gram-negative bacteria.
- Third-generation cephalosporins, which act primarily against gram-negative organisms, are the drugs of choice for infections caused by *Enterobacter*, *P. aeruginosa*, and anaerobic organisms.
- Fourth-generation cephalosporins are active against a wide range of gram-positive and gram-negative bacteria.

Drug interactions

Patients receiving cephalosporins who drink alcoholic beverages with or up to 72 hours after taking a dose may experience acute alcohol intolerance, with such signs and symptoms as headache, flushing, dizziness, nausea, vomiting, or abdominal cramps within 30 minutes of alcohol ingestion. This reaction can occur up to 3 days after discontinuing the antibiotic.

Advantageous interaction

Uricosurics (drugs to relieve gout), such as probenecid and sulfinpyrazone, can reduce kidney excretion of some cephalosporins. Sometimes, probenecid is used therapeutically to increase and prolong plasma cephalosporin concentrations.

Adverse reactions

Adverse reactions to cephalosporins include:
- confusion
- seizures
- bleeding
- nausea
- vomiting
- diarrhoea.

Bleed, indeed

Some cephalosporins, ceftriaxone in particular, may be associated with a decrease in PT and partial thromboplastin time, leading to an increased risk of bleeding. Populations at risk include elderly, debilitated, malnourished, and immunocompromised patients and those with renal impairment, hepatic disease, or impaired vitamin K synthesis or storage.

Systemically speaking

Hypersensitivity reactions are the most common systemic adverse reactions to cephalosporins and include:
- hives
- itching
- rash that appears like the measles
- serum sickness (reaction after injection of a foreign serum characterised by oedema, fever, hives, and inflammation of the blood vessels and joints)
- anaphylaxis (in rare cases).

Cephalosporins and alcohol don't mix. Acute alcohol intolerance can occur, even 3 days after stopping the drug.

Nursing process

These nursing process steps are appropriate for patients undergoing treatment with cephalosporins.

Assessment

- Review the patient's allergy history. Try to determine whether previous reactions were true hypersensitivity reactions or adverse effects (such as GI distress) that the patient interpreted as an allergy.
- Assess the patient continuously for possible hypersensitivity reactions or other adverse effects.
- Obtain a culture and sensitivity specimen before administering the first dose; therapy may begin pending test results. Check test results periodically to assess the drug's effectiveness.

Key nursing diagnoses

- Risk for infection related to superinfection.
- Risk for deficient fluid volume related to adverse GI reactions.
- Deficient knowledge related to drug therapy.

Planning outcome goals

- The patient's infection will resolve as evidenced by culture reports, temperature, and WBC counts.
- The patient will maintain adequate fluid volume.
- The patient and family will demonstrate an understanding of drug therapy.

Implementation

- Administer cephalosporins at least 1 hour before bacteriostatic antibacterial drugs (tetracyclines, erythromycins, and chloramphenicol); by decreasing cephalosporin uptake by bacterial cell walls, the antibacterial drugs inhibit bacterial cell growth.
- Refrigerate oral suspensions (stable for 14 days); shake well before administering to ensure correct dosage.
- Follow the manufacturers' directions for reconstitution, dilution, and storage of drugs; check expiration dates.
- Administer an I.M. dose deep into a large muscle mass (gluteal or midlateral thigh); rotate injection sites to minimise tissue injury.
- Don't add or mix other drugs with I.V. infusions, particularly aminoglycosides, which are inactivated if mixed with cephalosporins. If other drugs must be given I.V., temporarily stop infusion of the primary drug.
- Ensure adequate dilution of the I.V. infusion and rotate injection sites every 48 hours to help minimise local vein irritation; using a small-gauge needle in a larger available vein may be helpful.

Education edge

Teaching about cephalosporins

If cephalosporins are prescribed, review these points with the patient and caregivers:

- Take the drug exactly as prescribed for as long as prescribed. Follow the prescriber's instructions for maintaining an around-the-clock dosage.
- Take the oral form with food if GI irritation occurs.
- Review proper storage and disposal of the drug, and check the drug's expiration date before use.
- Watch for signs and symptoms of hypersensitivity (such as hives, itching, or rash) and other adverse reactions. Report any unusual effects.
- Report signs and symptoms of bacterial and fungal superinfection promptly.

- Eat yogurt or drink buttermilk to prevent intestinal superinfection resulting from the drug's suppression of normal intestinal flora.
- If diabetic and required to monitor urine glucose, use Diastix. Don't use Clinitest because results may be incorrect.
- Keep all follow-up appointments.
- Don't take other drugs, over-the-counter preparations, or herbal remedies without first consulting with the prescriber.

- Monitor renal function studies; dosages of certain cephalosporins must be lowered in patients with severe renal impairment. In patients with decreased renal function, monitor blood urea nitrogen (BUN) and creatinine levels and urine output for significant changes.
- Monitor PT and platelet counts, and assess the patient for signs of hypoprothrombinaemia, which may occur (with or without bleeding) during therapy with ceftriaxone.
- Monitor patients on long-term therapy for possible bacterial and fungal superinfection, especially elderly and debilitated patients and those receiving immunosuppressants or radiation therapy. Signs and symptoms include fever, malaise, muscular aches and pains, and oral ulcerations.
- Monitor susceptible patients receiving sodium salts of cephalosporins for possible fluid retention.

Evaluation
- Patient is free from infection.
- Patient maintains adequate hydration.
- Patient and family demonstrate understanding of drug therapy.
(See *Teaching about cephalosporins*.)

Tetracyclines

Tetracyclines are broad-spectrum antibacterial drugs. They may be classified as:
• intermediate-acting compounds, such as demeclocycline hydrochloride
• long-acting compounds, such as doxycycline hyclate and minocycline hydrochloride.

Pharmacokinetics

Tetracyclines are absorbed from the duodenum when taken orally. They're distributed widely into body tissues and fluids and concentrated in bile. The drug is calcium bound and should not be taken with or after meals, particularly those containing calcium-rich foods.

The way out

Tetracyclines are excreted primarily by the kidneys. Doxycycline is also excreted in faeces. Minocycline undergoes enterohepatic recirculation.

Tetracyclines inhibit bacteria growth or multiplication.

Pharmacodynamics

All tetracyclines are primarily bacteriostatic, meaning they inhibit the growth or multiplication of bacteria. They penetrate the bacterial cell by an energy-dependent process. Within the cell, they bind primarily to a subunit of the ribosome, inhibiting the protein synthesis required for maintaining the bacterial cell. (See *Tetracyclines: Tetracycline hydrochloride.*)

Packing more bacteriostatic action

The long-acting compounds doxycycline and minocycline provide more action against various organisms than other tetracyclines.

Pharmacotherapeutics

Tetracyclines provide a broad spectrum of activity, which means they cover a wide range of organisms, including:
• gram-positive and gram-negative aerobic and anaerobic bacteria
• spirochetes
• mycoplasmas
• rickettsiae
• chlamydiae
• some protozoa.
    Tetracyclines are particularly used to treat:
• Lyme disease

Prototype pro

Tetracyclines: Tetracycline hydrochloride

Actions

- Is bacteriostatic but may be bactericidal against certain organisms
- Binds reversibly to 30S and 50S ribosomal subunits, inhibiting bacterial protein synthesis

Indications

- Infection caused by susceptible organisms
- Gonorrhea

Nursing considerations

- Obtain a specimen for culture and sensitivity tests before giving the first dose. Therapy may begin pending results.
- Monitor the patient for adverse effects, such as nausea, vomiting, diarrhoea, haematologic disorders, Stevens-Johnson syndrome, intracranial hypertension, rash, photosensitivity, and hypersensitivity reactions.
- With large doses or prolonged treatment, monitor the patient for superinfections.

- nongonococcal urethritis caused by *Chlamydia* and *Ureaplasma urealyticum.*

Two-timing

Combination therapy with a tetracycline and streptomycin is the most effective treatment for brucellosis.

Faces are going clear up

Tetracyclines in low dosages effectively treat acne because they decrease the fatty acid content of sebum.

Drug interactions

Tetracyclines can reduce the effectiveness of hormonal contraceptives, which may result in breakthrough bleeding or ineffective contraception. Patients taking hormonal contraceptives should use a reliable, secondary method of contraception. Tetracyclines may also decrease the bactericidal action of penicillin.

Creating new pharmacodynamics

Other interactions commonly affect the ability of tetracyclines to move through the body:
- Aluminium, calcium, and magnesium antacids reduce the absorption of oral tetracyclines.

Low dosages of tetracyclines are used to treat acne.

- Iron salts, reduce the absorption of doxycycline, oxytetracycline, and tetracycline. Reduced absorption can be prevented by separating doses of tetracyclines and iron salts by 2 to 3 hours.
- Barbiturates, carbamazepine, and phenytoin increase the metabolism and reduce the antibiotic effect of doxycycline.

Be wary of dairy

Tetracyclines, with the exception of doxycycline and minocycline, may also interact with milk and milk products, which bind with the drugs and prevent their absorption. To prevent decreased absorption, administer the tetracycline 1 hour before or 2 hours after meals.

Adverse reactions
Tetracyclines produce many of the same adverse reactions as other antibacterials, including:
- superinfection (overgrowth of resistant organisms)
- nausea
- vomiting
- abdominal distress and distention
- diarrhoea.
  Other adverse reactions include:
- photosensitivity reactions (red rash on areas exposed to sunlight)
- hepatic toxicity
- renal toxicity.

Tetracyclines can also interact with milk!

Nursing process
These nursing process steps are appropriate for patients undergoing treatment with tetracyclines.

Assessment
- Assess the patient's allergy history.
- Assess the patient for adverse reactions.
- Obtain a specimen for culture and sensitivity tests before giving the first dose; therapy may being pending test results. Check cultures periodically to assess the drug's effectiveness.

Key nursing diagnoses
- Risk for infection related to altered immune status.
- Risk for deficient fluid volume related to adverse GI reactions.
- Deficient knowledge related to drug therapy.

Planning outcome goals
- The patient's infection will resolve as evidenced by culture reports, temperature, and WBC counts.

- The patient's fluid volume will remain within normal limits as evidenced by intake and output.
- The patient and family will demonstrate an understanding of drug therapy.

Implementation
- Give all oral tetracyclines (except doxycycline and minocycline) 1 hour before or 2 hours after meals for maximum absorption; don't give tetracyclines with food, milk, or other dairy products, sodium bicarbonate, iron compounds, or antacids, which may impair absorption.
- Give water with and after the patient takes the oral drug to facilitate passage to the stomach. Incomplete swallowing can cause severe oesophageal irritation.
- Don't give the drug within 1 hour of bedtime to prevent oesophageal reflux.
- Follow the manufacturer's directions for reconstituting and storing the drug; keep the drug refrigerated and away from light.
- Check the drug's expiration date before administration. Outdated tetracyclines may cause nephrotoxicity.
- Monitor the patient for bacterial and fungal superinfection, especially if the patient is elderly, debilitated, or receiving immunosuppressants or radiation therapy. Watch especially for oral candidiasis.
- Monitor I.V. injection sites and rotate them routinely to minimise local irritation. I.V. administration may cause severe phlebitis.

Evaluation
- Patient is free from infection.
- Patient maintains adequate hydration.
- Patient and family demonstrate understanding of drug therapy. (See *Teaching about tetracyclines*.)

Clindamycin

Clindamycin is a drug that is prescribed only when there's no therapeutic alternative because of its high potential for causing serious adverse effects. It's used for various gram-positive and anaerobic organisms.

Pharmacokinetics
When taken orally, clindamycin is absorbed well and distributed widely in the body. It's metabolised by the liver and excreted by the kidneys and biliary pathways.

Education edge

Teaching about tetracyclines

If tetracyclines are prescribed, review these points with the patient and caregivers:

- Take the drug exactly as prescribed for as long as prescribed.
- Keep all follow-up appointments.
- Don't take the drug with food, milk or other dairy products, sodium bicarbonate, or iron compounds because they may interfere with absorption.
- Wait 3 hours after taking a tetracycline before taking an antacid.
- Check the drug's expiration date before using and discard expired drug.
- Report adverse reactions promptly.
- Avoid direct exposure to sunlight and use a sunscreen to help prevent photosensitivity reactions.

Pharmacodynamics

Clindamycin inhibits bacterial protein synthesis and may also inhibit the binding of bacterial ribosomes. At therapeutic concentrations, clindamycin is primarily bacteriostatic against most organisms.

Pharmacotherapeutics

Because of its potential for causing serious toxicity and pseudomembranous colitis (characterised by severe diarrhoea, abdominal pain, fever, and mucus and blood in faeces), clindamycin is limited to a few clinical situations in which safer alternative antibacterials aren't available:

- It's potent against most aerobic gram-positive organisms, including staphylococci, streptococci (except *Enterococcus faecalis*), and pneumococci.
- It's effective against most of the clinically important anaerobes and is used primarily to treat anaerobic intra-abdominal, pleural, or pulmonary infections caused by *Bacteroides fragilis*. It's also used as an alternative to penicillin in treating *Clostridium perfringens* infections.
- It may be used as an alternative to penicillin in treating staphylococcal infections in patients who are allergic to penicillin.

Because of its high potential for causing serious adverse effects, clindamycin is a last resort, of sorts.

Drug interactions

Clindamycin has neuromuscular blocking properties and may enhance the neuromuscular blocking action of neuromuscular blockers. This can lead to profound respiratory depression.

Adverse reactions

Pseudomembranous colitis may occur with clindamycin use. This syndrome can be fatal and requires prompt discontinuation of the drug as well as aggressive fluid and electrolyte management. Although this is the most serious reaction to clindamycin and limits its use, other reactions may also occur, such as:

- diarrhoea
- stomatitis (mouth inflammation)
- nausea
- vomiting
- hypersensitivity reactions.

Nursing process

These nursing process steps are appropriate for patients undergoing treatment with clindamycin.

Assessment
- Assess the patient's infection before therapy and regularly throughout therapy.
- Obtain a specimen for culture and sensitivity tests before giving the first dose. Therapy may begin pending results.
- Monitor renal, hepatic, and haematopoietic functions during prolonged therapy.
- Assess for adverse reactions and drug interactions.
- Monitor the patient's hydration status if adverse GI reactions occur.
- Assess the patient's and family's knowledge about drug therapy.

Key nursing diagnoses
- Risk for infection related to altered immune status.
- Risk for deficient fluid volume related to adverse GI reactions.
- Deficient knowledge related to drug therapy.

Planning outcome goals
- The patient's infection will resolve as evidenced by culture reports, temperature, and WBC counts.
- Fluid volume will remain within normal limits as evidenced by intake and output.
- The patient and family will demonstrate an understanding of drug therapy.

Implementation
- Don't refrigerate a reconstituted oral solution because it will thicken. The drug is stable for 2 weeks at room temperature.
- Give the capsule form with a full glass of water to prevent dysphagia.
- Check the I.V. site daily for phlebitis and irritation. Follow the drug's dilution protocol and administer as directed.
- Inject the drug deeply I.M. and rotate sites. Warn the patient that I.M. injection may be painful. Doses over 600 mg per injection aren't recommended.
- Be aware that I.M. injection may raise creatine kinase levels in response to muscle irritation.
- Don't give opioid antidiarrhoeals to treat drug-induced diarrhoea; they may prolong and worsen diarrhoea.

Evaluation
- Patient is free from infection.
- Patient maintains adequate hydration.
- Patient and family demonstrate an understanding of drug therapy.

Don't refrigerate reconstituted oral clindamycin because it will thicken.

Macrolides

Macrolides are used to treat a number of common infections. They include erythromycin and its derivatives, such as:

- erythromycin
- erythromycin ethylsuccinate
- erythromycin lactobionate
- erythromycin stearate.
  Other macrolides include:
- azithromycin
- clarithromycin
- telithromycin.

Pharmacokinetics

Because erythromycin is acid-sensitive, it must be buffered or have an enteric coating to prevent destruction by gastric acid. Erythromycin is absorbed in the duodenum. It's distributed to most tissues and body fluids except, in most cases, cerebrospinal fluid (CSF). However, as a class, macrolides can enter the CSF when meninges are inflamed.

Following many paths

Erythromycin is metabolised by the liver and excreted in bile in high concentrations; small amounts are excreted in urine. It also crosses the placental barrier and is secreted in breast milk.

Something in common

Azithromycin is rapidly absorbed by the GI tract and is distributed throughout body. It readily penetrates cells but doesn't readily enter the CNS. Like erythromycin, azithromycin is excreted mostly in bile; small amounts are excreted in urine.

Different exits

Clarithromycin and telithromycin are rapidly absorbed and widely distributed; clarithromycin is excreted in urine, whereas dirithromycin is excreted in bile and urine.

Pharmacodynamics

Macrolides inhibit ribonucleic acid (RNA)–dependent protein synthesis by acting on a small portion of the ribosome, much like clindamycin.

> Being the acid-sensitive erythromycin I am, I must be buffered or have an enteric coating to prevent being destroyed by gastric acid.

Pharmacotherapeutics

Erythromycin has a range of therapeutic uses.
- It provides a broad spectrum of antimicrobial activity against gram-positive and gram-negative bacteria, including *Mycobacterium*, *Treponema*, *Mycoplasma*, and *Chlamydia*.
- It's effective against pneumococci and group A streptococci.
- *Staphylococcus aureus* is sensitive to erythromycin; however, resistant strains may appear during therapy.
- It's the drug of choice for treating *Mycoplasma pneumoniae* infections as well as pneumonia caused by *Legionella pneumophila*.

More tolerable

In patients who are allergic to penicillin, erythromycin is effective for infections produced by group A beta-haemolytic streptococci or *Streptococcus pneumoniae*. It may also be used to treat gonorrhea and syphilis in patients who can't tolerate benzylpenicillin or the tetracyclines. Erythromycin may also be used to treat minor staphylococcal infections of the skin. (See *Erythromycin therapy exception*.)

Applaud for the broads (spectrums, that is)

Each of these broad-spectrum antibacterial drugs (drugs that cover a wide range of organisms) has its own therapeutic actions:
- Azithromycin provides a broad spectrum of antimicrobial activity against gram-positive and gram-negative bacteria, including *Mycobacterium*, *S. aureus*, *Haemophilus influenzae*, *Moraxella catarrhalis*, and *Chlamydia*.
- Azithromycin is also effective against pneumococci and groups C, F, and G streptococci.
- Clarithromycin is active against gram-positive aerobes, such as *S. aureus*, *S. pneumoniae*, and *Streptococcus pyogenes*; gram-negative aerobes, such as *H. influenzae* and *M. catarrhalis*; and other aerobes such as *M. pneumoniae*.
- Clarithromycin has been used in combination with antacids, histamine-2 (H_2) blockers, and proton pump inhibitors to treat *Helicobacter pylori*–induced duodenal ulcer disease.
- Telithromycin should only be used to treat beta-haemolytic streptococcal pharyngitis and tonsillitis, sinusitis, community aquired pneumonia, and exacerbations of chronic bronchitis if caused by organisms resistant to beta-lactam antibacterial agents or macrolides, or if conventional therapies are contra-indicated.

Erythromycin therapy exception

The use of erythromycin to prevent bacterial endocarditis in patients who haven't previously received erythromycin therapy is no longer recommended However, erythromycin may still be used for prophylaxis in individual patients who have previously responded to the drug.

Drug interactions

Macrolides may cause these drug interactions:
• Erythromycin, azithromycin, and clarithromycin can increase theophylline levels in patients receiving high dosages of theophylline, increasing the risk of theophylline toxicity.
• Clarithromycin may increase the concentration of carbamazepine when the drugs are used together.

Adverse reactions

Although macrolides produces few adverse effects, they may produce:
• epigastric distress
• nausea and vomiting
• diarrhoea (especially with large doses)
• rashes
• fever
• eosinophilia (an increase in the number of eosinophils, a type of WBC)
• anaphylaxis.

Why me? Epigastric distress is an adverse effect of macrolides.

Nursing process

These nursing process steps are appropriate for patients undergoing treatment with macrolides.

Assessment

• Assess the patient's infection before therapy and regularly throughout therapy.
• Obtain a specimen for culture and sensitivity tests before giving the first dose. Therapy may begin pending results.
• Assess for adverse reactions and drug interactions.
• Assess the patient's and family's knowledge about drug therapy.

Key nursing diagnoses

• Risk for infection related to altered immune status.
• Risk for deficient fluid volume related to adverse GI reactions.
• Deficient knowledge related to drug therapy.

Planning outcome goals

• The patient's infection will resolve as evidenced by culture reports, temperature, and WBC counts.
• Fluid volume will remain within normal limits as evidenced by intake and output.
• The patient and family will demonstrate an understanding of drug therapy.

Implementation
- When giving the suspension, note the concentration.
- For best absorption, give the oral form with a full glass of water 1 hour before or 2 hours after meals.
- Coated tablets may be taken with meals.
- Tell the patient not to drink fruit juice with the drug.
- Chewable erythromycin tablets shouldn't be swallowed whole.
- Coated tablets or encapsulated pellets cause less GI upset; they may be more tolerable in patients who can't tolerate erythromycin.
- Reconstitute the drug according to the manufacturer's directions, and dilute each 250 mg in at least 100 ml of normal saline solution. Infuse over 1 hour.
- Don't give erythromycin lactobionate with other drugs.
- Monitor hepatic function (increased levels of alkaline phosphatase, alanine aminotransferase, aspartate aminotransferase, and bilirubin may occur). Be aware that all erythromycin derivatives have the potential to cause hepatotoxicity in adults. Patients who develop hepatotoxicity from estolate may react similarly to treatment with other erythromycin preparations.
- Monitor the patient's hydration status if adverse GI reactions occur.

Hold the fruit juice when giving a patient macrolides.

Evaluation
- Patient is free from infection.
- Patient maintains adequate hydration.
- Patient and family demonstrate understanding of drug therapy.

Vancomycin

Vancomycin hydrochloride is used increasingly to treat methicillin-resistant *S. aureus*, which has become a major concern in the developed world. Because of the emergence of vancomycin-resistant enterococci, vancomycin must be used judiciously. As a rule of thumb, it should be used only when culture and sensitivity test results confirm the need for it.

Pharmacokinetics
Because vancomycin is absorbed poorly from the GI tract, it must be given I.V. to treat systemic infections. An oral form of vancomycin is used to treat pseudomembranous colitis. Remember, however, that I.V. vancomycin can't be used in place of oral vancomycin and vice versa. The two forms aren't interchangeable.

Did you hear the news? Vancomycin must be given I.V. to treat systemic infections because it's absorbed poorly from the GI tract.

Flowing with fluids

Vancomycin diffuses well into pleural (around the lungs), pericardial (around the heart), synovial (joint), and ascitic (in the peritoneal cavity) fluids.

And then what happens?

The metabolism of vancomycin is unknown. Approximately 85% of the dose is excreted unchanged in urine within 24 hours. A small amount may be eliminated through the liver and biliary tract.

Pharmacodynamics

Vancomycin inhibits bacterial cell-wall synthesis, damaging the bacterial plasma membrane. When the bacterial cell wall is damaged, the body's natural defenses can attack the organism.

Pharmacotherapeutics

Vancomycin has several therapeutic uses:
* It's active against gram-positive organisms, such as *Staphylococcus aureus, S. epidermidis, S. pyogenes, Enterococcus,* and *S. pneumoniae.*
* The I.V. form is the therapy of choice for patients with serious resistant staphylococcal infections who are hypersensitive to penicillins.
* The oral form is used for patients with antibiotic-associated *Clostridium difficile* colitis who can't take or have responded poorly to metronidazole.
* When used with an aminoglycoside, vancomycin is also the treatment of choice for *E. faecalis* endocarditis in patients who are allergic to penicillin.

Drug interactions

Vancomycin may increase the risk of toxicity when administered with other drugs toxic to the kidneys and organs of hearing, such as aminoglycosides, amphotericin B, cisplatin, bacitracin, colistin, and polymyxin B.

Adverse reactions

Adverse reactions to vancomycin, although rare, include:
* hypersensitivity and anaphylactic reactions
* drug fever
* eosinophilia
* neutropenia (reduced number of neutrophils, a type of WBC)

- hearing loss (transient or permanent) especially in excessive doses as when it is given with other ototoxic drugs.

Slow it down!

Severe hypotension may occur with rapid I.V. administration of vancomycin and may be accompanied by a red rash with flat and raised lesions on the face, neck, chest, and arms (red man's syndrome). Dosages of less than or equal to 1 g should be given over 1 hour and doses greater than 1 g given over 1.5 to 2 hours.

Nursing process

These nursing process steps are appropriate for patients undergoing treatment with vancomycin.

Assessment
- Assess the patient's infection before therapy and regularly throughout therapy.
- Obtain a specimen for culture and sensitivity tests before giving the first dose. Therapy may begin pending results.
- Obtain hearing evaluation and kidney function studies before therapy and repeat during therapy.
- Monitor serum levels regularly, especially in geriatric patients, premature neonates, and those with decreased renal function.
- Assess for adverse reactions and drug interactions.
- Assess the patient's and family's knowledge about drug therapy.

Key nursing diagnoses
- Risk for infection related to altered immune status.
- Risk for deficient fluid volume related to adverse GI reactions.
- Deficient knowledge related to drug therapy.

Planning outcome goals
- The patient's infection will resolve as evidenced by culture reports, temperature, and WBC counts.
- Fluid volume will remain within normal limits as evidenced by intake and output.
- The patient and family will demonstrate an understanding of drug therapy.

Implementation
- Adjust the dosage for a patient with renal dysfunction.
- Know that the oral form of the drug is stable for 2 weeks if refrigerated.

- For I.V. infusion, dilute in 200 ml of saline–glucose injection solution, and infuse over 60 minutes.
- Check the I.V. site daily for phlebitis and irritation. Report the presence of pain at the infusion site. Watch for irritation and infiltration; extravasation can cause tissue damage and necrosis.
- Don't give the drug I.M.
- If red-neck or red man's syndrome occurs because drug is infused too rapidly, stop the infusion and report this finding to the prescriber.
- Refrigerate an I.V. solution after reconstitution and use it within 96 hours.
- When using vancomycin to treat staphylococcal endocarditis, give it for at least 4 weeks.

Evaluation
- Patient is free from infection.
- Patient maintains adequate hydration.
- Patient and family demonstrate understanding of drug therapy.

Carbapenems

Carbapenems are a class of beta-lactam antibacterials that includes:
- imipenem-cilastatin sodium (a combination drug)
- meropenem
- ertapenem.

Super-sized spectrum of activity

The antibacterial spectrum of activity for imipenem-cilastatin is broader than that of other antibacterial drugs studied to date. Because of this broad spectrum of activity, it's used for serious or life-threatening infection, especially gram-positive and gram-negative nosocomial infections.

Pharmacokinetics
The pharmacokinetic properties of carbapenems slightly vary.

Enabling imipenem's effects

Imipenem is given with cilastatin because imipenem alone is rapidly metabolised in the tubules of the kidneys, rendering it ineffective. After parenteral administration, imipenem-cilastatin is distributed widely. It's metabolised by several mechanisms and excreted primarily in urine.

Because of its broad spectrum of activity, imipenem-cilastatin is used for serious or life-threatening infection.

Follow the ertapenem road

Ertapenem is completely absorbed after I.V. administration and is more highly protein-bound than the other two carbapenems. It's metabolised by hydrolysis and excreted mainly in urine.

Sights on the CNS and elsewhere

After parenteral administration, meropenem is distributed widely, including to the CNS. Metabolism is insignificant; 70% of the drug is excreted unchanged in urine.

Pharmacodynamics

Imipenem-cilastatin, ertapenem, and meropenem are usually bactericidal. They exert antibacterial activity by inhibiting bacterial cell-wall synthesis.

Pharmacotherapeutics

Imipenem-cilastatin has the broadest spectrum of activity of currently available beta-lactam antibacterial drugs:
• It's effective against aerobic gram-positive species, such as *Streptococcus, Staphylococcus aureus*, and *S. epidermidis*.
• It inhibits most *Enterobacter* species.
• It inhibits *P. aeruginosa* (including strains resistant to piperacillin and ceftazidime) and most anaerobic species, including *B. fragilis*.
• It may be used to treat serious nosocomial infections and infections in immunocompromised patients caused by mixed aerobic and anaerobic organisms.

Meropenem marvels

Meropenem is indicated for treatment of intra-abdominal infections as well as for management of bacterial meningitis caused by susceptible organisms.

Enter ertapenem

Ertapenem's spectrum of activity includes intra-abdominal, skin, urinary tract, and gynaecologic infections as well as community-acquired pneumonias caused by various gram-positive, gram-negative, and anaerobic organisms.

Drug interactions

These drug interactions may occur with carbapenems:
• Taking probenecid with imipenem-cilastatin increases the serum concentration of cilastatin and slightly increases the serum concentration of imipenem.

- Probenecid may cause meropenem and ertapenem to accumulate to toxic levels.
- The combination of imipenem-cilastatin and an aminoglycoside acts synergistically against *E. faecalis*.

Adverse reactions

Common adverse reactions to imipenem-cilastatin, ertapenem, and meropenem include:
- nausea and vomiting
- diarrhoea
- hypersensitivity reactions such as rashes (particularly in patients with known hypersensitivity to penicillins).

Ertapenem extras

Ertapenem may also cause:
- seizures
- hypotension
- hyperkalaemia
- respiratory distress
- death.

What a pair! Imipenem-cilastatin is used with an aminoglycoside to fight *E. faecalis*.

Nursing process

These nursing process steps are appropriate for patients undergoing treatment with carbapenems.

Assessment
- Assess the patient's infection before therapy and regularly throughout therapy.
- Obtain a specimen for culture and sensitivity tests before giving the first dose. Therapy may begin pending results.
- Assess for adverse reactions and drug interactions.
- Assess the patient's and family's knowledge about drug therapy.

Key nursing diagnoses
- Risk for infection related to altered immune status.
- Risk for deficient fluid volume related to adverse GI reactions.
- Deficient knowledge related to drug therapy.

Planning outcome goals
- The patient's infection will resolve as evidenced by culture reports, temperature, and WBC counts.
- Fluid volume will remain within normal limits as evidenced by intake and output.
- The patient and family will demonstrate an understanding of drug therapy.

Implementation
- Don't give the drug by direct I.V. bolus injection; reconstitute it as directed. Infuse over 40 to 60 minutes. If nausea occurs, slow the infusion.
- When reconstituting the powder form, shake it until the solution is clear. Solutions may range from colourless to yellow; variations of colour within this range don't affect the drug's potency. After reconstitution, the solution is stable for 10 hours at room temperature and for 48 hours when refrigerated.
- Reconstitute the drug for an I.M. injection with 1% lidocaine hydrochloride without adrenaline (epinephrine) as directed.
- If seizures develop and persist despite using anticonvulsants, notify the prescriber, who may discontinue the drug and institute seizure precautions and protocols.
- Monitor the patient's hydration status if adverse GI reactions occur.
- In a patient with decreased or impaired renal function, the dose of carbapenems may need to be adjusted.

Evaluation
- Patient is free from infection.
- Patient maintains adequate hydration.
- Patient and family demonstrate understanding of drug therapy.

Monobactams

Monobactams are used when a patient is allergic to penicillin. They bind and inhibit enzymes like other antibacterial drugs, but their composition is slightly different. Aztreonam is the first member in this class of antibacterial drugs and the only one currently available. It's a synthetic monobactam with a narrow spectrum of activity that includes many gram-negative aerobic bacteria.

Pharmacokinetics
After parenteral administration, aztreonam is rapidly and completely absorbed and widely distributed. It's metabolised partially and excreted primarily in urine as unchanged drug.

Pharmacodynamics
Aztreonam's bactericidal activity results from inhibition of bacterial cell-wall synthesis. It binds to the PBP-3 of susceptible gram-negative bacteria, inhibiting cell-wall division and resulting in lysis.

Pharmacotherapeutics

Aztreonam is indicated in a range of therapeutic situations:
• It's effective against a variety of gram-negative aerobic organisms, including *P. aeruginosa*.
• It's effective against most strains of these organisms: *E. coli, Enterobacter, Klebsiella pneumoniae, K. oxytoca, Proteus mirabilis, Serratia marcescens, H. influenzae*, and *Citrobacter*.
• It's used to treat complicated and uncomplicated UTIs, septicaemia, and lower respiratory tract, skin and skin-structure, intra-abdominal, and gynaecologic infections caused by susceptible gram-negative aerobic bacteria.
• It's usually active against gram-negative aerobic organisms that are resistant to antibiotics hydrolysed by beta-lactamases. (Beta-lactamase is an enzyme that makes an antibacterial drug ineffective.)

When experience doesn't count

Aztreonam shouldn't be used alone as empiric therapy (treatment based on clinical experience rather than on medical data) in seriously ill patients who may have a gram-positive bacterial infection or a mixed aerobic-anaerobic bacterial infection.

Drug interactions

Aztreonam may interact with several other drugs:
• Probenecid increases serum levels of aztreonam by prolonging the tubular secretion rate of aztreonam in the kidneys.
• Synergistic or additive effects occur when aztreonam is used with aminoglycosides or other antibiotics, such as cefotaxime, clindamycin, and piperacillin.
• Potent inducers of beta-lactamase production (such as imipenem) may inactivate aztreonam. Concomitant use isn't recommended.
• Taking aztreonam with clavulanic acid–containing antibiotics (co-amoxiclav) may produce synergistic or antagonistic effects, depending on the organism involved.

Adverse reactions

Adverse reactions to aztreonam include:
• diarrhoea
• hypersensitivity and skin reactions
• hypotension
• nausea and vomiting
• transient electrocardiogram (ECG) changes (including ventricular arrhythmias)
• transient increases in serum liver enzymes.

Nursing process

These nursing process steps are appropriate for patients undergoing treatment with aztreonam.

Assessment
• Assess the patient's infection before therapy and regularly throughout therapy.
• Obtain a specimen for culture and sensitivity tests before giving the first dose. Therapy may begin pending results.
• Assess for adverse reactions and drug interactions.
• Assess the patient's and family's knowledge about drug therapy.

Key nursing diagnoses
• Risk for infection related to altered immune status.
• Risk for deficient fluid volume related to adverse GI reactions.
• Deficient knowledge related to drug therapy.

Planning outcome goals
• The patient's infection will resolve as evidenced by culture reports, temperature, and WBC counts.
• Fluid volume will remain within normal limits as evidenced by intake and output.
• The patient and family will demonstrate an understanding of drug therapy.

Implementation
• Although patients who are allergic to penicillins or cephalosporins may not be allergic to aztreonam, closely monitor patients who have had an immediate hypersensitivity reaction to these antibacterial drugs.
• To give an I.V. bolus dose, inject the drug slowly over 3 to 5 minutes, directly into a vein or I.V. tubing.
• Give infusions over 20 minutes to 1 hour.
• Give I.M. injections deep into a large muscle mass, such as the upper, outer quadrant of gluteus maximus or the lateral aspect of thigh.
• Give doses larger than 1 g by the I.V. route.
• Warn the patient receiving the drug I.M. that pain and swelling may develop at the injection site.

Evaluation
• Patient is free from infection.
• Patient maintains adequate hydration.
• Patient and family demonstrate understanding of drug therapy.

Evidence of infection can be found in the patient's culture reports, temperature, and WBC counts.

Fluoroquinolones

Fluoroquinolones are structurally similar synthetic antibacterial drugs. They're primarily administered to treat UTIs, upper respiratory tract infections, pneumonia, and gonorrhea. Examples of fluoroquinolones include:

- ciprofloxacin
- levofloxacin
- moxifloxacin hydrochloride
- norfloxacin
- ofloxacin.

Pharmacokinetics

After oral administration, fluoroquinolones are absorbed well. They aren't highly protein-bound, are minimally metabolised in the liver, and are excreted primarily in urine.

Pharmacodynamics

Fluoroquinolones interrupt deoxyribonucleic acid (DNA) synthesis during bacterial replication by inhibiting DNA gyrase, an essential enzyme of replicating DNA. As a result, the bacteria can't reproduce.

Pharmacotherapeutics

Fluoroquinolones can be used to treat a wide variety of UTIs. Each drug in this class also has specific indications:

- Ciprofloxacin is used to treat lower respiratory tract infections, infectious diarrhoea, and skin, bone, and joint infections.
- Levofloxacin is indicated for treatment of lower respiratory tract infections, skin infections, and UTIs.
- Moxifloxacin is used to treat acute bacterial sinusitis and mild to moderate community-acquired pneumonia.
- Norfloxacin is used to treat UTIs and prostatitis.
- Ofloxacin is used to treat selected sexually transmitted diseases, lower respiratory tract infections, skin and skin-structure infections, and prostatitis (inflammation of the prostate gland).

Drug interactions

Several drug interactions may occur with the fluoroquinolones:

- Administration with antacids that contain magnesium or aluminium hydroxide results in decreased absorption of the fluoroquinolone.

Who are you going to call when you need to treat a UTI? The fluoroquinolones!

• Some fluoroquinolones, such as ciprofloxacin, norfloxacin, and ofloxacin, interact with xanthine derivatives, such as aminophylline and theophylline, increasing the plasma theophylline concentration and the risk of theophylline toxicity.
• Giving ciprofloxacin or norfloxacin with probenecid results in decreased kidney elimination of these fluoroquinolones, increasing their serum concentrations and half-lives.
• Drugs that prolong the QT interval, such as antiarrhythmics, should be used cautiously during moxifloxacin therapy.

Adverse reactions

Fluoroquinolones are well tolerated by most patients, but some adverse effects may occur, including:
• dizziness
• nausea and vomiting
• diarrhoea
• abdominal pain.

Blister in the sun

Moderate to severe phototoxic reactions have occurred with direct and indirect sunlight and with artificial ultraviolet lights, both with and without sunscreen. These types of light should be avoided while the patient is on fluoroquinolone therapy and for several days after cessation of therapy.

Nursing process

These nursing process steps are appropriate for patients undergoing treatment with fluoroquinolones.

Assessment
• Assess the patient's infection before therapy and regularly throughout therapy.
• Obtain a specimen for culture and sensitivity tests before giving the first dose. Therapy may begin pending results.
• Assess for adverse reactions and drug interactions.
• Assess the patient's and family's knowledge about drug therapy.

Key nursing diagnoses
• Risk for infection related to altered immune status.
• Risk for deficient fluid volume related to adverse GI reactions.
• Deficient knowledge related to drug therapy.

Planning outcome goals
- The patient's infection will resolve as evidenced by culture reports, temperature, and WBC counts.
- Fluid volume will remain within normal limits as evidenced by intake and output.
- The patient and family will demonstrate an understanding of drug therapy.

Implementation
- Oral forms may be given 2 hours after meals, 2 hours before meals, or 6 hours after taking antacids, sucralfate, or products that contain iron (such as vitamins with mineral supplements).
- Dilute the drug for I.V. use as directed and monitor for adverse effects. Infuse slowly (over 1 hour) into a large vein.
- Adjust the dosage as necessary in a patient with impaired renal function.
- Monitor the patient's hydration status if adverse GI reactions occur.

Evaluation
- Patient is free from infection.
- Patient maintains adequate hydration.
- Patient and family demonstrate understanding of drug therapy. (See *Teaching about fluoroquinolones.*)

Education edge

Teaching about fluoroquinolones

If fluoroquinolones are prescribed, review these points with the patient and caregivers:

- Take oral form 2 hours after meals.
- Take prescribed antacids at least 2 hours after taking the drug.
- Drink plenty of fluids to reduce the risk of crystallurea.
- Avoid hazardous tasks that require alertness, such as driving, until the drug's central nervous system effects are known.

- Avoid caffeine while taking the drug; there's a potential for cumulative caffeine effects.
- Hypersensitivity reactions may occur even after the first dose. If a rash or other allergic reactions develop, stop the drug immediately and notify the prescriber.
- Stop breast-feeding during treatment or consult with the prescriber about taking a different drug.

Sulphonamides

Sulphonamides were the first effective systemic antibacterial drugs. They include:

- co-trimoxazole (sulfamethoxazole and trimethoprim)
- sulfadiazine.

The sulphonamides were the first effective systemic antibacterial drugs.

Pharmacokinetics

Most sulphonamides are well absorbed and widely distributed in the body. They're metabolised in the liver to inactive metabolites and excreted by the kidneys. Because crystalluria and subsequent stone formation may occur during the metabolic excretory phase, adequate fluid intake is highly recommended during oral sulphonamide therapy.

Pharmacodynamics

Sulphonamides are bacteriostatic drugs that prevent the growth of microorganisms by inhibiting folic acid production. The decreased folic acid synthesis decreases the number of bacterial nucleotides and inhibits bacterial growth.

Pharmacotherapeutics

Sulphonamides are commonly used to treat acute UTIs. With recurrent or chronic UTIs, the infecting organism may not be susceptible to sulphonamides. Therefore, the choice of therapy should be based on bacteria susceptibility tests.

Other targets

Sulphonamides also are used to treat infections caused by *Nocardia asteroides* and *Toxoplasma gondii*. In addition, sulphonamides exhibit a wide spectrum of activity against gram-positive and gram-negative bacteria.

Sulphonamides inhibit folic acid production. Less folic acid means less bacterial growth.

Winning combination

Co-trimoxazole (a combination of a sulfa drug and a folate antagonist) is used for various other infections, such as *Pneumocystis carinii* pneumonia, acute otitis media (due to *H. influenzae* and *S. pneumoniae*), and acute exacerbations of chronic bronchitis (due to *H. influenzae* and *S. pneumoniae*). (See *Sulphonamides: Co-trimoxazole.*)

Prototype pro

Sulphonamides: Co-trimoxazole

Actions

- Is bacteriostatic (mechanism of action correlates directly with the structural similarities it shares with para-aminobenzoic acid)
- Inhibits biosynthesis of folic acid, thus inhibiting susceptible bacteria that synthesise folic acid

Indications

- Infection of the urinary tract, respiratory tract, and ear caused by susceptible organisms
- Chronic bacterial prostatitis
- Prevention of recurrent urinary tract infection in women and of "travellers' diarrhoea"

Nursing considerations

- Obtain a specimen for culture and sensitivity tests before giving the first dose. Therapy may begin pending results.
- Monitor the patient for adverse effects such as seizures, nausea, vomiting, diarrhoea, haematologic disorders, Stevens-Johnson syndrome, toxic nephrosis, and hypersensitivity reactions.
- Reduced dosages are needed in patients with renal and hepatic impairment.
- With large doses or prolonged treatment, monitor the patient for superinfections.

Drug interactions

Sulphonamides have few significant interactions:

- They increase the hypoglycaemic effects of the sulphonylureas (oral antidiabetic drugs), which may decrease blood glucose levels.
- When taken with methenamine, they may lead to the development of crystals in the urine.
- Co-trimoxazole may increase the anticoagulant effect of coumarin anticoagulants.
- Co-trimoxazole plus ciclosporine increases the risk of kidney toxicity.

Adverse reactions

These adverse reactions may occur with sulphonamides:

- Excessively high doses of less water-soluble sulphonamides can produce crystals in the urine and deposits of sulphonamide crystals in the renal tubules; however, this complication isn't a problem with the newer water-soluble sulphonamides.
- Hypersensitivity reactions may occur and appear to increase as the dosage increases.
- A reaction that resembles serum sickness may occur, producing fever, joint pain, hives, bronchospasm, and leucopenia (reduced WBC count).
- Photosensitivity may occur.

> Patients with diabetes need to watch their glucose levels when taking sulphonamides. Sulphonamides increase the hypoglycaemic effects of oral antidiabetic drugs.

Nursing process

These nursing process steps are appropriate for patients undergoing treatment with sulphonamides.

Assessment

• Assess the patient's infection before therapy and regularly thereafter.

• Assess the patient's history of allergies, especially to sulphonamides or to drugs containing sulphur (such as thiazides, furosemide, and oral sulphonylureas).

• Assess the patient for adverse reactions and drug interactions; patients with acquired immunodeficiency syndrome (AIDS) have a much higher risk of adverse reactions.

• Obtain a specimen for culture and sensitivity tests before giving the first dose; treatment may begin pending test results. Check test results periodically to assess the drug's effectiveness.

• Monitor intake and output.

• Monitor urine cultures, full blood count (FBC), and urinalysis before and during therapy.

Before giving sulphonamides, confirm that the patient isn't allergic to drugs containing sulphur.

Key nursing diagnoses

• Risk for infection related to superinfection.

• Risk for deficient fluid volume related to adverse GI reactions.

• Deficient knowledge related to drug therapy.

Planning outcome goals

• The patient's infection will resolve as evidenced by culture reports, temperature, and WBC counts.

• Fluid volume will remain within normal limits as evidenced by intake and output.

• The patient and family will demonstrate an understanding of drug therapy.

Implementation

• Give an oral dose with 240 ml of water. Give 3 to 4 L of fluids daily, depending on the drug. Urine output should be at least 1,500 ml daily to ensure proper hydration. Inadequate urine output can lead to crystalluria or tubular deposits of the drug.

• Follow the manufacturers' directions for reconstituting, diluting, and storing drugs; check expiration dates.

• Shake oral suspensions well before administration to ensure correct dosage.

• During long-term therapy, monitor the patient for possible superinfection.

Education edge

Teaching about sulphonamides

If sulphonamides are prescribed, review these points with the patient and caregivers:

- Take the drug exactly as prescribed, complete the prescribed regimen, and keep follow-up appointments.
- Take the oral form with a full glass of water and drink plenty of fluids. The tablet may be crushed and swallowed with water to ensure maximal absorption.
- Report signs and symptoms of hypersensitivity and other adverse reactions, such as bloody urine, difficulty breathing, rash, fever, chills, or severe fatigue.
- Avoid direct sun exposure and use a sunscreen to help prevent photosensitivity reactions.
- Sulphonamides may increase the effects of oral hypoglycaemic drugs. Don't use Clinitest to monitor urine glucose levels.
- Sulphasalazine may cause an orange-yellow discoloration of urine or skin and may permanently stain soft contact lenses yellow.

Evaluation
- Patient is free from infection.
- Patient maintains adequate hydration.
- Patient and family demonstrate understanding of drug therapy.
(See *Teaching about sulphonamides*.)

Nitrofurantoin

Nitrofurantoin is a drug that has higher antibacterial activity in acid urine. It's commonly used to treat acute and chronic UTIs.

Pharmacokinetics

After oral administration, nitrofurantoin is absorbed rapidly and well from the GI tract. Taking the drug with food enhances its bioavailability.

Form facts

Nitrofurantoin is available in a microcrystalline form and a macrocrystalline form. The microcrystalline form is absorbed more slowly because of slower dissolution and thus causes less GI distress.

Oh where oh where does nitrofurantoin go?

Nitrofurantoin is 20% to 60% protein-bound. It crosses the placental barrier and is secreted in breast milk. It's also distributed in bile.

Nitrofurantoin is partially metabolised by the liver, and 30% to 50% is excreted unchanged in urine.

Pharmacodynamics

Usually bacteriostatic, nitrofurantoin may become bactericidal, depending on its urinary concentration and the susceptibility of the infecting organisms.

Zapping bacterial energy

Although its exact mechanism of action is unknown, nitrofurantoin appears to inhibit formation of acetyl coenzyme A from pyruvic acid, thereby inhibiting the energy production of the infecting organism. Nitrofurantoin also may disrupt bacterial cell-wall formation.

Pharmacotherapeutics

Because the absorbed drug concentrates in urine, nitrofurantoin is used to treat UTIs. Nitrofurantoin isn't effective against systemic bacterial infections. In addition, it isn't useful in treating pyelonephritis or perinephric (around the kidney) diseases.

Fortunately, nitrofurantoin has few significant drug interactions.

Drug interactions

Nitrofurantoin has few significant interactions:
• Probenecid and sulfinpyrazone inhibit the excretion of nitrofurantoin by the kidneys, reducing its efficacy and increasing its toxic potential.
• Magnesium salts and antacids containing magnesium can decrease the extent and rate of nitrofurantoin absorption.
• Nitrofurantoin may decrease the antibacterial activity of norfloxacin and nalidixic acid.

Adverse reactions

Adverse reactions to nitrofurantoin include:
• GI irritation
• anorexia
• nausea and vomiting
• diarrhoea
• dark yellow or brown urine
• abdominal pain
• chills
• fever
• joint pain
• anaphylaxis
• hypersensitivity reactions involving the skin, lungs, blood, and liver.

Nursing process

These nursing process steps are appropriate for patients undergoing treatment with nitrofurantoin.

Assessment
- Assess the patient's infection before therapy and regularly thereafter.
- Assess the patient's allergy history, especially allergies to sulphonamides or to drugs containing sulphur (such as thiazides, furosemide, and oral sulphonylureas).
- Assess the patient for adverse reactions and drug interactions.
- Obtain a specimen for culture and sensitivity tests before giving the first dose; treatment may begin pending results. Check these test results periodically to assess the drug's effectiveness.
- Assess the patient's and family's knowledge of drug therapy.

Key nursing diagnoses
- Risk for infection related to superinfection.
- Risk for deficient fluid volume related to adverse GI reactions.
- Deficient knowledge related to drug therapy.

Planning outcome goals
- The patient's infection will resolve as evidenced by culture reports, temperature, and WBC counts.
- Fluid volume will remain within normal limits as evidenced by intake and output.
- The patient and family will demonstrate an understanding of drug therapy.

Implementation
- Give the drug with food or milk to minimise GI distress.
- Monitor the patient for hypersensitivity, which can develop during drug therapy.
- Monitor urine cultures; treatment continues for 3 days after urine specimens become sterile.
- Monitor the patient's hydration status if adverse GI reactions occur.
- Monitor FBC and pulmonary status regularly.
- Monitor intake and output. This drug may turn urine brown or dark yellow.

Evaluation
- Patient is free from infection.
- Patient maintains adequate hydration.
- Patient and family demonstrate understanding of drug therapy.

Antiviral drugs

Antiviral drugs are used to prevent or treat viral infections ranging from influenza to human immunodeficiency virus (HIV). The major antiviral drug classes used to treat systemic infections include:

- synthetic nucleosides
- nucleoside analogue reverse transcriptase inhibitors (NRTIs)
- non-nucleoside reverse transcriptase inhibitors (NNRTIs)
- nucleotide analogue reverse transcriptase inhibitors
- protease inhibitors.

Synthetic nucleosides

Synthetic nucleosides are a group of drugs used to treat various viral syndromes that can occur in immunocompromised patients, including herpes simplex virus (HSV) and cytomegalovirus (CMV). Drugs in this class include:

- aciclovir
- famciclovir
- ganciclovir
- valaciclovir hydrochloride
- valganciclovir hydrochloride.

Pharmacokinetics

Each of these synthetic nucleosides travels its own route through the body:

- When given orally, absorption of aciclovir is slow and only 15% to 30% complete. It's distributed throughout the body and metabolised primarily inside the infected cells; most of the drug is excreted in urine.
- Famciclovir is less than 20% bound to plasma proteins. It's extensively metabolised in the liver and excreted in urine.
- Ganciclovir is administered I.V. because it's absorbed poorly from the GI tract. More than 90% of ganciclovir isn't metabolised and is excreted unchanged by the kidneys.
- Valaciclovir is converted to aciclovir during its metabolism and has pharmacokinetic properties similar to those of aciclovir.
- Valganciclovir is metabolised in the intestinal wall and liver to ganciclovir; however, interchanging the two drugs isn't effective.

Pharmacodynamics

The actions of these drugs also varies:

- Aciclovir enters virus-infected cells, where it's changed through a series of steps to aciclovir triphosphate. Aciclovir triphosphate

> Oral aciclovir metabolises primarily inside virus-infected cells.

inhibits virus-specific DNA polymerase, an enzyme necessary for viral growth, thus disrupting viral replication.
• On entry into virus-infected cells, ganciclovir is converted to ganciclovir triphosphate, which is thought to produce its antiviral activity by inhibiting viral DNA synthesis.
• Famciclovir enters viral cells (HSV types 1 and 2, varicella zoster), where it inhibits DNA polymerase, viral DNA synthesis and, thus, viral replication.
• Valaciclovir rapidly converts to aciclovir and aciclovir then becomes incorporated into viral DNA and inhibits viral DNA polymerase, thus inhibiting viral multiplication.
• Valganciclovir is converted to ganciclovir, which inhibits replication of viral DNA synthesis of CMV.

Pharmacotherapeutics

Aciclovir is an effective antiviral drug that causes minimal toxicity to cells. Oral aciclovir is used primarily to treat initial and recurrent HSV type 2 infections. (See *Antivirals: Aciclovir.*)

I.V. instances

Aciclovir I.V. is used to treat:
• severe initial HSV type 2 infections in patients with normal immune systems
• initial and recurrent skin and mucous membrane HSV type 1 and 2 infections in immunocompromised patients
• herpes zoster infections (shingles) caused by the varicella-zoster virus in immunocompromised patients
• disseminated varicella-zoster virus in immunocompromised patients
• varicella infections (chickenpox) caused by the varicella-zoster virus in immunocompromised patients.

Rounding out the group

Other synthetic nucleosides have their own therapeutic uses:
• Ganciclovir is used to treat CMV retinitis in immunocompromised patients, including those with AIDS, other CMV infections (such as encephalitis), and HSV.
• Famciclovir is used to treat acute herpes zoster, genital herpes, and recurrent herpes simplex in HIV-infected patients.
• Valganciclovir is used to treat CMV retinitis in AIDS patients.
• Valaciclovir is effective against herpes zoster, genital herpes, and herpes labialis.

Prototype pro

Antivirals: Aciclovir

Actions

• Interferes with deoxyribonucleic acid synthesis and inhibits viral multiplication

Indications

• Treatment of herpes simplex virus types 1 and 2
• Varicella

Nursing considerations

• Monitor the patient for adverse effects, such as malaise, headache, encephalopathy, renal failure, thrombocytopenia, and pain at the injection site.

Drug interactions

These drug interactions may occur with synthetic nucleosides:
• Probenecid reduces kidney excretion and increases blood levels of ganciclovir, valganciclovir, valaciclovir, famciclovir, and aciclovir, increasing the risk of toxicity.
• Taking ganciclovir with drugs that are damaging to tissue cells, such as dapsone, pentamidine isethionate, flucytosine, vincristine, vinblastine, doxorubicin, amphotericin B, and co-trimoxazole, inhibits replication of rapidly dividing cells in the bone marrow, GI tract, skin, and sperm-producing cells.
• Imipenem-cilastatin increases the risk of seizures when taken with ganciclovir or valganciclovir.
• Zidovudine increases the risk of granulocytopenia (reduced number of granulocytes, a type of WBC) when taken with ganciclovir.

Adverse reactions

Treatment with synthetic nucleosides drugs may cause these adverse reactions:
• Reversible kidney impairment may occur with rapid I.V. injection or infusion of aciclovir.
• Headache, nausea, vomiting, and diarrhoea are common reactions to oral aciclovir.
• Hypersensitivity reactions may occur with aciclovir.
• Granulocytopenia and thrombocytopenia are the most common adverse reactions to ganciclovir.
• Famciclovir and valaciclovir may cause headache and nausea.
• Valganciclovir may also cause seizures, retinal detachment, neutropenia, and bone marrow suppression.

Nursing process

These nursing process steps are appropriate for patients undergoing treatment with synthetic nucleosides.

Assessment
• Obtain a baseline assessment of the patient's viral infection; reassess regularly to monitor the drug's effectiveness.
• Assess for adverse reactions and drug interactions.
• Assess the patient's and family's knowledge of drug therapy.

Key nursing diagnoses
• Ineffective protection related to adverse haematologic reactions.
• Risk for deficient fluid volume related to adverse GI reactions.
• Deficient knowledge related to drug therapy.

Take it easy when giving aciclovir I.V. or by infusion. Although it's reversible, kidney impairment may occur.

Planning outcome goals
• The patient won't incur injury while receiving drug therapy.
• Fluid volume will remain within normal limits as evidenced by intake and output.
• The patient and family will demonstrate an understanding of drug therapy.

Implementation
• Monitor renal and hepatic function, CBC, and platelet count regularly.
• Monitor the patient's mental status when giving the drug I.V. Encephalopathic changes are more likely in patients with neurologic disorders or in those who have had neurologic reactions to cytotoxic drugs.
• Monitor the patient's hydration status if adverse GI reactions occur.
• Follow the manufacturers' guidelines for reconstituting and administering these drugs.
• Obtain a prescription for an antiemetic or antidiarrhoeal drug, if needed.
• Take safety precautions if the patient has adverse CNS reactions. For example, place the bed in a low position, raise the bed rails, and supervise ambulation and other activities.
• Notify the prescriber about serious or persistent adverse reactions.
• Instruct the patient on how to prevent spreading the infection.

Evaluation
• Patient doesn't incur injury while receiving drug therapy.
• Patient maintains adequate hydration.
• Patient and family demonstrate understanding of drug therapy. (See *Teaching about antiviral drug therapy*.)

Pyrophosphate analogues

Pyrophosphate analogues target pyrophosphate-binding sites of certain viruses. Foscarnet sodium is one such drug that's used to treat CMV retinitis in patients with AIDS. It's also used to treat aciclovir-resistant HSV infections in immunocompromised patients.

Pharmacokinetics
Foscarnet is poorly bound to plasma proteins. In patients with normal kidney function, the majority of foscarnet is excreted unchanged in the urine.

If a patient has adverse CNS reactions to an antiviral drug, take safety precautions such as supervising ambulation.

Education edge

Teaching about antiviral drug therapy

If antiviral drug therapy is prescribed, review these points with the patient and caregivers:

- Take the drug exactly as prescribed, even if signs and symptoms improve.
- Notify the prescriber promptly about severe or persistent adverse reactions.
- Keep appointments for follow-up care.
- The drug effectively manages viral infection but may not eliminate it or cure it.
- Report early signs and symptoms of infection, such as fever, pain, and itching.
- Maintain immunisations against viral infections as indicated.
- The drug won't prevent the infection from spreading to others. Use proper techniques to prevent the spread of infection. For example, avoid sexual intercourse when visible lesions are present, always wash hands after touching lesions, practice safer sex by using a condom, and avoid sharing I.V. needles.
- Maintain an adequate diet.
- Be sure to get adequate amounts of rest and exercise.

How retro

If the patient is taking antiretroviral drugs, review these additional points:

- Effective treatment of human immunodeficiency virus (HIV) requires drug therapy with several drugs and daily doses. Missing doses decreases blood levels of the drugs and results in increased HIV replication. This can result in drug-resistant viral strains.
- Don't take other drugs, over-the-counter products, or herbal preparations without first consulting the prescriber. They may make anti-HIV drugs less effective or more toxic.
- Adverse effects may vary depending on the specific drugs used; request information about the adverse effects and what to do if they occur.
- Have regular tests, such as viral load, CD4$^+$ cell count, full blood count, and renal and hepatic function, as indicated.

Pharmacodynamics

Foscarnet prevents viral replication by selectively inhibiting DNA polymerase (an enzyme that helps form DNA from a precursor substance that exists in DNA).

Pharmacotherapeutics

Foscarnet's primary therapeutic use is treating CMV retinitis in patients with AIDS. It's also used in combination therapy with ganciclovir for patients who have relapsed with either drug.

Drug interactions

Foscarnet has few drug interactions:
- Foscarnet and pentamidine together increase the risk of hypocalcaemia (low blood calcium levels) and toxicity to the kidneys.
- Using foscarnet along with other drugs that alter serum calcium levels may result in hypocalcaemia.

• The risk of kidney impairment increases when drugs toxic to the kidneys, such as amphotericin B and aminoglycosides, are taken with foscarnet. Because of the risk of kidney toxicity, patients should be aggressively hydrated during treatment.

Adverse reactions

Adverse reactions to foscarnet may include:
• fatigue
• depression
• fever
• confusion
• headache
• numbness and tingling
• dizziness
• seizures
• nausea and vomiting
• diarrhoea
• abdominal pain
• granulocytopenia
• leucopenia
• involuntary muscle contractions
• neuropathy
• difficult breathing
• rash
• altered kidney function.

Foscarnet may alter kidney function. Lucky me!

Nursing process

These nursing process steps are appropriate for patients undergoing treatment with foscarnet.

Assessment
• Obtain a baseline assessment of the patient's viral infection; reassess regularly to monitor the drug's effectiveness.
• Assess for adverse reactions and drug interactions.
• Assess the patient's and family's knowledge of drug therapy.

Key nursing diagnoses
• Ineffective protection related to adverse haematologic reactions.
• Risk for deficient fluid volume related to adverse GI reactions.
• Deficient knowledge related to drug therapy.

Planning outcome goals
• The patient won't incur injury while receiving drug therapy.
• Fluid volume will remain within normal limits as evidenced by intake and output.

- The patient and family will demonstrate an understanding of drug therapy.

Implementation
- Give the drug over at least 1 hour using an infusion pump. To minimise renal toxicity; ensure adequate hydration before and during the infusion.
- Monitor renal and hepatic function, CBC, and platelet count regularly.
- Monitor electrolyte levels (calcium, phosphate, magnesium, potassium).
- Monitor creatinine clearance two to three times weekly during induction and at least once every 1 to 2 weeks during maintenance.
- Monitor for tetany and seizures with abnormal electrolyte levels; the drug may cause dose-related transient decrease in ionised serum calcium, which may not be reflected in laboratory values.
- Monitor the patient's mental status. Encephalopathic changes are more likely in patients with neurologic disorders or in those who have had neurologic reactions to cytotoxic drugs.
- Follow the manufacturer's guidelines for reconstituting and administering the drug.
- Obtain a prescription for an antiemetic or antidiarrhoeal drug, if needed.
- Take safety precautions if the patient has adverse CNS reactions. For example, place the bed in a low position, raise the bed rails, and supervise ambulation and other activities.
- Notify the prescriber about serious or persistent adverse reactions.

To minimise renal toxicity, ensure adequate hydration before giving foscarnet.

Evaluation
- Patient doesn't incur injury while receiving therapy.
- Patient maintains adequate hydration.
- Patient and family demonstrate understanding of drug therapy.

Influenza A and syncytial virus drugs

Influenza A and syncytial virus drugs include:
- amantadine hydrochloride
- oseltamivir
- ribavirin.

Pharmacokinetics
After oral administration, amantadine and oseltamivir are well absorbed in the GI tract and widely distributed throughout the

body. Amantadine is eliminated primarily in urine; oseltamivir is extensively metabolised and then excreted in urine.

Take a deep breath

Ribavirin may be administered by nasal inhalation or by aerosol inhalation with a small-particle aerosol generator. The drug is well absorbed, but it has a limited, specific distribution, with the highest concentrations found in the respiratory tract and in red blood cells (RBCs).

Inhaled ribavirin is well absorbed but has limited distribution. Highest concentrations are found in the respiratory tract and in RBCs.

Swallow this

Ribavirin capsules are rapidly absorbed after administration and are distributed in plasma. Ribavirin is metabolised in the liver and by RBCs, and then excreted primarily by the kidneys, with some excreted in faeces.

Pharmacodynamics

Influenza A and syncytial virus drugs act in various ways:
* Although its exact mechanism of action is unknown, amantadine appears to inhibit an early stage of viral replication.
* Oseltamivir inhibits viral RNA and protein synthesis.
* The mechanism of action of ribavirin isn't known completely, but the drug's metabolites inhibit viral DNA and RNA synthesis, subsequently halting viral-replication.

Pharmacotherapeutics

Amantadine and oseltamivir are sometimes used to prevent and treat respiratory tract infections caused by strains of the influenza A virus. They can reduce the severity and duration of fever and other symptoms in patients already infected with influenza A.

Offering some protection

Amantadine and oseltamivir also protect patients who have received the influenza vaccine during the 2 weeks needed for immunity to develop as well as patients who can't take the influenza vaccine because of hypersensitivity.

Amantadine and oseltamivir can reduce the severity of symptoms in patients infected with influenza A. That's nothing to sneeze at!!

Tremor tamer

Amantadine is also used to treat parkinsonism and drug-induced extrapyramidal reactions (abnormal involuntary movements).

Ribavirin remedy

Ribavirin is used to treat respiratory syncytial virus in children as well as in combination with interferon alfa 2b to treat chronic hepatitis C in adults.

Drug interactions

These drug interactions may occur with amantadine:
- Taking anticholinergics with amantadine increases adverse anticholinergic effects.
- Amantadine given with the combination drug hydrochlorothiazide and triamterene results in decreased urine excretion of amantadine, resulting in increased amantadine levels.
- Amantadine and trimethoprim (co-trimoxazole) levels are increased when used together.

Not a troublemaker

No clinically significant drug interactions have been documented with rimantadine.

Adverse reactions

Adverse reactions with amantadine include:
- anorexia
- anxiety
- confusion
- depression
- fatigue
- forgetfulness
- hallucinations
- hypersensitivity reactions
- insomnia
- irritability
- nausea
- nervousness
- psychosis.

Ribavarin reactions

Adverse reactions to ribavirin include:
- apnea (lack of breathing)
- cardiac arrest
- hypotension
- pneumothorax (air in the pleural space, causing the lung to collapse)
- worsening of respiratory function.

Nursing process

These nursing process steps are appropriate for patients undergoing treatment with influenza A and syncytial virus drugs.

Assessment

- Obtain a baseline assessment of the patient's viral infection; reassess regularly to monitor the drug's effectiveness.
- Assess for adverse reactions and drug interactions.
- Assess the patient's and family's knowledge of drug therapy.

Key nursing diagnoses

- Ineffective protection related to adverse haematologic reactions.
- Risk for deficient fluid volume related to adverse GI reactions.
- Deficient knowledge related to drug therapy.

Planning outcome goals

- The patient won't incur injury while receiving drug therapy.
- Fluid volume will remain within normal limits as evidenced by intake and output.
- The patient and family will demonstrate an understanding of drug therapy.

Implementation

- Monitor renal and hepatic function, FBC, and platelet count regularly.
- Monitor the patient's hydration status if adverse GI reactions occur.
- If the patient has a history of heart failure, watch closely for exacerbation or recurrence during amantadine therapy.
- Follow the manufacturers' guidelines for reconstituting and administering these drugs.
- Obtain a prescription for an antiemetic or antidiarrhoeal drug, if needed.
- Take safety precautions if adverse CNS reactions occur. For example, place the bed in a low position, raise the bed rails, and supervise ambulation and other activities.
- Notify the prescriber about serious or persistent adverse reactions.
- Warn the patient with parkinsonism not to stop the drug abruptly; doing so could cause a parkinsonian crisis.

Patients with a history of heart failure should be watched for exacerbation or recurrence of the condition during amantadine therapy.

Well, of course!

Evaluation

- Patient doesn't incur injury while receiving drug therapy.
- Patient maintains adequate hydration.
- Patient and family demonstrate understanding of drug therapy.

Nucleoside analogue reverse transcriptase inhibitors

NRTIs are used to treat advanced HIV infections. Drugs in this class include:

- zidovudine
- didanosine
- abacavir sulphate
- lamivudine
- stavudine
- emtricitabine.

Leading the way

Zidovudine was the first drug to receive licence approval for treating AIDS and AIDS-related complex.

Pharmacokinetics

Each of the NRTIs has its own pharmacokinetic properties.

A familiar path

Zidovudine is well absorbed from the GI tract, widely distributed throughout the body, metabolised by the liver, and excreted by the kidneys.

Buffed up

Because didanosine is degraded rapidly in gastric acid, didanosine tablets and powder contain a buffering drug to increase pH. The exact route of metabolism isn't fully understood. Approximately one-half of an absorbed dose is excreted in urine.

Food for thought

Oral zalcitabine is well absorbed from the GI tract when administered on an empty stomach. Absorption is reduced when the drug is given with food. Zalcitabine penetrates the blood-brain barrier.

Abracad-abacavir

Abacavir is rapidly and extensively absorbed after oral administration. It's distributed in the extravascular space, and about 50% binds with plasma proteins. Abacavir is metabolised by the cytosolic enzymes and excreted primarily in urine with the remainder excreted in faeces.

Ride the rapids

Lamivudine and stavudine are both rapidly absorbed after administration and are excreted by the kidneys. Emtricitabine is rapidly and extensively absorbed after oral administration. It's also excreted by the kidneys.

Pharmacodynamics

NRTIs must undergo conversion to their active metabolites to produce their action:

* Zidovudine is converted by cellular enzymes to an active form, zidovudine triphosphate, which prevents viral DNA from replicating. (See *How zidovudine works*.)
* Didanosine undergoes cellular enzyme conversion to its active antiviral metabolites to block HIV replication.
* Abacavir is converted to an active metabolite that inhibits the activity of HIV-1 transcriptase by competing with a natural component and incorporating into viral DNA.
* Lamivudine and stavudine are converted in the cells to their active metabolites, which inhibit viral DNA replication.
* Emtricitabine inhibits the enzyme reverse transcriptase and thus inhibits viral DNA replication.

Pharmacotherapeutics

NRTIs are used to treat HIV and AIDS.

Common combinations

Lamivudine, stavudine, emtricitabine, and abacavir are used in combination with other antiretrovirals to treat HIV infection. For example, Combivir is a combination therapy that includes lamivudine and zidovudine. Trizivir is a combination therapy that includes abacavir, lamivudine, and zidovudine.

The vein game

The I.V. form of zidovudine is used as part of a multidrug regimen in hospitalised patients who can't take oral drugs. It's also used to prevent transmission of HIV from mother to foetus and to treat AIDS-related dementia.

Another option

Didanosine, in combination with other antiretrovirals, is an alternative initial treatment for HIV infection.

Pharm function

How zidovudine works

Zidovudine inhibits replication of human immunodeficiency virus (HIV). The first two illustrations show how HIV invades cells and then replicates itself. The bottom illustration shows how zidovudine blocks viral transformation.

Invade and replicate

HIV particle enters cell.

HIV uses reverse transcriptase to change its own ribonucleic acid (RNA) into deoxyribonucleic acid (DNA).

Virus-constructed DNA takes over cellular genetic mechanism.

Messenger RNA (mRNA) and other proteins form new HIV particle.

Blocked transformation

HIV particle enters cell.

Zidovudine mimics structure of reverse transcriptase so it can block viral transformation of RNA to DNA.

HIV particle
Host cell
DNA
Reverse transcriptase
RNA
Nucleus

Host cell
Nucleus
DNA
mRNA
Proteins
New HIV particle

Host cell
RNA
Reverse transcriptase
Nucleus

Drug interactions

NRTIs may be responsible for a number of drug interactions:

• Potentially fatal lactic acidosis (increased lactic acid production in the blood) and severe hepatomegaly (enlargement of liver) with steatosis (accumulation of fat) have occurred in patients taking NRTIs alone or with other antiretrovirals such as tenofovir. Most of these patients were women. Obesity and prolonged NRTI exposure may be additional risk factors.

• An increased risk of cellular and kidney toxicity occurs when zidovudine is taken with such drugs as dapsone, pentamidine isetionate, flucytosine, vincristine, vinblastine, doxorubicin, interferon, and ganciclovir.

• Taking zidovudine with probenecid, aspirin, paracetamol, indometacin, cimetidine, or lorazepam increases the risk of toxicity of either drug.

• Zidovudine plus aciclovir may produce profound lethargy and drowsiness.

• Didanosine may reduce the absorption of tetracyclines, and fluoroquinolones.

• Abacavir levels increase with alcohol consumption.

Lactic acidosis and severe hepatomegaly with steatosis can occur in patients taking NRTIs.

Bad combinations

Because of inhibition of phosphorylation (the process needed to form the active DNA-inhibiting metabolite), stavudine shouldn't be given in combination with zidovudine.

Plays well with others

Emtricitabine has no clinically significant drug interactions when used in combination with indinavir, stavudine, famciclovir, and tenofovir.

Adverse reactions

Adverse reactions to zidovudine and lamivudine include:

• blood-related reactions
• headache and fever
• dizziness
• muscle pain
• rash
• nausea and vomiting
• abdominal pain and diarrhoea.

Didanosine may cause:
- nausea and vomiting
- abdominal pain and constipation or diarrhoea
- stomatitis
- unusual taste or loss of taste
- dry mouth
- pancreatitis
- headache, peripheral neuropathy, or dizziness
- muscle weakness or pain
- rash and itchiness
- hair loss.

Stavudine may cause:
- peripheral neuropathy
- mouth ulcers
- nausea
- rash
- headache
- muscle pain
- fatigue.

Abacavir may cause potentially fatal hypersensitivity reactions. Emtricitabine may cause severe hepatomegaly and lactic acidosis.

Nursing process

These nursing process steps are appropriate for patients undergoing treatment with NRTIs.

Assessment
- Obtain a baseline assessment of the patient's viral infection; reassess regularly to monitor the drug's effectiveness.
- Assess for adverse reactions and drug interactions.
- Assess the patient's and family's knowledge of drug therapy.

Key nursing diagnoses
- Ineffective protection related to adverse haematologic reactions.
- Risk for deficient fluid volume related to adverse GI reactions.
- Deficient knowledge related to drug therapy.

Planning outcome goals
- The patient won't incur injury while receiving drug therapy.
- Fluid volume will remain within normal limits as evidenced by intake and output.
- The patient and family will demonstrate an understanding of drug therapy.

Implementation
- Monitor renal and hepatic function, CBC, and platelet count regularly.
- Monitor the patient's mental status when giving drugs I.V. Encephalopathic changes are more likely in patients with neurologic disorders or in those who have had neurologic reactions to cytotoxic drugs.
- Monitor the patient's hydration status if adverse GI reactions occur.
- Follow the manufacturers' guidelines for reconstituting and administering these drugs.
- Obtain a prescription for an antiemetic or antidiarrhoeal drug, if needed.
- Take safety precautions if adverse CNS reactions occur. For example, place the bed in a low position, raise the bed rails, and supervise ambulation and other activities.
- Notify the prescriber about serious or persistent adverse reactions.
- Dosages may need to be adjusted in a patient with kidney or liver disease.

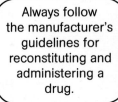

Always follow the manufacturer's guidelines for reconstituting and administering a drug.

Evaluation
- Patient doesn't incur injury while receiving drug therapy.
- Patient maintains adequate hydration.
- Patient and family demonstrate understanding of drug therapy.

(See *Teaching about zidovudine therapy*.)

Education edge

Teaching about zidovudine therapy

If zidovudine therapy is prescribed, review these points with the patient and caregivers:

- Blood transfusions may be needed during treatment because the drug commonly causes a low red blood cell count.
- Compliance with the every-4-hour dosage schedule is important. Use reminders, such as an alarm clock, to avoid missing doses.

- Don't take other drugs (including illicit drugs) without first consulting the prescriber. Other drugs, including other acquired immunodeficiency syndrome drugs, may interfere with zidovudine's effectiveness.
- For pregnant women infected with human immunodeficiency virus (HIV), drug therapy only reduces the risk of HIV transmission to neonates. Long-term risks to infants are unknown.

Non-nucleoside reverse transcriptase inhibitors

NNRTIs are used in combination with other antiretrovirals to treat HIV infection. Drugs in this class include:

- nevirapine
- efavirenz.

Pharmacokinetics

Efavirenz is a highly protein-bound after absorption and distribution. Nevirapine is widely distributed throughout the body. These drugs are metabolised by the cytochrome P-450 liver enzyme system and excreted in urine and faeces.

Pharmacodynamics

Nevirapine binds to the reverse transcriptase enzyme, preventing it from exerting its effect. This prevents HIV replication. Efavirenz competes for the enzyme through noncompetitive inhibition.

Pharmacotherapeutics

NNRTIs are used in combination with other antiretrovirals in HIV treatment; nevirapine is specifically indicated for patients whose clinical condition and immune status have deteriorated.

Drug interactions

These drug interactions may occur with NNRTIs:

- Nevirapine may decrease the activity of protease inhibitors and hormonal contraceptives; don't use these drugs together.
- Indinavir levels are decreased when administered with efavirenz.

Adverse reactions

Adverse reactions to NNRTIs include:

- headache
- dizziness
- asthenia
- nausea and vomiting
- diarrhoea.

Rash response

In addition, nevirapine has been associated with a severe rash that may be life-threatening. If a rash occurs, discontinue the drug.

Nursing process

These nursing process steps are appropriate for patients undergoing treatment with NNRTIs.

Assessment
- Obtain a baseline assessment of the patient's viral infection; reassess regularly to monitor the drug's effectiveness.
- Assess for adverse reactions and drug interactions.
- Assess the patient's and family's knowledge of drug therapy.

Key nursing diagnoses
- Ineffective protection related to adverse haematologic reactions.
- Risk for deficient fluid volume related to adverse GI reactions.
- Deficient knowledge related to drug therapy.

Planning outcome goals
- The patient won't incur injury while receiving drug therapy.
- Fluid volume will remain within normal limits as evidenced by intake and output.
- The patient and family will demonstrate an understanding of drug therapy.

Implementation
- Monitor renal and hepatic function, FBC, and platelet count regularly.
- Monitor the patient's mental status when giving the drug I.V. Encephalopathic changes are more likely in patients with neurologic disorders or in those who have had neurologic reactions to cytotoxic drugs.
- Monitor the patient's hydration status if adverse GI reactions occur.
- Follow the manufacturers' guidelines for reconstituting and administering these drugs.
- Obtain a prescription for an antiemetic or antidiarrhoeal drug, if needed
- Take safety precautions if adverse CNS reactions occur. For example, place the bed in a low position, raise the bed rails, and supervise ambulation and other activities.
- Notify the prescriber about serious or persistent adverse reactions.

Patients taking nevirapine may develop a severe, life-threatening rash. If this happens, stop the drug.

Evaluation
- Patient doesn't incur injury while receiving drug therapy.
- Patient maintains adequate hydration.
- Patient and family demonstrate understanding of drug therapy.

Nucleotide analogue reverse transcriptase inhibitors

The only drug in this class to date is tenofovir. It works similarly to the NRTIs.

Pharmacokinetics

Tenofovir is absorbed much better after a high-fat meal. It's then distributed in small amounts into plasma and serum proteins. Metabolism isn't thought to be mediated by cytochrome P-450 liver enzymes, and the drug is excreted by the kidneys.

Pharmacodynamics

Tenofovir competes with substrates and is subsequently incorporated into the DNA chain, thus halting HIV replication.

Pharmacotherapeutics

Tenofovir is used to treat HIV infection in combination with other drugs.

Drug interactions

These drug interactions may occur with tenofovir:
- Drugs that are eliminated through the kidneys or that decrease renal function may increase levels of tenofovir when given concurrently.
- Didanosine concentrations increase when given with tenofovir; watch for didanosine-based adverse effects.

Adverse reactions

Adverse reactions to tenofovir include:
- nausea and vomiting
- diarrhoea
- anorexia
- abdominal pain.

Tenofovir is absorbed better after a high-fat meal.

Handle with care

Potentially fatal lactic acidosis and severe hepatomegaly with steatosis have occurred in patients taking tenofovir alone or with other antiretrovirals. Most patients were women. Obesity and previous NRTI exposure may also be risk factors. Patients with preexisting liver disease should take this drug with caution. Suspend treatment if hepatotoxicity is suspected.

Nursing process

These nursing process steps are appropriate for patients undergoing treatment with tenofovir.

Assessment
• Obtain a baseline assessment of the patient's viral infection; reassess regularly to monitor the drug's effectiveness.
• Assess for adverse reactions and drug interactions.
• Assess the patient's and family's knowledge of drug therapy.

Key nursing diagnoses
• Ineffective protection related to adverse haematologic reactions.
• Risk for deficient fluid volume related to adverse GI reactions.
• Deficient knowledge related to drug therapy.

Planning outcome goals
• The patient won't incur injury while receiving drug therapy.
• Fluid volume will remain within normal limits as evidenced by intake and output.
• The patient and family will demonstrate an understanding of drug therapy.

Implementation
• Monitor renal and hepatic function, FBC, and platelet count regularly. Monitor for body changes in fat as well as for bone abnormalities and renal toxicity.
• Monitor the patient's mental status when giving the drug I.V. Encephalopathic changes are more likely in patients with neurologic disorders or in those who have had neurologic reactions to cytotoxic drugs.
• Monitor the patient's hydration status if adverse GI reactions occur.
• Follow the manufacturer's guidelines for reconstituting and administering antiviral drugs.
• Obtain a prescription for an antiemetic or antidiarrhoeal drug, if needed.
• Take safety precautions if adverse CNS reactions occur. For example, place the bed in a low position, raise the bed rails, and supervise ambulation and other activities.
• Notify the prescriber about serious or persistent adverse reactions.

Evaluation
- Patient doesn't incur injury while receiving drug therapy.
- Patient maintains adequate hydration.
- Patient and family demonstrate understanding of drug therapy.

Protease inhibitors

Protease inhibitors are drugs that act against the HIV enzyme protease, preventing it from dividing a larger viral precursor protein into the active smaller enzymes that the HIV virus needs to fully mature. The result is an immature, noninfectious cell. Drugs in this group include:
- saquinavir and saquinavir mesylate
- nelfinavir mesylate
- ritonavir
- indinavir sulphate
- lopinavir
- amprenavir
- atazanavir sulphate.

> Protease inhibitors prevent the HIV virus from fully maturing.

Pharmacokinetics

Protease inhibitors have different pharmacokinetic properties.

Saquinavir's story

Saquinavir and saquinavir mesylate are poorly absorbed from the GI tract. They're widely distributed, highly bound to plasma proteins, metabolised by the liver, and excreted mainly by the kidneys.

Nelfinavir notables

Nelfinavir's bioavailability (the degree to which it becomes available to target tissue after administration) isn't known. Food increases its absorption. It's highly protein-bound, metabolised in the liver, and excreted primarily in faeces.

Ritonavir review

Ritonavir is well absorbed, metabolised by the liver, and broken down into at least five metabolites. It's mainly excreted in faeces, with some elimination through the kidneys.

Inside indinavir

Indinavir sulphate is rapidly absorbed and moderately bound to plasma proteins. It's metabolised by the liver into seven metabolites. The drug is excreted mainly in faeces.

One boosts the other

Lopinavir is extensively metabolised by the liver's cytochrome P-450 system; ritonavir acts as an inhibitor of lopinavir. Lopinavir and ritonavir are used in combination because of their positive effects on HIV RNA levels and CD4+ counts. When given together, ritonavir inhibits the metabolism of lopinavir, leading to increased plasma lopinavir levels.

All about amprenavir

Amprenavir is metabolised in the liver to active and inactive metabolites and is minimally excreted in urine and faeces.

At last, atazanavir

Atazanavir is rapidly absorbed and is metabolised in the liver by the CYP3A pathway. The drug is excreted mainly in faeces and urine.

Pharmacodynamics

All of these drugs inhibit the activity of HIV protease and prevent the cleavage (division) of viral polyproteins.

Pharmacotherapeutics

Protease inhibitors are used in combination with other antiretroviral agents to treat HIV infection.

Drug interactions

Protease inhibitors may interact with many drugs. Here are some common interactions:
- Saquinavir's action may be reduced by phenobarbital, phenytoin, dexamethasone, and carbamazepine.
- Ritonavir may increase the effects of alpha-adrenergic blockers, antiarrhythmics, antidepressants, antiemetics, antifungals, antilipemics, antimalarials, antineoplastics, beta-adrenergic blockers, calcium channel blockers, cimetidine, corticosteroids, erythromycin, immunosuppressants, methylphenidate, pentoxifylline, phenothiazines, and warfarin.
- Indinavir sulphate inhibits the metabolism of midazolam, increasing the risk of potentially fatal events such as cardiac arrhythmias.
- Didanosine decreases gastric absorption of indinavir; give these drugs at least 1 hour apart.
- Rifampicin markedly reduces plasma concentrations of most protease inhibitors including atazanavir.

- Nelfinavir may greatly increase plasma levels of amiodarone, ergot derivatives, midazolam, and rifabutin.
- Carbamazepine, phenobarbital, and phenytoin may reduce the effectiveness of nelfinavir.
- Protease inhibitors may increase sildenafil concentrations and result in sildenafil-associated adverse reactions, including hypotension, vision changes, and priapism (a persistent, possibly painful erection).
- Atazanavir shouldn't be given with other drugs metabolised by the CYP3A pathway, such as HMG-CoA reductase inhibitors. Concurrent use may increase the risk of myopathy and rhabdomyolysis.
- Atazanavir may prolong the PR interval. Drugs that prolong the PR interval, such as calcium channel blockers (diltiazem, for example) and beta-adrenergic blockers (atenolol, for example) should be used cautiously with atazanavir.
- Atazanavir shouldn't be administered with such benzodiazepines as midazolam because of the potential for increased sedation or respiratory depression.
- Atazanavir shouldn't be administered with ergot derivatives, such as ergotamine, because life-threatening ergot toxicity can result, causing peripheral vasospasm and ischaemia of the extremities.
- St. John's wort may reduce plasma concentrations of atazanavir.
- Indinavir and ritonavir may increase plasma nelfinavir levels.

Adverse reactions

Adverse reactions depend on the type of protease inhibitor used:
- Saquinavir may cause diarrhoea, abdominal discomfort, or nausea.
- Ritonavir's adverse reactions include muscle weakness, nausea, diarrhoea, vomiting, anorexia, abdominal pain, and taste perversion.
- Adverse reactions to indinavir include abdominal pain, muscle weakness, fatigue, flank pain, nausea, diarrhoea, vomiting, acid reflux, anorexia, dry mouth, headache, insomnia, dizziness, taste perversion, and back pain.
- Nelfinavir may cause seizures, suicidal ideation, diarrhoea, pancreatitis, hepatitis, hypoglycaemia, or allergic reactions.
- Amprenavir may cause paraesthesia, nausea, vomiting, loose stools, hyperglycaemia, and rash.
- Reactions to combination therapy with lopinavir and ritonavir include encephalopathy, deep vein thrombosis, diarrhoea, nausea, haemorrhagic colitis, and pancreatitis.
- Atazanavir may cause hepatotoxicity, arrhythmias, or lactic acidosis.

Adverse reactions to protease inhibitors vary from drug to drug. Make sure you familiarise yourself with the specific reactions of the drug your patient is taking.

Nursing process

These nursing process steps are appropriate for patients undergoing treatment with protease inhibitors.

Assessment
• Obtain a baseline assessment of the patient's viral infection; reassess regularly to monitor the drug's effectiveness.
• Assess for adverse reactions and drug interactions.
• Assess the patient's and family's knowledge of drug therapy.

Key nursing diagnoses
• Ineffective protection related to adverse haematologic reactions.
• Risk for deficient fluid volume related to adverse GI reactions.
• Deficient knowledge related to drug therapy.

Planning outcome goals
• The patient won't incur injury while receiving drug therapy.
• Fluid volume will remain within normal limits as evidenced by intake and output.
• The patient and family will demonstrate an understanding of drug therapy.

Implementation
• Monitor renal and hepatic function, FBC, and platelet count regularly.
• Monitor the patient's mental status when giving the drug I.V. Encephalopathic changes are more likely in patients with neurologic disorders or in those who have had neurologic reactions to cytotoxic drugs.
• Monitor the patient's hydration status if adverse GI reactions occur.
• Follow the manufacturer's guidelines for reconstituting and administering antiviral drugs.
• Obtain a prescription for an antiemetic or antidiarrhoeal drug, if needed.
• Take safety precautions if adverse CNS reactions occur. For example, place the bed in a low position, raise the bed rails, and supervise ambulation and other activities.
• Notify the prescriber about serious or persistent adverse reactions.

Evaluation
• Patient doesn't incur injury while receiving drug therapy.
• Patient maintains adequate hydration.
• Patient and family demonstrate understanding of drug therapy.

Antitubercular drugs

Antitubercular drugs are used to treat tuberculosis (TB), which is caused by *Mycobacterium tuberculosis*. These drugs also are effective against less common mycobacterial infections caused by *M. kansasii*, *M. avium-intracellulare*, *M. fortuitum*, and related organisms. Although not always curative, these drugs can halt the progression of a mycobacterial infection.

Compliance can get complicated

Unlike most antibacterials, antitubercular drugs may need to be administered over many months. This creates such problems as patient noncompliance, the development of bacterial resistance, and drug toxicity. (See *Directly observable therapy for TB.*)

Tag team therapy

Traditionally, isoniazid, rifampicin, and ethambutol hydrochloride were the mainstays of multidrug TB therapy and successfully prevented the emergence of drug resistance.

Because of the current incidence of drug-resistant TB strains, however, a four-drug regimen is now recommended for initial treatment:
- isoniazid
- rifampicin
- pyrazinamide
- streptomycin sulphate or ethambutol

Times to modify

The antitubercular regimen should be modified if local testing shows resistance to one or more of these drugs. If local outbreaks of TB resistant to isoniazid and rifampicin are occurring in institutions (for example, health care or correctional facilities), then five-drug or six-drug regimens are recommended as initial therapy. (See *Other antitubercular drugs.*)

Pharmacokinetics

Most antitubercular drugs are administered orally. When administered orally, these drugs are well absorbed from the GI tract and widely distributed throughout the body. They're metabolised primarily in the liver and excreted by the kidneys.

Antitubercular drugs may need to be administered over many months.

Directly observable therapy for TB

Among infectious diseases, tuberculosis (TB) remains a frequent killer worldwide. Treatment is difficult because it requires long-term medical therapy—often as long as 6 to 9 months. The length of treatment commonly creates problems with patient compliance, and poor compliance contributes to reactivation of the disease and development of drug-resistant TB.

Prototype pro

Antituber-cular drugs: Isoniazid

Actions

- Appears to inhibit cell wall biosynthesis by interfering with lipid and deoxyribonucleic acid synthesis

Indications

- Tuberculosis

Nursing considerations

- Monitor the patient for adverse effects, such as peripheral neuropathy, seizures, haematologic disorders, hepatitis, and hypersensitivity reactions.
- Always give isoniazid with other antitubercular drugs to prevent the development of resistant organisms.

Pharmacodynamics

Antitubercular drugs are specific for mycobacteria. At usual doses, ethambutol and isoniazid are tuberculostatic, meaning that they inhibit the growth of *M. tuberculosis*. In contrast, rifampicin is tuberculocidal, meaning that it destroys the mycobacteria. Because bacterial resistance to isoniazid and rifampicin can develop rapidly, they should always be used with other antitubercular drugs.

Mysterious ways

The exact mechanism of action of ethambutol remains unclear, but it may be related to inhibition of cell metabolism, arrest of multiplication, and cell death. Ethambutol acts only against replicating bacteria.

Wall buster

Although isoniazid's exact mechanism of action isn't known, the drug is believed to inhibit the synthesis of mycolic acids, important components of the mycobacterium cell wall. This inhibition disrupts the cell wall. Only replicating, not resting, bacteria appear to be inhibited. (See *Antitubercular drugs: Isoniazid.*)

RNA repressor

Rifampicin inhibits RNA synthesis in susceptible organisms. The drug is effective primarily in replicating bacteria but may have some effect on resting bacteria as well.

Other antitubercular drugs

Several other drugs are used as antitubercular drugs in combination with first-line drugs. Because these drugs have a greater incidence of toxicity, they're used primarily when resistance or allergies to less toxic drugs exist.

Fluoroquinolones

Fluoroquinolones, such as ciprofloxacin and ofloxacin, are effective against *Mycobacterium tuberculosis.* Of these two drugs, ofloxacin is more potent and may be an initial choice in retreatment. These drugs are administered orally and are generally well tolerated. GI adverse reactions are most commonly reported. However, resistance to fluoroquinolones develops rapidly when these drugs are used alone or in insufficient doses.

Streptomycin

Streptomycin was the first drug recognised as effective in treating TB. Streptomycin is administered I.M. only. It appears to enhance the activity of oral antitubercular drugs and is of greatest value in the early weeks to months of therapy. However, I.M. administration limits its usefulness in long-term therapy. Rapidly absorbed from the I.M. injection site, streptomycin is excreted primarily by the kidneys as unchanged drug. Most patients tolerate streptomycin well, but those receiving large doses may exhibit eighth cranial nerve toxicity (ototoxicity).

Acid wash

The exact mechanism of action of pyrazinamide isn't known, but the antimycobacterial activity appears to be linked to the drug's conversion to the active metabolite pyrazinoic acid. Pyrazinoic acid, in turn, creates an acidic environment where mycobacteria can't replicate.

Pharmacotherapeutics

Isoniazid is usually used with ethambutol, rifampicin, or streptomycin. This is because combination therapy for TB and other mycobacterial infections can prevent or delay the development of resistance.

For simpler times

Ethambutol is used with isoniazid and rifampicin to treat patients with uncomplicated pulmonary TB. It's also used to treat infections resulting from *M. bovis* and most strains of *M. kansasii.*

Most antitubercular drugs act only against replicating bacteria, but rifampicin may have some effect on resting bacteria as well.

Preventive power

Although isoniazid is the most important drug for treating TB, bacterial resistance develops rapidly if it's used alone. However, resistance doesn't pose a problem when isoniazid is used alone to prevent TB in individuals who have been exposed to the disease, and no evidence exists of cross-resistance between isoniazid and other antitubercular drugs. Isoniazid is typically given orally, but may be given I.V., if necessary.

Rapid resistance

Rifampicin is used to treat pulmonary TB with other antitubercular drugs. It combats many gram-positive and some gram-negative bacteria but is seldom used for nonmycobacterial infections because bacterial resistance develops rapidly. It's used to treat asymptomatic carriers of *Neisseria meningitidis* when the risk of meningitis is high, but it isn't used to treat *N. meningitidis* infections because of the potential for bacterial resistance.

First in line

Pyrazinamide is currently recommended as a first-line TB drug in combination with ethambutol, rifampicin, and isoniazid. Pyrazinamide is a highly specific drug that's active only against *M. tuberculosis*. Resistance to pyrazinamide may develop rapidly when it's used alone.

Drug interactions

Antitubercular drugs may interact with a number of other drugs:
- Cycloserine and ethionamide may produce additive CNS effects, such as drowsiness, dizziness, headache, lethargy, depression, tremor, anxiety, confusion, and tinnitus (ringing in the ears), when administered with isoniazid.
- Isoniazid may increase levels of phenytoin, carbamazepine, diazepam, ethosuximide, primidone, theophylline, and warfarin.
- When corticosteroids and isoniazid are taken together, the effectiveness of isoniazid is reduced while the effects of corticosteroids are increased.
- Isoniazid may reduce the plasma concentration of ketoconazole, itraconazole, and oral antidiabetic drugs.
- When given together, the combination of rifampicin, isoniazid, ethionamide, and pyrazinamide increases the risk of hepatotoxicity.
- Pyrazinamide combined with phenytoin may increase phenytoin levels.

Adverse reactions

Adverse reactions to antitubercular drugs vary:
- Ethambutol may cause itching, joint pain, GI distress, malaise, leucopenia, headache, dizziness, numbness and tingling of the

extremities, and confusion. Although rare, hypersensitivity reactions to ethambutol may produce rash and fever. Anaphylaxis may also occur.
• Peripheral neuropathy is the most common adverse reaction to isoniazid. Severe and occasionally fatal hepatitis associated with isoniazid may occur even many months after treatment has stopped. Patients must be monitored carefully.
• The most common adverse reactions to rifampicin include epigastric pain, nausea, vomiting, abdominal cramps, flatulence, anorexia, and diarrhoea.
• Liver toxicity is the major limiting adverse reaction to pyrazinamide. GI disturbances include nausea, vomiting, and anorexia.

Liver toxicity is the major limiting adverse reaction to pyrazinamide.

Nursing process

These nursing process steps are appropriate for patients undergoing treatment with antitubercular drugs.

Assessment
• Assess the patient's infection before therapy.
• Monitor the patient for improvement, and evaluate culture and sensitivity tests.
• Assess for adverse reactions and drug interactions.
• Assess the patient's and family's knowledge of drug therapy.

Key nursing diagnoses
• Risk for infection related to underlying process.
• Disturbed sensory perception (tactile) related to drug-induced peripheral neuropathy.
• Deficient knowledge related to drug therapy.

Planning outcome goals
• The patient will be free from infection as evidenced by negative cultures and normal WBC counts.
• The patient will state that tactile sensations are normal.
• The patient and family will demonstrate an understanding of drug therapy.

Implementation
• Administer oral doses 1 hour before or 2 hours after meals to avoid decreased absorption.
• Follow protocol for I.M. dosage. Switch to oral form as soon as possible.
• Monitor the patient for paraesthesia of the hands and feet, which usually precedes peripheral neuropathy, especially in patients who are malnourished, alcoholic, or diabetic.
• Monitor hepatic function closely for changes.

Education edge

Teaching about antitubercular drugs

If antitubercular drugs are prescribed, review these points with the patient and caregivers:

- Take the drug as prescribed; don't stop the drug without the prescriber's consent. Treatment may last for months or years.
- Take the drug with food if GI irritation occurs.
- Avoid alcohol during drug therapy.

- Avoid certain foods, including fish (particularly sardines and tuna) and products containing tyramine (such as aged cheese, beer, and chocolate), because the drug has some monoamine-oxidase inhibitor activity.
- Notify the prescriber immediately if symptoms of liver impairment occur (loss of appetite, fatigue, malaise, jaundice, or dark urine).

Evaluation
- Patient is free from infection.
- Patient maintains normal peripheral nervous system function.
- Patient and family demonstrate understanding of drug therapy.
(See *Teaching about antitubercular drugs*.)

Antifungal drugs

Antifungal, or antimycotic, drugs are used to treat fungal infections. They include:
- polyenes
- flucytosine
- ketoconazole
- synthetic triazoles
- glucan synthesis inhibitors
- terbinafine hydrochloride. (See *Other antifungal drugs*.)

Polyenes

The polyenes include amphotericin B and nystatin. The potency of amphotericin B has made it the most widely used antifungal drug for severe systemic fungal infections. Nystatin is used only topically or orally to treat local fungal infections because it's extremely toxic when administered parenterally.

Other antifungal drugs

Several other antifungal drugs offer alternative forms of treatment for topical fungal infections.

Clotrimazole

An imidazole derivative, clotrimazole is used:

- topically to treat dermatophyte and *Candida albicans* infections
- orally to treat oral candidiasis
- vaginally to treat vaginal candidiasis.

Griseofulvin

Griseofulvin is used to treat fungal infections of the:

- skin (tinea corporis)
- feet (tinea pedis)
- groin (tinea cruris)
- beard area of the face and neck (tinea barbae)
- nails (tinea unguium)
- scalp (tinea capitis).

Use with extreme prejudice

To prevent a relapse, griseofulvin therapy must continue until the fungus is eradicated and the infected skin or nails are replaced.

Miconazole

Available as miconazole or miconazole nitrate, this imidazole derivative is used to treat local fungal infections, such as vaginal and vulvar candidiasis, and topical fungal infections, such as chronic candidiasis of the skin and mucous membranes.

Delivery options

Miconazole may be administered:

- I.V. or intrathecally (into the subarachnoid space) to treat fungal meningitis
- I.V. or in bladder irrigations to treat fungal bladder infections
- locally to treat vaginal infections
- topically to treat topical infections.

Other topical antimycotic drugs

Econazole nitrate, tioconazole, tolnaftate, sulconazole nitrate, are available only as topical drugs.

Pharmacokinetics

After I.V. administration, amphotericin B is distributed throughout the body and excreted by the kidneys. Its metabolism isn't well defined.

Not much circulation

Oral nystatin undergoes little or no absorption, distribution, or metabolism. It's excreted unchanged in faeces. Topical nystatin isn't absorbed through intact skin or mucous membranes.

Pharmacodynamics

Amphotericin B works by binding to sterol (a lipid) in the fungal cell membrane, altering cell permeability (ability to allow a substance to pass through) and allowing intracellular components to leak out.

Fungi town

Amphotericin B usually acts as a fungistatic drug (inhibiting fungal growth and multiplication) but can become fungicidal (destroying fungi) if it reaches high concentrations in the fungi.

Manipulating membranes

Nystatin binds to sterols in fungal cell membranes and alters the permeability of the membranes, leading to loss of cell components. Nystatin can act as a fungicidal or fungistatic drug, depending on the organism present.

Pharmacotherapeutics

Amphotericin B is usually administered to treat severe systemic fungal infections and meningitis caused by fungi sensitive to the drug. It's never used for noninvasive forms of fungal disease because it's highly toxic. It's usually the drug of choice for severe infections caused by *Candida*, *Paracoccidioides brasiliensis*, *Blastomyces dermatitidis*, *Coccidioides immitis*, *Cryptococcus neoformans*, and *Sporothrix schenckii*. It's also effective against *Aspergillus fumigatus*, *Microsporum audouinii*, *Rhizopus*, *Candida glabrata*, *Trichophyton*, and *Rhodotorula*.

Know the limits

Because amphotericin B is highly toxic, its use is limited to patients who have a definitive diagnosis of life-threatening infection and are under close medical supervision.

Canning candidal infections

Different forms of nystatin are available for treating different types of candidal infections:
• Topical nystatin is used to treat candidal skin or mucous membrane infections, such as oral thrush, nappy rash, vaginal and vulvar candidiasis, and candidiasis between skin folds.
• Oral nystatin is used to treat GI infections.

Drug interactions

Amphotericin B may have significant interactions with many drugs:
• Because of the synergistic effects between flucytosine and amphotericin B, these two drugs are commonly combined in therapy for candidal or cryptococcal infections, especially for cryptococcal meningitis.
• The risk of kidney toxicity increases when amphotericin B is taken with aminoglycosides, ciclosporine, or aciclovir.
• Corticosteroids, extended-spectrum penicillins, and digoxin may worsen hypokalaemia (low blood potassium levels) produced by amphotericin B, possibly leading to heart problems. Moreover, the risk of digoxin toxicity is increased.

- Amphotericin B increases muscle relaxation when given with nondepolarising skeletal muscle relaxants (such as pancuronium bromide).
- Electrolyte solutions may inactivate amphotericin B when diluted in the same solution. Amphotericin B preparations must be mixed with D_5W; they can't be mixed with saline solutions.
- Magnesium and potassium levels and renal function must be monitored frequently in patients receiving amphotericin.

Don't mix amphotericin B preparations with saline solutions! They must be mixed with 5% glucose in water.

A wallflower

Nystatin doesn't interact significantly with other drugs.

Adverse reactions

Almost all patients receiving I.V. amphotericin B, particularly at the beginning of low-dose therapy, experience:
- chills
- fever
- nausea and vomiting
- anorexia
- muscle and joint pain
- indigestion.

Watch those RBCs

Most patients also develop normochromic (adequate haemoglobin in each RBC) or normocytic anaemia (too few RBCs) that significantly decreases haematocrit.

Altered electrolytes and ECGs

Hypomagnesaemia and hypokalaemia may occur, causing ECG changes requiring replacement electrolyte therapy.

Losing concentration

Up to 80% of patients may develop some degree of kidney toxicity, causing the kidneys to lose their ability to concentrate urine.

The higher the dosage, the harder they react

Reactions to nystatin seldom occur, but high dosages may produce:
- diarrhoea
- nausea and vomiting
- abdominal pain
- a bitter taste
- hypersensitivity reactions
- skin irritation (topical form).

Nursing process

These nursing process steps are appropriate for patients undergoing treatment with polyenes.

Assessment

- Obtain a history of the fungal infection as well as a specimen for culture and sensitivity tests before giving the first dose. Reevaluate the patient's condition during therapy.
- Assess for adverse reactions and drug interactions.
- Assess the patient's and family's knowledge of drug therapy.

Key nursing diagnoses

- Risk for infection related to the underlying condition.
- Risk for injury related to drug-induced adverse reactions.
- Deficient knowledge related to drug therapy.

Planning outcome goals

- The patient's infection will resolve as evidenced by culture reports, temperature, and WBC counts.
- The patient won't incur injury while receiving drug therapy.
- The patient and family will demonstrate an understanding of drug therapy.

Implementation

- The lozenge form of drug should be dissolved slowly.
- Parenteral I.V. use is for hospitalised patients only after diagnosis of potentially fatal fungal infection is confirmed. The initial dose is usually a test dose and administered over 20 to 30 minutes.
- Use an infusion pump and in-line filter with a mean pore diameter larger than 1 micron. Infuse over 2 to 6 hours; rapid infusion may cause cardiovascular collapse.
- Give antibacterials separately; don't mix them or give them piggyback with other drugs.
- Monitor the patient's pulse, respiratory rate, temperature, and blood pressure every 30 minutes for at least 4 hours after giving the drug I.V.; fever, shaking chills, anorexia, nausea, vomiting, headache, tachypnea, and hypotension may appear 1 to 3 hours after the start of an I.V. infusion. Symptoms are usually more severe with initial doses.
- Monitor BUN, creatinine (or creatinine clearance), and electrolyte levels; FBC; and liver function test results at least weekly. If BUN exceeds 40 mg/dl, or if creatinine level exceeds 3 mg/dl, the prescriber may reduce or stop the drug until renal function improves.
- Monitor for rhinocerebral phycomycosis, especially in a patient with uncontrolled diabetes. Leucoencephalopathy may also occur. Monitor pulmonary function. Acute reactions are characterised by dyspnea, hypoxaemia, and infiltrates.

Take the patient's blood pressure every 30 minutes for at least 4 hours after giving polyenes I.V.

- If the patient has severe adverse infusion reactions to the initial dose, stop the infusion and notify the prescriber, who may prescribe antipyretics, antihistamines, antiemetics, or small doses of corticosteroids. To prevent reactions during subsequent infusions, premedicate with these drugs or give amphotericin B on an alternate-day schedule.

Evaluation
- Patient is free from fungal infection.
- Patient doesn't experience injury as a result of drug-induced adverse reactions.
- Patient and family demonstrate understanding of drug therapy.

Flucytosine

Flucytosine, a fluorinated pyrimidine analogue, is the only antimetabolite (a substance that closely resembles one required for normal physiologic functioning and that exerts its effect by interfering with metabolism) that acts as an antifungal, it's a purine and pyrimidine inhibitor.

Pharmacokinetics
After oral administration, flucytosine is well absorbed from the GI tract and widely distributed. It undergoes little metabolism and is excreted primarily by the kidneys.

Pharmacodynamics
Flucytosine penetrates fungal cells, where it's converted to its active metabolite fluorouracil. Fluorouracil is then incorporated into the RNA of the fungal cells, altering their protein synthesis and causing cell death.

Pharmacotherapeutics
Flucytosine is used primarily with another antifungal drug, such as amphotericin B, to treat systemic fungal infections. For example, although amphotericin B is effective in treating candidal and cryptococcal meningitis alone, flucytosine is given with it to reduce the dosage and the risk of toxicity. This combination therapy is the treatment of choice for cryptococcal meningitis.

Memory jogger

If a drug is *fungicidal,* it destroys the fungus—*cidus* is a Latin term for "killing." If it's *fungistatic,* it prevents fungal growth and multiplication—*stasis* is a Greek term for "halting."

Flucytosine reduces the risk of amphotericin B toxicity when the drugs are given together.

Drug interactions

Cytarabine may antagonise the antifungal activity of flucytosine, possibly by competitive inhibition. Haematologic, kidney, and liver function must be closely monitored during flucytosine therapy because of the drug's serious risk of toxicity.

Adverse reactions

Flucytosine may produce unpredictable adverse reactions, including:
- confusion
- headache
- drowsiness
- vertigo
- hallucinations
- difficulty breathing
- respiratory arrest
- rash
- nausea and vomiting
- abdominal distention
- diarrhoea
- anorexia.

Nursing process

These nursing process steps are appropriate for patients undergoing treatment with flucytosine.

Assessment
- Assess the patient's fungal infection before therapy and regularly throughout therapy.
- Before therapy, obtain haematologic tests and renal and liver function studies. Make sure susceptibility tests showing that the organism is flucytosine-sensitive are included on the chart.
- Assess for adverse reactions and drug interactions.
- Assess the patient's and family's knowledge of drug therapy.

Key nursing diagnoses
- Risk for infection related to the underlying condition.
- Risk for deficient fluid volume related to adverse GI reactions.
- Deficient knowledge related to drug therapy.

Planning outcome goals
- The patient's infection will resolve as evidenced by culture reports, temperature, and WBC counts.

Before starting therapy, make sure susceptibility tests showing that the organism is flucytosine-sensitive are included on the patient's chart.

- Fluid volume will remain within normal limits as evidenced by intake and output.
- The patient and family will demonstrate an understanding of drug therapy.

Implementation
- Give capsules over 15 minutes to reduce adverse GI reactions.
- Monitor the patient for adverse CNS reactions.
- Monitor blood, liver, and renal function studies frequently; obtain susceptibility tests weekly to monitor drug resistance.
- If possible, regularly perform blood level assays of the drug to maintain flucytosine at therapeutic level (25 to 120 mcg/ml). Higher blood levels may be toxic.
- Monitor the patient's hydration status if adverse GI reactions occur.

Evaluation
- Patient is free from infection.
- Patient maintains adequate hydration.
- Patient and family demonstrate understanding of drug therapy

Ketoconazole

Ketoconazole, a synthetic imidazole derivative is an effective oral antifungal drug with a broad spectrum of activity.

Pharmacokinetics
When given orally, ketoconazole is absorbed variably and distributed widely. It undergoes extensive liver metabolism and is excreted in bile and faeces.

Pharmacodynamics
Within the fungal cells, ketoconazole interferes with sterol synthesis, damaging the cell membrane and increasing its permeability. This leads to a loss of essential intracellular elements and inhibition of cell growth.

Inhibits and destroys

Ketoconazole usually produces fungistatic effects but can also produce fungicidal effects under certain conditions.

Pharmacotherapeutics

Ketoconazole is used to treat topical and systemic infections caused by susceptible fungi, which include dermatophytes and most other fungi.

Drug interactions

Ketoconazole may have significant interactions with other drugs:
- Ketoconazole use with drugs that decrease gastric acidity, such as cimetidine, ranitidine, famotidine, nizatidine, antacids, and anticholinergic drugs, may decrease absorption of ketoconazole and reduce its antimycotic effects. If the patient must take these drugs, delay administration of ketoconazole by at least 2 hours.
- Taking ketoconazole with phenytoin may alter metabolism and increase blood levels of both drugs.
- When taken with theophylline, ketoconazole may decrease the serum theophylline level.
- Use with other hepatotoxic drugs may increase the risk of liver disease.
- Combined with ciclosporine therapy, ketoconazole may increase ciclosporine and serum creatinine levels.
- Ketoconazole increases the effect of oral anticoagulants and can cause haemorrhage.
- Ketoconazole can inhibit metabolism (and possibly increase concentrations) of sulphonylureas, carbamazepine, and protease inhibitors.
- Ketoconazole shouldn't be given with rifampicin because serum ketoconazole concentrations may decrease.

Help! We need antifungal activity!

Adverse reactions

The most common adverse reactions to ketoconazole are nausea and vomiting. Less frequent reactions include:
- anaphylaxis
- joint pain
- chills
- fever
- tinnitus
- impotence
- photophobia
- hepatotoxicity (rare; reversible when the drug is stopped).

Nursing process

These nursing process steps are appropriate for patients undergoing treatment with ketoconazole.

Assessment
- Assess the patient's fungal infection before therapy and regularly throughout therapy.
- Assess for adverse reactions and drug interactions.
- Assess the patient's and family's knowledge of drug therapy.

Key nursing diagnoses
- Risk for infection related to the underlying condition.
- Risk for deficient fluid volume related to adverse GI reactions.
- Deficient knowledge related to drug therapy.

Planning outcome goals
- The patient's infection will resolve as evidenced by culture reports, temperature, and WBC counts.
- Fluid volume will remain within normal limits as evidenced by intake and output.
- The patient and family will demonstrate an understanding of drug therapy.

Implementation
- Because of the risk of serious hepatotoxicity, the drug shouldn't be used for less serious conditions, such as fungal infections of the skin or nails.
- To minimise nausea, divide the daily amount into two doses and give the drug with meals.
- Monitor the patient's hydration status if adverse GI reactions occur.

Evaluation
- Patient is free from infection.
- Patient maintains adequate hydration.
- Patient and family demonstrate understanding of drug therapy.

Synthetic triazoles

The synthetic triazoles include fluconazole, itraconazole, and voriconazole.

Pharmacokinetics

After oral administration, fluconazole is about 90% absorbed. It's distributed into all body fluids, and more than 80% of the drug is excreted unchanged in urine.

With and without food

Oral bioavailability is greatest when itraconazole is taken with food; voriconazole is more effective if taken 1 hour before or after a meal. Both itraconazole and voriconazole are bound to plasma proteins and extensively metabolised in the liver into a large number of metabolites. They're minimally excreted in faeces.

Pharmacodynamics

Fluconazole inhibits fungal cytochrome P-450, an enzyme responsible for fungal sterol synthesis, causing fungal cell walls to weaken. Itraconazole and voriconazole interfere with fungal cell-wall synthesis by inhibiting the formation of ergosterol and increasing cell-wall permeability, making the fungus susceptible to osmotic instability.

Pharmacotherapeutics

The synthetic triazoles treat various infections:
- Fluconazole is used to treat mouth, throat, and oesophageal candidiasis and serious systemic candidal infections, including UTIs, peritonitis, and pneumonia. It's also used to treat cryptococcal meningitis.
- Itraconazole is used to treat blastomycosis, nonmeningeal histoplasmosis, candidiasis, aspergillosis, and fungal nail disease.
- Voriconazole is used to treat invasive aspergillosis and serious fungal infections caused by *Scedosporium apiospermum* and *Fusarium* species.

Synthetic triazoles either cause fungal cell walls to weaken or interfere with cell wall synthesis.

Drug interactions

Fluconazole may have these drug interactions:
- Use with warfarin may increase the risk of bleeding.
- It may increase levels of phenytoin and ciclosporine.
- It may increase the plasma concentration of oral antidiabetic drugs, such as tolbutamide, and glipizide, increasing the risk of hypoglycaemia.
- Rifampicin and cimetidine enhance the metabolism of fluconazole, reducing its plasma level.
- It may increase the activity of zidovudine.
  Itraconazole and voriconazole have these drug interactions:
- Both may increase the risk of bleeding when combined with oral anticoagulants.
- Antacids, H_2-receptor antagonists, phenytoin, and rifampicin lower plasma itraconazole levels.

- Voriconazole may inhibit the metabolism of phenytoin, benzodiazepines, calcium channel blockers, sulphonylureas, and tacrolimus.
- Voriconazole is contraindicated with sirolimus and ergot alkaloids because voriconazole may increase plasma concentrations of these drugs.
- Voriconazole is contraindicated with pimozide because of the risk of prolonged QT interval and, rarely, torsades de pointes.

Adverse reactions

Adverse reactions to fluconazole and voriconazole include:
- abdominal pain
- diarrhoea
- dizziness
- headache
- increase in liver enzymes
- nausea and vomiting
- rash.

Adverse reactions to itraconazole include:
- dizziness
- headache
- hypertension
- impaired liver function
- nausea.

Nursing process

These nursing process steps are appropriate for patients undergoing treatment with synthetic triazoles.

Assessment

- Assess the patient's fungal infection before therapy and regularly throughout therapy.
- Periodically monitor liver function during prolonged therapy. Although adverse hepatic effects are rare, they can be serious.
- Assess for adverse reactions and drug interactions.
- Assess the patient's and family's knowledge of drug therapy.

Key nursing diagnoses

- Risk for infection related to the underlying condition
- Risk for deficient fluid volume related to adverse GI reactions
- Deficient knowledge related to drug therapy

Planning outcome goals
- The patient's infection will resolve as evidenced by culture reports, temperature, and WBC counts.
- Fluid volume will remain within normal limits as evidenced by intake and output.
- The patient and family will demonstrate an understanding of drug therapy.

Implementation
- Don't remove protective overwraps from I.V. bags of fluconazole until just before use to ensure product sterility.
- Give by continuous infusion with an infusion pump at a rate of no more than 200 mg/hour. To prevent air embolism, don't give the drug in a series with other infusions.
- Don't add other drugs to the solution.
- If the patient develops a mild rash, monitor him closely. Stop the drug if lesions progress, and notify the prescriber.
- Monitor the patient's hydration status if adverse GI reactions occur.

Evaluation
- Patient is free from infection.
- Patient maintains adequate hydration.
- Patient and family demonstrate understanding of drug therapy.

Glucan synthesis inhibitors

Caspofungin acetate is a drug in a new class known as *glucan synthesis inhibitors* (also known as *echinocandins*). Caspofungin is primarily used in patients who haven't been successful with other antifungal therapies.

Pharmacokinetics
Given I.V., caspofungin is highly protein-bound, with little distribution into RBCs. The drug is slowly metabolised and excreted in urine and faeces.

Pharmacodynamics
Caspofungin inhibits the synthesis of beta (1,3)-D-glucan, an integral component of the fungal cell wall.

Caspofungin is called into the ring when other antifungal therapies have failed.

Pharmacotherapeutics

Caspofungin is used to treat invasive aspergillosis in patients who have failed to respond to, or can't tolerate, other antifungals, such as amphotericin B or itraconazole. It hasn't been studied as an initial treatment for invasive aspergillosis.

Drug interactions

Caspofungin is known to cause these drug interactions:
• Patients taking caspofungin and tacrolimus may need higher doses of tacrolimus because caspofungin decreases the blood tacrolimus level.
• Inducers of drug clearance, such as phenytoin, carbamazepine, efavirenz, nevirapine, and nelfinavir, may lower caspofungin clearance.
• Concurrent use of caspofungin and ciclosporine may result in elevated liver enzyme levels and decreased caspofungin clearance; use together isn't recommended.

Adverse reactions

Adverse reactions to caspofungin include:
• paraesthesia
• tachycardia
• tachypnea
• nausea and vomiting
• diarrhoea
• rash
• facial swelling.

Nursing process

These nursing process steps are appropriate for patients undergoing treatment with glucan synthesis inhibitors such as caspofungin.

Assessment

• Assess the patient's hepatic function before starting drug therapy.
• Observe the patient for histamine-mediated reactions (rash, facial swelling, pruritus, sensation of warmth).
• Assess the patient's and family's knowledge of drug therapy.

Key nursing diagnoses

• Risk for infection and risk for impaired skin integrity related to adverse effects of I.V. drug administration.

Patients taking caspofungin may experience histamine-mediated reactions, including rash, facial swelling, pruritus, and a sensation of warmth.

- Ineffective health maintenance related to the underlying disease process and immunocompromised state.
- Deficient knowledge related to aspergillosis infection and drug therapy.

Planning outcome goals
- The patient's infection will resolve as evidenced by culture reports, temperature, and WBC counts.
- The patient will maintain adequate health status throughout drug therapy.
- The patient and family will demonstrate an understanding of drug therapy.

Implementation
- Dilute drugs as directed and administer slowly via I.V. infusion over 1 hour.
- Keep in mind that the dosage may need to be adjusted if the patient has hepatic insufficiency.
- Monitor the I.V. site carefully for phlebitis.
- Monitor the patient's laboratory test results carefully for an increase in liver function test values.

Evaluation
- Patient is free from infection.
- Patient responds positively to antifungal drug therapy.
- Patient and family demonstrate understanding of drug therapy.

Terbinafine

Terbinafine is a synthetic allylamine antifungal. It inhibits fungal cell growth by inhibiting an enzyme responsible for manufacturing ergosterol.

Pharmacokinetics
Terbinafine is well absorbed and distributed, especially if taken with food. It's extensively metabolised; more than two-thirds of the drug is excreted in urine.

Pharmacodynamics
Terbinafine is thought to inhibit squalene epoxidase, which blocks the biosynthesis of ergosterol, an essential component of fungal cell membranes.

Pharmacotherapeutics

Terbinafine is used to treat tinea unguium (fungal infection of the toenail or fingernail).

Drug interactions

The clearance of terbinafine is decreased by cimetidine and increased by rifampicin. Terbinafine also increases plasma concentrations of caffeine and dextromethorphan and decreases concentrations of ciclosporine.

Adverse reactions

Adverse reactions to terbinafine include:
- headache
- vision disturbances
- nausea
- diarrhoea
- abdominal pain
- neutropenia
- Stevens-Johnson syndrome.

Terbinafine can cause liver failure. Avoid using this drug in patients with suspected liver disease.

Look out, liver!

Rare cases of liver failure have occurred with terbinafine use, even in patients with no known history of liver disease. Avoid using this drug if you suspect liver disease, and obtain baseline liver enzyme test results before use.

Nursing process

These nursing process steps are appropriate for patients undergoing treatment with terbinafine.

Assessment
- Assess the patient's fungal infection before therapy and regularly throughout therapy.
- Assess for adverse reactions and drug interactions.
- Assess the patient's and family's knowledge of drug therapy.

Key nursing diagnoses
- Risk for infection related to the underlying condition.
- Risk for deficient fluid volume related to adverse GI reactions.
- Deficient knowledge related to drug therapy.

Planning outcome goals
• The patient's infection will resolve as evidenced by culture reports, temperature, and WBC counts.
• Fluid volume will remain within normal limits as evidenced by intake and output.
• The patient and family will demonstrate an understanding of drug therapy.

Implementation
• Give the drug as prescribed.
• Monitor blood, liver, and renal function studies frequently; obtain susceptibility tests weekly to monitor drug resistance.
• Monitor the patient's hydration status if adverse GI reactions occur.

Evaluation
• Patient is free from infection.
• Patient maintains adequate hydration.
• Patient and family demonstrate understanding of drug therapy.

Quick quiz

1. What's an adverse reaction to aminoglycosides?
    A. Peripheral nerve toxicity
    B. Cardiotoxicity
    C. Hepatic toxicity
    D. Toxic megacolon

Answer: A. Adverse reactions to aminoglycosides include neuromuscular reactions, ranging from peripheral nerve toxicity to neuromuscular blockade, ototoxicity, and renal toxicity.

2. Which food should the patient receiving isoniazid therapy avoid?
    A. Red wine
    B. Chocolate
    C. Coffee
    D. Eggs

Answer: B. The patient taking isoniazid should avoid fish (particularly skipjack and tuna) and products containing tyramine (such as aged cheese, beer, and chocolate) because the drug has some monoamine oxidase inhibitor activity.

3. Which implementation step is appropriate for a patient who's taking zidovudine for an HIV infection?
- A. Anticipate the need for dosage adjustment for impaired hepatic function.
- B. Administer the drug every 4 hours, around the clock.
- C. Administer one dose daily.
- D. Monitor the patient's cardiac status.

Answer: B. Zidovudine is usually administered over 1 hour at a constant rate and is given every 4 hours around the clock.

Scoring

☆☆☆ If you answered three questions correctly, impeccable! You're privy to the pills that pounce those pesky pathogens.

☆☆ If you answered two questions correctly, magnificent! Those malicious microorganisms are marked now that you're on the scene.

☆ If you answered fewer than two questions correctly, don't get in a funk. You'll be fluent in antifungals and all the rest before you know it.

⑫ Anti-inflammatory and immuno-modulating drugs

Just the facts

In this chapter, you'll learn:

♦ classes of drugs that modify immune or inflammatory responses

♦ uses and varying actions of these drugs

♦ absorption, distribution, metabolism, and excretion of these drugs

♦ drug interactions and adverse reactions to these drugs.

Drugs and the immune system

Immune and inflammatory responses protect the body from invading foreign substances. Certain classes of drugs can modify these responses:
- *Antihistamines* block the effects of histamine on target tissues.
- *Corticosteroids* suppress immune responses and reduce inflammation.
- *Immunosuppressants (noncorticosteroid)* prevent rejection of transplanted organs and can be used to treat autoimmune disease.
- *Uricosurics* control the occurrence of gouty arthritis attacks.

Antihistamines

Antihistamines primarily act to block histamine effects that occur in an immediate (type I) hypersensitivity reaction, commonly called an *allergic reaction*. They're available alone or in combination products and may be obtained by prescription or over the counter.

Histamine-1 receptor antagonists

The term *antihistamine* refers to drugs that act as histamine-1 (H_1) receptor antagonists; that is, they compete with histamine for H_1-receptor sites throughout the body. However, they don't displace histamines already bound to receptors.

It's all about chemistry

Antihistamines are categorised into major classes based on their chemical structures:
- *Ethanolamines* include fumarate and dimenhydrinate.
- *Alkylamines* include chlorphenamine.
- *Phenothiazines* include promethazine hydrochloride.
- *Piperidines* include cetirizine, cyproheptadine hydrochloride, desloratadine, fexofenadine, and loratadine.
- Miscellaneous drugs, such as hydroxyzine hydrochloride and hydroxyzine pamoate, also act as antihistamines.

Pharmacokinetics

H_1-receptor antagonists are absorbed well after oral or parenteral administration. Some can also be given rectally. With the exception of loratadine and desloratadine, antihistamines are distributed widely throughout the body and central nervous system (CNS).

On the alert

Fexofenadine, desloratadine, and loratadine are nonsedating antihistamines. Because these drugs only minimally penetrate the blood-brain barrier, they aren't widely distributed throughout the CNS. As a result, they produce fewer sedative effects than other antihistamines.

Antihistamines are metabolised by liver enzymes and excreted in urine, with small amounts secreted in breast milk. Fexofenadine, mainly excreted in faeces, is an exception. Cetirizine undergoes hepatic metabolism.

Pharmacodynamics

H_1-receptor antagonists compete with histamine for H_1 receptors on effector cells (the cells that cause allergic symptoms), blocking histamine from producing its effects. (See *How chlorphenamine stops allergic response.*)

Come on, histamine! I can take you on.

Pharm function

How chlorphenamine stops allergic response

Although chlorphenamine can't reverse symptoms of an allergic response, it can stop its progression. Here's what happens.

Release the mediators

When sensitised to an antigen, a mast cell reacts to repeated antigen exposure by releasing chemical mediators. One of these mediators, histamine, binds to histamine-1 (H_1) receptors found on effector cells (the cells responsible for allergic symptoms). This initiates the allergic response that typically affects the respiratory, cardiovascular, GI, endocrine, and integumentary systems.

The first one there wins

Chlorphenamine acts by competing with histamine for H_1-receptor sites on the effector cells. By attaching to these sites first, the drug prevents histamine from binding to the effector cells, inhibiting additional systemic responses, as shown below.

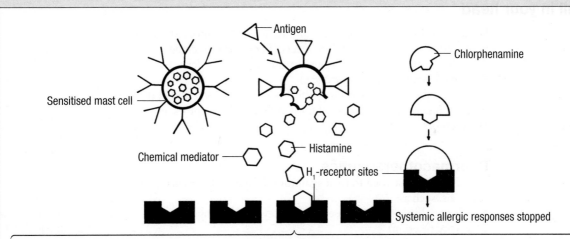

Effector cells

Respiratory responses	*Cardiovascular responses*	*GI responses*	*Endocrine responses*	*Integumentary responses*
• Bronchial constriction and bronchospasm • Decreased vital capacity • Itchy nose and throat • Rhinorrhea (runny nose) • Sneezing	• Decreased blood pressure • Elevated heart rate • Increased vasodilation • Increased capillary permeability	• Increased parietal cell secretion • Increased smooth-muscle contraction	• Increased release of adrenaline (epinephrine) and noradrenaline (norepinephrine)	• Angioedema (hives and swelling of skin, mucous membranes, or internal organs) • Flushing • Itching

Antagonising line of attack

H_1-receptor antagonists produce their effects by:
- blocking the action of histamine on small blood vessels
- decreasing arteriole dilation and tissue engorgement
- reducing leakage of plasma proteins and fluids out of the capillaries (capillary permeability), thereby lessening oedema
- inhibiting most smooth-muscle responses to histamine (in particular, blocking the constriction of bronchial, GI, and vascular smooth muscle)
- relieving symptoms by acting on the terminal nerve endings in the skin that flare and itch when stimulated by histamine
- suppressing adrenal medulla stimulation, autonomic ganglia stimulation, and exocrine gland secretion, such as lacrimal and salivary secretion.

Memory jogger

Anti- is a familiar prefix that means *opposing*. And that's exactly what antihistamines do: they oppose histamine effects (or allergic reactions).

It's all in your head

Several antihistamines have a high affinity for H_1 receptors in the brain and are used for their CNS effects. These drugs include dimenhydrinate, promethazine, and various piperidine derivatives. (See *Antihistamines: Dimenhydrinate.*)

H_1-receptor antagonists don't affect parietal cell secretion in the stomach because the receptors of these cells are H_2 receptors, not H_1 receptors.

Pharmacotherapeutics

Antihistamines are used to treat symptoms of type I hypersensitivity reactions, such as:
- allergic rhinitis (runny nose and itchy eyes caused by a local sensitivity reaction)
- vasomotor rhinitis (rhinitis not caused by allergy or infection)
- allergic conjunctivitis (inflammation of the eye membranes)
- urticaria (hives)
- angioedema (submucosal swelling in the hands, face, and feet).

Antihistamines relieve the symptoms of an allergic reaction. However, they don't give the body immunity to the allergy itself.

Beyond the obvious

Antihistamines have other therapeutic uses as well. Many are used primarily as antiemetics (to control nausea and vomiting). They can also be used as adjunctive therapy to treat an anaphylactic reaction after serious symptoms are controlled. Because of its antiserotonin qualities, cyproheptadine may be used to treat Cushing's disease, serotonin-associated diarrhoea, vascular cluster headaches, and anorexia nervosa.

Prototype pro

Antihistamines: Dimenhydrinate

Actions

- Competes with histamine for H_1-receptor sites on the smooth muscle of the bronchi, GI tract, uterus, and large blood vessels, binding to the cellular receptors and preventing access and subsequent activity of histamine
- Antagonises the action of histamine that causes increased capillary permeability and resultant oedema and suppresses flare and pruritus associated with endogenous release of histamine (doesn't directly alter histamine or prevent its release)

Indications

- Rhinitis
- Allergy symptoms
- Motion sickness
- Parkinson's disease

Nursing considerations

- Monitor for adverse effects, such as drowsiness, sedation, seizures, nausea, dry mouth, thrombocytopenia, agranulocytosis, thickening of secretions, and anaphylactic shock.
- Use with extreme caution in patients with prostatic hyperplasia, asthma, chronic obstructive pulmonary disease, hyperthyroidism, cardiovascular disease, or hypertension.

Drug interactions

Antihistamines interact with many other drugs, sometimes with life-threatening consequences. Here are a few examples:

- Antihistamines may block or reverse the vasopressor effects of adrenaline (epinephrine), producing vasodilation, increased heart rate, and dangerously low blood pressure.
- Antihistamines may mask toxic signs and symptoms of ototoxicity (a detrimental effect on hearing) associated with aminoglycosides or large doses of salicylates.
- Antihistamines may increase the sedative and respiratory depressant effects of CNS depressants, such as tranquillisers and alcohol.
- Loratadine may cause serious cardiac effects when taken with macrolide antibiotics (such as erythromycin), fluconazole, ketoconazole, itraconazole, miconazole, cimetidine, ciprofloxacin, and clarithromycin.

Beware of the possibility of serious, even life-threatening, drug interactions when giving antihistamines.

Adverse reactions

The most common adverse reaction to antihistamines (with the exception of fexofenadine and loratadine) is CNS depression. Other CNS reactions include:

- dizziness
- fatigue
- disturbed coordination
- muscle weakness.

Gut reactions

GI reactions may include:

- epigastric distress
- loss of appetite
- nausea and vomiting
- constipation
- diarrhoea
- dryness of the mouth, nose, and throat.

Cardiac concerns

Cardiovascular reactions may include:

- hypotension
- hypertension
- rapid heart rate
- arrhythmias.

A sensitive issue

Sensitivity reactions can also occur.

Nursing process

These nursing process steps are appropriate for patients undergoing treatment with antihistamines.

Assessment

- Obtain a history of the patient's underlying condition before therapy and reassess regularly thereafter.
- Monitor the patient for adverse reactions and drug interactions.
- Monitor blood counts during long-term therapy; watch for signs of blood dyscrasia as these drugs may induce thrombocytopenia or leucopenia.
- Evaluate the patient's and family's knowledge of drug therapy.

Key nursing diagnoses

- Ineffective health maintenance related to the underlying condition.
- Risk for injury related to drug-induced adverse CNS reactions.
- Deficient knowledge related to drug therapy.

Planning outcome goals
- An improvement in the patient's underlying condition will be exhibited.
- The risk of injury to the patient will be minimised.
- The patient and family will demonstrate an understanding of drug therapy.

Implementation
- Reduce GI distress by giving antihistamines with food.
- Follow the manufacturer's guidelines for I.V. administration.
- If administering the drug I.M., alternate injection sites to prevent irritation. Give I.M. injections into large muscles.
- Provide sugarless gum or ice cubes to relieve dry mouth.
- Increase the patient's fluid intake (if allowed) or humidify the air to decrease thickened secretions.
- Notify the prescriber if tolerance is observed because the patient may require a substitute antihistamine.

Evaluation
- Patient shows improvement in underlying condition.
- Patient sustains no injury from result of therapy.
- Patient and family state an understanding of drug therapy.
(See *Teaching about antihistamines*.)

Education edge

Teaching about antihistamines

If antihistamine therapy is prescribed, review these points with the patient and caregivers:

- Take the drug with meals or snacks to prevent GI upset.
- Drinking coffee or tea may reduce drowsiness.
- Use warm water rinses, artificial saliva, ice cubes, or sugarless gum to relieve dry mouth. Avoid overuse of mouthwash, which may worsen dryness and destroy normal flora.
- If you're using the medication to prevent motion sickness, take the drug 30 minutes before travel.
- Avoid hazardous activities, such as driving, until the full central nervous system effects of the drug are known.

- Seek medical approval before using alcohol, tranquillisers, sedatives, pain relievers, or sleeping medications.
- Stop taking antihistamines 4 days before diagnostic skin tests to preserve the accuracy of test results.
- Notify your prescriber if tolerance develops because a different antihistamine may need to be prescribed.
- Be aware that the drug may cause photosensitivity. Use sunblock or protective clothing.
- Avoid using other products containing diphenhydramine, including topical forms, because of the risk of adverse reactions.

Corticosteroids

Corticosteroids suppress immune responses and reduce inflammation. They're available as natural or synthetic steroids.

Nature's bounty

Natural corticosteroids are hormones produced by the adrenal cortex; most corticosteroid drugs are synthetic forms of these hormones.

Natural and synthetic corticosteroids are classified according to their biological activities:

- *Glucocorticoids*, such as cortisone acetate and dexamethasone, affect carbohydrate and protein metabolism.
- *Mineralocorticoids*, such as fludrocortisone acetate, regulate electrolyte and water balance.

> Glucocorticoids exert anti-inflammatory, metabolic, or immunosuppressant effects.

Glucocorticoids

Most glucocorticoids are synthetic analogues of hormones secreted by the adrenal cortex. They exert anti-inflammatory, metabolic, and immunosuppressant effects. Drugs in this class include:

- beclomethasone
- betamethasone
- cortisone
- dexamethasone
- hydrocortisone
- methylprednisolone
- prednisolone
- triamcinolone.

Pharmacokinetics

Glucocorticoids are well absorbed when administered orally. After I.M. administration, they're completely absorbed.

Glucocorticoids are bound to plasma proteins and distributed through the blood. They're metabolised in the liver and excreted by the kidneys.

Pharmacodynamics

Glucocorticoids suppress hypersensitivity and immune responses through a process that isn't entirely understood.

Prototype pro

Corticosteroids: Prednisolone

Actions

- Decreases inflammation by stabilising leucocyte lysosomal membranes, suppressing immune response, stimulating bone marrow, and influencing protein, fat, and carbohydrate metabolism

Indications

- Severe inflammation
- Immunosuppression

Nursing considerations

- Monitor for adverse effects, such as euphoria, insomnia, seizures, heart failure, arrhythmias, thromboembolism, peptic ulcers, pancreatitis, and acute adrenal insufficiency.
- Monitor the patient's weight, blood pressure, and serum electrolytes.
- The drug may mask signs of infection.
- The dose must be gradually reduced after long-term therapy.

The research suggests...

Researchers believe that glucocorticoids inhibit immune responses by:
- suppressing or preventing cell-mediated immune reactions
- reducing levels of leucocytes, monocytes, and eosinophils
- decreasing the binding of immunoglobulins to cell surface receptors
- inhibiting interleukin synthesis.

Oh so soothing

Glucocorticoids suppress the redness, oedema, heat, and tenderness associated with the inflammatory response. They start on the cellular level by stabilising the lysosomal membrane (a structure within the cell that contains digestive enzymes) so that it doesn't release its store of hydrolytic enzymes into the cells. (See *Corticosteroids: Prednisolone.*)

A job well done

Glucocorticoids prevent leakage of plasma from capillaries, suppress the migration of polymorphonuclear leucocytes (cells that kill and digest microorganisms), and inhibit phagocytosis (cellular ingestion and destruction of solid substances).

To ensure a job well done, glucocorticoids decrease antibody formation in injured or infected tissues and disrupt histamine

Pharm function

How methylprednisolone works

Tissue trauma normally leads to tissue irritation, oedema, inflammation, and production of scar tissue. Methylprednisolone counteracts the initial effects of tissue trauma, promoting healing.

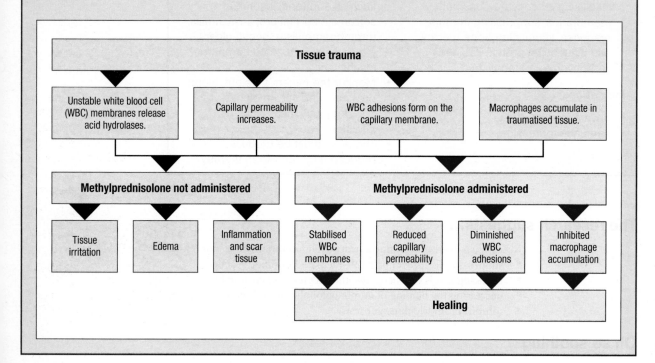

synthesis, fibroblast development, collagen deposition, capillary dilation, and capillary permeability. (See *How methylprednisolone works.*)

Pharmacotherapeutics

Glucocorticoids are used as replacement therapy for patients with adrenocortical insufficiency. They're also prescribed for immunosuppression (such as in allergic reactions) and disorders requiring treatment by reduction of inflammation (such as arthritis). They're also prescribed for their effects on the blood and lymphatic systems and as such are useful in counteracting shock.

Drug interactions

These drug interactions can occur with glucocorticoids:
- Barbiturates, phenytoin, rifampicin, and aminoglutethimide may reduce the effects of glucocorticoids.
- Amphotericin B, chlortalidone, furosemide, and thiazide diuretics may enhance glucocorticoids' potassium-wasting effects.
- Erythromycin may increase the effects of glucocorticoids by reducing their metabolism.
- Glucocorticoids reduce the serum concentration and effects of salicylates.
- The risk of peptic ulcers associated with nonsteroidal anti-inflammatory drugs and salicylates is increased when these agents are taken with corticosteroids.
- The response to vaccines and toxoids may be reduced in a patient taking glucocorticoids.
- Oestrogen and hormonal contraceptives that contain oestrogen increase the effects of glucocorticoids.
- The effects of antidiabetic drugs may be reduced, resulting in increased blood glucose levels.

Adverse reactions

Glucocorticoids affect almost all body systems. Their widespread adverse effects include:
- insomnia
- increased sodium and water retention
- increased potassium excretion
- suppressed immune and inflammatory responses
- osteoporosis
- intestinal perforation
- peptic ulcers
- impaired wound healing.

Glucocorticoids affect almost all body systems. You might say we're all-inclusive.

Endocrine system

Endocrine system reactions may include:
- diabetes mellitus
- hyperlipidaemia
- adrenal atrophy
- hypothalamic-pituitary axis suppression
- cushingoid signs and symptoms (such as buffalo hump, moonface, and elevated blood glucose levels).

Nursing process

These nursing process steps are appropriate for patients undergoing treatment with glucocorticoids.

Assessment

- Assess the patient's condition before therapy and regularly thereafter.
- Establish baseline blood pressure, fluid and electrolyte status, and weight; reassess regularly.
- Watch for depression or psychotic episodes, especially at high doses.
- Monitor the glucose levels of a patient with diabetes closely; increased insulin may be needed.
- Monitor the patient's stress level; dosage adjustment may be needed.
- Closely monitor the patient for adverse reactions and drug interactions.
- Evaluate the drug's effectiveness at regular intervals.
- Evaluate the patient's and family's knowledge of drug therapy.

Key nursing diagnoses

- Ineffective protection related to drug-induced adverse reactions.
- Risk for infection related to immunosuppression.
- Deficient knowledge related to drug therapy.

Planning outcome goals

- The patient won't experience adverse reactions.
- The patient will be free from infection as evidenced by normal temperature, cultures, and white blood cell (WBC) counts.
- The patient and family will demonstrate an understanding of drug therapy.

Implementation

- Give the drug early in the day to mimic circadian rhythm.
- Give the drug with food to prevent GI irritation.
- Take precautions to avoid exposing the patient to infection.
- Expect to increase the drug dosage during times of physiologic stress, such as surgery, trauma, or infection.
- Don't stop the drug abruptly. (See *Pitfalls of abrupt withdrawal*.)
- Avoid prolonged use of corticosteroids, especially in children.
- Notify the prescriber of severe or persistent adverse reactions.
- Unless contraindicated, offer a low-sodium diet that's high in potassium and protein. Administer potassium supplements as needed.

Evaluation

- Patient shows no evidence of adrenal insufficiency.
- Patient is free from infection.

> Glucocorticoids can reduce the effects of antidiabetic drugs. Monitor glucose levels of a patient with diabetes closely.

Pitfalls of abrupt withdrawal

If corticosteroids are rapidly withdrawn, abrupt withdrawal symptoms can occur. These include rebound inflammation, fatigue, weakness, arthralgia, fever, dizziness, lethargy, depression, fainting, orthostatic hypotension, dyspnea, anorexia, and hypoglycaemia. After long-term therapy, increased stress or abrupt withdrawal may cause acute adrenal insufficiency. Sudden withdrawal after prolonged therapy can be fatal.

Education edge

Teaching about corticosteroid therapy

If corticosteroid therapy is prescribed, review these points with the patient and caregivers:

- Take the drug exactly as prescribed, and never stop the drug suddenly. If you miss a dose, don't double the next dose. Continue with your regular dosing schedule and follow-up with your prescriber. Missed doses or suddenly stopping the drug may result in complications (especially if you're on long-term corticosteroid therapy). It's important to notify your prescriber of a change in your regular dosing schedule.
- Notify your prescriber if your stress level increases; the dosage may need to be temporarily adjusted.
- Take the oral form of the drug with food.
- Report sudden weight gain, swelling, slow healing, black tarry stools, bleeding, bruising, blurred vision, emotional changes, or other unusual effects.
- If receiving long-term therapy, ask your prescriber about vitamin D or calcium supplements, and have periodic eye examinations.

- Wear or carry medical identification at all times, indicating the need for systemic glucocorticoids during stress.
- If receiving long-term therapy, watch for cushingoid symptoms (weight gain, swelling of the face) and report them immediately.
- Be aware of early signs of adrenal insufficiency, including fatigue, muscular weakness, joint pain, fever, anorexia, nausea, dyspnea, dizziness, and fainting.
- Keep regular medical checkups to help detect early adverse reactions, evaluate disease status, and assess drug response. Dosage adjustments may be needed.
- Don't take other medications, over-the-counter preparations, or herbal remedies without first consulting your prescriber.
- Ask your physician about activity or exercise needed to help prevent or delay osteoporosis, a common adverse reaction.
- Report signs of infection to your prescriber.

- Patient and family state an understanding of drug therapy. (See *Teaching about corticosteroid therapy*.)

Mineralocorticoids

Mineralocorticoids affect electrolyte and water balance. These drugs include:
- fludrocortisone acetate, a synthetic analogue of hormones secreted by the adrenal cortex.

Pharmacokinetics

Fludrocortisone acetate is absorbed well and distributed to all parts of the body. It's metabolised in the liver to inactive metabolites and excreted by the kidneys.

Pharmacodynamics

Fludrocortisone acetate affects fluid and electrolyte balance by acting on the distal renal tubule to increase sodium reabsorption and potassium and hydrogen secretion.

Pharmacotherapeutics

Fludrocortisone acetate is used as replacement therapy for patients with adrenocortical insufficiency (reduced secretion of glucocorticoids, mineralocorticoids, and androgens).

A balancing act

Fludrocortisone acetate may also be used to treat salt-losing congenital adrenogenital syndrome (characterised by a lack of cortisol and deficient aldosterone production) after the patient's electrolyte balance has been restored.

Drug interactions

The drug interactions associated with mineralocorticoids are similar to those associated with glucocorticoids.

Adverse reactions

The adverse reactions associated with mineralocorticoids are similar to those associated with glucocorticoids.

Nursing process

These nursing process steps are appropriate for patients undergoing treatment with mineralocorticoids.

Assessment
* Assess the patient's condition before therapy and regularly thereafter.
* Establish baseline blood pressure, fluid and electrolyte status, and weight; reassess regularly.
* Monitor the patient closely for adverse reactions and drug interactions.
* Evaluate the drug's effectiveness at regular intervals.
* Evaluate the patient's and family's knowledge of drug therapy.

Key nursing diagnoses
* Risk for injury related to drug-induced adverse reactions.
* Excess fluid volume related to drug-induced adverse effects.
* Deficient knowledge related to drug therapy.

Planning outcome goals
- The patient won't experience adverse reactions.
- The patient's fluid volume status will remain within normal limits as evidenced by intake and output and vital signs.
- The patient and family will demonstrate an understanding of drug therapy.

Implementation
- Administer the drug as prescribed, and monitor for adverse reactions and drug interactions.
- Notify the prescriber of severe or persistent adverse reactions.
- Notify the prescriber if hypertension occurs.
- Monitor the patient's electrolyte levels; potassium supplements may be needed. Assess for hypokalaemia, such as muscle cramps and electrocardiogram changes.

Evaluation
- Patient's health is improved.
- Patient doesn't develop sodium and water insufficiency.
- Patient and family demonstrate an understanding of drug therapy.

Immunosuppressants

Several drugs used for their immunosuppressant effects in patients undergoing allograft transplantation (a transplant between two people who aren't identical twins) are also used experimentally to treat autoimmune diseases (diseases resulting from an inappropriate immune response directed against the self). They include:

- azathioprine
- anakinra
- basiliximab
- ciclosporine
- daclizumab
- mycophenolate mofetil
- sirolimus
- tacrolimus.

Pharmacokinetics
Immunosuppressants take different paths through the body:
- When administered orally, azathioprine is absorbed from the GI tract readily, whereas the absorbtion of ciclosporin is varied and incomplete.

- Anakinra, basiliximab, and daclizumab are administered only by I.V. injection.
- The distributions of azathioprine, daclizumab, and basiliximab aren't fully understood.
- Ciclosporine is distributed widely throughout the body.
- Azathioprine and ciclosporine cross the placental barrier.
- Distribution of tacrolimus depends on several factors, with 75% to 99% being protein bound. Sirolimus is 97% protein bound.

How it all adds up...

Azathioprine and ciclosporine are metabolised in the liver. Mycophenolate is metabolised in the liver to mycophenolate acid, an active metabolite, and then further metabolised to an inactive metabolite, which is excreted in urine and bile. Concentrations of mycophenolate and acyclovir may be increased in the presence of nephrotoxicity. Azathioprine, and anakinra are excreted in urine; ciclosporine is excreted principally in bile.

...and out

Tacrolimus is extensively metabolised and primarily excreted in bile; less than 1% is excreted unchanged in urine. Sirolimus is metabolised by a mixed function oxidase system, primarily cytochrome P-450 3A4; 91% is excreted in faeces and 2% in urine. Metabolism and excretion of basiliximab and daclizumab isn't understood.

Pharmacodynamics

It's unknown how certain immunosuppressants achieve their desired effects.

The jury's still out...

For example, the exact mechanisms of action of azathioprine and ciclosporine is unknown; however, these drugs may undergo these processes:
- Azathioprine antagonises the metabolism of the amino acid purine and, therefore, inhibits ribonucleic acid and deoxyribonucleic acid structure and synthesis. It may also inhibit coenzyme formation and function.
- Ciclosporine is thought to inhibit helper T cells and suppressor T cells through a modulation of interleukin and cytokine inflammatory mediators.

...but this much is known

In a patient receiving a kidney allograft, azathioprine suppresses cell-mediated hypersensitivity reactions and produces various alterations in antibody production.

Anakinra, basiliximab, and daclizumab block the activity of interleukin. Mycophenolate inhibits responses of T- and B-lymphocytes, suppresses antibody formation by B-lymphocytes, and may inhibit the recruitment of leucocytes into sites of inflammation and graft rejection. Sirolimus is an immunosuppressant that inhibits T-lymphocyte activation and proliferation that occurs in response to antigenic and cytokine stimulation; it also inhibits antibody formation.

Although the exact actions of immunosuppressants aren't fully understood, we're certainly involved.

Pharmacotherapeutics

Immunosuppressants are mainly used to prevent rejection in patients undergoing organ transplantation. (See *Ciclosporine: Miracle drug or death sentence?*)

Crusader against cancer

Cyclophosphamide, classified as an alkylating drug, is primarily used to treat cancer. However, it can also be used as an immunosuppressant.

Anakinra is indicated for adults with moderate to severely active rheumatoid arthritis who have taken at least one disease-modifying antirheumatic drug.

Cyclosporine: Miracle drug or death sentence?

Organ transplantation can save a life. However, ciclosporine, an immunosuppressant used to reduce the risk of organ rejection, may also cause cancer.

Does ciclosporine encourage cells to become cancerous?

It has long been believed that when the immune system is weakened by immunosuppressant drugs, it loses its ability to fight and kill cancerous cells. Research suggests that ciclosporine may also encourage abnormal cells to become cancerous and, in addition, perhaps even grow aggressively.

A double-edged sword

This research has raised obvious concern about the use of ciclosporine in organ transplantation. However, this concern needs to be balanced against the life-threatening risk of organ rejection. Scientists are now looking for ways to block this tumour-promoting effect of ciclosporine.

Drug interactions

Drug interactions with this class commonly involve other immunosuppressant and anti-inflammatory drugs or various antibiotic and antimicrobial drugs:

- Allopurinol increases the blood levels of azathioprine.
- Verapamil increases the blood levels of sirolimus.
- Levels of ciclosporine may be increased by ketoconazole, calcium channel blockers, cimetidine, anabolic steroids, hormonal contraceptives, erythromycin, and metoclopramide.
- Coadministration of voriconazole and sirolimus is contraindicated because of the inhibition of cytochrome P-450 3A4 enzymes by voriconazole, which increase sirolimus levels.
- The absorption of mycophenolate is decreased when taken with antacids or colestyramine. Coadministration of mycophenolate with acyclovir may increase concentrations of both drugs, especially in a patient with renal impairment.
- The risk of toxicity to the kidneys increases when ciclosporine is taken with acyclovir, aminoglycosides, or amphotericin B.
- The risk of infection and lymphoma (neoplasm of the lymph tissue, most likely malignant) is increased when ciclosporine or sirolimus is taken with other immunosuppressants (except corticosteroids).
- Barbiturates, rifampicin, phenytoin, sulphonamides, and trimethoprim decrease plasma ciclosporine and sirolimus levels.
- Serum digoxin levels may be increased when ciclosporine is taken with digoxin.
- Anakinra, basiliximab and daclizumab with other immunosuppressant drugs increases the risk of infection and lymphoma. Anakinra therapy shouldn't be initiated in a patient with an active infection or neutropenia.

Adverse reactions

All immunosuppressants can cause hypersensitivity reactions. Listed here are adverse reactions to individual drugs.

Azathioprine

Adverse reactions to azathioprine include:
- bone marrow suppression
- nausea and vomiting
- liver toxicity.

Ciclosporine
Adverse reactions to ciclosporine include:
- kidney toxicity
- hyperkalaemia
- infection
- liver toxicity
- nausea and vomiting.

Daclizumab
Adverse reactions to daclizumab include:
- GI disorders
- hypertension or hypotension
- chest pain
- tachycardia
- oedema
- dyspnea
- pulmonary oedema
- thrombosis
- bleeding
- renal tubular necrosis.

Mycophenolate
Adverse reactions to mycophenolate include:
- nausea
- diarrhoea
- leucopenia
- headache
- tremors
- weakness
- chest pain
- urinary tract infection
- liver function test abnormalities
- skin rash.

Sirolimus
Adverse reactions to sirolimus include:
- tremors
- anaemia
- leucopenia
- thrombocytopenia
- hyperlipidaemia

- hypertension
- arthralgia
- myalgia
- urinary frequency.

Tacrolimus

Adverse reactions to tacrolimus include:
- nausea and vomiting
- diarrhoea or constipation
- tremors
- leucopenia
- hypertension
- nephrotoxicity
- hepatotoxicity.

Nursing process

These nursing process steps are appropriate for patients undergoing treatment with other immunosuppressants.

Assessment
- Obtain a history of the patient's immune status before therapy.
- Monitor the drug's effectiveness by observing the patient for signs of organ rejection. Therapeutic response usually occurs within 8 weeks.
- Watch for adverse reactions and drug interactions.
- Monitor haemoglobin, haematocrit, and WBC and platelet counts at least once monthly; monitor them more often at the beginning of treatment.
- Evaluate the patient's and family's knowledge of drug therapy.

Key nursing diagnoses
- Ineffective protection related to threat of organ rejection.
- Risk for infection related to drug-induced immunosuppression.
- Deficient knowledge related to drug therapy.

Planning outcome goals
- The patient's vital signs will be within normal limits and assessment findings will be normal.
- No signs of infection will be present as evidenced by normal WBC and temperature and negative culture results.
- The patient and family will demonstrate an understanding of drug therapy.

Implementation
- Administer the medication as prescribed; reconstitute according to policy and procedure.
- Monitor the patient's reaction to the medication and watch for adverse reactions.
- Monitor WBC counts; the medication may need to be stopped if the patient's WBC count is less than $3,000/mm^3$. Notify the prescriber.
- To prevent bleeding, avoid I.M. injections when the platelet count is below $100,000/mm^3$.
- Monitor the patient for signs of infection and report fever, sore throat, and malaise because the drug is a potent immunosuppressant.
- Instruct a female patient to avoid conception during therapy and for 4 months after stopping therapy.
- Warn the patient that hair thinning may occur.
- Tell the patient that medication can take up to 12 weeks to be effective.

You shouldn't become pregnant while taking immunosuppressant drugs and for 4 months after stopping therapy.

Evaluation
- Patient exhibits no signs of organ rejection.
- Patient demonstrates no signs and symptoms of infection.
- Patient and family state understanding of drug therapy.

Uricosurics

Uricosurics and other antigout drugs exert their anti-inflammatory actions through their effects on uric acid. Increased uric acid in the blood (hyperuricaemia) results in gout, a specific form of acute arthritis.

Uricosuric drugs

The two major uricosurics are probenecid and sulfinpyrazone.

Out with the gout

Uricosurics act by increasing uric acid excretion in urine. The primary goal in using uricosurics is to prevent or control the frequency of gouty arthritis attacks.

Pharmacokinetics

Uricosurics are absorbed from the GI tract. Distribution of the two drugs is similar, with 75% to 95% of probenecid and 98% of sulfinpyrazone being protein bound. Metabolism of the drugs occurs in the liver, and excretion occurs primarily through the kidneys. Only small amounts of these drugs are excreted in faeces.

Pharmacodynamics

Probenecid and sulfinpyrazone reduce the reabsorption of uric acid at the proximal convoluted tubules of the kidneys. This results in excretion of uric acid in urine, reducing serum urate levels.

Pharmacotherapeutics

Probenecid and sulfinpyrazone are indicated for the treatment of:
*   chronic gouty arthritis
*   tophaceous gout (the deposition of tophi or urate crystals under the skin and into joints).

Outbound action

Probenecid is also used to promote uric acid excretion in patients experiencing hyperuricaemia.

When acute, substitute

Probenecid and sulfinpyrazone shouldn't be given during an acute gouty attack. If taken at that time, these drugs prolong inflammation. Because these drugs may increase the chance of an acute gouty attack when therapy begins and whenever the serum urate level changes rapidly, colchicine is administered during the first 3 to 6 months of therapy.

Drug interactions

Many drug interactions, some potentially serious, can occur with uricosuric drugs:
*   Probenecid can significantly increase and prolong the effects of cephalosporins, penicillins, and sulphonamides.
*   Serum urate levels may be increased when probenecid is taken with antineoplastic drugs.
*   Probenecid increases the serum concentration of dapsone, aminosalicylic acid, and methotrexate, causing toxic reactions.
*   Sulfinpyrazone increases the effectiveness of warfarin, increasing the risk of bleeding.
*   Salicylates reduce the effects of sulfinpyrazone.
*   Sulfinpyrazone may increase the effects of oral antidiabetic agents, increasing the risk of hypoglycaemia.

During an acute gouty attack, probenecid and sulfinpyrazone shouldn't be "in the game" because they can prolong inflammation and the duration of the attack.

Adverse reactions

Adverse reactions to uricosurics include uric acid stone formation and blood abnormalities.

Probenecid

Additional adverse reactions to probenecid include:
* headache
* anorexia
* nausea and vomiting
* hypersensitivity reactions.

Sulfinpyrazone

Additional adverse reactions to sulfinpyrazone include:
* nausea
* indigestion
* GI pain
* GI blood loss.

Nursing process

These nursing process steps are appropriate for patients undergoing treatment with uricosurics.

Assessment
* Assess the patient's condition before therapy and regularly thereafter.
* Periodically monitor blood urea nitrogen levels and renal function tests in long-term therapy. Note that the drug is ineffective in patients with chronic renal insufficiency (glomerular filtration rate less than 30 ml/minute).
* Be alert for adverse reactions and drug interactions.
* Monitor the patient's hydration status if adverse GI reactions occur.
* Evaluate the patient's and family's knowledge of drug therapy.

Key nursing diagnoses
* Ineffective health maintenance related to the underlying condition.
* Risk for deficient fluid volume related to adverse GI reactions.
* Deficient knowledge related to drug therapy.

Planning outcome goals
* Assessment parameters will be within normal limits.
* The patient will exhibit adequate hydration as demonstrated by intake and output.
* The patient and family will demonstrate an understanding of drug therapy.

Implementation

- Give the medication with milk, food, or antacids to minimise GI distress. Continued disturbances may indicate a need to lower the dosage.
- Encourage the patient to drink fluids to maintain a minimum daily output of 2 L of water per day. Sodium bicarbonate or potassium citrate may be needed to alkalinise urine. These measures prevent haematuria, renal colic, urate stone development, and costovertebral pain.
- Begin therapy when an acute attack subsides. Keep in mind that the drug contains no analgesic or anti-inflammatory agents and isn't useful during acute gout attacks.
- Be aware that the drug may increase the frequency, severity, and duration of acute gout attacks during the first 12 months of therapy. Prophylactic colchicine or another anti-inflammatory is given during the first 3 to 6 months.
- Instruct the patient to avoid drugs that contain aspirin, which may precipitate gout.
- Tell the patient to avoid alcohol during drug therapy because it increases the urate level.
- Advise the patient to limit intake of foods high in purine, such as anchovies, liver, sardines, kidneys, peas, and lentils.

Evaluation

- Patient responds positively to therapy.
- Patient maintains adequate hydration.
- Patient and family state an understanding of drug therapy.

Other antigout drugs

Other antigout drugs include allopurinol and colchicine. Allopurinol is used to reduce uric acid production, preventing gouty attacks, and colchicine is used to treat acute gouty attacks.

Other antigout drugs include allopurinol and colchicine.

Pharmacokinetics

Allopurinol and colchicine take somewhat different paths through the body.

All aboard allopurinol

When given orally, allopurinol is absorbed from the GI tract. Allopurinol and its metabolite oxypurinol are widely distributed throughout the body except in the brain, where drug concentrations are less than those found in the rest of the body. It's metabolised by the liver and excreted in urine.

"Tracting" colchicine's course

Colchicine is also absorbed from the GI tract. Colchicine is partially metabolised in the liver. The drug and its metabolites then reenter the intestinal tract through biliary secretions. After reabsorption from the intestines, colchicine is distributed to various tissues. The drug is excreted primarily in faeces and to a lesser degree in urine.

Pharmacodynamics

Allopurinol and its metabolite oxypurinol inhibit xanthine oxidase, the enzyme responsible for the production of uric acid. By reducing uric acid formation, allopurinol eliminates the hazards of hyperuricuria.

WBCs, don't go there!

Colchicine appears to reduce the inflammatory response to monosodium urate crystals deposited in joint tissues. Colchicine may produce its effects by inhibiting migration of WBCs to the inflamed joint. This reduces phagocytosis and lactic acid production by WBCs, decreasing urate crystal deposits and reducing inflammation.

Pharmacotherapeutics

Allopurinol treats primary gout, hopefully preventing acute gouty attacks. It can be prescribed with uricosurics when smaller dosages of each drug are directed. It's used to:
* treat gout or hyperuricaemia that may occur with blood abnormalities and during treatment of tumours or leukaemia
* treat primary or secondary uric acid nephropathy (with or without the accompanying symptoms of gout)
* treat and prevent recurrent uric acid stone formation
* treat patients who respond poorly to maximum dosages of uricosurics or who have allergic reactions or intolerance to uricosuric drugs.

What a relief!

Colchicine is used to relieve the inflammation of acute gouty arthritis attacks. If given promptly, it's especially effective in relieving pain. Also, giving colchicine during the first several months of allopurinol, probenecid, or sulfinpyrazone therapy may prevent the acute gouty attacks that sometimes accompany the use of these drugs.

Drug interactions

Colchicine doesn't interact significantly with other drugs. When allopurinol is used with other drugs, the resulting interactions can be serious:
* Allopurinol potentiates the effect of oral anticoagulants.
* Allopurinol increases the serum concentrations of mercaptopurine and azathioprine, increasing the risk of toxicity.

- Angiotensin-converting enzyme inhibitors increase the risk of hypersensitivity reactions to allopurinol.
- Allopurinol increases serum theophylline levels.
- The risk of bone marrow depression increases when cyclophosphamide is taken with allopurinol.

Adverse reactions

The most common adverse reaction to allopurinol is a rash. Prolonged administration of colchicine may cause bone marrow suppression.

Allopurinol and colchicine commonly cause:
- nausea and vomiting
- diarrhoea
- intermittent abdominal pain.

Nursing process

These nursing process steps are appropriate for patients undergoing treatment with other antigout drugs.

Assessment
- Assess the patient's condition before therapy and regularly thereafter.
- Assess the patient's uric acid level, joint stiffness, and pain before and during therapy. Optimal benefits may require 2 to 6 weeks of therapy.
- Monitor the patient's complete blood count and hepatic and renal function at the start of therapy and periodically during therapy.
- Be alert for adverse reactions and drug interactions.
- Monitor the patient's fluid intake and output. Daily urine output of at least 2 L and maintenance of neutral or slightly alkaline urine are desirable.
- Evaluate the patient's and family's knowledge of drug therapy.

Key nursing diagnoses
- Acute pain related to the underlying condition.
- Risk for infection related to drug-induced agranulocytosis.
- Deficient knowledge related to drug therapy.

Planning outcome goals
- The patient will state that pain is decreased.
- Assessment parameters will be within normal limits.
- The patient and family will demonstrate an understanding of drug therapy.

Implementation
- Give medication with meals or immediately after to minimise GI distress.
- Encourage the patient to drink fluids while taking the drug, unless contraindicated.
- Notify the prescriber if renal insufficiency occurs during treatment; this usually warrants a dosage reduction.
- Give colchicine with allopurinol, if prescribed. This combination prophylactically treats acute gout attacks that may occur in the first 6 weeks of therapy.
- Advise the patient to refrain from driving or performing hazardous tasks requiring mental alertness until the CNS effects of the drug are known.
- Advise the patient taking allopurinol for treatment of recurrent calcium oxalate stones to reduce intake of animal protein, sodium, refined sugars, oxalate-rich foods, and calcium.
- Stop the drug at the first sign of a rash, which may precede severe hypersensitivity or other adverse reaction. A rash is more common in patients taking diuretics and those with renal disorders. Tell the patient to report all adverse reactions immediately.
- Tell the patient to avoid alcohol during drug therapy because it increases urate level.

Give colchicine with allopurinol for a 1-2 punch against gout.

Evaluation
- Patient expresses relief from joint pain.
- Patient is free from infection.
- Patient and family state an understanding of drug therapy.

Quick quiz

1. Which class of drugs suppresses immune response and reduces inflammation?
    A. Antihistamines
    B. Corticosteroids
    C. Immunosuppressants
    D. Uricosurics

Answer: B. Corticosteroids suppress immune responses and reduce inflammation.

2. During the nursing assessment, the patient states that he's taking digoxin, furosemide, a tranquilliser, and amoxicillin. Which medication would cause a drug interaction with the antihistamine the physician prescribed?
    A. Digoxin
    B. Furosemide
    C. Tranquiliser
    D. Amoxicillin

Answer: C. Antihistamines can interact with many drugs, sometimes with life-threatening consequences. They may increase the sedative and respiratory depressant effects of CNS depressants, such as tranquilisers and alcohol.

3. The nurse is monitoring a patient receiving prednisolone. For which adverse reaction should the nurse monitor the patient?
   A. Somnolence
   B. Hyperglycaemia
   C. Hyperkalaemia
   D. Hypoglycaemia

Answer: B. Corticosteroids affect almost all body systems. Endocrine system reactions may include decreased glucose tolerance, resulting in hyperglycaemia and possibly precipitating diabetes mellitus.

4. The nurse is assessing a patient who's receiving an immunosuppressant. The patient is hypotensive, experiencing chest pain, and tachycardic. These signs indicate an adverse reaction to which immunosuppressant?
   A. Azathioprine
   B. Ciclosporine
   C. Tacrolimus
   D. Daclizumab

Answer: D. Daclizumab may cause GI disorders, hypertension, hypotension, chest pain, tachycardia, oedema, dyspnea, pulmonary oedema, thrombosis, bleeding, and renal tubular necrosis.

5. Which medication interacts with allopurinol?
   A. Oral anticoagulants
   B. Antihistamines
   C. Cardiac glycosides
   D. Antidiabetic agents

Answer: A. Allopurinol potentiates the effects of oral anticoagulants.

Scoring

☆☆☆ If you answered all five questions correctly, extraordinary! You certainly aren't allergic to smarts!

☆☆ If you answered four questions correctly, congratulations! You're taking the sting out of learning!

☆ If you answered fewer than four questions correctly, keep trying! With continued improvement, the next chapter should have you feeling better!

13 Antineoplastic drugs

Just the facts

In this chapter, you'll learn:

♦ classes of drugs used to treat cancer

♦ uses and varying actions of these drugs

♦ absorption, distribution, metabolism, and excretion of these drugs

♦ drug interactions and adverse reactions to these drugs.

Drugs and cancer

In the 1940s, antineoplastic (chemotherapeutic) drugs were developed to treat cancer. However, these agents commonly caused serious adverse reactions.

A change for the good

Today, many of these drugs have lower toxicity levels so they aren't as devastating to the patient. With modern chemotherapy, childhood malignancies, such as acute lymphoblastic leukaemia, and adult cancers, such as testicular cancer, are curable in most cases. Novel therapeutic strategies, such as using monoclonal antibodies or targeting specific proteins, are further improving the time that a patient's cancer can remain in remission. In addition, other drugs, such as interferons, are being used to treat patients with cancer.

Alkylating drugs

Alkylating drugs, given alone or with other drugs, effectively act against various malignant neoplasms. These drugs are categorised into one of six classes:
- nitrogen mustards
- alkyl sulphonates
- nitrosoureas
- triazenes
- ethylenimines
- alkylating-like drugs.

Unfazed at any phase

Alkylating drugs produce their antineoplastic effects by damaging deoxyribonucleic acid (DNA). They halt DNA's replication process by cross-linking its strands so that amino acids don't pair up correctly. Alkylating drugs are cell cycle–phase nonspecific. This means that their alkylating actions may take place at any phase of the cell cycle.

Nitrogen mustards

Nitrogen mustards represent the largest group of alkylating drugs. They include:
- chlorambucil
- cyclophosphamide
- estramustine
- ifosfamide
- mechlorethamine hydrochloride
- melphalan.

The opening act

Mechlorethamine hydrochloride was the first nitrogen mustard introduced and is rapid acting.

Pharmacokinetics

As with most alkylating drugs, the absorption and distribution of nitrogen mustards vary widely. Nitrogen mustards are metabolised in the liver and excreted by the kidneys.

Before you can say 1-2-3

Mechlorethamine undergoes metabolism so rapidly that, after a few minutes, no active drug remains. Most nitrogen mustards possess more intermediate half-lives than mechlorethamine.

Pharm function

How alkylating drugs work

Alkylating drugs can attack deoxyribonucleic acid (DNA) in two ways, as shown in the illustrations below.

Bifunctional alkylation

Some drugs become inserted between two base pairs in the DNA chain, forming an irreversible bond between them. This is called *bifunctional alkylation,* which causes cytotoxic effects capable of destroying or poisoning cells.

Monofunctional alkylation

Other drugs react with just one part of a pair, separating it from its partner and eventually causing it and its attached sugar to break away from the DNA molecule. This is called *monofunctional alkylation,* which eventually may cause permanent cell damage.

Pharmacodynamics

Nitrogen mustards form covalent bonds with DNA molecules in a chemical reaction known as alkylation. Alkylated DNA can't replicate properly, thereby resulting in cell death. Unfortunately, cells may develop resistance to the cytotoxic effects of nitrogen mustards. (See *How alkylating drugs work.*)

Pharmacotherapeutics

Because they produce leucopenia (a reduced number of white blood cells [WBCs]), the nitrogen mustards are effective in treating malignant neoplasms, such as Hodgkin's disease (cancer causing painless enlargement of the lymph nodes, spleen, and lymphoid tissues) and leukaemia (cancer of the blood forming tissues) that can have an associated elevated WBC count.

Alkylating drugs deactivate my DNA, cutting my life short.

Nitrogen bomb

Nitrogen mustards also prove effective against malignant lymphoma (cancer of the lymphoid tissue), multiple myeloma (cancer of the marrow plasma cells), melanoma (malignancy that arises from melanocytes), and cancer of the breast, ovaries, uterus, lung, brain, testes, bladder, prostate, and stomach.

Drug interactions

Nitrogen mustards interact with several other drugs:
- Calcium-containing drugs and foods, such as antacids and dairy products, reduce absorption of estramustine.
- Taking cyclophosphamide with cardiotoxic drugs produces additive cardiac effects.
- Cyclophosphamide can reduce serum digoxin levels.
- An increased risk of ifosfamide toxicity exists when the drug is taken with allopurinol, barbiturates, chloral hydrate, or phenytoin.
- Corticosteroids reduce the effects of ifosfamide.
- The lung toxicity threshold of carmustine may be reduced when taken with melphalan.
- Interferon alpha may reduce the serum concentration of melphalan.

Adverse reactions

Many patients experience fatigue during nitrogen mustard therapy. Other adverse reactions include:
- bone marrow suppression, leading to severe leucopenia and thrombocytopenia
- nausea and vomiting from central nervous system (CNS) irritation
- stomatitis
- reversible hair loss.

Handle with care

Because nitrogen mustards are powerful local vesicants (blistering drugs), direct contact with these drugs or their vapours can cause severe reactions, especially to the skin, eyes, and respiratory tract.

Direct contact with nitrogen mustards can cause severe skin, eye, and respiratory reactions.

Nursing process

These nursing process steps are appropriate for patients undergoing treatment with nitrogen mustard drugs.

Assessment
- Assess the patient's underlying neoplastic disorder before therapy and reassess regularly throughout therapy.
- Perform a complete assessment before therapy begins.
- Monitor for adverse reactions and drug interactions throughout therapy.

- Monitor haematocrit, platelet, and total and differential leucocyte counts, and blood urea nitrogen (BUN), alanine aminotransferase (ALT), aspartate aminotransferase (AST), lactate dehydrogenase (LD), serum bilirubin, serum creatinine, uric acid, and other levels as needed.
- Monitor the patient's vital signs and catheter or I.V. line patency throughout drug administration.
- Evaluate the patient's and family's knowledge of drug therapy.

Key nursing diagnoses
- Ineffective health maintenance related to the presence of neoplastic disease.
- Ineffective protection related to drug-induced haematologic adverse reactions.
- Deficient knowledge related to drug therapy.

Planning outcome goals
- The patient will demonstrate an improvement in assessments and diagnostic testing.
- The patient will be free from infection as evidenced by normal temperature, cultures, and WBC counts.
- The patient and family will demonstrate an understanding of drug therapy.

Implementation
- Follow established procedures for safe and proper handling, administration, and disposal of chemotherapeutic drugs.
- Treat extravasation promptly.
- Keep adrenaline (epinephrine), corticosteroids, and antihistamines available during administration. Anaphylactoid reactions may occur.
- Administer the medications as prescribed and monitor for effects.
- Administer adequate hydration and monitor intake and output.
- Administer an antiemetic for nausea and vomiting caused by drug use.
- Follow facility policy for infection control in immunocompromised patients whose WBC counts fall below 2,000/mm^3 or granulocyte counts fall below 1,000/mm^3.

Evaluation
- Patient shows an improvement in underlying neoplastic condition on follow-up diagnostic tests.
- Patient remains free from infection and doesn't bleed abnormally.
- Patient and family state an understanding of drug therapy. (See *Teaching about chemotherapy with alkylating drugs*.)

Education edge

Teaching about chemotherapy with alkylating drugs

If chemotherapy with alkylating drugs is prescribed, review these points with the patient and caregivers:

- Avoid people with bacterial or viral infections because chemotherapy can increase susceptibility. Watch for signs of infection (fever, sore throat, fatigue) and bleeding (easy bruising, nosebleeds, bleeding gums, melena). Take your temperature daily and report signs of infection promptly.
- Use proper oral hygiene, including cautious use of toothbrush, dental floss, and toothpicks.
- Complete dental work before therapy begins or delay it until your blood counts are normal.
- Be aware that you may bruise easily because of the drug's effect on your blood count.
- Don't take over-the-counter (OTC) products, medications, or herbal remedies without first consulting your prescriber.

- Avoid OTC products that contain aspirin.
- Take medications as directed.
- Keep all appointments for chemotherapy, blood tests, and check-ups.
- Maintain an adequate intake of nutritious food and fluids; consult with a dietitian to help design a diet that meets your needs.
- Use an electric razor to help minimise bleeding.
- Be prepared for hair loss.
- Inform any other physician, dentist, or health care provider, before any treatment, that you are receiving chemotherapy.
- If you are of childbearing age, effective contraception should be carried out during, and for a few months after, chemotherapy.

Alkyl sulphonates

The alkyl sulfonate busulfan has historically been used to treat chronic myelogenous leukaemia, polycythaemia vera (increased red blood cell [RBC] mass and an increased number of WBCs and platelets), and other myeloproliferative (pertaining to overactive bone marrow) disorders. Busulfan is used at high doses to treat leukaemia during bone marrow transplantation.

Pharmacokinetics
Busulfan is absorbed rapidly and well from the GI tract. Little is known about its distribution. Busulfan is metabolised extensively in the liver before urinary excretion. Its half-life is 2 to 3 hours.

Pharmacodynamics
As an alkyl sulphonate, busulfan forms covalent bonds with the DNA molecules in alkylation.

Pharmacotherapeutics

Busulfan primarily affects granulocytes (a type of WBC) and, to a lesser degree, platelets. Because of its action on granulocytes, it has been used for treating chronic myelogenous leukaemia and in conditioning regimens for bone marrow transplantation.

To a screeching halt

Busulfan is also effective in treating polycythaemia vera. However, other drugs are usually used to treat polycythaemia vera because busulfan can cause severe myelosuppression (halting of bone marrow function).

Drug interactions

There's an increased risk of bleeding when busulfan is taken with anticoagulants or aspirin. Concurrent use of busulfan and tioguanine may cause liver toxicity, oesophageal varices (enlarged, swollen veins in the oesophagus), or portal hypertension (increased pressure in the portal vein of the liver).

Adverse reactions

The major adverse reaction to busulfan is bone marrow suppression, producing severe leucopenia, anaemia, and thrombocytopenia (reduced WBCs, RBCs, and platelets, respectively), which is usually dose related and reversible.

A latecomer

Pulmonary fibrosis may occur as late as 4 to 6 months after treatment. Seizures are also a concern. (See *Busulfan warning*.)

Nursing process

These nursing process steps are appropriate for patients undergoing treatment with alkyl sulphonates.

Assessment
- Assess the patient's underlying neoplastic disorder before therapy and reassess regularly throughout therapy.
- Perform a complete assessment before therapy begins.
- Monitor for adverse reactions and drug interactions throughout therapy.

Going down

- Monitor the patient's WBC count and platelet counts weekly during therapy. The WBC count falls about 10 days after the start

Before you give that drug!

Busulfan warning

Seizures can occur as an adverse reaction to I.V. infusion of busulfan. The patient may be premedicated with phenytoin to decrease the risk of seizures.

of therapy and continues to fall for 2 weeks after stopping the drug.
• Monitor the patient's uric acid level.
• Monitor the patient's vital signs and catheter or I.V. line patency throughout drug administration.
• Monitor the drug's effectiveness by noting results of follow-up diagnostic tests and the patient's overall physical status. Note his response (increased appetite and sense of well-being, decreased total WBC count, and reduced size of spleen), which usually begins within 1 to 2 weeks.
• Evaluate the patient's and family's knowledge of drug therapy.

Key nursing diagnoses
• Ineffective health maintenance related to the presence of neoplastic disease.
• Risk for infection related to drug-induced immunosuppression.
• Deficient knowledge related to drug therapy.

Planning outcome goals
• An improvement in the patient's underlying condition will be exhibited.
• No signs of infection will be present as evidenced by normal WBC count and temperature and negative cultures.
• The patient and family will demonstrate an understanding of drug therapy.

Implementation
• Follow established procedures for safe and proper handling, administration, and disposal of chemotherapeutic drugs.
• Give the drug at the same time each day.
• Treat extravasation promptly.
• Administer the medications as prescribed and monitor for effects.
• Administer adequate hydration and monitor intake and output.
• The dosage is adjusted based on the patient's weekly WBC count, and the prescriber may temporarily stop drug therapy if severe leucocytopenia develops. Therapeutic effects are commonly accompanied by toxicity.
• The drug is usually given with allopurinol in addition to adequate hydration to prevent hyperuricaemia with resulting uric acid nephropathy.
• Advise a breast-feeding patient to stop during drug therapy because of the possible risk of infant toxicity.

Evaluation
• Patient shows an improvement in the underlying neoplastic condition on follow-up diagnostic tests.

Handle all chemotherapeutic drugs with care! Be sure to follow established procedures for safe and proper handling, administration, and disposal of these drugs.

- Patient remains free from infection.
- Patient and family state an understanding of drug therapy.

Nitrosoureas

Nitrosoureas are alkylating agents that halt cancer cell reproduction. They include:
- carmustine
- lomustine.

Pharmacokinetics

When administered I.V., carmustine achieves a steady-state volume of distribution. With oral administration, lomustine is absorbed adequately, although incompletely.

The fat of the matter is...

Nitrosoureas are lipophilic (attracted to fat) drugs, and are distributed to fatty tissues and cerebrospinal fluid (CSF). They're metabolised extensively before urine excretion.

Pharmacodynamics

During a process called bifunctional alkylation, nitrosoureas interfere with amino acids, purines, and DNA needed for cancer cells to divide, thus halting their reproduction.

Pharmacotherapeutics

The nitrosoureas are highly lipid (fat) soluble, which allows them or their metabolites to easily cross the blood-brain barrier. Because of this ability, nitrosoureas are used to treat brain tumours and meningeal leukaemias.

Drug interactions

Each of the nitrosoureas has its own interactions with other drugs:
- Cimetidine may increase carmustine's bone marrow toxicity. (See *Carmustine warning*.)
- Lomustine used with anticoagulants or aspirin increases the risk of bleeding; avoid using these drugs together.

Before you give that drug!

Carmustine warning

Obtain baseline pulmonary function tests before therapy because pulmonary toxicity appears to be related to the dosage. Be sure to evaluate results of liver, renal, and pulmonary function tests periodically thereafter.

Adverse reactions

All of the nitrosoureas can produce severe nausea and vomiting.

Bad to the bone

Carmustine and lomustine produce bone marrow suppression that begins 4 to 6 weeks after treatment and lasts 1 to 2 weeks.

Kidney concerns

Kidney toxicity and kidney failure may also occur with patients taking nitrosoureas. High-dose carmustine may produce reversible liver toxicity.

Pulmonary problems

Carmustine may cause lung toxicity characterised by lung infiltrates or fibrosis (scarring).

Nursing process

These nursing process steps are appropriate for patients undergoing treatment with nitrosoureas.

Assessment
- Assess the patient's underlying neoplastic disorder before therapy and reassess regularly throughout therapy.
- Perform a complete assessment before therapy begins.
- Obtain baseline pulmonary function tests before therapy because pulmonary toxicity appears to be dose related. Be sure to evaluate the results of liver, renal, and pulmonary function tests periodically thereafter.
- Monitor for adverse reactions and drug interactions throughout therapy.
- Monitor the patient's complete blood count (CBC) and uric acid level.
- Monitor the patient's vital signs and catheter or I.V. line patency throughout drug administration.
- Evaluate the patient's and family's knowledge of drug therapy.

Key nursing diagnoses
- Ineffective health maintenance related to the presence of neoplastic disease.
- Risk for injury related to drug-induced adverse reactions.
- Deficient knowledge related to drug therapy.

Planning outcome goals
- An improvement in the patient's underlying condition will be exhibited.
- The risk of injury to the patient will be minimised.
- The patient and family will demonstrate an understanding of drug therapy.

Implementation
- Follow established procedures for safe and proper handling, administration, and disposal of chemotherapeutic drugs.
- Give an antiemetic before giving the drug to reduce nausea.
- Administer the medications per facility policy for reconstitution, mixing, storage, and administration. Monitor for effects.
- Use carmustine only in glass containers. The solution is unstable in plastic I.V. bags. Avoid contact with skin because carmustine will cause a brown stain. If skin contact occurs, wash it off thoroughly.
- Use double gloves when handling carmustine wafer in the treatment room.
- Administer adequate hydration and monitor the patient's intake and output.
- Allopurinol may be used with adequate hydration to prevent hyperuricaemia and uric acid nephropathy.
- Advise a breast-feeding patient to stop during therapy because of possible infant toxicity.
- Repeat lomustine administration only when CBC results reveal safe haematologic parameters.
- Institute infection control and bleeding precautions.

Be sure to follow your facility's policy for reconstituting, mixing, storing, and administering chemotherapeutic drugs.

Evaluation
- Patient shows an improvement in the underlying neoplastic condition on follow-up diagnostic tests.
- Patient doesn't experience injury from drug-induced adverse reactions.
- Patient and family state an understanding of drug therapy.

Triazenes

The triazene, dacarbazine, functions as an alkylating drug only after it has been activated by the liver.

Pharmacokinetics

After I.V. injection, dacarbazine is distributed throughout the body and metabolised in the liver. Within 6 hours, 30% to 45% of a dose is excreted by the kidneys (half is excreted unchanged; the other half is excreted as one of the metabolites).

Dysfunction junction

In a patient with kidney or liver dysfunction, the drug's half-life may increase to 7 hours.

Pharmacodynamics

Dacarbazine first must be metabolised in the liver to become an alkylating drug. It seems to inhibit ribonucleic acid (RNA) and protein synthesis. Like other alkylating drugs, dacarbazine is cell cycle–nonspecific.

Pharmacotherapeutics

Dacarbazine is used primarily to treat patients with malignant melanoma. It's also used with other drugs to treat patients with Hodgkin's disease.

Drug interactions

No significant drug interactions have been reported with dacarbazine.

After I.V. injection, dacarbazine must be metabolised by the liver before it becomes an antineoplastic drug.

Adverse reactions

Dacarbazine use may cause the following adverse reactions:
- leucopenia
- thrombocytopenia
- nausea and vomiting (which begin within 1 to 3 hours after administration in most cases and may last up to 12 hours)
- phototoxicity
- flu-like syndrome
- hair loss.

Nursing process

These nursing process steps are appropriate for patients undergoing treatment with triazenes.

Assessment
- Assess the patient's underlying neoplastic disorder before therapy and reassess regularly throughout therapy.
- Perform a complete assessment before therapy begins.

- Monitor for adverse reactions and drug interactions throughout therapy.
- Monitor the patient's CBC, platelet count, and liver enzyme levels.
- Monitor the patient's vital signs and catheter or I.V. line patency throughout drug administration.
- Evaluate the patient's and family's knowledge of drug therapy.

Key nursing diagnoses
- Ineffective health maintenance related to the presence of neoplastic disease.
- Risk of injury related to drug-induced adverse reactions.
- Deficient knowledge related to drug therapy.

Planning outcome goals
- The patient will demonstrate an improvement in assessments and diagnostic testing.
- The risk for injury to the patient will be minimised.
- The patient and family will demonstrate an understanding of drug therapy.

Implementation
- Follow established procedures for safe and proper handling, administration, and disposal of chemotherapeutic drugs.
- Administer the medications as prescribed and monitor for effects.
- Administer adequate hydration and monitor the patient's intake and output.
- Administer an antiemetic before giving dacarbazine to help decrease nausea. Nausea and vomiting may subside after several doses.
- Reconstitute the drug according to facility policy. During infusion, protect the bag from direct sunlight to avoid drug breakdown. The solution may be diluted further or the infusion slowed to decrease pain at the infusion site.
- Discard the drug if the solution turns pink; this is a sign of decomposition.
- Take care to avoid extravasation during infusion. If the I.V. site infiltrates, discontinue the infusion immediately, apply ice to the area for 24 to 48 hours, and notify the prescriber.
- Advise the patient to avoid sunlight and sunlamps for the first 2 days after treatment.
- Reassure the patient that flu-like syndrome may be treated with mild antipyretics such as paracetamol.

Evaluation
- Patient shows an improvement in underlying neoplastic condition on follow-up diagnostic tests.
- Patient remains free from infection and doesn't bleed abnormally.
- Patient and family state an understanding of drug therapy.

Ethylenimines

Thiotepa, an ethylenimine derivative, is a multifunctional alkylating drug.

Pharmacokinetics

After I.V. administration, thiotepa is 100% bioavailable. Significant systemic absorption may occur when it's administered into pleural (around the lungs) or peritoneal (abdominal) spaces to treat malignant effusions or instilled into the bladder. Thiotepa crosses the blood-brain barrier and is metabolised extensively in the liver. Thiotepa and its metabolites are excreted in urine.

Pharmacodynamics

Thiotepa exerts its cytotoxic activity by interfering with DNA replication and RNA transcription. Ultimately, it disrupts nucleic acid function and causes cell death.

Pharmacotherapeutics

Thiotepa is used to treat bladder cancer. This alkylating drug is also prescribed for palliative (symptom relief) treatment of lymphomas and ovarian or breast carcinomas.

Talk about a good return on your investment. After I.V. administration, thiotepa is 100% bioavailable.

And there's more

Thiotepa is used to treat intracavitary effusions (fluid accumulation in a body cavity). It may also prove useful in the treatment of lung cancer.

Drug interactions

Thiotepa may interact with other drugs:
- Concurrent use of thiotepa, anticoagulants, and aspirin may increase the risk of bleeding.
- Taking thiotepa with neuromuscular blocking drugs may prolong muscular paralysis.

• Concurrent use of thiotepa and other alkylating drugs or radiation therapy may intensify toxicity rather than enhance the therapeutic response.

It'll take your breath away

When used with suxamethonium, thiotepa may cause prolonged respirations and apnea (periods of not breathing). Thiotepa appears to inhibit the activity of cholinesterase, the enzyme that deactivates suxamethonium.

Adverse reactions

The major adverse reactions to thiotepa are blood related and include leucopenia, anaemia, thrombocytopenia, and pancytopenia (deficiency of all cellular elements of the blood), which may be fatal. Other adverse reactions include:
• nausea and vomiting (commonly)
• stomatitis and ulceration of the intestinal mucosa (especially at bone marrow transplant doses)
• hives, rash, and pruritus (occasionally).

Nursing process

These nursing process steps are appropriate for patients undergoing treatment with ethylenimines.

Assessment
• Assess the patient's underlying neoplastic disorder before therapy and reassess regularly throughout therapy.
• Perform a complete assessment before therapy begins.
• Monitor the patient for adverse reactions and drug interactions throughout therapy.
• Monitor the patient's CBC weekly for at least 3 weeks after the last dose.
• Monitor the patient's uric acid level.
• Adverse GI reactions are reversible in 6 to 8 months.
• Monitor the patient's vital signs and catheter or I.V. line patency throughout drug administration.
• Evaluate the patient's and family's knowledge of drug therapy.

Key nursing diagnoses
• Ineffective health maintenance related to the presence of neoplastic disease.
• Ineffective protection related to drug-induced haematologic adverse reactions.
• Deficient knowledge related to drug therapy.

Planning outcome goals
- An improvement in the patient's underlying condition will be exhibited.
- No signs of infection will be present as evidenced by normal WBC count and temperature and negative culture results.
- The patient and family will demonstrate an understanding of drug therapy.

Implementation
- Follow established procedures for safe and proper handling, administration, and disposal of chemotherapeutic drugs.
- Reconstitute the drug per facility policy for I.V. administration. The drug may be given by rapid I.V. administration in doses of 0.3 to 0.4 mg/kg at intervals of 1 to 4 weeks.
- If intense pain occurs with I.V. administration, use a local anaesthetic at the injection site. If pain occurs at the insertion site, dilute the solution further or use a local anaesthetic. Make sure that the drug doesn't infiltrate.
- Discard if the I.V. solution appears grossly opaque or contains precipitate. The solutions should be clear to slightly opaque.
- Administer the medications as prescribed and monitor for effects.
- Thiotepa may be used for bladder instillation. (See *Thiotepa warning*.)
- For neoplastic effusions, thiotepa may be administered intracavitarily by mixing the drug with 2% procaine hydrochloride or adrenaline (epinephrine) hydrochloride 1:1,000. The drug can be given by all parenteral routes, including direct injection into the tumour.
- Refrigerate and protect dry powder from direct sunlight.
- Report a WBC count below 3,000/mm^3 or a platelet count below 150,000/mm^3 and stop the drug.
- To prevent hyperuricaemia with resulting uric acid nephropathy, allopurinol may be used with adequate hydration.
- Advise a breast-feeding patient to stop during therapy because of the risk of infant toxicity.

Evaluation
- Patient shows an improvement in underlying neoplastic condition on follow-up diagnostic tests.
- Patient remains free from infection and doesn't bleed abnormally.
- Patient and family state an understanding of drug therapy.

Alkylating-like drugs

Carboplatin, oxaliplatin, and cisplatin are heavy metal complexes that contain platinum. Because their action resembles that of a

Before you give that drug!

Thiotepa warning

Thiotepa can be used for intracavitary use. For neoplastic effusions, mix the drug with 2% procaine hydrochloride or adrenaline (epinephrine) hydrochloride 1:1,000. The drug can be given by all parenteral routes, including direct injection into the tumour.

bifunctional alkylating drug, these drugs are referred to as *alkylating-like drugs.*

Pharmacokinetics

The distribution and metabolism of carboplatin aren't clearly defined. After I.V. administration, carboplatin is eliminated primarily by the kidneys.

By and bi

The elimination of carboplatin is biphasic. It has an initial half-life of 1 to 2 hours and a terminal half-life of 2.5 to 6 hours. Oxaliplatin is 70% to 90% bound to plasma proteins and is eliminated primarily by the kidneys. When administered intrapleurally (into the pleural space around the lung) or intraperitoneally (into the peritoneum), cisplatin may exhibit significant systemic absorption.

Reaching new heights

Highly protein bound, cisplatin reaches high concentrations in the kidneys, liver, intestines, and testes, but has poor CNS penetration. The drug undergoes some liver metabolism, followed by excretion through the kidney.

Going platinum

Platinum is detectable in tissue for at least 4 months after administration.

Pharmacodynamics

Like alkylating drugs, carboplatin, oxaliplatin, and cisplatin are cell cycle–nonspecific and inhibit DNA synthesis. They act like bifunctional alkylating drugs by cross-linking strands of DNA and inhibiting DNA synthesis. (See *Alkylating drugs: Cisplatin.*)

Pharmacotherapeutics

These alkylating-like drugs are used to treat several cancers:
• Carboplatin is used primarily to treat ovarian and lung cancer.
• Cisplatin is prescribed to treat bladder and metastatic ovarian and testicular cancers.
• Cisplatin may also be used to treat head, neck, and lung cancer.
• Oxaliplatin is used in combination with other agents in colorectal cancer.

Prototype pro

Alkylating drugs: Cisplatin

Actions

- Probably cross-links strands of cellular deoxyribonucleic acid and interferes with ribonucleic acid transcription, causing growth imbalance that leads to cell death
- Kills selected cancer cells

Indications

- Adjunct therapy in metastatic testicular and ovarian cancer
- Advanced bladder and oesophageal cancer
- Head and neck cancer
- Cervical cancer
- Non-small-cell lung cancer
- Brain tumour
- Osteogenic sarcoma or neuroblastoma

Nursing considerations

- Monitor for adverse reactions, such as peripheral neuritis, seizures, tinnitus, hearing loss, nausea and vomiting, severe renal toxicity, myelosuppression, leucopenia, thrombocytopenia, anaemia, and anaphylactoid reaction.
- Assess the underlying neoplastic disease before therapy and reassess regularly throughout therapy.

Drug interactions

These alkylating-like drugs interact with a few other drugs:
- When carboplatin, cisplatin, or oxaliplatin are administered with an aminoglycoside, the risk of toxicity to the kidney increases.
- Taking carboplatin or cisplatin with bumetanide, and furosemide increase the risk of ototoxicity (damage to the organs of hearing and balance).
- Cisplatin may reduce serum phenytoin levels.

Adverse reactions

Carboplatin and cisplatin produce many of the same adverse reactions as the alkylating drugs:
- Carboplatin can produce bone marrow suppression.
- Kidney toxicity can occur with cisplatin, usually after multiple courses of therapy. Carboplatin is less toxic to the kidneys.
- With long-term cisplatin therapy, neurotoxicity can occur. Neurotoxicity is less common with carboplatin.
- Tinnitus (ringing in the ears) and hearing loss, which is usually permanent, may occur with cisplatin. It's much less common with carboplatin.
- Cisplatin can also produce marked nausea and vomiting.

Nursing process

These nursing process steps are appropriate for patients undergoing treatment with alkylating-like drugs.

Assessment
• Assess the patient's underlying neoplastic disorder before therapy and reassess regularly throughout therapy.
• Perform a complete assessment before therapy begins.
• Monitor the patient for adverse reactions and drug interactions throughout therapy.
• Monitor the patient's CBC, electrolyte levels (especially potassium and magnesium), platelet count, and renal function studies before initial and subsequent dosages.
• To detect permanent hearing loss, obtain audiometry test results before initial dose and subsequent courses.
• Evaluate the patient's and family's knowledge of drug therapy.

Key nursing diagnoses
• Ineffective health maintenance related to the presence of neoplastic disease.
• Ineffective protection related to drug-induced haematologic adverse reactions.
• Deficient knowledge related to drug therapy.

Planning outcome goals
• The patient will demonstrate an improvement in assessments and diagnostic testing.
• No signs of infection will be present as evidenced by normal WBC count and temperature and negative culture results.
• The patient and family will demonstrate an understanding of drug therapy.

Implementation
• Follow established procedures for safe and proper handling, administration, and disposal of chemotherapeutic drugs. (See *Cisplatin warning*.)
• Administer the medications as prescribed and monitor for effects.
• Administer adequate hydration and monitor intake and output.
• Dilute the medication as directed; cisplatin infusions are most stable in chloride-containing solutions. Don't use needles or I.V. administration sets that contain aluminium because it will displace platinum, causing a loss of potency and formation of black precipitate.
• Monitor the patient's renal function because renal toxicity is cumulative. Their renal function must return to normal before the next dose can be given.

Before you give that drug!

Cisplatin warning

Follow facility policy to reduce risks. Preparation and administration of parenteral forms of a chemotherapeutic drug, such as cisplatin, is linked to carcinogenic, mutagenic, and teratogenic risks for personnel.

Mannitol or furosemide is given before and with cisplatin infusion to maintain diuresis of 100 to 400 ml/hour during and for 24 hours after therapy. Prehydration and diuresis may reduce renal toxicity and ototoxicity significantly.

- The dosage shouldn't be repeated unless the patient's platelet count is more than 100,000/mm³, WBC count is over 4,000/mm³, creatinine level is under 1.5 mg/dl, or BUN level is under 25 mg/dl.
- Check current protocol with drug administration. Some clinicians use I.V. sodium thiosulphate to minimise toxicity.
- Administer an antiemetic, as prescribed; nausea and vomiting may be severe and protracted (up to 24 hours). Provide I.V. hydration until the patient can tolerate adequate oral intake. Ondansetron, granisetron, and high-dose metoclopramide have been used effectively to prevent and treat nausea and vomiting. Some clinicians combine metoclopramide with dexamethasone and antihistamines or ondansetron or granisetron with dexamethasone.
- Delayed vomiting (3 to 5 days after treatment) has been reported. The patient may need prolonged antiemetic treatment.
- To prevent hypokalaemia, potassium chloride (10 to 20 mmol/l) is commonly added to I.V. fluids before and after cisplatin therapy.
- Immediately give adrenaline (epinephrine), corticosteroids, or antihistamines for anaphylactoid reactions.
- Tell the patient to report tinnitus immediately as well as oedema or a decrease in urine output (if recording intake and output at home).

Evaluation

- Patient shows an improvement in underlying neoplastic condition on follow-up diagnostic tests.
- Patient remains free from infection and doesn't bleed abnormally.
- Patient and family state an understanding of drug therapy.

Antimetabolite drugs

Because antimetabolite drugs structurally resemble DNA base pairs, they can become involved in processes associated with DNA base pairs—that is, the synthesis of nucleic acids and proteins.

Getting specific

Antimetabolites differ significantly from the DNA base pairs in how they interfere with this synthesis. Because the antimetabolites are cell cycle–specific and primarily affect cells that actively synthesise DNA, they're referred to as S phase–specific. Normal cells that are reproducing actively as well as the cancer cells are affected by the antimetabolites.

> The antimetabolite drugs are cell cycle–specific. They're referred to as S phase–specific because they primarily affect cells that actively synthesise DNA.

Each according to its metabolite

These drugs are subclassified according to the metabolite affected and include:
- folic acid analogues
- pyrimidine analogues
- purine analogues.

Folic acid analogues

Although researchers have developed many *folic acid analogues*, the early compound methotrexate remains the most commonly used.

Pharmacokinetics

Methotrexate is absorbed well and distributed throughout the body. It can accumulate in any fluid collection, such as ascites or pleural or pericardial effusion. This can result in prolonged elimination and higher than expected toxicity, especially myelosuppression.

Do not enter

At usual dosages, methotrexate doesn't enter the CNS readily. (See *Antimetabolite drugs: Methotrexate.*) Although methotrexate is metabolised partially, it's excreted primarily unchanged in urine.

A disappearing act

Methotrexate exhibits a three-part disappearance from plasma; the rapid distributive phase is followed by a second phase, which reflects kidney clearance. The last phase, the terminal half-life, is 3 to 10 hours for a low dose and 8 to 15 hours for a high dose.

Pharmacodynamics

Methotrexate reversibly inhibits the action of the enzyme dihydrofolate reductase. This blocks normal folic acid processing, which inhibits DNA and RNA synthesis. The result is cell death.

Pharmacotherapeutics

Methotrexate is especially useful in treating:
- acute lymphoblastic leukaemia (abnormal growth of lymphocyte precursors, the lymphoblasts), the most common leukaemia in children
- acute lymphocytic leukaemia (abnormal growth of lymphocytes), and may be given as treatment and prophylaxis for meningeal leukaemia

Prototype pro

Antimetabolite drugs: Methotrexate

Actions

- Prevents the reduction of folic acid to tetrahydrofolate by binding to dihydrofolate reductase
- Kills certain cancer cells and reduces inflammation

Indications

- Trophoblastic tumours (chori-ocarcinoma, hydatidiform mole)
- Acute lymphoblastic and lymphatic leukaemia, meningeal leukaemia
- Burkitt's lymphoma (stage I or stage II)
- Lymphosarcoma (stage III)
- Osteosarcoma

Nursing considerations

- Monitor for adverse reactions, such as stomatitis, diarrhoea, intestinal perforation, nausea, vomiting, renal failure, anaemia, leucopenia, thrombocytopenia, acute hepatic toxicity, pulmonary fibrosis, urticaria, and sudden death.
- Assess the underlying neoplastic disease before therapy and reassess regularly throughout therapy.
- Follow facility policy for reconstitution and administration.

- CNS diseases (given intrathecally)
- choriocarcinoma (cancer that develops from the chorionic portions of the products of conception)
- osteogenic sarcoma (bone cancer)
- malignant lymphomas
- carcinomas of the head, neck, bladder, testis, and breast.

Unconventional treatment

The drug is also prescribed in low doses to treat severe psoriasis, graft-versus-host disease, and rheumatoid arthritis that fail conventional therapy.

Drug interactions

Methotrexate interacts with several other drugs:
- Probenecid decreases methotrexate excretion, increasing the risk of methotrexate toxicity, including fatigue, bone marrow suppression, and stomatitis (mouth inflammation).

• Salicylates and nonsteroidal anti-inflammatory drugs (NSAIDs), especially diclofenac, ketoprofen, indomethacin, and naproxen, also increase methotrexate toxicity.
• Colestyramine reduces the absorption of methotrexate from the GI tract.
• Concurrent use of alcohol and methotrexate increases the risk of liver toxicity.
• Taking co-trimoxazole with methotrexate may produce blood cell abnormalities.
• Penicillin decreases renal tubular secretion of methotrexate, increasing the risk of methotrexate toxicity.

Adverse reactions

Adverse reactions to methotrexate include:
• bone marrow suppression
• stomatitis
• pulmonary toxicity, exhibited as pneumonitis or pulmonary fibrosis
• skin reactions, such as photosensitivity and hair loss.

To the rescue

Kidney toxicity can also occur with high doses of methotrexate. During high-dose therapy, calcium folinate may be used to minimise adverse reactions. This process is known as folinate rescue.

Intrathecal threats

Adverse reactions to intrathecal administration (through the dura into the subarachnoid space) of methotrexate may include seizures, paralysis, and death. Other less severe adverse reactions may also occur, such as headaches, fever, neck stiffness, confusion, and irritability.

Nursing process

These nursing process steps are appropriate for patients undergoing treatment with folic acid analogues.

Assessment
• Perform a complete assessment before therapy begins. Assess the patient's condition before therapy and regularly thereafter.
• Monitor the patient for adverse reactions and drug interactions.
• Monitor the patient's fluid intake and output daily.
• Monitor the patient's vital signs and catheter or I.V. line patency throughout drug administration.

- Monitor haematocrit; ALT, AST, LD, serum bilirubin, serum creatinine, uric acid, and BUN levels; platelet and total and differential leucocyte counts; and other values, as required.
- Evaluate the patient's and family's knowledge of drug therapy.

Key nursing diagnoses
- Ineffective protection related to drug-induced adverse reactions.
- Risk of infection related to immunosuppression.
- Deficient knowledge related to drug therapy.

Planning outcome goals
- The risk for injury to the patient will be minimised.
- No signs of infection will be present as evidenced by normal WBC count and temperature and negative cultures.
- The patient and family will demonstrate an understanding of drug therapy.

Implementation
- Follow the established procedures for safe and proper handling, administration, and disposal of drugs.
- Try to ease anxiety in the patient and family before treatment.
- Give an antiemetic before giving the drug to lessen nausea.
- Give cytarabine with allopurinol to decrease the risk of hyperuricaemia. Promote a high fluid intake.
- Provide diligent mouth care to prevent stomatitis with cytarabine, fluorouracil, or methotrexate therapy.
- Anticipate the need for folinate rescue with high-dose methotrexate therapy.
- Treat extravasation promptly.
- Tell the patient to defer immunisations if possible until haematologic stability is confirmed.
- Anticipate diarrhoea, possibly severe, with prolonged fluorouracil therapy.

Evaluation
- Patient develops no serious bleeding complications.
- Patient remains free from infection.
- Patient and family state an understanding drug therapy. (See *Teaching about antimetabolite drugs.*)

Education edge

Teaching about antimetabolite drugs

If antimetabolite drugs are prescribed, review these points with the patient and caregivers:

- Use proper oral hygiene, including cautious use of toothbrush, dental floss, and toothpicks. Chemotherapy can increase the risk of microbial infection, delayed healing, and bleeding gums.
- Complete dental work before therapy begins or delay it until blood counts are normal.
- Be aware that you may bruise easily because of the drug's effect on platelets.
- Avoid close contact with persons who have taken oral poliovirus vaccine and who have been exposed to persons with bacterial or viral infection because chemotherapy may increase susceptibility. Notify your prescriber promptly if you develop signs or symptoms of infection.

- Report redness, pain, or swelling at the injection site. Local tissue injury and scarring may result from tissue infiltration at the infusion site.
- Be aware of the expected adverse effects of the drug, especially nausea, vomiting, diarrhoea, and hand-foot syndrome (pain, swelling, and redness of the hands or feet). Patient-specific dose adaptations during therapy are expected and needed. Stop taking the drug and contact your prescriber immediately if adverse effects occur.
- If you miss a dose, don't take the missed dose and don't double the next one. Continue with your regular dosing schedule and check with your prescriber.
- Don't take over-the-counter medications, other medicines, or herbal preparations without first consulting your prescriber.

Pyrimidine analogues

Pyrimidine analogues are a diverse group of drugs that inhibit production of pyrimidine nucleotides necessary for DNA synthesis. They include:
- capecitabine
- cytarabine
- fluorouracil
- gemcitabine.

Pharmacokinetics

Because pyrimidine analogues are absorbed poorly when given orally, they're usually administered by other routes. With the exception of cytarabine, pyrimidine analogues are distributed well throughout the body, including the CSF. They're metabolised extensively in the liver and are excreted in urine. Intrathecal cytarabine may be given with or without cranial radiation to treat CNS leukaemia.

How pyrimidine analogues work

To understand how pyrimidine analogues work, it helps to consider the basic structure of deoxyribonucleic acid (DNA).

Climbing the ladder to understanding

DNA resembles a ladder that has been twisted. The rungs of the ladder consist of pairs of nitrogenous bases: adenine always pairs with thymine, and guanine always pairs with cytosine. Cytosine and thymine are pyrimidines; adenine and guanine are purines.

One part sugar...

The basic unit of DNA is the nucleotide. A nucleotide is the building block of nucleic acids. It consists of a sugar, a nitrogen-containing base, and a phosphate group. It's on these components that pyrimidine analogues do their work.

In the guise of a nucleotide

After pyrimidine analogues are converted into nucleotides, they're incorporated into DNA, where they may inhibit DNA and ribonucleic acid synthesis as well as other metabolic reactions necessary for proper cell growth.

Pharmacodynamics

Pyrimidine analogues kill cancer cells by interfering with the natural function of pyrimidine nucleotides. (See *How pyrimidine analogues work*.)

Pharmacotherapeutics

Pyrimidine analogues may be used to treat many types of tumours. However, they're primarily indicated in the treatment of:
- acute leukaemias
- GI tract adenocarcinomas, such as colorectal, pancreatic, oesophageal, and stomach cancers
- carcinomas of the breast and ovaries
- malignant lymphomas.

Drug interactions

No significant drug interactions occur with most of the pyrimidine analogues; however, several are possible with capecitabine:
- Capecitabine may have increased absorption when coadministered with antacids.

- Capecitabine can increase the pharmacodynamic effects of warfarin, thereby increasing the risk of bleeding.
- Capecitabine may increase serum phenytoin levels.

Adverse reactions

Like most antineoplastic drugs, pyrimidine analogues can cause:
- fatigue
- inflammation of the mouth, oesophagus, and throat, leading to painful ulcerations and tissue sloughing
- bone marrow suppression
- nausea
- anorexia.

High-dose cytarabine can cause severe cerebellar neurotoxicity, chemical conjunctivitis, diarrhoea, fever, and hand-foot syndrome (numbness, paraesthesia, tingling, painless or painful swelling, erythema, desquamation, blistering, and severe pain of hands or feet). Crab erythema can be seen with high-dose cytarabine and continuous infusions of fluorouracil. Other adverse reactions with fluorouracil include diarrhoea and hair loss.

Nursing process

These nursing process steps are appropriate for patients undergoing treatment with pyrimidine analogues.

Assessment
- Perform a complete assessment before therapy begins and regularly thereafter.
- Monitor the patient for adverse reactions and drug interactions.
- Monitor the patient's daily fluid intake and output.
- Monitor the patient's vital signs and catheter or I.V. line patency throughout drug administration.
- Monitor the patient for hand-foot syndrome, hyperbilirubinaemia, and severe nausea. Drug therapy will need to be immediately adjusted.
- Evaluate the patient's and family's knowledge of drug therapy.

Key nursing diagnoses
- Ineffective protection related to drug-induced adverse reactions.
- Risk of infection related to immunosuppression.
- Deficient knowledge related to drug therapy.

Planning outcome goals
- The risk for injury to the patient will be minimised.
- No signs of infection will be present as evidenced by normal WBC count and temperature and negative cultures.
- The patient and family will demonstrate an understanding of drug therapy.

Implementation
- Follow established procedures for safe and proper handling, administration, and disposal of drugs.
- Try to ease anxiety in the patient and family before treatment.
- Give an antiemetic before giving the drug to lessen nausea.
- Give cytarabine with allopurinol to decrease the risk of hyperuricaemia.
- Promote a high fluid intake.
- Provide diligent mouth care to prevent stomatitis with cytarabine, fluorouracil, or methotrexate therapy.
- Treat extravasation promptly.
- Tell the patient to defer immunisations if possible until haematologic stability is confirmed.
- Anticipate diarrhoea, possibly severe, with prolonged fluorouracil therapy.

Evaluation
- Patient develops no serious bleeding complications.
- Patient remains free from infection.
- Patient and family state an understanding of drug therapy.

Purine analogues

Purine analogues are incorporated into DNA and RNA, interfering with nucleic acid synthesis and replication. They include:
- cladribine
- fludarabine phosphate
- mercaptopurine
- pentostatin
- tioguanine.

Pharmacokinetics
The pharmacokinetics of purine analogues aren't defined clearly. They're largely metabolised in the liver and excreted in urine.

Pharmacodynamics
As with the other antimetabolites, fludarabine, mercaptopurine, and tioguanine first must undergo conversion via phosphorylation to the nucleotide level to be active. The resulting nucleotides are then incorporated into DNA, where they may inhibit DNA and RNA synthesis as well as other metabolic reactions necessary for proper cell growth. Cladribine responds in a similar fashion. Pentostatin inhibits adenosine deaminase, causing an increase in intracellular

levels of deoxyadenosine triphosphate. This leads to cell damage and death. The greatest activity of adenosine deaminase is in cells of the lymphoid system, especially malignant T cells.

Analogous to pyrimide analogues

This conversion to nucleotides is the same process that pyrimidine analogues experience but, in this case, it's purine nucleotides that are affected. Purine analogues are cell cycle–specific as well, exerting their effect during that same S phase.

Pharmacotherapeutics

Purine analogues are used to treat acute and chronic leukaemias and may be useful in the treatment of lymphomas.

Drug interactions

No significant interactions occur with cladribine or tioguanine.

A serious flub with fludarabine

Taking fludarabine and pentostatin together may cause severe pulmonary toxicity, which can be fatal. Taking pentostatin with allopurinol may increase the risk of rash.

No bones about it

Concomitant administration of mercaptopurine and allopurinol may increase bone marrow suppression by decreasing mercaptopurine metabolism.

Adverse reactions

Purine analogues can produce:
- bone marrow suppression
- nausea and vomiting
- anorexia
- mild diarrhoea
- stomatitis
- rise in uric acid levels (a result of the breakdown of purine).

High-dose horrors

Fludarabine, when used at high doses, may cause severe neurologic effects, including blindness, coma, and death.

Nursing process

These nursing process steps are appropriate for patients undergoing treatment with purine analogues.

Assessment
• Perform a complete assessment before therapy begins and regularly thereafter.
• Monitor the patient for adverse reactions and drug interactions.
• Monitor the patient's fluid intake and output daily.
• Monitor the patient's vital signs and catheter or I.V. line patency throughout drug administration.
• Careful haematologic monitoring, especially of neutrophil and platelet counts, is needed. Bone marrow suppression can be severe.
• Evaluate the patient's and family's knowledge of drug therapy.

Key nursing diagnoses
• Ineffective protection related to drug-induced adverse reactions.
• Risk for infection related to immunosuppression.
• Deficient knowledge related to drug therapy.

Planning outcome goals
• The risk of injury to the patient will be minimised.
• No signs of infection will be present as evidenced by normal WBC count and temperature and negative cultures.
• The patient and family will demonstrate an understanding of drug therapy.

Implementation
• Follow established procedures for safe and proper handling, administration, and disposal of drugs. Follow the facility's policy to reduce risks. Preparation and administration of parenteral forms create mutagenic, teratogenic, and carcinogenic risks for staff.
• Prepare the medication according to the facility policy regarding reconstitution and administration.
• Try to ease anxiety in the patient and family before treatment.
• Give an antiemetic before giving the drug to lessen nausea.
• Treat extravasation promptly.
• Tell the patient to defer immunisations if possible until haematologic stability is confirmed.

Evaluation
• Patient develops no serious bleeding complications.
• Patient remains free from infection.
• Patient and family state an understanding of drug therapy.

Antibiotic antineoplastic drugs

Antibiotic antineoplastic drugs are antimicrobial products that produce tumouricidal (tumour-destroying) effects by binding with DNA. These drugs inhibit the cellular processes of normal and malignant cells. They include:

- anthracyclines (daunorubicin, doxorubicin, and idarubicin)
- bleomycin
- dactinomycin
- mitomycin
- mitoxantrone.

Pharmacokinetics

Because antibiotic antineoplastic drugs are usually administered I.V., no absorption occurs. They're considered 100% bioavailable.

Direct delivery

Some of the drugs are also directly administered into the body cavity being treated. Bleomycin, doxorubicin, and mitomycin are sometimes given as topical bladder instillations where significant systemic absorption doesn't occur. When bleomycin is injected into the pleural space for malignant effusions, up to one-half of the dose is absorbed. (See *Antibiotic antineoplastic drugs: Doxorubicin hydrochloride.*)

Distribution of antibiotic antineoplastic drugs throughout the body varies as does their metabolism and elimination.

Because antibiotic antineoplastic drugs are usually administered I.V., no absorption occurs.

Pharmacodynamics

With the exception of mitomycin, antibiotic antineoplastic drugs intercalate, or insert themselves, between adjacent base pairs of a DNA molecule, physically separating them.

Worming their way in

Remember, DNA looks like a twisted ladder with the rungs made up of pairs of nitrogenous bases. Antibiotic antineoplastic drugs insert themselves between these nitrogenous bases. Then, when the DNA chain replicates, an extra base is inserted opposite the intercalated antibiotic, resulting in a mutant DNA molecule. The overall effect is cell death.

Breaking the chain

Mitomycin is activated inside the cell to a bifunctional or trifunctional alkylating drug. It produces single-strand breakage of DNA, cross-links DNA, and inhibits DNA synthesis.

Prototype pro

Antibiotic antineoplastic drugs: Doxorubicin hydrochloride

Actions

- Thought to interfere with deoxyribonucleic acid-dependent ribonucleic acid synthesis by intercalation (chemical effect unknown)
- Hinders or kills certain cancer cells

Indications

- Bladder, breast, lung, ovarian, stomach, testicular, and thyroid cancers
- Hodgkin's disease
- Acute lymphoblastic and myeloblastic leukaemia
- Wilms' tumour

- Neuroblastoma
- Lymphoma
- Sarcoma

Nursing considerations

- Monitor for adverse reactions, such as arrhythmias, leucopenia, thrombocytopenia, myelosuppression, alopecia, and anaphylaxis.
- Assess the underlying neoplastic disease before therapy and reassess regularly throughout therapy.
- Follow facility policy for reconstitution and administration.

Pharmacotherapeutics

Antibiotic antineoplastic drugs act against many cancers, including:
- Hodgkin's disease and malignant lymphomas
- testicular carcinoma
- squamous cell carcinoma of the head, neck, and cervix
- Wilms' tumour (a malignant neoplasm of the kidney, occurring in young children)
- osteogenic sarcoma and rhabdomyosarcoma (malignant neoplasm composed of striated muscle cells)
- Ewing's sarcoma (a malignant tumour that originates in bone marrow, typically in long bones or the pelvis) and other soft-tissue sarcomas
- breast, ovarian, bladder, and lung cancer
- melanoma
- carcinomas of the GI tract
- choriocarcinoma
- acute leukaemia.

Drug interactions

Antibiotic antineoplastic drugs interact with many other drugs:
- Concurrent therapy with fludarabine and idarubicin isn't recommended because of the risk of fatal lung toxicity.
- Bleomycin may decrease serum digoxin and serum phenytoin levels.

- Doxorubicin may reduce serum digoxin levels.
- Combination chemotherapies enhance leucopenia and thrombocytopenia (reduced number of platelets).
- Mitomycin and vinca alkaloids may cause acute respiratory distress.

Adverse reactions

The primary adverse reaction to antibiotic antineoplastic drugs is bone marrow suppression. Irreversible cardiomyopathy and acute electrocardiogram (ECG) changes can also occur as well as nausea and vomiting.

Running hot and cold

An antihistamine and antipyretic should be given before bleomycin to prevent fever and chills. An anaphylactic reaction can occur in patients receiving bleomycin for lymphoma, so test doses should be given first.

Seeing red...or blue-green

Doxorubicin may colour urine red; mitoxantrone may colour it blue-green.

Nursing process

These nursing process steps are appropriate for patients undergoing treatment with antibiotic antineoplastic drugs.

Assessment
- Perform a complete assessment before therapy begins.
- Obtain a history of the patient's neoplastic disorder before therapy, and reassess regularly thereafter.
- Assess ECG results before treatment with doxorubicin.
- Monitor the patient for adverse reactions.
- Monitor the patient's vital signs and catheter or I.V. line patency.
- Monitor haemoglobin, haematocrit, platelet, and total and differential leukocyte counts, ALT, AST, LDH, bilirubin, creatinine, uric acid, and BUN levels.
- Monitor pulmonary function tests in a patient receiving bleomycin. Assess lung function regularly.
- Monitor ECG before and during treatment with daunorubicin and doxorubicin.

Key nursing diagnoses
- Ineffective health maintenance related to the presence of neoplastic disease.
- Risk for infection related to immunosuppression.
- Deficient knowledge related to drug therapy.

Planning outcome goals
- An improvement in the patient's underlying condition will be exhibited.
- No signs of infection will be present as evidenced by normal WBC count and temperature and negative cultures.
- The patient and family will demonstrate an understanding of drug therapy.

Implementation
- Follow established procedures for safe and proper handling, administration, and disposal of chemotherapeutic drugs.
- Try to ease anxiety in the patient and family before treatment.
- Keep adrenaline (epinephrine), corticosteroids, and antihistamines available during therapy. Anaphylactoid reactions may occur.
- Treat extravasation promptly.
- Ensure adequate hydration during idarubicin therapy.
- Discontinue procarbazine and notify the prescriber if the patient becomes confused or neuropathies develop.

Evaluation
- Patient exhibits an improvement of health.
- Patient remains free from infection.
- Patient and family state an understanding of drug therapy. (See *Teaching about antibiotic antineoplastic drugs*.)

Education edge

Teaching about antibiotic antineoplastic drugs

If antibiotic antineoplastic therapy is prescribed, review these points with the patient and caregivers:

- Avoid close contact with individuals who have received the oral poliovirus vaccine.
- Avoid exposure to persons with bacterial or viral infections because chemotherapy increases susceptibility. Report signs of infection immediately.
- Use proper oral hygiene, including cautious use of toothbrush, dental floss, and toothpicks. Chemotherapy can increase the risk of microbial infection, delayed healing, and bleeding gums.

- Complete dental work before therapy begins or delay it until blood counts are normal.
- Be aware that you may bruise easily.
- Report redness, pain, or swelling at the injection site immediately. Local tissue injury and scarring may result if I.V. infiltration occurs.
- If you're taking daunorubicin, doxorubicin, or idarubicin, your urine may turn orange or red for 1 to 2 days after therapy begins.

Hormonal antineoplastic drugs and hormone modulators

Hormonal antineoplastic drugs and hormone modulators are prescribed to alter the growth of malignant neoplasms or to manage and treat their physiologic effects. These drugs fall into six classes:
* aromatase inhibitors
* antioestrogens
* androgens
* antiandrogens
* progestins
* gonadotropin-releasing hormone analogues.

Hitting them where it hurts

Hormonal therapies and hormone modulators prove effective against hormone-dependent tumours, such as cancers of the prostate, breast, and endometrium. Lymphomas and leukaemias are usually treated with therapies that include corticosteroids because of their potential for affecting lymphocytes.

Aromatase inhibitors

Aromatase inhibitors prevent androgen from being converted into oestrogen in postmenopausal women. This blocks oestrogen's ability to activate cancer cells by limiting the amount of oestrogen reaching the cancer cells to promote growth. Aromatase inhibitors may be type 1 steroidal inhibitors, such as the drug exemestane, or type 2 nonsteroidal inhibitors, such as anastrozole and letrozole.

Pharmacokinetics

Aromatase inhibitors are taken orally in pill form and are well tolerated by most women. Steady state plasma levels after daily doses are reached in 2 to 6 weeks. Inactive metabolites are excreted in urine.

Pharmacodynamics

In postmenopausal women, oestrogen is produced through aromatase, an enzyme that converts hormone precursors into oestrogen. Aromatase inhibitors work by lowering the body's production of the female hormone oestrogen. In up to half of all patients with breast cancer, the tumours are dependent on this hormone to grow.

After the pause

Aromatase inhibitors are used in postmenopausal women because they lower the amount of oestrogen that's produced outside the ovaries in muscle and fat tissue. Because they induce oestrogen deprivation, bone thinning and osteoporosis may develop in time.

What's your type?

Type 1 inhibitors irreversibly inhibit the aromatase enzyme, whereas type 2 inhibitors reversibly inhibit the aromatase enzyme. It has also been suggested that type 1 aromatase inhibitors might have some effect after the failure of a type 2 aromatase inhibitor.

Exemestane selectively inhibits oestrogen synthesis and doesn't affect synthesis of adrenocorticosteroid, aldosterone, or thyroid hormones. Anastrozole and letrozole act by competitively binding to haem of cytochrome P450 subunit of aromatase, leading to decreased biosynthesis of oestrogen in all tissues. They don't affect synthesis of adrenocorticosteroid, aldosterone, or thyroid hormones.

Pharmacotherapeutics

Aromatase inhibitors are indicated primarily for postmenopausal women with metastatic breast cancer. It may be administered alone or with other agents such as tamoxifen.

Drug interactions

- Certain drugs may decrease the effectiveness of anastrozole, including tamoxifen and oestrogen-containing drugs.
- Exemestane given in combination with cytochrome P450 isoenzyme 3A4 inducers, may result in decreased serum exemestane concentrations.

Adverse reactions

Adverse reactions to aromatase inhibitors are rare but may include dizziness, mild nausea, mild muscle and joint aches, and hot flushes. They can also affect cholesterol levels; anastrazole may elevate high-density lipoprotein and low-density lipoprotein levels.

Nursing process

These nursing process steps are appropriate for patients undergoing treatment with aromatase inhibitors.

Aromatase inhibitors lower the amount of oestrogen that's produced outside the ovaries, in muscle and fat tissue. They're primarily used for postmenopausal women with metastatic breast cancer.

Assessment
- Assess the patient's breast cancer before therapy and regularly thereafter.
- Monitor the patient for adverse reactions and drug interactions.
- Monitor the patient's hydration status if adverse GI reactions occur.
- Evaluate the patient's and family's knowledge of drug therapy.

Key nursing diagnoses
- Ineffective health maintenance related to the presence of breast cancer.
- Ineffective protection related to adverse drug effects.
- Deficient knowledge related to drug therapy.

Planning outcome goals
- An improvement in the patient's underlying condition will be exhibited.
- The risk of injury to the patient will be minimised.
- The patient and her family will demonstrate an understanding of drug therapy.

Implementation
- Administer the agent per facility protocol to postmenopausal women.
- Don't give the drug with oestrogen-containing drugs because doing so could interfere with the drug's intended action.
- Monitor the patient for adverse effects and drug interactions.
- Continue the treatment until tumour progression is evident.
- Administer the drug after meals.

Evaluation
- Patient responds well to drug therapy.
- Patient doesn't experience adverse effects.
- Patient and her family state an understanding of drug therapy.

Antioestrogens

Antioestrogens bind to oestrogen receptors and block oestrogen action. The antioestrogens include tamoxifen citrate, toremifene citrate and fulvestrant. Tamoxifen and toremifene are nonsteroidal oestrogen agonist-antagonists. Fulvestrant is a pure oestrogen antagonist.

Pharmacokinetics

After oral administration, tamoxifen is absorbed well and undergoes extensive metabolism in the liver before being excreted in faeces. I.M. injection of fulvestrant yields peak serum levels within 7 to 9 days and has a half-life of 40 days. Toremifene is well absorbed and isn't influenced by food.

Pharmacodynamics

The exact antineoplastic action of these agents is unknown. However, it's known that they act as oestrogen antagonists. Oestrogen receptors, found in the cancer cells of 50 percent of premenopausal and 75 percent of postmenopausal women with breast cancer, respond to oestrogen to induce tumour growth.

It's bound to inhibit growth

Tamoxifen, toremifene, and fulvestrant bind to the oestrogen receptors and inhibit oestrogen-mediated tumour growth in breast tissue. Tamoxifen can retain oestrogen against activity at other tissue such as bone. The inhibition may result because tamoxifen binds to receptors at the nuclear level or because the binding reduces the number of free receptors in the cytoplasm. Ultimately, DNA synthesis and cell growth are inhibited.

Pharmacotherapeutics

The antioestrogen tamoxifen citrate is used alone and as adjuvant treatment with radiation therapy and surgery in women with negative axillary lymph nodes and in postmenopausal women with positive axillary nodes.

At a later stage

It's also used for advanced breast cancer involving oestrogen receptor–positive tumours in postmenopausal women that's oestrogen receptor–positive. Tumours in postmenopausal women are more responsive to tamoxifen than those in premenopausal women.

Tamoxifen may also be used to reduce the incidence of breast cancer in women at high risk. Toremifene is used to treat metastatic breast cancer in postmenopausal women with oestrogen receptor–positive tumours. Fulvestrant is used in postmenopausal women with receptor-positive metastatic breast cancer with disease progression after treatment with tamoxifen.

Drug interactions

- There are no known drug interactions with fulvestrant.
- Tamoxifen and toremifene may increase the effects of warfarin sodium, increase the prothrombin time (PT; a test to measure clotting factors), and increase the risk of bleeding.
- Bromocriptine increases the effects of tamoxifen.

Adverse reactions

Adverse reactions to antioestrogens vary by drug.

Tamoxifen

Tamoxifen is a relatively nontoxic drug. The most common adverse reactions include:
- hot flushes
- nausea and vomiting
- diarrhoea
- fluid retention
- leucopenia or thrombocytopenia (reduced WBCs and platelets, respectively)
- hypercalcaemia (elevated serum calcium levels) in patients with bone metastasis.

Toremifene

Adverse reactions to toremifene include:
- hot flushes
- sweating
- nausea and vomiting
- vaginal discharge or bleeding
- oedema.

Fulvestrant

Adverse reactions to fulvestrant include:
- hot flushes
- nausea and vomiting
- diarrhoea or constipation
- abdominal pain
- headache
- back pain
- pharyngitis.

Adverse reactions to toremifene include hot flushes, sweating, nausea, vomiting, vaginal discharge or bleeding, and oedema.

Nursing process

These nursing process steps are appropriate for patients undergoing treatment with antioestrogens.

Assessment

- Assess the patient's breast cancer before therapy and regularly thereafter.
- Monitor CBC closely in the patient with leucopenia or thrombocytopenia.
- Monitor lipid levels during long-term therapy in patients with hyperlipidaemia.
- Monitor the patient's calcium level. The drug may compound hypercalcaemia related to bone metastases during the initiation of therapy.

- Monitor the patient for adverse reactions.
- Monitor the patient's hydration status if adverse GI reactions occur.
- Evaluate the patient's and family's knowledge of drug therapy.

Key nursing diagnoses
- Ineffective health maintenance related to the presence of breast cancer.
- Risk for deficient fluid volume related to drug-induced adverse GI reactions.
- Deficient knowledge related to drug therapy.

Planning outcome goals
- An improvement in the patient's underlying condition will be exhibited.
- Fluid volume will remain within normal limits as evidenced by the patient's vital signs and intake and output.
- The patient and her family will demonstrate an understanding of drug therapy.

Implementation
- Administer the medication as prescribed and monitor for effects.
- Make sure that the patient swallows enteric-coated tablets whole.
- Monitor the patient for adverse effects and drug interactions.

Evaluation
- Patient responds well to drug therapy.
- Patient maintains adequate hydration.
- Patient and her family state an understanding of drug therapy.
(See *Teaching about tamoxifen*.)

Androgens

Androgens are synthetic derivatives of naturally occurring testosterone. They include:
- testosterone enantate
- testosterone propionate.

Pharmacokinetics
The pharmacokinetic properties of therapeutic androgens resemble those of naturally occurring testosterone.

Specific design

Testosterone enantate and testosterone propionate, are designed specifically for slow absorption after I.M. injection. Androgens are distributed well throughout the body, metabolised extensively in the liver, and excreted in urine.

Education edge

Teaching about tamoxifen

If tamoxifen therapy is prescribed, review these points with the patient and caregivers:

- Report symptoms of a pulmonary embolism (chest pain, difficulty breathing, rapid breathing, sweating, or fainting).
- Report symptoms of a stroke, including headache, vision changes, confusion, difficulty speaking or walking, and weakness in the face, arm or leg, especially on one side of the body.
- Take an analgesic for pain. Acute bone pain during drug therapy usually means that the drug will produce a good response.
- Have regular gynaecologic examinations because of an increased risk of uterine cancer.

- If you're taking the drug to reduce the risk of breast cancer, use the proper technique of self-breast examination. Review this with your health care provider.
- It's important to keep appointments for clinical breast examinations, annual mammograms, and gynaecologic examinations.
- If you're premenopausal, use a barrier form of contraception because short-term therapy induces ovulation.
- If you are of childbearing age, avoid pregnancy during therapy and consult with your prescriber before becoming pregnant.

Checking the suspension

The duration of parenterally administered androgens is longer because the oil suspension is absorbed slowly. Parenteral androgens are administered one to three times per week.

Pharmacodynamics

Androgens probably act by one or more mechanisms. They may reduce the number of prolactin receptors or may bind competitively to those that are available.

Keeping its' sister hormone in check

Androgens may inhibit oestrogen synthesis or competitively bind at oestrogen receptors. These actions prevent oestrogen from affecting oestrogen-sensitive tumours. However, they have been largely superseded by other drugs for the treatment of breast cancer.

Pharmacotherapeutics

Androgens are indicated for the palliative treatment of advanced breast cancer, particularly in postmenopausal women with bone metastasis.

Drug interactions

Androgens may alter dose requirements in patients receiving insulin, oral antidiabetic drugs, or oral anticoagulants. Taking these drugs with other drugs that are toxic to the liver increases the risk of liver toxicity.

Adverse reactions

Nausea and vomiting are the most common adverse reactions to androgens. Fluid retention caused by sodium retention may also occur as well as paraesthesia and peripheral neuropathy.

In females

Women taking androgens may develop:

- acne
- clitoral hypertrophy
- deeper voice
- increased facial and body hair
- increased sexual desire
- menstrual irregularity.

In males

Males taking androgens may experience these effects as a result of conversion of steroids to female sex hormone metabolites:

- gynaecomastia
- prostatic hypertrophy
- testicular atrophy.

In children

Children taking androgens may develop:

- premature epiphyseal closure
- secondary sex characteristics (especially boys).

Children taking androgens may develop premature epiphyseal closure and secondary sex characteristics, especially boys.

Nursing process

These nursing process steps are appropriate for patients undergoing treatment with androgens.

Assessment

- Assess the patient's breast cancer before therapy and regularly thereafter.
- Monitor fluid and electrolyte levels, especially calcium level.
- Monitor the patient for adverse reactions and drug interactions.
- Evaluate the patient's and family's knowledge of drug therapy.

Key nursing diagnoses
- Ineffective health maintenance related to the presence of cancer.
- Disturbed sensory perception (tactile) related to drug-induced paraesthesia and peripheral neuropathy.
- Deficient knowledge related to drug therapy.

Planning outcome goals
- The patient will demonstrate an improvement in assessments and diagnostic testing.
- The patient won't experience injury from disturbed sensory perception.
- The patient and her family will demonstrate an understanding of drug therapy.

Implementation
- Encourage the patient to drink fluids to aid calcium excretion.
- Encourage the patient to exercise to prevent hypercalcaemia.
- Administer the drug according to facility guidelines.
- Monitor the patient for effects and adverse reactions. Inform her that therapeutic response may not be immediate; it may take up to 3 months for the benefit to be noted.

Evaluation
- Patient responds well to drug therapy.
- Patient lists ways to protect against the risk of injury caused by diminished tactile sensation.
- Patient and her family state an understanding of drug therapy.

Antiandrogens

Antiandrogens are used as an adjunct therapy with gonadotropin-releasing hormone analogues in treating advanced prostate cancer. These drugs include:
- flutamide
- cyproterone acetate
- bicalutamide.

Pharmacokinetics
After oral administration, antiandrogens are absorbed rapidly and completely. They're metabolised rapidly and extensively and excreted primarily in urine.

Pharmacodynamics

Flutamide, cyproterone acetate, and bicalutamide exert their antiandrogenic action by inhibiting androgen uptake or preventing androgen binding in cell nuclei in target tissues.

Pharmacotherapeutics

Antiandrogens are used with a gonadotropin-releasing hormone analogue, such as leuprorelin acetate, to treat metastatic prostate cancer.

A flare for their work

Concomitant administration of antiandrogens and a gonadotropin-releasing hormone analogue may help prevent the disease flare that occurs when the gonadotropin-releasing hormone analogue is used alone.

Drug interactions

Antiandrogens don't interact significantly with other drugs. However, flutamide and bicalutamide may affect the PT in a patient receiving warfarin.

Adverse reactions

When an antiandrogen is used with a gonadotropin-releasing hormone analogue, the most common adverse reactions are:
- hot flushes
- decreased sexual desire
- impotence
- diarrhoea
- nausea and vomiting
- breast enlargement.

Nursing process

These nursing process steps are appropriate for patients undergoing treatment with antiandrogens.

Assessment
- Assess the patient's prostate cancer before therapy.
- Monitor liver function tests periodically.
- Monitor the patient for adverse reactions.
- Monitor the patient's hydration status if adverse GI reactions occur.
- Evaluate the patient's and family's knowledge of drug therapy.

Key nursing diagnoses
- Ineffective health maintenance related to the presence of prostate cancer.
- Risk for deficient fluid volume related to adverse GI reactions.
- Deficient knowledge related to drug therapy.

Planning outcome goals
- The patient will demonstrate an improvement in assessments and diagnostic testing.
- The patient's fluid volume will remain within normal limits as exhibited by vital signs and intake and output.
- The patient and family will demonstrate an understanding of drug therapy.

Implementation
- Administer medication per facility policy. The drug may be given without regard to meals.
- Administer flutamide with a luteinising hormone (LH)-releasing antagonist such as leuprorelin acetate.
- Tell the patient that flutamide must be taken continuously with a drug used for medical castration, such as leuprolide acetate, to allow for the full benefit of therapy. Leuprorelin suppresses testosterone production while flutamide inhibits testosterone action at the cellular level. Together they can impair the growth of androgen-responsive tumours. Advise the patient not to discontinue either drug.
- Monitor the patient for adverse effects and drug interactions.

Evaluation
- Patient responds well to drug therapy.
- Patient maintains adequate hydration throughout drug therapy.
- Patient and family state an understanding of drug therapy.

Progestins

Progestins are hormones used to treat various forms of cancer and include:
- medroxyprogesterone acetate
- megestrol acetate
- norethisterone.

Pharmacokinetics
When taken orally, megestrol acetate and norethistrone are absorbed well. After I.M. injection in an aqueous or oil suspension, medroxyprogesterone is absorbed slowly from its deposit site.

Fat chance

These drugs are distributed well throughout the body and may sequester in fatty tissue. Progestins are metabolised in the liver and excreted as metabolites in urine.

Pharmacodynamics

The mechanism of action of progestins in treating tumours isn't completely understood. Researchers believe that the drugs bind to a specific receptor to act on hormonally sensitive cells.

Keeping the numbers down

Because progestins don't exhibit a cytotoxic activity (destroying or poisoning cells), they're considered cytostatic (they keep cells from multiplying).

Pharmacotherapeutics

Progestins are used for the palliative treatment of advanced endometrial, breast, and renal cancers. Of these drugs, megestrol is used most often.

Drug interactions

No drug interactions have been identified for megestrol. However, other progestins do have significant interactions with other drugs:
- Barbiturates, carbamazepine, and rifampicin reduce progestin effects.
- Norethisterone and medroxyprogesterone may interfere with bromocriptine's effects, causing menstruation to stop.
- Taking norethisterone with dantrolene and other drugs toxic to the liver increases the risk of liver toxicity.
- Aminoglutethimide and rifampicin may reduce the progestin effects of medroxyprogesterone.

Adverse reactions

Mild fluid retention is probably the most common reaction to progestins. Other adverse reactions include:
- thromboemboli
- breakthrough bleeding, spotting, and changes in menstrual flow
- breast tenderness
- liver function abnormalities.

Progestins are cytostatic drugs. That means we prevent cancer cells from multiplying.

Nursing process

These nursing process steps are appropriate for patients undergoing treatment with progestins.

Assessment
- Assess the patient's condition before therapy and regularly thereafter.
- Monitor the patient for adverse reactions and drug interactions.
- Evaluate the patient's and family's knowledge of drug therapy.

Key nursing diagnoses
- Ineffective health maintenance related to the presence of prostate cancer.
- Risk for imbalanced fluid volume related to adverse GI reactions.
- Deficient knowledge related to drug therapy.

Planning outcome goals
- The patient will demonstrate an improvement in assessments and diagnostic testing.
- The fluid volume will remain within normal limits as exhibited by the patient's vital signs and intake and output.
- The patient and family will demonstrate an understanding of drug therapy.

Implementation
- Administer the medication per facility policy.
- Monitor the patient for adverse effects and drug interactions.
- Instruct the patient to avoid caffeine and smoking during drug therapy.
- Teach a female patient how to perform routine monthly breast self-examinations.

Evaluation
- Patient responds well to drug therapy.
- Patient maintains adequate hydration throughout drug therapy.
- Patient and family state an understanding of drug therapy.

Gonadotropin-releasing hormone analogues

Gonadotropin-releasing hormone analogues are used to treat advanced prostate cancer. They include:
- goserelin acetate
- leuprorelin acetate
- triptorelin pamoate.

Pharmacokinetics

Goserelin is absorbed slowly for the first 8 days of therapy and rapidly and continuously thereafter. After subcutaneous injection, leuprorelin is absorbed well. The distribution, metabolism, and excretion of these drugs isn't clearly defined. Triptorelin has peak serum levels within 1 week of I.M. injection with serum levels being detectable for 4 weeks.

Pharmacodynamics

Goserelin and leuprorelin act on the male's pituitary gland to increase LH secretion, which stimulates testosterone production.

The rise...

The peak testosterone level is reached about 72 hours after daily administration. Triptorelin is a potent inhibitor of gonadotropin secretion. After the first dose, levels of LH, follicle-stimulating hormone (FSH), testosterone, and estradiol surge transiently.

...and fall...

After long-term continuous administration, LH and FSH secretion steadily declines and testicular and ovarian steroidogenesis decreases. In men, testosterone declines to a level typically seen in surgically castrated men. As a result, tissues and functions that depend on these hormones become quiescent.

and reverse

With long-term administration, however, goserelin and leuprorelin inhibit LH release from the pituitary gland and subsequently inhibit testicular release of testosterone. Because prostate tumour cells are stimulated by testosterone, the reduced testosterone level inhibits tumour growth.

Pharmacotherapeutics

Goserelin, triptorelin, and leuprorelin are used for the palliative treatment of metastatic prostate cancer. These drugs lower the testosterone level without the adverse psychological effects of castration or the adverse cardiovascular effects of diethylstilbestrol.

Drug interactions

No drug interactions have been identified with goserelin, triptorelin, or leuprorelin.

Adverse reactions

Hot flushes, impotence, and decreased sexual desire are commonly reported reactions to goserelin and leuprorelin. Other adverse reactions include:
- peripheral oedema
- nausea

- vomiting
- constipation
- anorexia.

On the rise

Disease symptoms and pain may worsen or flare during the first
2 weeks of goserelin or leuprorelin therapy. The flare can be fatal in
patients with bony vertebral metastasis.

Nursing process

These nursing process steps are appropriate for patients undergoing
treatment with gonadotropin-releasing hormone analogues.

Assessment
- Assess the patient's condition before therapy and regularly
thereafter.
- When used for prostate cancer, LH-RH analogues, such as
goserelin, may initially worsen symptoms because the drug initially
increases testosterone levels. Some patients may have increased
bone pain. Rarely, disease (spinal cord compression or ureteral
obstruction) may worsen.
- Monitor the patient for adverse reactions.
- Evaluate the patient's and family's knowledge of drug therapy.

Key nursing diagnoses
- Ineffective health maintenance related to the underlying
condition.
- Acute pain related to drug-induced adverse reactions.
- Deficient knowledge related to drug therapy.

Planning outcome goals
- An improvement in the patient's underlying condition will be
exhibited.
- The patient's pain will decrease.
- The patient and family will demonstrate an understanding of
drug therapy.

Implementation
- The drug should be given under supervision of the prescriber.
Administer medication according to facility policy. (See *Goserelin
warning*.)
- To avoid the need for a new syringe and injection site, don't
aspirate after inserting the needle.
- Implant comes in a preloaded syringe for goserelin. If the
package is damaged, don't use the syringe. Make sure that the drug
is visible in the translucent chamber.

**Before
you give
that drug!**

Goserelin warning

Administer goserelin
into the upper
abdominal wall using
aseptic technique.
After cleaning the
area with an alcohol
swab and injecting
a local anaesthetic,
stretch the patient's
skin with one hand
while grasping the
barrel of syringe
with the other.
Insert the needle
into subcutaneous
fat; then change
the direction of
the needle so that
it parallels the
abdominal wall. The
needle should then
be pushed in until
the hub touches the
patient's skin and
then withdrawn about
3/8″ (1 cm) (this
creates a gap for the
drug to be injected)
before depressing
the plunger
completely.

- After implantation, withdraw the needle and apply a bandage to the area.
- Be prepared to schedule the patient for an ultrasound to locate goserelin implants if they require removal.
- Notify the prescriber of adverse reactions and provide supportive care, as indicated and prescribed.

Reporting as required

- Advise the patient to report every 28 days for a new implant. A delay of a few days is permissible.
- Tell the patient to call the prescriber if menstruation persists or if breakthrough bleeding occurs. Menstruation should stop during treatment. After therapy ends, inform the patient that they may experience delayed return of menses. Persistent amenorrhea is rare.
- If the patient is to continue subcutaneous injection of leuprorelin at home, instruct with respect to correct technique and advise them to use only syringes provided by the manufacturer.

Evaluation
- Patient responds well to drug therapy.
- Patient has no pain.
- Patient and family state an understanding of drug therapy.

Natural antineoplastic drugs

A subclass of antineoplastic drugs known as *natural products* includes:
- vinca alkaloids
- podophyllotoxins.

Vinca alkaloids

Vinca alkaloids are nitrogenous bases derived from the periwinkle plant. These drugs are cell cycle–specific for the M phase and include:
- vinblastine
- vincristine
- vinorelbine.

Pharmacokinetics
After I.V. administration, the vinca alkaloids are distributed well throughout the body. They undergo moderate liver metabolism before being eliminated through different phases, primarily in faeces with a small percentage eliminated in urine.

Pharmacodynamics

Vinca alkaloids may disrupt the normal function of the microtubules (structures within cells that are associated with the movement of DNA) by binding to the protein tubulin in the microtubules.

Separation anxiety

With the microtubules unable to separate chromosomes properly, the chromosomes are dispersed throughout the cytoplasm or arranged in unusual groupings. As a result, formation of the mitotic spindle is prevented, and the cells can't complete mitosis (cell division).

Under arrest

Cell division is arrested in metaphase, causing cell death. Therefore, vinca alkaloids are cell cycle, M phase–specific. Interruption of the microtubule function may also impair some types of cellular movement, phagocytosis (engulfing and destroying microorganisms and cellular debris), and CNS functions.

I.V. administration gets vinca alkaloids where they need to go!

Pharmacotherapeutics

Vinca alkaloids are used in several therapeutic situations:
• Vinblastine is used to treat metastatic testicular carcinoma, lymphomas, Kaposi's sarcoma (the most common acquired immunodeficiency syndrome [AIDS]-related cancer), neuroblastoma (a highly malignant tumour originating in the sympathetic nervous system), breast carcinoma, and choriocarcinoma.
• Vincristine is used in combination therapy to treat Hodgkin's disease, non-Hodgkin's lymphoma, Wilms' tumour, rhabdomyosarcoma, and acute lymphocytic leukaemia.
• Vinorelbine is used to treat non-small-cell lung cancer. It may also be used in the treatment of metastatic breast carcinoma, cisplatin-resistant ovarian carcinoma, and Hodgkin's disease.

Drug interactions

Vinca alkaloids interact in many ways with other drugs:
• Erythromycin may increase the toxicity of vinblastine.
• Vinblastine decreases the plasma levels of phenytoin.
• Vincristine reduces the effects of digoxin.
• Asparaginase decreases liver metabolism of vincristine, increasing the risk of toxicity.
• Calcium channel blockers enhance vincristine accumulation, increasing the tendency for toxicity.

Adverse reactions

Vinca alkaloids may cause the following adverse reactions:
• nausea and vomiting
• constipation
• stomatitis (mouth inflammation).

Vinblastine and vinorelbine toxicities occur primarily as bone marrow suppression. Neuromuscular abnormalities frequently occur with vincristine and vinorelbine and occasionally with vinblastine therapy.

A stinging sensation

Vinblastine may produce tumour pain described as an intense stinging or burning in the tumour bed, with an abrupt onset 1 to 3 minutes after drug administration. The pain usually lasts 20 minutes to 3 hours.

Hair scare

Reversible alopecia occurs in up to one-half of patients receiving vinca alkaloids; it's more likely to occur with vincristine than vinblastine.

Nursing process
These nursing process steps are appropriate for patients undergoing treatment with natural antineoplastic drugs.

Assessment
- Assess the patient's condition before therapy and regularly thereafter.
- Monitor the patient for the development of life-threatening acute bronchospasm after drug administration. This reaction is most likely if the patient also receives mitomycin.
- Monitor the patient for adverse reactions and drug interactions.
- Assess for numbness and tingling in the patient's hands and feet. Assess his gait for early evidence of footdrop. Vinblastine is less neurotoxic than vincristine.
- Monitor the patient for hyperuricaemia, especially if he has leukaemia or lymphoma.
- With vincristine, check for depression of the Achilles tendon reflex, numbness, tingling, footdrop or wristdrop, difficulty in walking, ataxia, and slapping gait. Also check the patient's ability to walk on their heels.
- Monitor the patient's bowel function. Constipation may be an early sign of neurotoxicity when administering vincristine.
- Evaluate the patient's and family's knowledge of drug therapy.

Key nursing diagnoses
- Ineffective health maintenance related to the presence of neoplastic disease.
- Ineffective protection related to drug-induced adverse reactions.
- Deficient knowledge related to drug therapy.

Planning outcome goals
- The patient will demonstrate an improvement in assessments and diagnostic testing.

- The risk of injury to the patient will be minimised.
- The patient and family will demonstrate an understanding of drug therapy.

Implementation
- Give an antiemetic before giving the drug.
- Follow facility policy to reduce risks. Preparation and administration of the parenteral form of the drug are linked to carcinogenic, mutagenic, and teratogenic risks for personnel.
- Reconstitute the drug as prescribed and administer per facility policy.
- If extravasation occurs, stop the infusion immediately and notify the prescriber. (See *More on vinblastine and vincristine.*)
- If acute bronchospasm occurs after administration, notify the prescriber immediately.
- Make sure that the patient maintains adequate fluid intake to facilitate excretion of uric acid.
- Be prepared to stop the drug and notify the prescriber if stomatitis occurs.
- The dosage shouldn't be repeated more frequently than every 7 days because severe leucopenia can develop.
- Anticipate a decrease in the dosage by 50% if the bilirubin level is greater than 3 mg/dl.
- Fluid restriction may be needed if syndrome of inappropriate diuretic hormone develops.

Evaluation
- Patient responds well to drug therapy.
- Patient doesn't develop serious complications from adverse haematologic reactions.
- Patient and family state an understanding of drug therapy.

Podophyllotoxins

Podophyllotoxins are semisynthetic glycosides that are cell cycle–specific and act during the G2 and late S phases of the cell cycle. This class of drug includes etoposide.

Pharmacokinetics
When taken orally, podophyllotoxins are only moderately absorbed. Although the drugs are distributed widely throughout the body, they achieve poor CSF levels. Podophyllotoxins undergo liver metabolism and are excreted primarily in urine.

Pharmacodynamics
Although their mechanism of action isn't completely understood, podophyllotoxins produce several biochemical changes in tumour cells.

More on vinblastine and vincristine

Manufacturers recommend that moderate heat be applied to an area of leakage or extravasation of vinblastine or vincristine. Local injection of hyaluronidase may help disperse the drug. Some clinicians prefer to apply ice packs on and off every 2 hours for 24 hours, with local injection of hydrocortisone or normal saline solution. Don't inject the drug into a limb with compromised circulation.

Vinblastine and vincristine are fatal if given intrathecally; they're for I.V. use only.

The highs and lows

At low concentrations, these drugs block cells at the late S or G2 phase. At higher concentrations, they arrest the cells in the G2 phase.

Breaking the mould

Podophyllotoxins can also break one of the strands of the DNA molecule. These drugs can also inhibit nucleotide transport and incorporation into nucleic acids.

Pharmacotherapeutics

Etoposide is used to treat testicular cancer and small-cell lung cancer.

Drug interactions

Podophyllotoxins have few significant interactions with other drugs:
• Etoposide may increase the risk of bleeding in a patient taking warfarin.

Adverse reactions

Most patients receiving podophyllotoxins experience hair loss. Other adverse reactions include:
• nausea and vomiting
• anorexia
• stomatitis
• bone marrow suppression, causing leucopenia and, less commonly, thrombocytopenia
• acute hypotension (if a podophyllotoxin is infused too rapidly by the I.V. route).

Nursing process

These nursing process steps are appropriate for patients undergoing treatment with podophyllotoxins.

Assessment

• Assess the patient's condition before therapy and regularly thereafter.
• Monitor the patient for adverse reactions and drug interactions.
• Obtain the patient's baseline blood pressure before therapy and monitor blood pressure at 30-minute intervals during infusion.
• Monitor the drug's effectiveness by noting results of follow-up diagnostic tests and overall physical status and by regularly checking tumour size and rate of growth through appropriate studies.

- Monitor the patient's CBC. Observe him for signs of bone marrow suppression.
- Evaluate the patient's and family's knowledge of drug therapy.

Key nursing diagnoses
- Ineffective health maintenance related to the presence of neoplastic disease
- Ineffective protection related to drug-induced adverse reactions
- Deficient knowledge related to drug therapy

Planning outcome goals
- The patient will demonstrate an improvement in assessments and diagnostic testing.
- The risk of injury to the patient will be minimised.
- The patient and family will demonstrate an understanding of drug therapy.

Implementation
- Follow facility policy to reduce risks. Preparation and administration of the parenteral form of the drug are linked to carcinogenic, mutagenic, and teratogenic risks for personnel.
- Reconstitute the drug as prescribed and administer per facility policy.
- Store oral capsules in the refrigerator.
- I.V. infusion is given slowly, over at least 30 minutes, to prevent severe hypotension.
- If the patient's systolic blood pressure falls below 90 mm Hg, stop infusion and notify the prescriber.
- Don't give the drug through a membrane-type in-line filter because the diluent may dissolve filter.
- Keep hydrocortisone, adrenaline (epinephrine), and necessary emergency equipment available to establish airway in case of anaphylaxis.
- Monitor the patient for signs of infection and bleeding. Teach them how to take infection-control and bleeding precautions.
- Tell the patient that hair loss is possible, but reversible.
- Instruct the patient to report discomfort, pain, or burning at the I.V. insertion site.

Store oral capsules in the refrigerator.

Evaluation
- Patient responds well to drug therapy.
- Patient doesn't develop serious complications from adverse haematologic reactions.
- Patient and family state an understanding of drug therapy.

Monoclonal antibodies

Recombinant DNA technology has allowed for the development of monoclonal antibodies directed at targets, such as other immune cells, or the cancer cells. They include:
- alemtuzumab
- rituximab
- trastuzumab.

Pharmacokinetics

The monoclonal antibodies, by virtue of their large protein molecule structure, aren't absorbed orally. They may have a limited volume of distribution as well as a long half-life, sometimes measured in weeks.

Pharmacodynamics

The monoclonal antibodies bind to target receptor or cancer cells and can cause tumour death via several mechanisms. They can induce programmed cell death and recruit other elements of the immune system to attack the cancer cell. They can also be used to deliver toxic chemotherapy drugs or radiation dose to the site of the tumour.

Pharmacotherapeutics

Monoclonal antibodies have demonstrated activity in solid tumours and haematologic malignancies, such as:
- non-Hodgkin's lymphoma—rituximab (target CD20 or malignant B lymphocytes)
- chronic lymphocytic leukaemia—alemtuzumab (target CD52 antigen or B cells)
- breast cancer—trastuzumab (target HER-2 protein in breast cancer cells).

Drug interactions
- There are no known drug interactions with alemtuzumab.
- Trastuzumab increases the cardiac toxicity associated with anthracycline administration.
- Retuximab should similarly be used with caution in patients receiving cardiotoxic chemotherapy.

Adverse reactions

All monoclonal antibodies are associated with infusion-related toxicities, such as fever, chills, shortness of breath, low blood pressure, and anaphylaxis. Fatalities have been reported. In addition, the following adverse reactions can occur:
* Alemtuzumab is associated with myelosuppression and an increased risk of opportunistic infections, such as pneumocystitis, pneumonia, and fungal and viral infections.
* Retuximab has been associated with severe cytokine release syndrome.

Nursing process

These nursing process steps are appropriate for patients undergoing treatment with monoclonal antibodies.

Assessment
* Assess the patient's condition before therapy and regularly thereafter.
* Monitor the patient for adverse reactions and drug interactions.
* Obtain the patient's baseline blood pressure before therapy and monitor him for hypotensive symptoms during drug administration.
* Monitor the drug's effectiveness by noting results of follow-up diagnostic tests and overall physical status and by regularly checking tumour size and rate of growth through appropriate studies.
* Obtain a baseline CBC and platelet count before starting therapy; assess weekly during therapy and more frequently if anaemia, neutropenia, or thrombocytopenia worsens.
* Monitor the patient's haematologic studies carefully during therapy. Even with normal dosages, he may experience signs and symptoms of haematologic toxicity, including myelosuppression, bone marrow dysplasia, and thrombocytopenia.
* After treatment, monitor the patient's CD4$^+$ count until it reaches 200 cells/mm^3 or more.
* Evaluate the patient's and family's knowledge of drug therapy.

Key nursing diagnoses
* Risk for infection related to an immunocompromised state.
* Fatigue due to drug therapy.
* Deficient knowledge related to drug therapy.

Planning outcome goals
- No signs of infection will be present as evidenced by normal WBC count and temperature and negative cultures.
- The patient will exhibit less fatigue.
- The patient and family will demonstrate an understanding of drug therapy.

Implementation
- Reconstitute the drug as prescribed and administer per facility policy. (See *Alemtuzumab warning*.)
- Don't use the solution if it's discoloured or contains precipitate. Filter with a sterile, low-protein-binding, 5-micron filter before dilution.
- Irradiate blood if transfusions are needed to protect against graft-versus-host disease.
- Don't immunise with live viral vaccines.
- If therapy is stopped for more than 7 days, restart with a gradual dose increase.
- I.V. infusion is given slowly, over at least 2 hours.
- Tell women of childbearing age and men to use effective contraceptive methods during therapy and for at least 6 months following the completion of therapy.

Evaluation
- Patient remains free from infection.
- Patient doesn't develop serious complications from adverse reactions.
- Patient and family state an understanding of drug therapy.

Topoisomerase I inhibitors

Topoisomerase I inhibitors inhibit the enzyme topoisomerase enzyme I. These agents are derived from a naturally occurring alkaloid from the Chinese tree *Camptotheca acuminata*. Currently available drugs include:
- irinotecan
- topotecan.

Pharmacokinetics
Irinotecan and topotecan are minimally absorbed and must be given I.V. Irinotecan undergoes metabolic changes to become the active metabolite SN-38. The half-life of SN-38 is approximately 10 hours, and it's eliminated through biliary excretion. Topotecan

Before you give that drug!

Alemtuzumab warning

Before administering monoclonal antibodies, such as alemtuzumab, premedicate the patient with a non-sedating antihistamine and paracetamol before the initial infusion and before each dose increase. Hydrocortisone may be given to decrease severe infusion-related adverse effects. Give anti-infective prophylaxis while the patient is receiving therapy. Prophylaxis should continue for 2 months or until the CD4$^+$ count is 200 cells/mm^3 or more, whichever occurs later.

is metabolised hepatically although renal excretion is a significant elimination pathway.

Pharmacodynamics

These agents excrete their cytotoxic effect by inhibiting topoisomerase I enzyme, an essential enzyme that mediates the relaxation of supercoiled DNA. Topoisomerase inhibitors bind to the DNA topoisomerase I complex and prevent resealing, thereby causing DNA strand breaks, resulting in impaired DNA synthesis.

Pharmacotherapeutics

Topoisomerase I inhibitors are active against solid tumours and haematologic malignancies. Topotecan is administered in ovarian cancer, small cell lung cancer, and acute myeloid leukaemia. Irinotecan is administered to patients with colorectal cancer or small cell lung cancer.

Drug interactions

Topoisomerase I inhibitors are associated with drug interactions, particularly irinotecan.
• Ketoconazole can significantly increase SN-38 serum concentrations, increasing the risk of associated toxicities.
• Concurrent administration of diuretics may exacerbate dehydration caused by irinotecan-induced diarrhoea.
• Concurrent administration of laxatives with irinotecan can induce diarrhoea.
• Prochlorperazine administered with irinotecan can increase the incidence of extrapyramidal toxicities.

Adverse reactions

Diarrhoea is the most common adverse reaction to topoisomerase I inhibitors, especially with irinotecan, which is cholinergically mediated; this can be reversed with atropine.

Delayed reaction

Later-onset diarrhoea, which may persist for up to 1 week, can present itself several days after chemotherapy has been administered. Treat with scheduled loperamide every 2 hours until stools become formed.

The more common adverse reactions to topoisomerase I inhibitors, particularly irinotecan, include:
• increased sweating and saliva production
• watery eyes
• abdominal cramps

- nausea and vomiting
- loss of appetite
- fatigue
- hair loss or thinning.
  Occasionally, these reactions may occur:
- mouth sores and ulcers
- muscle cramps
- temporary effect on liver function tests
- rashes, which may be itchy.
  These reactions rarely occur but are more serious:
- Both drugs are associated with significant myelosuppression, especially topotecan.
- Irinotecan has been associated with thromboembolic events, namely myocardial infarction and stroke, when given with 5-fluoroacil and leucovorin, which have resulted in death.

Nursing process

These nursing process steps are appropriate for patients undergoing treatment with topoisomerase I inhibitors.

Assessment

- Assess the patient's condition before therapy and regularly thereafter.
- Monitor the patient for adverse reactions and drug interactions.
- Obtain a baseline neutrophil count; it must be greater than 1,500 cells/mm³ and platelet count greater than 100,000 cells/mm³ before therapy can start.
- Frequent monitoring of peripheral blood cell count is critical. Don't give repeated doses until the neutrophil count is greater than 1,000 cells/mm³, platelet count is greater than 100,000 cells/mm³, and haemoglobin is greater than 9 mg/dl.
- Evaluate the patient's and family's knowledge of drug therapy.

Key nursing diagnoses

- Ineffective health maintenance related to the presence of neoplastic disease.
- Ineffective protection related to drug-induced adverse reactions.
- Deficient knowledge related to drug therapy.

Planning outcome goals

- The patient will demonstrate an improvement in assessments and diagnostic testing.
- The risk of injury to the patient will be minimised.
- The patient and family will demonstrate an understanding of drug therapy.

Frequent monitoring of peripheral blood cell count is critical.

Implementation
• Prepare the drug under a vertical laminar flow hood while wearing gloves and protective clothing. If the drug contacts skin, wash immediately and thoroughly with soap and water. If mucous membranes are affected, flush with water.
• Reconstitute the drug as prescribed. Dilute and administer the drug per facility policy.
• I.V. infusion is given slowly, over at least 30 minutes.
• Protect unopened vials of the drug from light.
• Monitor the patient for signs of infection, such as sore throat, fever, chills, or unusual bleeding or bruising, and report them promptly.
• Tell a female patient of childbearing age to avoid pregnancy and breast-feeding during treatment.

Evaluation
• Patient responds well to drug therapy.
• Patient doesn't develop serious complications from adverse haematologic reactions.
• Patient and family state an understanding of drug therapy.

Targeted therapies

A groundbreaking approach to anticancer therapies is to target proteins associated with the growth patterns for a specific type of cancer. These new drugs include:
• gefitinib
• imatinib
• bortezomib.

Pharmacokinetics
Gefitinib is available in an oral dosage form in which approximately half the dose is absorbed. The drug is widely distributed in tissues. It undergoes hepatic metabolism with minimal urinary excretion.

Imatinib is available in an oral dosage form, which is almost completely absorbed. It's 95% bound to plasma proteins and extensively metabolised by the liver. The half-life is approximately 15 hours.

Bortezomib isn't absorbed orally and must be given I.V. It's extensively distributed into body tissues and hepatically metabolised.

Pharmacodynamics

Gefitinib inhibits the epidermal growth factor receptor-1 tyrosine kinase, which is overexpressed with certain cancers, such as non-small cell lung cancer. This blocks signalling pathways for the growth, survival, and metastasis of cancer.

In a bind

Imatinib binds to the ATP binding domain of the BCR-ABL protein, which stimulates other tyrosine kinase proteins to result in abnormally high production of WBCs in chronic myeloid leukaemia. This binding of imatinib effectively shuts down the abnormal WBC production.

Bortezomib inhibits proteosomes, which are involved in integral cell cycle function, which promote tumour growth. Proteolysis by bortezomib results in disruption of the normal homeostatic mechanisms and leads to cell death.

Pharmacotherapeutics

Gefitinib is used as a single agent for patients with non-small cell lung cancer that have failed two previous standard chemotherapy regimens. Imatinib is used to treat chronic myeloid leukaemia, acute lymphoid leukaemia, and GI stomal tumours. Bortezomib is used to treat multiple myeloma that has relapsed after standard chemotherapy.

Drug interactions

Bortezomib, gefitinab, and imatinib have been associated with some drug interactions:
• Bortezomib, when taken with drugs that are inhibitors or inducers of the cytochrome P-450 CYP3A4, could cause either toxicities or reduced efficacy of these drugs. Inhibitors of CYP3A4 include amiodarone, cimetidine, erythromycin, diltiazem, fluoxetine, grapefruit juice, verapamil and zafirlukast. Inducers of CYP3A4 include amiodarone, carbamazepine, nevirapine, phenobarbital, phenytoin, and rifampicin.
• Bortezomib, when taken with oral hypoglycaemics, could cause hypoglycaemia or hyperglycaemia in patients with diabetes.
• Plasma levels of gefitinib and imatinib are reduced, sometimes substantially, when these drugs are given with carbamazepine, dexamethasone, phenobarbital, phenytoin, rifampicin, or St. John's wort.
• High doses of ranitidine with sodium bicarbonate when taken with gefitinib reduce gefitinib levels.

- Administration of gefitinib or imatinib with warfarin causes elevations in the International Normalised Ratio, increasing the risk of bleeding.
- Drugs that inhibit the CYP3A4 family (such as clarithromycin, erythromycin, itraconazole, and ketoconazole) when taken with imatinib may increase the imatinib plasma levels.
- Imatinib administered with CYP3A4 inducers (carbamazepine, dexamethasone, phenobarbital, phenytoin, and rifampicin) may increase metabolism of imatinib and decrease imatinib level.
- Imatinib given with simvastatin increases simvastatin levels about threefold.
- Imatinib increases plasma levels of other CYP3A4-metabolised drugs, such as triazolo-benzodiazepines, dihydropyridine, calcium channel blockers, and certain HMG-CoA reductase inhibitors.

Adverse reactions

Toxicities have occurred from administration of targeted therapies. Patients should avoid becoming pregnant during administration of these agents as a result of animal studies having shown that they cross the placental barrier and have resulted in foetal harm and death.

Gefitinib

Adverse reactions to gefitinib include:
- skin rash
- diarrhoea
- abnormal eyelash growth
- lung and liver damage.

Imatinib

Adverse reactions to imatinib include:
- oedema (periorbital and lower limb), which may result in pulmonary oedema, effusions, and heart or renal failure. Management includes treatment with diuretics and supportive measures such as decreasing the dose.
- nausea, vomiting, liver function abnormalities, and myelosuppression (especially neutropenia and thrombocytopenia).

Bortezomib

The most common adverse reactions to bortezomib include:
- asthenic conditions (fatigue, malaise, and weakness), nausea, diarrhoea, appetite loss (anorexia), constipation, pyrexia, and vomiting.

Other reactions include:
- peripheral neuropathy, headache, low blood pressure, liver toxicity, thrombocytopenia, and renal toxicity
- cardiac toxicity (arrhythmias, such as bradycardia, ventricular tachycardia, atrial fibrillation and atrial flutter; heart failure; myocardial ischaemia and infarction; pulmonary oedema; and pericardial effusion).

Depending on the severity of the reactions, the dosage may need to be reduced or withheld until the toxicity resolves. With severe reactions, the medication is discontinued.

Nursing process

These nursing process steps are appropriate for patients undergoing treatment with targeted therapies.

Assessment
- Assess the patient's condition before therapy and regularly thereafter.
- Monitor the patient for adverse reactions and drug interactions.
- Obtain a baseline weight before therapy, and weigh the patient daily throughout therapy. Evaluate and treat unexpected and rapid weight gain.
- Evaluate the patient's and family's knowledge of drug therapy.

Key nursing diagnoses
- Ineffective health maintenance related to the presence of neoplastic disease.
- Risk for falls related to drug-induced adverse reactions.
- Deficient knowledge related to drug therapy.

Planning outcome goals
- The patient will demonstrate an improvement in assessments and diagnostic testing.
- The risk of injury to the patient will be minimised.
- The patient and family will demonstrate an understanding of drug therapy.

Implementation
- Reconstitute the drug as prescribed and administer per facility policy.
- Monitor the patient closely for fluid retention, which can be severe.
- Monitor the patient's CBC weekly for the first month, monitor biweekly for the second month, and then periodically thereafter.

- Because GI irritation is common, give the drug with food, as appropriate.
- Monitor liver function tests carefully because hepatotoxicity (occasionally severe) may occur. Decrease the dosage as needed.
- Because the long-term safety of the drug isn't known, monitor renal and liver toxicity and immunosuppression carefully.

Evaluation
- Patient responds well to drug therapy.
- Patient doesn't develop serious complications from adverse reactions.
- Patient and family state an understanding of drug therapy.

Unclassified antineoplastic drugs

Many other antineoplastic drugs can't be included in existing classifications. These drugs include:
- aldesleukin
- arsenic trioxide
- asparaginase
- hydroxyurea
- interferons
- procarbazine
- taxanes (paclitaxel and docetaxel).

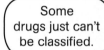

Some drugs just can't be classified.

Aldesleukin

Aldesleukin is a human recombinant interleukin-2 derivative that's used to treat metastatic renal cell carcinoma.

Pharmacokinetics
After I.V. administration of aldesleukin, about 30% is absorbed into the plasma and about 70% is absorbed rapidly by the liver, kidneys, and lungs. The drug is excreted primarily by the kidneys.

Pharmacodynamics
The exact antitumour mechanism of action of aldesleukin is unknown. The drug may stimulate an immunologic reaction against the tumour.

Pharmacotherapeutics

Aldesleukin is used to treat metastatic renal cell carcinoma. It may also be used in the treatment of Kaposi's sarcoma and metastatic melanoma.

Drug interactions

Aldesleukin will interact with other drugs:
• Concomitant administration of aldesleukin and drugs with psychotropic properties (such as opioids, analgesics, antiemetics, sedatives, and tranquillisers) may produce additive CNS effects.
• Glucocorticoids may reduce aldesleukin's antitumour effects.
• Antihypertensive drugs may potentiate aldesleukin's hypotensive effects.
• Concurrent therapy with drugs that are toxic to the kidneys (such as aminoglycosides), bone marrow (such as cytotoxic chemotherapy drugs), heart (such as doxorubicin), or liver (such as methotrexate or asparaginase) may increase toxicity to these organs.

Adverse reactions

During clinical trials, more than 15% of patients developed adverse reactions to aldesleukin. These include:
• pulmonary congestion and difficulty breathing
• anaemia, thrombocytopenia, and leucopenia
• elevated bilirubin, transaminase, and alkaline phosphatase levels
• hypomagnesaemia and acidosis
• reduced or absent urinary output
• elevated serum creatinine level
• stomatitis
• nausea and vomiting.

Nursing process

These nursing process steps are appropriate for patients undergoing treatment with aldesleukin.

Assessment
• Assess the patient's condition before therapy and regularly thereafter.
• Monitor the patient for adverse reactions and drug interactions.
• Monitor blood studies, as appropriate.
• Evaluate the patient's and family's knowledge of drug therapy.

Key nursing diagnoses
• Ineffective health maintenance related to the presence of neoplastic disease.

- Risk for injury related to drug-induced adverse reactions.
- Deficient knowledge related to drug therapy.

Planning outcome goals
- The patient will demonstrate an improvement in assessments and diagnostic testing.
- The risk of injury to the patient will be minimised.
- The patient and family will demonstrate an understanding of drug therapy.

Implementation
- Administer the medication according to facility protocol.
- Assess the patient for effects of medication as well as drug interactions.
- Notify the prescriber of severe adverse reactions, which may require dosage reduction or discontinuation.

Evaluation
- Patient responds well to drug therapy.
- Patient doesn't develop serious complications from adverse reactions.
- Patient and family state an understanding of drug therapy.

Asparaginases

Asparaginases are cell cycle specific and act during the G1 phase.

Pharmacokinetics

Asparaginase is administered parenterally. It's considered 100% bioavailable when administered I.V. and about 50% bioavailable when administered I.M.

After administration, asparaginase remains inside the blood vessels, with minimal distribution elsewhere. The metabolism of asparaginase is unknown; only trace amounts appear in urine.

Pharmacodynamics

Asparaginase capitalises on the biochemical differences between normal and tumour cells.

Eat your asparagines, or else

Most normal cells can synthesise asparagine, but some tumour cells depend on other sources of asparagine for survival. Asparaginase helps to degrade asparagine to aspartic acid and ammonia. Deprived of their supply of asparagine, the tumour cells die.

Pharmacotherapeutics

Asparaginase is used primarily to induce remission in patients with acute lymphocytic leukaemia in combination with standard chemotherapy.

Drug interactions

Asparaginase may interact with other drugs. The drug can reduce the effectiveness of methotrexate. Concurrent use of asparaginase with prednisone or vincristine increases the risk of adverse reactions.

Adverse reactions

Many patients receiving asparaginase develop nausea and vomiting. Fever, headache, abdominal pain, pancreatitis, coagulopathy, and liver toxicity can also occur.

Raising the risk

Asparaginase can cause anaphylaxis, which is more likely to occur with intermittent I.V. dosing than with daily I.V. dosing or I.M. injections. The risk of a reaction rises with each successive treatment. Hypersensitivity reactions may also occur.

Asparaginases can cause anaphylaxis, especially with intermittent I.V. dosing. And the risk increases with each successive treatment.

Nursing process

These nursing process steps are appropriate for patients undergoing treatment with asparaginase.

Assessment
• Assess the patient's condition before therapy and regularly thereafter.
• Monitor the patient for adverse reactions and drug interactions.
• Monitor the drug's effectiveness by noting results of follow-up diagnostic tests and overall physical status.
• Monitor the patient's CBC and bone marrow function test results. Bone marrow regeneration may take 5 to 6 weeks.
• Evaluate the patient's and family's knowledge of drug therapy.

Key nursing diagnoses
• Ineffective health maintenance related to the presence of neoplastic disease
• Ineffective protection related to drug-induced adverse reactions
• Deficient knowledge related to drug therapy

Planning outcome goals
- The patient will demonstrate an improvement in assessments and diagnostic testing.
- The risk of injury to the patient will be minimised.
- The patient and family will demonstrate an understanding of drug therapy.

Implementation
- Follow facility policy to reduce risks. Preparation and administration of the parenteral form of the drug are linked to carcinogenic, mutagenic, and teratogenic risks for personnel.
- Reconstitute the drug as prescribed and administer per facility policy. The drug is given in a hospital under close supervision. (See *Asparaginase warning*.)
- Prevent tumour lysis, which can result in uric acid nephropathy, by increasing fluid intake. Allopurinol should be started before therapy begins.
- Limit the dose at a single injection site to 2 ml when administering the drug I.M.
- I.V. infusion is given slowly, over at least 30 minutes.
- Keep diphenhydramine, adrenaline (epinephrine), and I.V. corticosteroids available for treating anaphylaxis.
- Refrigerate unopened dry powder. Reconstituted solution is stable for 8 hours if refrigerated.
- If the drug contacts skin or mucous membranes, wash with copious amounts of water for at least 15 minutes.

Before you give that drug!

Asparaginase warning

The risk of hypersensitivity reactions increases with repeated doses of asparaginase. An intradermal skin test should be performed before the initial dose and repeated after an interval of a week or more, between doses, as prescribed. Observe the injection site for at least 1 hour for erythema or a wheal, which indicates a positive response. An allergic reaction to the drug may still develop in a patient with a negative skin test.

A desensitisation dose may be prescribed. The dose is doubled every 10 minutes if no reaction occurs, until the total amount given equals the patient's total dose for that day.

- Because of vomiting, administer parenteral fluids for 24 hours or until the patient can tolerate oral fluids.

Evaluation
- Patient responds well to drug therapy.
- Patient doesn't develop serious complications from adverse haematologic reactions.
- Patient and family state an understanding of drug therapy.

Hydroxyurea

Hydroxyurea is used most commonly for patients with chronic myelogenous leukaemia. Hydroxyurea is also used for solid tumours and head and neck cancer.

Pharmacokinetics
Hydroxyurea is absorbed readily and distributed well into CSF after oral administration. It reaches a peak serum level 2 hours after administration.

Half and half

About half of a dose is metabolised by the liver to carbon dioxide, which is excreted by the lungs, or to urea, which is excreted by the kidneys. The remaining half is excreted unchanged in urine.

Pharmacodynamics
Hydroxyurea exerts its effect by inhibiting the enzyme ribonucleotide reductase, which is necessary for DNA synthesis.

Divide and conquer

Hydroxyurea kills cells in the S phase of the cell cycle and holds other cells in the G1 phase, when they're most susceptible to irradiation.

Pharmacotherapeutics
Hydroxyurea is used to treat selected myeloproliferative disorders. It may produce temporary remissions in some patients with metastatic malignant melanomas as well.

When your neck is on the line

Hydroxyurea also is used in combination therapy with radiation to treat carcinomas of the head, neck, and lung.

Drug interactions

Cytotoxic drugs and radiation therapy enhance the toxicity of hydroxyurea.

Adverse reactions

Treatment with hydroxyurea leads to few adverse reactions. Those that do occur include:
- bone marrow suppression
- drowsiness
- headache
- nausea and vomiting
- anorexia
- elevated uric acid levels, which require some patients to take allopurinol to prevent kidney damage.

Nursing process

These nursing process steps are appropriate for patients undergoing treatment with hydroxyurea.

Assessment
- Assess the patient's condition before therapy and regularly thereafter.
- Monitor the patient for adverse reactions and drug interactions.
- Monitor CBC, BUN, uric acid, and creatinine levels.
- Monitor the patient's renal function. Auditory and visual hallucinations and haematologic toxicity increase with decreased renal function.
- Evaluate the patient's and family's knowledge of drug therapy.

Remember to monitor the patient's CBC, BUN, uric acid, and creatinine levels. An elevated uric acid level may require allopurinol.

Key nursing diagnoses
- Ineffective health maintenance related to the presence of neoplastic disease
- Ineffective protection related to drug-induced adverse haematologic reactions
- Deficient knowledge related to drug therapy

Planning outcome goals
- The patient will demonstrate an improvement in assessments and diagnostic testing.
- The risk of injury to the patient will be minimised.
- The patient and family will demonstrate an understanding of drug therapy.

Implementation
- Encourage fluids to hydrate the patient, as appropriate.
- Monitor the patient for signs of infection (such as fever, sore throat, and fatigue) and bleeding (easy bruising, nosebleeds, bleeding gums, melena). Tell him to take his temperature daily and report elevations.
- Administer the medication according to facility protocol.
- If the patient can't swallow capsules, empty contents of capsules into water and have him drink it immediately.
- Advise a woman of childbearing age not to become pregnant during therapy, and to consult with her prescriber before becoming pregnant.

Evaluation
- Patient responds well to drug therapy.
- Patient doesn't develop serious complications from adverse reactions.
- Patient and family state an understanding of drug therapy.

Interferons

A family of naturally occurring glycoproteins, called *interferons*, are so named because of their ability to interfere with viral replication. These drugs have anticancer activity as well as activity against condylomata acuminata (soft, wartlike growths on the skin and mucous membranes of the genitalia caused by a virus).

The three types of interferons are:

alfa interferons derived from leucocytes

beta interferons derived from fibroblasts (connective tissue cells)

gamma interferons derived from fibroblasts and lymphocytes.

And one stands alone

Alfa interferons (alfa-2a, alfa-2b, and alfa-n3) are the most commonly used. The beta and gamma interferons tend to be limited to investigational use.

Pharmacokinetics
After I.M. or subcutaneous administration, alfa interferons are usually absorbed well. Information about their distribution is unavailable. Alfa interferons are filtered by the kidneys, where they're degraded. Liver metabolism and biliary excretion of interferons are negligible.

Pharmacodynamics

Although their exact mechanism of action is unknown, alfa interferons appear to bind to specific membrane receptors on the cell surface. When bound, they initiate a sequence of intracellular events that includes the induction of certain enzymes.

Running interference

This process may account for the ability of interferons to:
- inhibit viral replication
- suppress cell proliferation
- enhance macrophage activity (engulfing and destroying microorganisms and other debris)
- increase cytotoxicity of lymphocytes for target cells.

Interferons can put a stop to viral replication.

Pharmacotherapeutics

Alfa interferons have shown their most promising activity in treating blood malignancies, especially hairy cell leukaemia. Their approved indications currently include:
- hairy cell leukaemia
- AIDS-related Kaposi's sarcoma
- condylomata acuminata.

Alfa interferons also demonstrate some activity against chronic myelogenous leukaemia, malignant lymphoma, multiple myeloma, melanoma, and renal cell carcinoma.

Drug interactions

Interferons interact with other drugs:
- They may enhance the CNS effects of CNS depressants and substantially increase the half-life of methylxanthines (including theophylline and aminophylline).
- Concurrent use with a live virus vaccine may potentiate replication of the virus, increasing the adverse effects of the vaccine and decreasing the patient's antibody response.
- Bone marrow suppression may be increased when an interferon is used with radiation therapy or a drug that causes blood abnormalities or bone marrow suppression.
- Alfa interferons increase the risk of kidney failure from interleukin-2.

Adverse reactions

Blood toxicity occurs in up to one-half of patients taking interferons and may produce leucopenia, neutropenia, thrombocytopenia, and anaemia. Adverse GI reactions include anorexia, nausea, and diarrhoea.

Alfa concerns

The most common adverse reaction to alfa interferons is a flu-like syndrome that may produce fever, fatigue, muscle pain, headache, chills, and joint pain.

It catches your breath

Coughing, difficulty breathing, hypotension, oedema, chest pain, and heart failure have also been associated with interferon therapy.

Nursing process

These nursing process steps are appropriate for patients undergoing treatment with interferons.

Assessment
- Assess the patient's condition before therapy and regularly thereafter.
- Monitor the patient for adverse reactions and drug interactions.
- Obtain an allergy history. The drug contains phenol as a preservative and serum albumin as a stabiliser.
- At the beginning of therapy, assess the patient for flu-like symptoms, which tend to diminish with continued therapy.
- Monitor blood studies. Any effects are dose-related and reversible. Recovery occurs within several days or weeks after withdrawal.
- Evaluate the patient's and family's knowledge of drug therapy.

Key nursing diagnoses
- Ineffective health maintenance related to the presence of neoplastic disease.
- Risk for injury related to drug-induced adverse reactions.
- Deficient knowledge related to drug therapy.

Planning outcome goals
- The patient will demonstrate an improvement in assessments and diagnostic testing.
- The risk of injury to the patient will be minimised.
- The patient and family will demonstrate an understanding of drug therapy.

Implementation
- Premedicate the patient with paracetamol to minimise flu-like symptoms.
- Give the drug at bedtime to minimise daytime drowsiness.
- Make sure that the patient is well hydrated, especially during the initial stages of treatment.

- Administer the medication according to facility protocol and monitor for effects.
- The subcutaneous administration route is used in a patient whose platelet count is below 50,000/mm^3.
- Intralesional use may be used with interferon alfa-2b; dilute and reconstitute per facility policy. The drug may be given in evening with paracetamol.
- Refrigerate the drug.
- Notify the prescriber of severe adverse reactions, which may require a dosage reduction or discontinuation.

Evaluation
- Patient responds well to drug therapy.
- Patient doesn't develop serious complications from adverse reactions.
- Patient and family state an understanding of drug therapy. (See *Teaching about interferons*.)

Procarbazine

Procarbazine hydrochloride, a methylhydrazine derivative with MAO-inhibiting properties, is used to treat Hodgkin's disease, primary and metastatic brain tumours, and lymphoma. It is cell cycle–phase specific and acts on the S phase.

Pharmacokinetics
After oral administration, procarbazine is absorbed well. It readily crosses the blood-brain barrier and is well distributed into CSF.

Procarbazine is metabolised rapidly in the liver and must be activated metabolically by microsomal enzymes. It's excreted in urine, primarily as metabolites. Respiratory excretion of the drug occurs as methane and carbon dioxide gas.

Pharmacodynamics
An inert drug, procarbazine must be activated metabolically in the liver before it can produce various cell changes. It can cause chromosomal damage, suppress mitosis, and inhibit DNA, RNA, and protein synthesis. Cancer cells can develop resistance to procarbazine quickly.

Drug interactions
Interactions with procarbazine can be significant:
- Procarbazine produces an additive effect when administered with CNS depressants.
- Taken with pethidine, it may result in severe hypotension and death.

Education edge

Teaching about interferons

If interferon therapy is prescribed, review these points with the patient and caregivers:

- Know that laboratory tests will be performed before and periodically during therapy. Tests include complete blood count with differential, platelet count, blood chemistry and electrolyte studies, liver function tests and, if you have a cardiac disorder or advanced stages of cancer, electrocardiograms.
- Proper oral hygiene is important during your treatment because interferon use may lead to microbial infection, delayed healing, gingival bleeding, and decreased salivary flow. Brush frequently (after meals and at bedtime) with a soft-bristled toothbrush and clean the toothbrush daily (may use hydrogen peroxide). Avoid toothpicks and water pressure gum cleaners that can traumatise the mucosa. Rinse your mouth with water or saline. Avoid commercial mouthwashes that contain alcohol, which may cause irritation.
- Follow your prescriber's instructions about taking and recording your temperature. Take paracetamol as directed for the treatment of adverse drug effects (fever, arthralgia, myalgia). Report adverse effects to your prescriber.
- If you miss a dose, check with your prescriber for instructions.

- The drug may cause temporary hair loss; it should grow back when therapy ends.
- Make sure that you understand the proper procedure to prepare and administer the drug, including proper hand-washing technique and injection technique. Dispose of used needles in a recommended container. Store the drug according to the manufacturer's recommendations.
- Take the drug at bedtime to minimise flu symptoms.
- Review the information provided by the drug manufacturer included with your prescription. If you have any questions regarding this information, contact your prescriber. If you don't receive this information, contact your pharmacist.
- You're at an increased risk for infection during therapy. Don't receive any immunisation without getting approval from your prescriber and avoid contact with people who have taken oral polio vaccine.
- If you're a woman of childbearing age, know that interferon poses danger to a foetus. Notify your prescriber promptly if you become pregnant during therapy.
- Avoid alcohol during drug therapy.
- Report signs of depression.
- Don't take over-the-counter products, herbal remedies, or prescription medications without first talking to your prescriber.

Mirroring MAO

Because of procarbazine's MAO-inhibiting properties, hypertensive reactions may occur when it's administered concurrently with sympathomimetics, antidepressants, and tyramine-rich foods.

Adverse reactions

Late-onset bone marrow suppression is the most common dose-limiting toxicity associated with procarbazine. Interstitial pneumonitis (lung inflammation) and pulmonary fibrosis (scarring) may also occur.

Off to a bad start

Initial procarbazine therapy may induce a flu-like syndrome, including fever, chills, sweating, lethargy, and muscle pain.

A gut feeling

GI reactions include nausea, vomiting, stomatitis, and diarrhoea.

Nursing process

These nursing process steps are appropriate for patients undergoing treatment with procarbazine.

Assessment
• Assess the patient's condition before therapy and regularly thereafter.
• Monitor the patient for adverse reactions and drug interactions.
• Monitor the patient's CBC and platelet counts.
• Evaluate the patient's and family's knowledge of drug therapy.

Key nursing diagnoses
• Ineffective health maintenance related to the presence of neoplastic disease.
• Ineffective protection related to drug-induced adverse reactions.
• Deficient knowledge related to drug therapy.

Planning outcome goals
• The patient will demonstrate an improvement in assessments and diagnostic testing.
• The risk of injury to the patient will be minimised.
• The patient and family will demonstrate an understanding of drug therapy.

Implementation
• Give the drug at bedtime to lessen nausea. It's usually given in divided doses.
• Monitor the patient for signs of infection (such as fever, sore throat, fatigue) and bleeding (easy bruising, nosebleeds, bleeding gums, melena). Ask the patient to take his temperature daily and report elevations.
• Stop the drug and notify the prescriber if the patient becomes confused or if paraesthesia or other neuropathies develop.
• Warn the patient to avoid alcohol during drug therapy.

- Stop the drug and notify the prescriber if a disulfiram-like reaction occurs (chest pain, rapid or irregular heartbeat, severe headache, stiff neck).
- Warn the patient to avoid hazardous activities until the CNS effects of the drug are known.
- Advise a woman of childbearing age not to avoid pregnancy during therapy and to consult with her prescriber before becoming pregnant.

Evaluation
- Patient responds well to drug therapy.
- Patient doesn't develop serious complications from adverse reactions.
- Patient and family state an understanding of drug therapy.

Taxanes may be used to treat ovarian or breast cancer if chemotherapy fails.

Taxanes

Taxane antineoplastics are used to treat metastatic ovarian and breast carcinoma after chemotherapy has failed. They include:
- paclitaxel
- docetaxel.

Pharmacokinetics

After I.V. administration, paclitaxel is highly bound to plasma proteins. Docetaxel is administered I.V. with a rapid onset of action. Paclitaxel is metabolised primarily in the liver with a small amount excreted unchanged in urine. Docetaxel is excreted primarily in faeces.

Pharmacodynamics

Paclitaxel and docetaxel exert their chemotherapeutic effect by disrupting the microtubule network that's essential for mitosis and other vital cellular functions.

Pharmacotherapeutics

Paclitaxel is used when first-line or subsequent chemotherapy has failed in treating metastatic ovarian carcinoma as well as metastatic breast cancer. The taxanes may also be used for to treat head and neck cancer, prostate cancer, and non–small-cell lung cancer.

Drug interactions

Taxanes have few interactions with other drugs:
- Concomitant use of paclitaxel and cisplatin may cause additive myelosuppressive effects.
- Cyclosporine, ketoconazole, erythromycin, and troleandomycin may modify docetaxel metabolism.
- Phenytoin may decrease paclitaxel serum concentration leading to a loss of efficacy.
- Quinupristin with dalfopristin may increase paclitaxel serum concentrations, increasing the risk of toxicity.

Adverse reactions

During clinical trials, 25% or more patients experienced these adverse reactions to paclitaxel:
- bone marrow suppression
- hypersensitivity reactions
- abnormal EEG tracings
- peripheral neuropathy
- muscle and joint pain
- nausea and vomiting
- diarrhoea
- mucous membrane inflammation
- hair loss.

Docetaxel

Adverse reactions to docetaxel include:
- hypersensitivity reactions
- fluid retention
- leucopenia, neutropenia, or thrombocytopenia
- hair loss
- mouth inflammation
- numbness and tingling
- pain
- weakness and fatigue.

Nursing process

These nursing process steps are appropriate for patients undergoing treatment with taxanes.

Assessment

- Assess the patient's condition before therapy and regularly thereafter.
- Continuously monitor the patient for the first 30 minutes of infusion and closely monitor throughout infusion.

- Monitor the patient's blood counts and liver function test results frequently during therapy.
- Monitor the patient for adverse reactions and drug interactions.
- Evaluate the patient's and family's knowledge of drug therapy.

Key nursing diagnoses
- Ineffective health maintenance related to cancer.
- Ineffective protection related to drug-induced adverse haematologic reactions.
- Deficient knowledge related to drug therapy.

Planning outcome goals
- The patient will demonstrate an improvement in assessments and diagnostic testing.
- The risk of injury to the patient will be minimised.
- The patient and family will demonstrate an understanding of drug therapy.

Implementation
- To reduce severe hypersensitivity, expect to pretreat the patient with corticosteroids, such as dexamethasone and antihistamines.
- Follow facility protocol for safe handling, preparation, and use of chemotherapy drugs. Preparation and administration of the parenteral form of the drug are linked to carcinogenic, mutagenic, and teratogenic risks for personnel.
- Mark all waste materials with chemotherapy hazard labels.
- Dilute concentrations and administer according to facility protocol.
- Prepare and store infusion solutions in glass containers.
- Take care to avoid extravasation.
- Monitor the patient for signs of bleeding, infection, and peripheral neuropathy (tingling, burning, or numbness in limbs).
- Warn the patient that alopecia occurs in up to 82% of patients.
- Advise female patients of childbearing age to avoid pregnancy during therapy. Also recommend consulting with her prescriber before becoming pregnant.

Evaluation
- Patient responds well to drug therapy.
- Patient develops no serious complications from drug-induced adverse haematologic reactions.
- Patient and family state an understanding of drug therapy.

Quick quiz

1. The patient is being administered nitrogen mustard chemotherapy and is taking antacids, hydrochlorothiazide, diphenhydramine, and diazepam. Which medication might cause a drug interaction with nitrogen mustards?

    A. Antacids
    B. Hydrochlorothiazide
    C. Diphenhydramine
    D. Diazepam

Answer: A. Nitrogen mustards interact with many other drugs. Calcium-containing drugs and foods, such as antacids and dairy products, reduce absorption of estramustine.

2. The nurse is observing the patient for adverse reactions to dacarbazine. Which adverse reaction may be caused by dacarbazine drug therapy?

    A. Rash
    B. Hypotension
    C. Flu-like syndrome
    D. Tachycardia

Answer: C. Dacarbazine use may cause some adverse reactions. These include leucopenia, thrombocytopenia, nausea and vomiting (which begin within 1 to 3 hours after administration in most cases and may last up to 12 hours), phototoxicity, flu-like syndrome, and hair loss.

3. Which action should the nurse perform before treatment with asparaginase?

    A. Monitoring blood pressure
    B. Assessing ECG
    C. Obtaining allergy history
    D. Performing an intradermal skin test

Answer: D. The risk of a hypersensitivity reaction increases with repeated doses of asparaginase. An intradermal skin test should be performed before the initial dose and repeated after an interval of 1 week or more, between doses.

Scoring

☆☆☆ If you answered all three questions correctly, extraordinary! You really mowed down the malignant neoplasms!

☆☆ If you answered two questions correctly, congratulations! You're competent to combat cancer.

☆ If you answered fewer than two questions correctly, give it another shot. Remember, this is your last crack at a quick quiz!

Appendices and index

Glossary

acetylcholinesterase inhibitor: drug that increases parasympathetic activity and blocks the action of acetylcholinesterase, an enzyme that inhibits the action of acetylcholine

action potential: electrical impulse across nerve or muscle fibers that have been stimulated

adrenergic agonist: drug that mimics the effects of the sympathetic nervous system

adrenergic blocking drug: drug that interferes with transmission of nerve impulses to adrenergic receptors, allowing a parasympathetic response

agranulocytosis: severe and acute decrease in granulocytes (basophils, eosinophils, and neutrophils) as an adverse reaction to a drug or radiation therapy; results in high fever, exhaustion, and bleeding ulcers of the throat, mucous membranes, and GI tract

allergen: substance that induces an allergy or a hypersensitivity reaction

anaphylaxis: severe allergic reaction to a foreign substance

angioedema: life-threatening reaction causing sudden swelling of tissues around the face, neck, lips, tongue, throat, hands, feet, genitals, or intestines

antibody: immunoglobulin molecule that reacts only with the specific antigen that induced its formation in the lymph system

anticoagulant drug: drug that prevents clot formation or extension but doesn't speed dissolution of preexisting clots

antigen: foreign substance (such as bacteria or toxins) that induces antibody formation

antipyretic: pertaining to a substance or procedure that reduces fever

ataxia: incoordination of voluntary muscle action, particularly in such activities as walking and reaching for objects

automaticity: ability of a cardiac cell to initiate an impulse on its own

bactericidal: causing death of bacteria

bioavailability: rate and extent to which a drug enters the circulation, thereby gaining access to target tissue

blood-brain barrier: barrier separating the parenchyma of the central nervous system from the circulating blood, preventing certain substances from reaching the brain or cerebrospinal fluid

body surface area (BSA): area covered by a person's external skin that's calculated in square metres (m^2) according to height and weight; used to calculate safe paediatric dosages for all drugs and safe dosages for adult patients receiving extremely potent drugs or drugs requiring great precision, such as antineoplastic and chemotherapeutic agents

bradykinesia: abnormally slow body movement

bronchospasm: narrowing of the bronchioles resulting from an increase in smooth muscle tone that causes wheezing

cerebral oedema: increased fluid content in the brain; may result from correcting hypernatraemia too rapidly

chemoreceptor trigger zone: region of the medulla of the brain that controls vomiting

conduction: transmission of electrical impulses through the myocardium

conductivity: ability of one cardiac cell to transmit an electrical impulse to another cell

contractility: ability of a cardiac cell to contract after receiving an impulse

cross-sensitivity: hypersensitivity or allergy to a drug in a particular class (for example, penicillin) that may cause an allergic reaction to another drug in the same class

cytotoxic: destructive to cells

debriding drug: drug used to remove foreign material and dead or damaged tissue from a wound or burn

depolarisation: response of a myocardial cell to an electrical impulse that causes movement of ions across the cell membrane, triggering myocardial contraction

diastole: phase of the cardiac cycle when both atria (atrial diastole) or both ventricles (ventricular diastole) are at rest and filling with blood

diplopia: double vision

dosage: the amount, frequency, and number of doses of a drug

dose: the amount of a drug to be given at one time

drip factor: number of drops to be delivered per millilitre of solution in an I.V. administration set; measured in gtt/ml (drops per millilitre); listed on the package containing the I.V. tubing administration set

drip rate: number of drops of I.V. solution to be infused per minute; based on the drip factor and calibrated for the selected I.V. tubing

emesis: vomiting

extrapyramidal symptoms: symptoms caused by an imbalance in the extrapyramidal portion of the nervous system; typically include pill-rolling motions, drooling, tremors, rigidity, and shuffling gait

excitability: ability of a cardiac cell to respond to an electrical stimulus

extravasation: leakage of intravascular fluid into surrounding tissue; can be caused by such medications as chemotherapeutic drugs, dopamine, and calcium solutions that produce blistering and, eventually, tissue necrosis

flow rate: the number of millilitres of I.V. fluid to administer over 1 hour; based on the total volume to be infused in millilitres and the amount of time for the infusion

hepatotoxicity: quality of being toxic to or capable of destroying liver cells

hirsutism: excessive growth of dark, coarse body hair in a masculine distribution

histamine-2 receptors: cells in the gastric mucosa that respond to histamine release by increasing gastric acid secretion

inhalation drug: drug that affects the respiratory tract locally; may be administered by handheld nebuliser, intermittent positive pressure breathing apparatus, nasal spray, or nose drops

insomnia: inability to sleep, sleep interrupted by periods of wakefulness, or sleep that ends prematurely

intramuscular route (I.M.): drug administration into a muscle

intradermal route: drug administration into the dermis of the skin

intravenous route (I.V.): drug administration into a vein

ischaemia: decreased blood supply to a body organ or tissue

leucocytosis: abnormal increase in circulating white blood cells

leucopenia: abnormal decrease in white blood cells to fewer than 5,000 cells/mm^3

lipid regulating drug: drug used to prevent or treat increased accumulation of fatty substances (lipids) in the blood

lipodystrophy: thickening of tissues and accumulation of fat at an injection site; results from too-frequent injection of insulin in the same site

millimole (mmol): A millimole is 1/1,000 of a mole. A mole is an amount of a substance that contains a certain number of molecules or atoms.; used to measure electrolytes

mydriasis: dilation of the pupil

necrotic: pertaining to localised tissue death

nephrotoxicity: quality of being toxic to or capable of destroying kidney cells

neutropenia: abnormal decrease in circulating neutrophils

nonparenteral drug: drug administered by the oral, topical, or rectal route

nystagmus: constant involuntary eye movement

oral route (P.O.): drug administration through the mouth

ototoxicity: potentially irreversible damage to the auditory and vestibular branches of the eighth cranial nerve; may cause hearing or balance loss

pancytopenia: abnormal decrease in erythrocytes, white blood cells, and platelets; also known as *aplastic anaemia*

paraesthesia: abnormal sensations (including numbness, prickling, and tingling) with no known cause

parasympatholytic drug: drug that blocks the effects of the parasympathetic nervous system, allowing a sympathetic response

parasympathomimetic drug: drug that mimics the effects of the parasympathetic nervous system

parenteral route: drug administration through a route other than the digestive tract, such as intravenously, intramuscularly, and subcutaneously

paroxysmal: episode of an arrhythmia that starts and stops suddenly

peak and trough drug concentration levels: serum drug concentration levels measured to determine whether the dosing regimen is therapeutic or toxic. Blood for peak concentration level is drawn immediately after the dose is administered; blood for trough concentration level is drawn just before the next dose is administered

phlebitis: inflammation of a vein

photosensitivity reaction: increased reaction of the skin to sunlight; may result in oedema, papules, urticaria, or acute burns

potentiate: to increase the action of another drug so that the combined effect of both drugs is greater than the sum of the effect of either drug alone

pruritus: itching

rhabdomyolysis: acute and potentially fatal skeletal muscle disease

rectal route: drug administration (usually by suppository) through the rectum

refractory period: period of relaxation after muscle excitement

renin: enzyme produced by the kidneys in response to an actual or perceived decline in extracellular fluid volume; important part of blood pressure regulation

repolarisation: recovery of the myocardial cells after depolarisation during which the cell membrane returns to its resting potential

sedative-hypnotic drug: drug that exerts a soothing or tranquillising effect while dulling the senses or inducing sleep

serotonin: neurotransmitter that acts as a powerful vasoconstrictor and is thought to be involved in sleep and sensory perception

serum drug level: amount of a drug present in the blood at a given moment

status epilepticus: rapid succession of seizures without intervals of consciousness; constitutes a medical emergency

stomatitis: inflammation and possible ulceration of the mucous membranes of the mouth

subcutaneous route: drug administration into the subcutaneous tissue

superinfection: new infection that's in addition to one that's already present

sympatholytic drug: drug that inhibits sympathetic activity; may block receptors or prevent release of noradrenaline (norepinephrine)

sympathomimetic drug: drug that mimics the effects of the sympathetic nervous system

systole: phase of the cardiac cycle during which both of the atria (atrial systole) or the ventricles (ventricular systole) are contracting

tardive dyskinesia: disorder characterised by involuntary repetitious movements of the muscles of the face, limbs, and trunk; most commonly results from extended periods of treatment with phenothiazine drugs

teratogenic: pertaining to the production of physical defects in an embryo or a foetus

thrombocytopenia: abnormal decrease in platelets, predisposing the patient to bleeding

thrombolytic drug: drug that dissolves a thrombus by activating plasminogen and converting it to plasmin

topical route: drug administration through the skin (after absorption

through the skin's layers, the drug enters circulation); usually in cream, ointment, or transdermal patch form

transdermal route: drug administration through the skin by which the drug is absorbed continuously and enters the systemic system

urticaria: itchy skin inflammation characterised by pale wheals with well-defined red edges; usually an allergic response to insect bites, food, or certain drugs; also called *hives*

vasopressor: drug that stimulates contraction of the muscular tissue of the capillaries and arteries

viscosity: state of being glutinous or sticky

withdrawal symptoms: unpleasant and sometimes life-threatening physiologic changes occurring when certain drugs are withdrawn after prolonged, regular use

Ophthalmic and dermatologic drugs

This chart reviews the major actions, pharmacotherapeutics, and adverse reactions of ophthalmic and dermatologic drugs.

Ophthalmic drugs

Drug	Action	Treatment uses	Adverse reactions
Antiallergic agents			
Antazoline sulphate Azelastine Emedastine Epinastine hydrochloride Ketotifen Lodoxamide Olopatadine	• Decrease irritation	• To treat allergic conjunctivitis • To treat seasonal conjunctivitis • To treat keratitis	• Tearing
Anaesthetics			
Oxybuprocaine Proxymetacaine Tetracaine	• Prevent initiation and transmission of nerve impulses	• To anaesthetise the cornea, allowing application of instruments for measuring IOP or removing foreign bodies • To prepare for suture removal, conjunctival or corneal scraping, and tear duct manipulation	• Corneal inflammation • Corneal opacities • Delayed corneal healing • Eye pain and redness • Loss of visual acuity • Scarring
Anti-infectives			
Ciprofloxacin Erythromycin Fusidic acid Gentamicin Levofloxacin Neomycin sulphate Ofloxacin Polymyxin B sulphate Propamidine isetionate Tobramycin	• Kill bacteria or inhibit growth of bacteria or viruses	• To treat corneal ulcers or conjunctivitis caused by bacteria, fungus, or virus (each drug is specific to particular organisms)	• Secondary eye infections (with prolonged use) • Severe hypersensitivity reactions

Ophthalmic drugs

Drug	Action	Treatment uses	Adverse reactions
Anti-inflammatories			
Steroidal anti-inflammatories Betamethasone Dexamethasone Fluorometholone Hydrocortisone Prednisolone Rimexolone	• Decrease leucocyte infiltration at inflammation sites, causing reduced oozing of fluids and reduced oedema, redness, and scarring	• To treat inflammatory disorders and hypersensitivity-related conditions of the cornea, iris, conjunctiva, sclera, and anterior uvea	• Corneal ulceration • Delayed corneal healing • Increased susceptibility to viral or fungal corneal infection
Nonsteroidal anti-inflammatories Diclofenac Flurbiprofen Ketorolac	• Decreases inflammation and itching	• To inhibit pupil constriction during surgery (flurbiprofen) • To reduce itching due to seasonal allergies (ketorolac) • To treat inflammation after surgery	• Tearing • Discomfort
Lubricants			
Acetylcysteine Hydroxyethylcellulose Polyvinyl alcohol	• Act as artificial tears • Moisten cornea	• To protect cornea during diagnostic procedures • To moisten contact lenses	• None
Miotics			
Pilocarpine	• Stimulate and contract the sphincter muscle of the iris, constricting the pupil • Improve aqueous outflow	• To treat open-angle glaucoma, acute and chronic angle-closure glaucoma, and certain cases of secondary glaucoma resulting from increased IOP	• Blurred vision • Bronchospasm • Cataract formation • Eye pain • Photosensitivity • Reversible iris cysts • Confusion • Dry skin • Flushing • Impaired ability to coordinate movement • Irritation • Rapid heart rate • Transient burning sensations

Ophthalmic drugs

Drug	Action	Treatment uses	Adverse reactions
Mydriatics and cycloplegics Atropine sulfate Cyclopentolate hydrochloride Homatropine hydrobromide Tropicamide	• Act on the ciliary body of the eye to paralyze the fine-focusing muscles (thereby preventing accommodation for near vision)	• To perform refractive eye examinations in children before and after ophthalmic surgery • To treat conditions involving the iris	• Blurred vision • Confusion • Dry skin • Flushing • Impaired ability to coordinate movement • Irritation • Rapid heart rate • Transient burning sensations
Other drugs to lower IOP			
Adrenergic blockers (topical) Apraclonidine Betaxolol Brimonidine Carteolol Levobunolol Metipranolol Timolol maleate	• May reduce aqueous humor formation and slightly increase aqueous humor outflow	• To prevent and control elevated IOP, chronic open-angle glaucoma, and secondary glaucoma	• Bronchospasm • Fatigue • Headaches • Slow heart rate
Carbonic anhydrase inhibitors Acetazolamide Brinzolamide Dorzolamide	• Inhibit action of carbonic anhydrase, thus decreasing aqueous humor production	• To treat chronic open-angle glaucoma, acute angle-closure episodes, and secondary glaucoma	• Haemolytic or aplastic anaemia • Hypokalaemia • Leucopenia • Nausea and vomiting
Osmotic agents Glycerol Mannitol	• Reduce volume of vitreous humor • Decrease IOP	• To prepare for intraocular surgery • To treat acute glaucoma	• Hypokalaemia • Diuresis
Prostaglandin analogs Bimatoprost Latanoprost Travoprost	• Decrease IOP	• To treat glaucoma	• Irritation • Tearing

Dermatologic drugs

Drug	Action	Treatment uses	Adverse reactions
Anti-infectives			
Antibacterials Azelaic acid Bacitracin Clindamycin Erythromycin Metronidazole Mupirocin Neomycin Silver sulfadiazine Tetracycline	• Kill or inhibit the growth of bacteria	• To treat infections caused by bacteria (each drug is specific to particular organisms; combination products may also be used)	• Contact dermatitis • Rash • Skin burning, itching, redness, and dryness • Stinging
Antifungals Amphotericin B Butenafine Ciclopirox Clotrimazole Econazole Ketoconazole Miconazole Nystatin Sulconazole Terbinafine	• Kill or inhibit the growth of fungi	• To treat infections caused by fungi (each drug is specific to particular organisms)	• Same as for antibacterials
Antivirals Aciclovir Penciclovir	• Inhibit the growth of the herpes virus	• To treat herpes genitalis or herpes labialis	• Same as for antibacterials

Dermatologic drugs

Drug	Action	Treatment uses	Adverse reactions
Anti-inflammatories			
Alclometasone dipropionate Betamethasone Clobetasol Dexamethasone Fluocinolone Fluocinonide Fluticasone Hydrocortisone Mometasone Triamcinolone acetonide	• Suppress inflammation by binding to intracellular corticosteroid receptors, initiating a cascade of anti-inflammatory mediators • Cause vasoconstriction in inflamed tissue and prevent macrophages and leucocytes from moving into the area	• To relieve inflammation and itching in topical steroid–responsive disorders, such as eczema, psoriasis, angioedema, contact dermatitis, seborrheic dermatitis, atopic dermatitis, and urticaria	• Adrenal hormone suppression • Stretch marks and epidermal atrophy (after 3 to 4 weeks of use)
Hair growth stimulants			
Minoxidil	• Stimulate hair growth by causing vasodilation, which increases blood flow to the skin (exact mechanism of action is unknown)	• To treat male and female pattern baldness	• Fluid retention • Rapid heart rate • Weight gain
Topical antiacne drugs			
Keratolytics Acitretin Adapalene Isotretinoin Tazarotene Tretinoin	• Produce antibacterial effects • Reduce inflammation	• To treat mild acne, oily skin, and acne vulgaris (oral antibiotic therapy used as needed for deep acne)	• Burning • Urticaria • Rash • Scaling, blistering, and peeling • Skin dryness and irritation • Superinfection (with prolonged use)

Dermatologic drugs

Drug	Action	Treatment uses	Adverse reactions
Topical antiacne drugs (continued)			
Counterirritants Azelaic acid Benzoyl peroxide	• Produce antibacterial effects • Reduce inflammation	• To treat mild acne, oily skin, and acne vulgaris (oral antibiotic therapy used as needed for deep acne)	• Same as for keratolytics
Antimicrobials Clindamycin Doxycycline Erythromycin Lymecycline Minocycline Tetracycline	• Produce antibacterial effects • Reduce inflammation	• To treat mild acne, oily skin, and acne vulgaris (oral antibiotic therapy used as needed for deep acne)	• Same as for keratolytics • Hypersensitivity reactions (oral) • Candidal vaginitis (oral) • Gram-negative pustular folliculitis (oral)
Scabicides and pediculicides			
Benzyl benzoate Carbaryl Dimeticone Lindane Malathion Permethrin Phenothrin	• Act on parasite nerve cell membranes to disrupt the sodium channel current, causing paralysis (some are also ovicidal)	• To treat scabies and lice	• Contact dermatitis • Hypersensitivity reactions • Respiratory allergy symptoms

Abbreviations to avoid

The use of abbreviations remains an area for concern in all aspects of pharmacology in that they frequently contribute to medication error. As such, the use of abbreviations is actively discouraged with legislation currently being introduced to actively prohibit their use within the healthcare system. In the meantime, local policies determine which abbreviations may be permitted and under what circumstances. However, there are some abbreviations that should never be used.

Abbreviation	Potential problem	Preferred handling
U (for unit)	Mistaken as zero, four, or cc	Write the word unit.
IU (for international unit)	Mistaken as IV (intravenous) or 10 (ten)	Write the words international unit.
Q.D., Q.O.D. (Latin abbreviation for once daily and every other day)	Mistaken for one another; the period after the Q can be mistaken for an "I" and the "O" can be mistaken for "I"	Write the words daily and every other day.
Trailing zero (X.0 mg), Lack of leading zero (.X mg)	Dosage errors caused by missed decimal point	Never write a zero by itself after a decimal point (X mg), and always use a zero before a decimal point (0.X mg).
MS, MSO_4, $MgSO_4$	Mistaken for one another; can mean morphine sulphate or magnesium sulphate	Write the words morphine sulphate or magnesium sulphate.

Selected references

Publications

Aschenbrenner, S.D., and Venable, S.J. Drug Therapy in Nursing. 2nd ed. Philadelphia: Lippincott Williams & Wilkins, 2007.

Conroy, S., et al. Interventions to reduce dosing errors in children: a systematic review of the literature. Drug Safety, 30: 1111–1125, 2007.

Karch, A.M. Focus on Nursing Pharmacology. 4th ed. Philadelphia: Lippincott Williams & Wilkins, 2007.

Lehne, R.A. Pharmacology for Nursing Care, 6th ed. Philadelphia: W.B. Saunders, 2007.

Nursing 2008 Drug Handbook, 28th ed. Philadelphia: Lippincott Williams & Wilkins, 2007.

Pharmacology: A 2-in-1 Reference for Nurses. Philadelphia: Lippincott Williams & Wilkins, 2004.

Roach, S.S., and Ford, S.M. Introductory Clinical Pharmacology, 8th ed. Phiadelphia: Lippincott Williams & Wilkins, 2007.

Springhouse Nurse's Drug Guide 2005, 6th ed. Philadelphia: Lippincott Williams & Wilkins, 2004.

Straight A's in Nursing Pharmacology, 2nd ed. Philadelphia: Lippincott Williams & Wilkins, 2003.

Additional resources

British National Formulary
www.bnf.org

National Institute for Health and Clinical Excellence
www.nice.org.uk

Paediatric Drug Information Advisory Line
Tel: 015 1252 5837

National Poisons Information Service
Tel: 084 4892 0111

Index

A

Abacavir, 520, 521
Abciximab, 371
Absorption, 8–10
Acarbose, 390, 391, 397
Acebutolol, 200, 230, 231
Acetazolamide, 49, 673t
Acetylcholine, 25–29
Acetylcysteine, 672
Aciclovir, 510–511, 674
Activated charcoal, 316–318, 317
Active transport, 8
Acute therapy, 16
Additive effect, 18
Adenosine, 208–210
Administration routes, 4
Adrenaline (epinephrine), 44–46
Adrenergic blocking drugs, 51–63
Adrenergic drugs, 42–51
Adrenocorticotropics, 405
Adsorbent drugs, 316–319
Adverse drug reactions, 20–22
Agonist, 14
Albendazole, 19
Aldesleukin, 649–651
Aldosterone, 224–225, 243
Alemtuzumab, 640, 641, 642
Alfa interferons, 656
Aliphatics, 455–460
Alkylamines, 558
Alkylating drugs, 586–604
Alkylating-like drugs, 600–604
Alkyl sulphonates, 590–593
Allopurinol, 580, 581, 582
Almotriptan, 131
Alpha-adrenergic blockers, 52–56
    as antihypertensive drugs, 228–230
Alpha-glucosidase inhibitors, 390, 393
Alprazolam, 420, 422
Aluminium carbonate gel, 304

Aluminium-magnesium complex, 304
Amantadine
    as antiparkinsonian drug, 86–95
    as influenza A virus drug, 88
Amide anaesthetics, 175
Amikacin, 469
Amiloride, 252, 253
Aminoglycosides, 467–471
1 (aminomethyl) cyclohexane acetic
        acid, 116–118
Aminophylline, 282
Amiodarone, 202–204
Amitriptyline, 160
Amlodipine, 219
Amobarbital, 424
Amoxicillin, 301, 302
Amphetamine salts, mixed, 460
Amphotericin B, 540–542, 674
Ampicillin, 471, 473
Amprenavir, 531, 532
Amylase, 320, 321
Anakinra, 571–574
Anastrozole, 619–620
Androgens, 624–627
Anaesthetic drugs, 168–178
Angiotensin-converting enzyme
        inhibitors, 223–227
Angiotensin II receptor blocking
        agents, 228–230
Anhydrous theophylline, 282
Animals as drug source, 3–4
Antacids, 304–316
Antagonist, 157–168
Antagonistic effects, 195
Anterior pituitary drugs, 405–408
Anthracyclines, 615
Antiandrogens, 627–629
Antianginal drugs, 211–223
Antianxiety drugs, 431–435
Antiarrhythmic drugs, 187–210
Antibacterial drugs, 466–509

Antibiotic antineoplastic drugs, 615–618
Antibiotic antiulcer drugs. *See also*
        Antiulcer drugs.
Anticholinergic drugs
    as antiparkinsonian drugs, 86–95
    as autonomic nervous system
            drugs, 25–64
    as respiratory drugs, 269–298
Anticholinesterase drugs, 29–34
Anticoagulant drugs, 361–377
Anticonvulsant drugs, 99–130
Antidepressant drugs, 435–460
Antidiabetic drugs, 383–394
Antidiarrhoeal drugs, 323–328
Antidiuretic hormone, 408, 412
Antiemetics, 342–345
Antioestrogens, 621–624
Antiflatulent drugs, 319–320
Antifungal drugs, 539–555
Antihistamines
    as antiemetics, 342–345
    as anti-inflammatory and
            immunomodulating
            drugs, 557–584
Antihypertensive drugs, 223–244
Anti-infective drugs, 464–556
Anti-inflammatory drugs, 557–584
Antimetabolite drugs, 604–614
Antimigraine drugs, 130–138
Antimycotic drugs, topical, 539, 540
Antineoplastic drugs, 585–666
Antiparkinsonian drugs, 84–95
Antiplatelet drugs *See also* Anticoagulant
        drugs. 361–377
Antipsychotic drugs, 453
Antipyretics, 141–148
Antithyroid drugs, 401–404
Antitubercular drugs, 534–539
Antitussives, 289–291
Antiulcer drugs, 299–304
Antiviral drugs, 510–533

679